616
D0332344

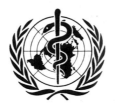

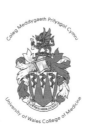

The Sir Herbert Duthie Library
University of Wales College of Medicine
Heath Park, Cardiff
Tel: (029) 2074 2875

This loan may be renewed

SI5 99407/PPP

World Health Organization Classification of Tumours

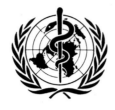

WHO   OMS

International Agency for Research on Cancer (IARC)

Pathology and Genetics of
Tumours of Endocrine Organs

Edited by

Ronald A. DeLellis

Ricardo V. Lloyd

Philipp U. Heitz

Charis Eng

IARCPress

Lyon, 2004

World Health Organization Classification of Tumours

| Series Editors | Paul Kleihues, M.D. |
| | Leslie H. Sobin, M.D. |

Pathology and Genetics of Tumours of Endocrine Organs

Editors	Ronald A. DeLellis, M.D.
	Ricardo V. Lloyd, M.D.
	Philipp U. Heitz, M.D.
	Charis Eng, M.D., Ph.D.

| Coordinating Editors | Wojciech Biernat, M.D. |
| | Janice Sych, Ph.D. |

Editorial Assistants	Isabelle Forcier
	Voichita Meyronein
	Agnès Meneghel

Layout	Vanessa Meister
	Marlen Grassinger
	Sibylle Söring

| Illustrations | Thomas Odin |

| Printed by | Team Rush |
| | 69603 Villeurbanne, France |

Publisher	IARCPress
	International Agency for
	Research on Cancer (IARC)
	69008 Lyon, France

This volume was produced in collaboration with the

International Academy of Pathology (IAP)

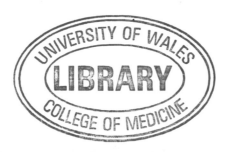

The WHO Classification of Tumours of Endocrine Organs
presented in this book reflects the views of a Working Group that
convened for an Editorial and Consensus Conference in Lyon, France,
April 23-26, 2003

Members of the Working Group are indicated
in the List of Contributors on page 263

Published by IARC Press, International Agency for Research on Cancer,
150 cours Albert Thomas, F-69008 Lyon, France

© International Agency for Research on Cancer, 2004

Publications of the World Health Organization enjoy copyright protection in
accordance with the provisions of Protocol 2 of the Universal Copyright Convention.
All rights reserved.

The International Agency for Research on Cancer welcomes
requests for permission to reproduce or translate its publications, in part or in full.
Requests for permission to reproduce figures or charts from this publication should be directed to
the respective contributor (see section Source of Charts and Photographs).

The designations used and the presentation of the material in this publication do not imply the
expression of any opinion whatsoever on the part of the Secretariat of the
World Health Organization concerning the legal status of any country, territory, city,
or area or of its authorities, or concerning the delimitation of its frontiers or boundaries.

The mention of specific companies or of certain manufacturers' products does not imply
that they are endorsed or recommended by the World Health Organization in preference to others
of a similar nature that are not mentioned. Errors and omissions excepted,
the names of proprietary products are distinguished by initial capital letters.

The authors alone are responsible for the views expressed in this publication.

Enquiries should be addressed to the
Communications Unit, International Agency for Research on Cancer, 69008 Lyon, France,
which will provide the latest information on any changes made to the text and plans for new editions.

Format for bibliographic citations:
DeLellis R.A., Lloyd R.V., Heitz P.U., Eng C. (Eds.): World Health Organization
Classification of Tumours. Pathology and Genetics of Tumours of Endocrine Organs.
IARC Press: Lyon 2004

IARC Library Cataloguing in Publication Data

Pathology and genetics of tumours of endocrine organs /
        editors R.A. DeLellis... [et al.]

    (World Health Organization classification of tumours ; 8)

    1. Pituitary gland neoplasms - genetics 2. Pituitary gland neoplasms - pathology
    3. Thyroid neoplasms - genetics 4. Thyroid neoplasms, - pathology
    5. Endocrine pancreas neoplasms - genetics 6. Endocrine pancreas neoplasms - pathology
    7. Adrenal neoplasms – genetics 8. Adrenal neoplasms - pathology
    I. DeLellis Ronald A. II. Series

    ISBN 92 832 2416 7 (NLM Classification: WJ 160)

Contents

CHAPTER 1

Tumours of the Pituitary Gland

The vast majority of neoplasms located in the sella turcica are benign pituitary adenomas derived from adenohypophysial cells. In many cases, they can be successfully removed by minimally invasive transsphenoidal surgery. However, their biology is complex and they can cause a variety of endocrine syndromes and disorders.

The immunohistochemical characterization of functional pituitary adenomas is mandatory for patient management, although it does not necessarily predict systemic hormone levels.

Pituitary tumours: Introduction

R.V. Lloyd
K. Kovacs
W.F. Young Jr.
W.E. Farrell
S.L. Asa

J. Trouillas
G. Kontogeorgos
T. Sano
B.W. Scheithauer
E. Horvath

Definition

Pituitary tumours are defined as neoplasms located in the sella turcica. The vast majority are pituitary adenomas derived from adenohypophysial cells with only a very small percentage of these tumours representing pituitary carcinomas. Other lesions located in the sella include mesenchymal, neural or epithelial tumours and metastases.

WHO Classification

Pituitary adenoma	
Typical adenoma	8272/0
Atypical adenoma	8272/1
Pituitary carcinoma	8272/3

Morphology codes of the International Classification of Diseases for Oncology (ICD-O) {664} and the Systematized Nomenclature of Medicine SNOMED (http://snomed.org). Behaviour is coded /0 for benign tumours, /3 for malignant tumours, and /1 for borderline or uncertain behaviour.

Epidemiology

Pituitary tumours constitute about 10 to 15 percent of intracranial neoplasms. Small incidental adenomas may occur in up to 27% of pituitary glands examined at autopsy {268,420,2254} and up to one fifth of the population has a pituitary abnormality on MRI {376,804}. Pituitary adenomas are uncommon in the paediatric population, representing about 2% of all pituitary adenomas {399,1032, 1179, 1695}. As with pituitary tumours in adults, PRL producing adenomas are the most common hormone-secreting tumours in the paediatric population, and ACTH producing adenomas are more common in children than in adults.
Pituitary adenomas are classified with functional classifications using histology, immunohistochemistry, ultrastructural features as well as biochemical, imaging and surgical findings {1159}. Historically, they have been divided into two groups, which include adenomas and carcinomas {919,1159,1961}.

Clinical features

Signs and symptoms

Patients with pituitary adenomas may present with features of hormone excess. These are detailed in the following sections. However, there are common features of mass effects that apply to many macroadenomas. These include symptoms of an intracranial mass such as headache, loss of normal anterior pituitary hormone production (by compressing the normal portion of the gland), visual field disturbances and mild hyperprolactinemia (usually < 200 ng/ml) due to pituitary stalk compression known as "stalk section effect" {1351,2468}. Visual impairment caused by compression of

Table 1.01
Pituitary adenoma types in an unselected surgical series of 2091 biopsies. From E. Horvath et al. {919}.

Adenoma Type	Frequency	M/F ratio	Immunoprofile
Sparsely granulated PRL cell adenoma	27.0	1/2.5	PRL
Densely granulated PRL cell adenoma	0.4	-	PRL
Sparsely granulated GH cell adenoma	7.6	1/1.2	GH, α-SU, PRL
Densely granulated GH cell adenoma	7.1	1/0.7	GH, α-SU, PRL, TSH, (LH,FSH)
Mixed (GH cell-PRL cell) adenoma	3.5	1/1.1	GH, PRL, α-SU, TSH
Mammosomatotroph cell adenoma	1.2	1/1.1	GH, PRL, α-SU, TSH
Acidophil stem cell adenoma	1.6	1/1.5	PRL, GH
Corticotroph cell adenoma	9.6	1/5.4	ACTH, (LH, α-SU)
Thyrotroph cell adenoma	1.1	1/1.3	TSH,α-SU, (GH, PRL)
Gonadotroph cell adenoma*	9.8	1/0.8	FSH, LH, α-SU, (ACTH)
Silent corticotroph adenoma, subtype I	2.0	1/0.2	ACTH
Silent corticotroph adenoma, subtype 2	1.5	1/1.7	β-Endorphin, ACTH
Silent adenoma, subtype 3	1.4	1/1.1	None
Null cell adenoma*	12.4	1/0.7	FSH, LH, α-SU, TSH
Oncocytoma*	13.4	1/0.5	FSH, LH, α-SU, TSH
Unclassified	1.8	NA	NA

NA—not applicable
* The incidence of these tumour types varies in different series, due to different classification criteria.

the optic chiasm usually progresses from superior lateral quadranopia to bilateral hemianopia, and eventually, blindness. In contrast, signs and symptoms of hypopituitarism are frequent but, being of insidious onset, patients rarely seek medical advice for symptoms of gonadal, thyroid, or adrenal failure. However, diabetes insipidus is extremely rare in patients with pituitary adenomas and other types of parasellar lesions should be considered in patients with this condition. They can also invade downwards into the paranasal sinuses, laterally into the cavernous sinuses (to compress cranial nerves resulting in ophthalmoplegias) and upwards into the parenchyma of the brain.

Imaging

A radiologic classification of pituitary tumours has designated small tumours less than or equal to 10 mm as microadenomas while larger tumours are macroadenomas. Tumours >4 cm are termed giant adenomas and are very uncommon. Microadenomas have been graded radiologically as grade 0 for intrasellar microadenomas with a normal sellar appearance or- grade I for intrasellar adenomas with slight sellar enlargement {833}. Macroadenomas are graded from II to IV with grade II tumours having diffuse sellar enlargement without bone erosion, grade III tumours having focal bone erosion, and grade IV tumours having extensive bone erosion including the skull base and extrasellar structures.

Accurate tumour dimensions and extent of invasion can be established by magnetic resonance imaging (MRI) {833,1480}. Pituitary diagnostic imaging is the domain of cross-sectional imaging. With its multiplanar capability and dramatic soft tissue contrast MRI is the superior modality {1376,1409,1500,1755, 1903,2113,2415}. Typically, MRI of the pituitary consists of coronal 3 mm T1 weighted images pre- and post-administration of intravenous gadolinium contrast {537,2204}. Additional sagittal pre- and post-contrast imaging is occasionally useful. Computed tomography (CT) of the pituitary can be performed but is less sensitive and specific than MRI due to difficulties with patient positioning, artifact from adjacent bone and lesser soft tissue contrast among others. The normal pituitary on T1 weighted MRI has homogeneous signal isointense to corti-

cal grey matter with the neurohypophysis demonstrating uniformly bright T1 signal thought to be related to phospholipid vacuoles {908}. Pituitary morphology at MRI is characterized by a midline infundibulum and a gentle upwardly convex superior surface.

Histopathology

Although descriptive terminology based

Table 1.02
Functional classification of pituitary adenomas.

1. Endocrine hyperfunction* - Clinical or biochemical evidence of serum hormone elevation.
> Acromegaly/gigantism - elevated serum GH/IGF1 levels
> Hyperprolactinemia and sequelae
> Cushing disease with elevated ACTH and cortisol levels
> Hyperthyroidism with inappropriate TSH secretion
> Significantly elevated FSH/LH and/or alpha subunit levels
> Multiple hormone overproduction from plurihormonal tumours or double adenomas
2. Clinically nonfunctioning
> No known hormone produced or released
> Hormones or hormone fragments produced which may not cause clinical manifestation - FSH, LH, and or alpha subunit
> Hormone normally causes clinical signs and symptoms is produced but without clinical or biological manifestations - silent ACTH or GH producing adenomas
> Biological inactive hormone fragment or a hormone product
3. Functional status indeterminate
*Pituitary hormone excess may also be due to ectopic hormone production, e.g. production of hypothalamic releasing hormones by neuroendocrine neoplasm; pituitary hyperplasia with or without adenoma; production of pituitary hormones by extrapituitary tumours. See reference {1961}

on tinctorial properties such as acidophils, basophils, and chromophobe tumours are used for diagnosing pituitary adenomas, these terms do not usually correlate with the functional or immunohistochemical findings and should be discouraged.

The majority of pituitary adenomas are composed of monomorphic proliferations of cells with uniform round nuclei, deli-

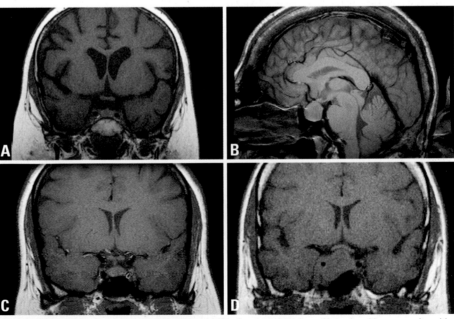

Fig. 1.01 Pituitary images. **A** Coronal T1-weighted MRI of a normal pituitary. Note signal homogeneity within the gland. **B** GH macroadenoma. Sagittal pregadolinium T1 weighted images show superior extension into the suprasellar cistern and smooth expansion of the sella. Note calvarial thickening associated with acromegaly. **C** Left pituitary PRL microadenoma. Coronal T1-weighted image demonstrates low signal at the left aspect of the pituitary. Note convexity at the left superior border of the gland, and deviation of the infundibular stalk to the right. **D** Right pituitary PRL macroadenoma. Coronal T1-weighted image demonstrates isointense mass at the right aspect of the sella.

Table 1.03
Possible etiologic factors implicated in pituitary tumour development and progression {1480}.

Inherited
MEN-1 with involvement of 11q13
Carney complex with involvement of 2p16 and 17q
Familial acromegaly with involvement of 11q13 and other loci
McCune-Albright syndrome with involvement of 20q13.2

Hypothalamic
Excess GHRH, CRH, TRH, or GnRH production

Pituitary
Hormone receptor abnormality
Signal transduction alterations (Gsp, CREB)
    Growth factors and receptors - FGF, FGFR, NGF, NGFR, EGF, EGFR, VEGF, VEGFR, TGFα and β
    Activated oncogenes/cell cycle defects - PTTG, Ras, p27, p18, p16, cyclins
    Loss of tumour suppressor gene function (11q13)

Peripheral
Target organ failure with feedback disruption, e.g. adrenal, thyroid and gonads

Environmental
None to date

CRH -   Corticotropin releasing hormone
EGF -   Epidermal growth factor
FGF -   Fibroblast growth factor
GHRH - Growth hormone releasing hormone
GnRH - Gonadotropin hormone releasing hormone
NGF -   Nerve growth factor
PTTG - Pituitary tumour transforming gene
TGF –   Transforming growth factor
TRH –   Thyrotropin releasing hormone
VEGF – Vascular endothelial growth factor

---

cate stippled chromatin, inconspicuous nucleoli, and moderate quantities of cytoplasm. As a rule, mitoses are uncommon in most adenomas. Ki-67 antigen (clone MIB-1) labeling indices are usually less than 3%. Some adenomas have atypical morphologic features suggestive of aggressive behaviour such as invasive growth. Other features include an elevated mitotic index and a Ki-67 labeling index greater than 3%, as well as extensive nuclear staining for p53 immunoreactivity. These features are usually lacking in noninvasive adenomas and are present in nearly all pituitary carcinomas. Tumours with these features that have no documented metastases can be designated as "atypical" adenomas.

Growth patterns
Expansive growth. Radiographically, grossly, and histologically apparent with a demarcated interface between the tumour and surrounding tissues. These tumours are usually not encapsulated.

Invasive growth — Involvement of bone, nerve, vessels, etc., which is seen radiographically, grossly or histologically. Note that microscopic invasion such as dural invasion is common and is not considered a reliable indicator of aggressive tumour behaviour {1966}.
Pituitary carcinoma. These tumours must show metastasis {1961}. There may be craniospinal or systemic metastases. Brain invasion as a criterion of malignancy is at present controversial.

Immunoprofile
This includes consistent positivity for synaptophysin, with a lower percentage of immunostaining for chromogranin A and low molecular weight keratins {1337}. Hormone profiles, transcription factor expression and ultrastructural features allow classification of these tumours as detailed in the following sections.

Etiology
The etiologic factors contributing to pituitary adenomas are largely derived from

epidemiologic evidence {1480}. Genetic factors, physiological alterations at the hypothalamic, pituitary, and peripheral level as well as environmental factors may contribute to the development of pituitary tumours {84,1480,1709,1710, 2413}. A great deal of information has been derived from experimental work with animal models as well as from molecular analyses of human pituitary tumours.

Somatic genetics
The various oncogenes and tumour suppressor genes implicated in pituitary tumourigenesis are largely cell type specific {882,1708}. For example, Gsp mutations have been detected mainly in GH producing adenomas while hypermethylation of p16 is present in gonadotroph and null cell tumours but not in GH producing adenomas {2056}.
Unlike in rodent models, mutations of the retinoblastoma (*RB*) gene have not been identified in human pituitary adenomas {437}, but the *RB1* promoter has been described to be silenced via methylation at a CpG island in tumour cells associated with diminished protein levels {2058}. Alternatively, loss of RB function and/or a closely linked tumour suppressor gene may occur through loss of heterozygosity (LOH) at the 13q site.
Similarly, mouse models of deficiency of cyclin-dependent kinases (CDKs) and their inhibitors result in pituitary adenomas, but in human tumours there is no evidence of alterations of these genes. Instead, p16ink4A may be silenced by extensive promoter methylation {2413}. Despite the well-recognized role of p27kip1 in the pathogenesis and prognosis of several human malignancies {1334}, the p27kip1 gene is structurally intact in human pituitary tumours {2189}. However, p27 expression is reduced in ACTH producing adenomas {1006, 1334}. Recurrent human pituitary adenomas, including null cell adenomas, exhibit lower p27 protein levels than their non-recurrent counterparts {117,1572}.
The pituitary is an abundant source of a number of growth factors. Of these, members of the fibroblast growth factor/receptor (FGFR) family have received the widest attention because of their putative role in tumour pathogenesis. A truncated kinase-containing variant of the fibroblast growth factor receptor 4 (*FGFR4*) with an alternative initiation site

was noted in primary human pituitary tumours {598}. Expression of this pituitary tumour-derived (ptd) kinase (ptd-FGFR4) results in cell transformation *in vitro* and *in vivo*. More significantly, pituitary-targeted expression of ptd-FGFR4 in transgenic mice recapitulates the morphologic features of invasive human pituitary adenomas {598}.

Other factors possibly implicated in the pathogenesis of pituitary tumours include the putative oncogenes *PTTG* and *Cyclin D1*. Adenohypophysiotropic hormones and growth factors such as fibroblast growth factors (FGF) 2 and 4, nerve growth factor (NGF), epidermal growth factor (EGF), transforming growth factors (TGF) α and β, and vascular endothelial growth factor (VEGF) have been implicated in tumour progression.

Therapy and prognosis
Surgical treatment
Surgical management is the main modality of treatment for patients with pituitary tumours {540,2221}. The usual approach is a transsphenoidal minimally invasive procedure. Surgery is especially indicated in (1) tumours with progressive mass effect, e.g. visual loss., (2) hyperfunctioning tumours in Cushing disease, acromegaly, or hyperthyroidism {539}, (3) failure of prior treatment such as medical therapy, and (4) massive acute haemorrhagic necrosis of an adenoma (pituitary apoplexy) {2221}.

Medical treatment
Medical therapy is often used as the initial treatment for many patients with PRL producing adenomas and some patients with GH producing adenomas {1226}.
Dopamine agonists are used to treat PRL producing adenomas. These drugs reduce hyperprolactinemia and tumour size {1526}.

Table 1.04
Putative oncogenes and tumour suppressor genes implicated in pituitary tumourigenesis.

Oncogenes
Gsp {2104}
CREB {181}
Ras {1041,1710}
PTTG {83,1708}
Cyclin D1 (*CCND1*) {882,1328}
ptd-FGFR4 {598}

Tumour Suppressor Genes
MEN 1 {13,92}
RB {1709,2059}
TP53 {1284}
ZAC {1674}
GADD45 {2489}
p16/CDKN2A {610,853,2056,2412,2413}
p27/KIP1 {1332,1334}

See also references {83,84,1480}

Long acting somatostatin analogues are mainly used to treat GH producing adenomas {1526,2009}. These drugs interact with pituitary somatostatin receptors to decrease pituitary GH secretion; in contrast to dopamine agonists, these drugs do not cause a significant reduction of tumour volume. They also partially inhibit GH-induced IGF-1 generation by liver, kidney, heart, and lungs leading to decreased plasma IGF-1 levels {2009}. A GH receptor antagonist may also be used to treat patients with GH producing pituitary tumours by normalizing serum IGF-I levels. In a study with patients treated for 12 months or more, 97% achieved normal IGF-I levels {2292}.
The medical treatment of Cushing disease has been generally unsuccessful {540}. Drugs such as dopamine agonists and cyproheptadine generally fail to reduce ACTH secretion. Ketoconazole, mitotane, and metyrapone have been used to reduce adrenal steroid hormone production, but surgery remains the most effective treatment {1526}. Somatostatin analogues have been used to treat TSH producing adenomas {1526}.
Clinically nonfunctioning tumours have been treated with dopamine agonists, somatostatin analogues, or gonadotrophin-releasing hormone analogues and antagonists with variable results.

Radiation therapy
Before the advent of transsphenoidal pituitary surgery, radiotherapy was more common. Today it is used to treat patients with incompletely excised or recurrent tumours, for patients medically unfit for surgical intervention, or for secretory tumours uncontrolled by other therapy {236,323,639,928,1548,2284}. The development of hypopituitarism, the prolonged delay in achieving a therapeutic effect and the risk of delayed radiation-induced glioma or sarcoma made conventional radiation a suboptimal therapeutic choice.
Gamma knife stereotactic radiosurgery has been used with increasing frequency in both paediatric and adult populations {831,1758,2027,2237}, but its precise role in the management of pituitary tumours is still evolving. The general recommendation is that the dose to the optic apparatus be kept below 8 Gy to decrease the level of complications {1548}. Novel therapeutic approaches may achieve tumour control in residual or recurrent nonfunctioning pituitary adenomas {2027} and pituitary carcinomas {831}.

Growth hormone producing adenoma

G. Kontogeorgos
R.E. Watson Jr.
E.P. Lindell

A.L. Barkan
W.E. Farrell
R.V. Lloyd

Definition

Pituitary adenomas secreting growth hormone (GH) in excess are clinically associated with either gigantism or acromegaly, depending on patient age at onset of disease. Well-documented nonfunctioning cases are very rare.

Pure GH producing tumours, solely consisting of somatotrophs, are separated into two well-defined types: densely granulated and sparsely granulated somatotroph adenomas.

Mixed GH-PRL cell adenomas and mammosomatotroph adenomas produce excess GH and prolactin (PRL); acidophil stem cell adenomas are typically associated with hyperprolactinemia in the absence of stigmata of acromegaly.

ICD-O code   8272/0

Synonyms and historical annotation

Pierre Marie described the syndrome of acromegaly in 1886 {1407} and Minkowski noted its association with pituitary adenoma in 1887 {1508}. According to various classifications, these tumours are referred to as somatotroph adenomas, somatotrophinomas, or GH cell adenomas. Mammosomatotroph adenomas are infrequently called somatomammotroph or somatolactotroph adenomas.

Epidemiology

Mammosomatotroph adenomas are the most common cause of gigantism, occurring in younger patients. Sparsely granulated somatotroph and acidophil stem cell adenomas show slight predominance in younger men. Signs of acromegaly usually appear between the ages of 25 and 35 years. However, due to a rather insidious clinical course, diagnosis and treatment are often delayed for 6 to 12 years.

GH producing tumours account for approximately 25-30% of all surgically removed pituitary adenomas. However, in clinical series the incidence is lower due to the inclusion of medically treated tumours. They are primarily solitary although multiple adenomas have been reported. In one series, two thirds of double adenomas identified in surgical material represented GH producing adenomas; most of them were densely granulated and exhibited a plurihormonal immunophenotype {1144}. In contrast, among multiple adenomas incidentally found in autopsy series, GH producing adenomas are very rare {1140}.

Localization

Microadenomas (≤10mm) are enclosed within the sella and located in one of the lateral wings {109}. Macroadenomas (> 10 mm) representing the majority of GH producing adenomas exhibit gradual ballooning enlargement of the sella turcica, and commonly show upward and/or lateral extension.

Clinical features

Clinical manifestations of GH producing adenomas consist of 3 distinct syndromes: effects of GH/IGF-I excess, mass effects of the tumour and the tumour-induced adenohypophysial hypofunction {595,1479,2238,2341}. The clinical picture is also heavily influenced by the age at which the tumour develops. Prepubertal onset is accompanied by an unrestrained somatic growth, gigantism. Postpubertal onset is primarily manifested as enlargement of acral parts of the body, acromegaly. Patients with gigantism usually present with at least some degree of acromegalic features and invariably develop them during ensuing years. Many growth promoting effects of GH are mediated by circulating and autocrine/paracrine IGF-I. IGF-I excess is manifest as enlargement of soft tissues and bone growth. Typically, the patient presents with enlargement of hands and feet that is mostly due to soft tissue

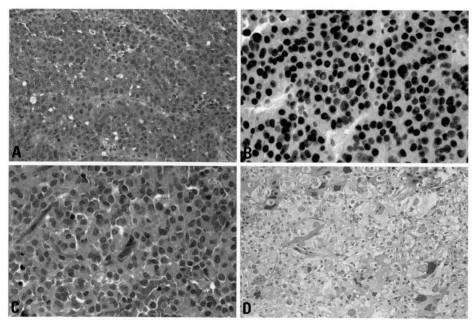

Fig. 1.02 A This densely granulated somatotroph adenoma is the classical "acidophilic" adenoma usually associated with acromegaly or gigantism. The tumour cells form solid nests and have abundant strongly acidophilic cytoplasm due to the storage of numerous GH-containing secretory granules. **B** Nuclear staining for Pit-1 is strong in GH-producing adenomas. In this densely granulated adenoma the nuclei are more regular than in sparsely granulated somatotroph adenomas. **C** A sparsely granulated somatotroph adenoma is composed of round, moderately discohesive cells that exhibit nuclear pleomorphism, mainly characterized by nuclear indentations by homogeneous acidophilic fibrous bodies. **D** Pleomorphic tumour cells are prominent in this case.

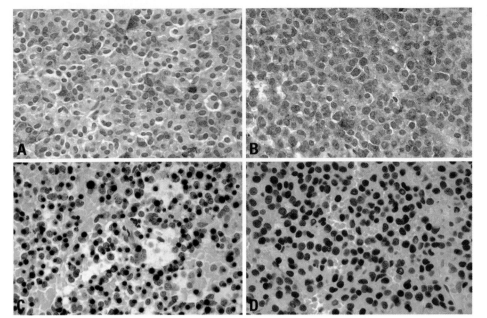

Fig. 1.03 GH adenoma. **A** Densely granulated somatotroph adenomas usually exhibit cytoplasmic staining for α-subunit of glycoprotein hormones that is found with variable distribution and intensity in tumour cells. **B** A sparsely granulated somatotroph adenoma has scant immunoreactivity for growth hormone. **C** The fibrous bodies of a sparsely granulated somatotroph adenoma are decorated by the Cam 5.2 antibody that identifies cytokeratins 8 and 18. This characteristic globular cytoplasmic positivity is the hallmark of this tumour type. **D** Nuclear staining for Pit-1 is strong in GH-producing adenomas and highlights the nuclear irregularities of this sparsely granulated somatotroph adenoma.

hypertrophy. Coarse facial features with large nose, thick lips and prominent nasolabial furrows are usually obvious at presentation. Overgrowth of skeletal tissues may be manifest as enlargement of lower jaw, widening of interdental spaces and prognathism. Enlargement of the sinuses leads to frontal bossing. The skin is thick and sweaty and usually there is obvious growth of skin tags in the neck and axillae. Large tongue and uvula often result in obstructive sleep apnea. Entrapment neuropathies, most often carpal and tarsal, are present in about 20-30% of the patients. Visceral hypertrophy may be symptomless (goiter and large salivary glands), but left ventricular hypertrophy leads to cardiomyopathy and life-threatening arrhythmias. A significant proportion of patients have diabetes mellitus. Overgrowth of the intraarticular cartilage leads to peripheral arthropathy in 70% of the patients. Radiologically and anatomically acromegalic arthropathy is indistinguishable from degenerative osteoarthritis. Some patients develop axial arthropathy that in advanced cases may cause severe kyphosis. Large pituitary tumours may exert pressure on the optic apparatus causing segmental loss of visual fields. Larger tumours extending

to 3rd ventricle may cause obstructive hydrocephalus. Apoplexy of the tumour that invaded cavernous sinuses may result in III, IV, or VI nerve ophthalmoplegia. The degree of hypopituitarism depends on the size of the original tumour. Co-secretion of prolactin or TSH causes specific syndromes of amenorrhea/galactorrhea or hyperthyroidism.

The biochemical diagnosis is best established by demonstrating high plasma IGF-I concentrations (age and sex adjusted). Plasma GH level may fluctuate from normal to grossly elevated. Oral glucose tolerance test does not suppress plasma GH <1 mg/L in the majority of patients with active disease, although it may decrease it as low as 0.4 mg/L in treated patients or in those with very mild disease. Other dynamic tests (TRH, GnRH or GHRH) are of limited diagnostic value.

Imaging

Magnetic resonance imaging (MRI) is the superior modality for pituitary diagnostic imaging {1376,1409,1500,1755,1903, 2113,2415} and allows clear resolution of tumour margins to define its size and invasiveness. Typically, MRI of the pituitary consists of coronal 3 mm T1 weight-

ed images pre- and post-administration of IV gadolinium contrast {537,2204}. Additional sagittal pre- and post-contrast imaging is occasionally useful. Computed tomography (CT) of the pituitary is less sensitive and specific. The normal pituitary on T1 weighted MRI has homogeneous signal isointense to cortical grey matter with the neurohypophysis demonstrating uniformly bright T1 signal thought to be related to phospholipid vacuoles {908}.

GH producing microadenomas on pre-gadolinium coronal T1 MRI are generally hypointense relative to the surrounding pituitary. Following gadolinium administration, microadenomas typically have less initial contrast enhancement than the surrounding normal pituitary.

Extension of GH producing adenomatous tissue beyond the sella can be identified on MRI. Critical regions to evaluate include the cavernous sinuses and their contents and the suprasellar cistern with attention to the optic chiasm. With extension into the cavernous sinus, it is important to determine the relationship of the macroadenoma to the carotid arteries. Macroadenomas are relatively soft tumours and rarely narrow the carotid arteries. In contrast to microadenomas, macroadenomas are generally characterized by robust contrast enhancement.

Macroscopy

GH producing adenomas are soft and white to grey-red. Microadenomas are well demarcated. Macroadenomas can infiltrate the meninges and the cavernous sinuses. They may invade the bone of the sella turcica and the sphenoid sinus; in rare instances they may protrude as polyps to the nasal cavity.

Histopathology
Densely granulated somatotroph adenomas

These consist of medium size, round or polyhedral acidophilic cells with granular cytoplasm showing a diffuse pattern of growth. The nuclei are round with finely dispersed chromatin, often exhibiting distinct nucleoli. They show strong, uniform and diffuse cytoplasmic immunoreactivity for GH. About half of tumours contain α-subunit of glycoprotein hormones. By electron microscopy, the cells are similar to normal somatotrophs. They display well developed Golgi apparatus and RER. The secretory granules are

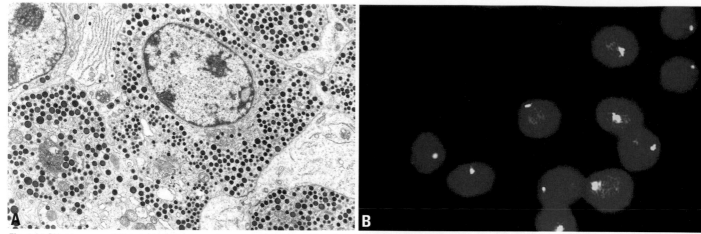

Fig. 1.04 GH adenoma. **A** This typical electron micrograph shows well developed Golgi apparatus and RER, and abundant large secretory granules. **B** FISH using an alpha-centromere specific probe for chromosome 11. Monosomy 11 in a patient with a mixed GH/PRL adenoma associated with MEN 1.

abundant, round and regular, randomly dispersed throughout the cytoplasm, measuring 300-450 nm.

Sparsely granulated somatotroph adenomas

These are cellular chromophobic tumours composed of small, round, partly irregular cells harbouring a round nucleus with conspicuous nucleoli. A fibrous body, namely a pale acidophilic, spherical inclusion, representing a diagnostic feature of this variant, often occupies the paranuclear cytoplasmic area. Fibrous bodies produce peripheral displacement of the nucleus, often with crescent formation. Nuclear pleomorphism and lobulated or multinucleated bizarre cells are frequent. Immunoreactivity for GH is variable and usually scant. Fibrous bodies are strongly reactive for low molecular weight cytokeratins, particularly keratin 8 {1931}. Electron microscopy reveals a cell type not present in the normal pituitary. The RER is variably developed and usually displays scattered to abundant parallel arrays. The fibrous bodies consist of concentric aggregates of intermediate filaments. The secretory granules are scarce and small measuring 100-250 nm.

Mixed somatotroph-lactotroph adenomas

These uncommon tumours consist of somatotrophs and lactotrophs. Histologically, the adenoma consists of two variably admixed acidophilic and chromophobic cell populations corresponding to somatotrophs and lactotrophs. GH and PRL immunostaining is localised

in each particular cell type.

Mammosomatotroph adenomas

These tumours consist of a single cell type producing both GH and PRL. By histology, the cells are polyhedral, strong acidophilic with a diffuse pattern of growth and they contain a round nucleus with a conspicuous nucleolus. By immunohistochemistry, GH and PRL are localised in the same cells. Electron microscopy reveals typical features of mammosomatotroph cells similar to those occurring in a normal pituitary. The cells resemble densely granulated somatotrophs and contain abundant and large secretory granules reaching up to 1500 nm. Misplaced exocytosis, a characteristic feature of PRL secreting cells, is also evident {1154,1963}.

Acidophil stem cell adenomas

These monomorphous tumours comprise less than 1% of all adenomas. They are chromophobic with some degree of acidophilia and show a diffuse pattern of growth. They may exhibit nuclear pleomorphism with coarse chromatin and prominent nucleoli. Large cytoplasmic vacuoles reaching the size of the nucleus and fibrous bodies may be noted. Immunohistochemistry shows reactivity for PRL, whereas GH is faint or negative. Cytokeratins of low molecular weight are present in fibrous bodies. Electron microscopy reveals mitochondrial accumulation, with giant mitochondria, a diagnostic hallmark not present in any other adenoma type. In addition, it demonstrates accumulated intermediate filaments forming fibrous bodies, and it

shows misplaced exocytosis. The secretory granules are sparse and small, measuring 150-200 nm. See also under PRL producing adenomas.

Plurihormonal GH producing adenomas

Plurihormonality, the production of more than one hormone by a tumour, is common in GH producing adenomas. About half of tumours, particularly densely granulated and mammosomatroph adenomas, contain PRL, α-SU, less commonly β-TSH, and exceptionally β-FSH and β-LH {1142}. These hormonal combinations are usually not clinically relevant.

Drug effects on GH producing adenomas

Total tumour removal is the objective of the surgery for GH producing adenomas, although medical therapy is widely used, particularly in case of surgical failure {1139}. In some centers, medical therapy is administered preoperatively to reduce complications and improve surgical outcome. Long-acting somatostatin analogues are known to inhibit GH secretion. Somatostatin administration ameliorates signs and symptoms of GH hypersecretion; however, slight to moderate reduction of tumour volume is evident only in a minority of cases. Morphologic changes are variable and inconsistent. In some cases, there is an increase in the size and number of secretory granules and presence of many lysosomes. Mild to moderate stromal fibrosis and hyalinisation are frequently observed {593,1139}. Somatostatin treated GH producing adenomas, particularly macroadenomas, show a slightly increased apoptotic index, as compared to non-treated tumours, although no significant differences were observed {1143,1176}.

Growth fraction / Ki-67 index
Morphometric studies show that pituitary adenomas have a slow growth rate with a low S-fraction. In particular, the S-fraction of somatotroph adenomas is 2.26 in diploid tumours and somewhat higher (2.86) in aneuploid tumours with no significant differences {1137}. Recent studies, using antibodies against the MIB-1 clone of Ki-67, confirm the low proliferation rate of GH-producing adenomas with a labeling index which is generally less than 3%. Sparsely granulated GH producing tumours have a higher mean labeling index, whereas mammosomatotroph adenomas have a lower mean index {2219}. It has been proposed that adenomas with growth fraction of more that 3% might have an aggressive biological behaviour.

Precursor lesions
Hyperplasia of somatotroph cells occurs in ectopic production of GHRH by endocrine tumours and in patients with McCune-Albright syndrome {1963}. An overlapping of GH producing adenoma with somatotroph hyperplasia may be present in some cases, particularly in the Carney complex. Transformation of hyperplasia to adenoma, which is evident in transgenic animals overexpressing GHRH {88}, remains poorly documented in humans {1929}.

Histogenesis
GH producing adenomas derive from the acidophil cell line. This lineage comprising somatotroph, lactotroph, and thyrotroph cells is controlled by a common transcription factor named PIT-1. This factor is localized in somatotrophs, lactotrophs and thyrotrophs and activates the GH, PRL and the β-TSH subunit genes {90,1867}. This transcription factor may explain the frequent plurihormonality of these tumours.

Somatic genetics
Cytogenetics and CGH
Studies at putative or candidate gene loci show frequent aberrations at 10q {133,206}, 11q {133,206,272,2216} and 13q {133,206,1709,2059}, where losses at some or all of these loci show signifi-

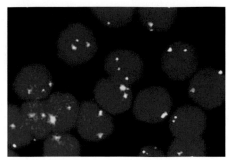

Fig. 1.05 GH adenoma. FISH using an alpha-centromere specific probe for chromosome 11. Several nuclei with three fluorescent signals in a sparsely granulated somatotroph adenoma.

cant increase from non-invasive to invasive adenoma and to pituitary carcinoma {133,206,1709}. Allelic imbalance, indicative of gene amplification of the *CCND1* locus on 11q has also been described using a microsatellite approach {882}.

Genome wide cytogenetic investigations have employed conventional karyotyping and fluorescent in situ hybridisation (FISH) to the study of pituitary adenoma including the GH producing adenoma subtype. These studies have shown aneuploidy for different chromosomes in pituitary adenoma subtypes including GH producing adenoma. One study showed trisomies of chromosomes 3,5,7,11,12,13,17, and 19 in a single tumour {499}, another trisomy of chromosome 12 in 2 GH producing adenoma {2189} . CGH studies have shown chromosomal imbalances that target multiple

chromosomes in pituitary tumours including GH producing adenomas {604, 628,832,935,1488,2259}. In general, aberrations appear more frequent in functioning adenomas than their non-functioning counterparts, and are more common in invasive/recurrent tumours than their more benign counterparts. Reported chromosomal imbalances range from 48% {1488} and 80% of adenomas {935}. The most common gains appear to be of chromosomes 9 and 17 {935} as well as losses of chromosome 18 {935}, 1 and 2 {832} and 11 {832, 1488}. Multiple other gains, in particular on chromosomes 5, 19 and 22, or losses involving either whole chromosomes, for example chromosome 1, or individual arms (13q) have also been reported.

GSP oncogene
One of the earliest molecular defects described in GH producing tumours were mutations in the α-subunit of the Gs protein leading to a constitutively active subunit termed the gsp oncogene {1373, 2286}. The *gsp* oncogene has varying geographic distribution in frequency {2104,2446,2460}. A downstream mediator in this pathway, the cAMP-responsive nuclear transcription factor (CREB), is also found in its phosphorylated (active) form in GH producing tumours irrespective of gsp status {181}. GH producing tumours also show increased expression and activity of the intracellular mediator protein kinase C (PKC) {44}. A conserved mutation in the α-subunit of PKC was

Table 1.05
Comparative genomic hybridization analyses of GH producing adenomas.

N	Abnormality	Losses	Gains	Reference
7	4/7	1p,11	4q,5,7,8q,7p,10p,13,X	{1488}
6	4/10	1p,6p,11q,13q,16q	3,6p,7,9q,11q,12q,14q,17,19,20	{604}
10	5/10	3p,10q,15	1q,5,6,8,9,12,13,14,15,16,17,19,20,X	{2259}
2	2/2	1p,2,11,13	1q,7q	{935}
10	8/10	1p,2q,4,5q,6q,13q,18	1p,3,5p,5q,9p.9q11,12,14,16p, 17p,19q,19,21q,22	{935}
6	1/6*	5,8	–	{628}
8	**8/8	11	11	{1136}

*Cytogenetic and Interphase FISH
**Interphase FISH

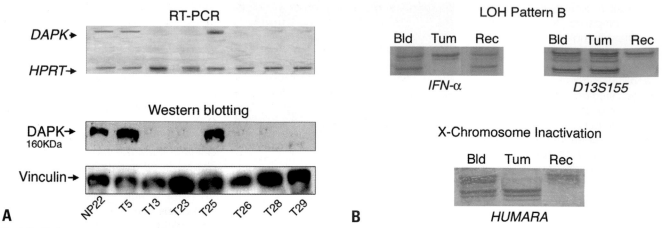

Fig. 1.06 Pituitary adenomas genetics. **A** RT-PCR and Western blot analysis for Death Associated Protein Kinase (DAPK). The figure shows post-mortem normal pituitary and representative sporadic pituitary adenomas. Normal pituitary (NP22) and some tumours show a DAPK transcript (T5, T25) whereas the remaining tumours do not. Alls specimens showed successful amplification of the housekeeping gene HPRT. Western blotting showed an identical pattern of expression to that observed by RT-PCR analysis. Both normal pituitary and all of the adenomas expressed vinculin as control for protein loading and integrity. Methylation of the DAPK genes CpG island, or promoter deletion were significantly associated with loss of expression (see text for details). **B** Clonality of pituitary adenomas as determined by LOH and X-chromosome inactivation analysis in an initial and a recurrent pituitary adenoma. The LOH (pattern B) shows that the patient is informative for the microsatellite markers IFNa and D13S155, since two alleles can be seen in the matched blood sample (Bld). For the marker IFNa the initial adenoma (Tum) shows LOH since the lower allele is absent. However, in the recurrence (from the same patient) there is no LOH. The converse is seen for the microsatellite marker D13S155, in this case the initial adenoma shows retention of heterozygosity and the recurrence shows LOH. These results suggest that both the initial and recurrent clones are mono-clonal but that they represent "different" clones. These conclusion are further supported by X-chromosome inactivation analysis by HUMARA analysis. The blood DNA shows that the patient is informative since two alleles are present. In the initial adenoma (Tum) and its recurrence (Rec) the opposite X-chromosomes are inactivated, however both specimens are monoclonal. Taken together (LOH and X-chromosome inactivation) show that and initial and recurrent adenomas from the same patient may show different clonal origins.

associated with invasive adenomas {43}, however, this was not confirmed in a subsequent report {1970}.

Promoter methylation
CpG island (CGI) methylation, an epigenetic change, is associated with or causal in gene silencing. Methylation-associated inactivation of the cell cycle regulatory molecules p16 (*CDKN2A*), is present with varying frequencies in GH producing tumours {990,1882,2000, 2056,2412}. Methylation or discrete homozygous deletion of the *RB1* gene CGI is also significantly associated with loss of pRb protein in GH producing tumours {2058}. A single report also describes methylation (or homozygous deletion) associated loss of the pro-apoptotic molecule Death Associated Protein Kinase (*DAPK*) in invasive GH producing tumours and nonfunctioning adenomas; methylation was infrequent in their non-invasive counterparts {2057}.

Expression profiles and proteomics
GH producing tumours show inappropriate expression profiles for growth factors and/or their receptors where the intrinsic molecular defects have not been elucidated. The growth stimulatory factor

GHRH and its receptor are expressed by GH producing tumour {842,1015, 1285,2220}. Increased expression of GHRH is seen in aggressive adenomas {2220} and some adenomas preferentially express a truncated nonfunctioning receptor {842}. Single reports have shown inappropriate expression of a functional TRH receptor {2438}, GnRH and its receptor {1926}. Somatostatin (SS) and its receptors (SSTRs) are expressed by GH producing tumours {1015,1063,1287,1501,1711,1712,1816} and SS levels are reduced in large invasive adenomas {1287}. Some studies have shown a relationship between SSTR density on GH producing tumours and secretory response to the somatostatin analogues {1816}. More recent reports show that the effect of SS and its analogues on tumour-cell proliferation and its ability to inhibit GH secretion are dissociated in this tumour type {451}. The epidermal growth factor (EGF), and vascular endothelial growth factor (VEGF) and their receptors are expressed by GH producing tumours and receptor levels correlate with aggressiveness {988,1279}. GH producing tumours also elaborate various isoforms of basic fibroblast growth factor (bFGF known as FGF2)

and its receptor {6,596,1293}. Very recently a pituitary tumour derived FGF4 receptor (ptdFGF4-R) was described that is constitutively active (phosphorylated). This oncogenic receptor is found in most pituitary adenoma subtypes including GH producing tumours {598}. The mechanisms responsible for its postulated alternate promoter usage and/or splicing are not currently known. A single report has shown an inverse relationship between expression of the purine- binding factor nm23 H2 and cavernous sinus invasion in GH producing tumours {2183}.

Several cell cycle regulatory molecules are subject to dysregulated expression in GH producing tumours. The pituitary tumour-transforming gene (PTTG) is overexpressed in the majority of pituitary adenoma subtypes including GH producing tumours and expression appears to correlate with invasion {2488}. Overexpression of p53 is also seen in some invasive adenomas and carcinomas, although as with PTTG the responsible molecular mechanisms have not been identified {2222}. Some studies have described overexpression of cyclin D1 in GH producing adenoma {882, 1013}, loss or reduced expression of p27

{570,1006,1297,1334,1781} in pituitary adenomas including GH producing adenoma. Although the mechanism responsible for reduced expression is not yet apparent it is postulated to occur through a proteosome-ubiquitin pathway {1297}. Very recently loss of the cell cycle regulatory molecule GADD45γ as determined by RT-PCR was described in the majority of pituitary tumour subtypes investigated including GH producing adenoma {2489}. A single study has employed microarray analysis of approximately 7000 genes {585}. In GH producing adenoma 30 genes were differentially expressed with an equal number showing overexpression as those showing reduced expression levels. For selected genes expression levels were confirmed by quantitative RT-PCR.

Genetic susceptibility

Most GH producing adenomas are sporadic; however, a small number occur with a familial aggregation. They may be components of multiple endocrine neoplasia type 1 (MEN1) due to mutation of the tumour suppressor gene MENIN on chromosome 11q13 {351}. Carney complex, an autosomal dominant disorder characterized by cardiac myxomas, endocrine overactivity including GH hypersecretion and other features, is due to germline mutations of the protein kinase A regulatory subunit (PRKAR1) gene on 2p16 {1094}. Rarely they occur as familial GH producing adenomas. Pituitary adenomas are present in 13-60% of patients with MEN1 (reviewed in {674}) and GH producing adenomas range from 0-37% {674}. GH producing adenomas are present in 10-21% of patients with Carney complex (reviewed in {674}). A single study has investigated pituitary tissue from patients with Carney complex and in all cases more than one adenoma was present within the gland, and where extratumoural tissue was excised there was evidence of hyperplasia surrounding the adenoma {1671}. This study also described CGH analysis of pituitary tissue associated with Carney complex; although no alterations were found in microadenomas, a macroadenoma exhibited multiple genetic changes. Isolated familial GH producing adenoma, not a component of Carney complex or MEN1, is a rare occurrence with approximately 20 families appearing in the literature since 1974. While some of these tumours show LOH at 11q13 (the MEN1 locus) no germ line mutations in this gene or its exon-intron boundaries were found {2188, 2208} implying that a gene in this region, distinct from MEN-1, is responsible for familial GH producing adenomas. Somatotroph, mammosomatotroph and mixed GH-PRL producing adenomas frequently show aberrations of chromosome 11, often with increased copy number involving 8-24% of adenoma cell population. Monosomy 11 was reported only in a patient with mixed GH-PRL producing adenoma. {1135,1136}. CGH showed cytogenetic changes in an aggressive invasive macroadenoma. Genomic aberrations involved several chromosomal regions, including loss of chromosome 11 {2149}.

Prognosis and predictive factors

DNA ploidy. Approximately 20% of all somatotroph and mammosomatotroph adenomas are aneuploid {1137,2119}. About half of the cases with chromosome 11 aberrations are associated with aneuploid histograms {1136,1138}.

Prolactin producing adenoma

W. Saeger
E. Horvath
K. Kovacs
V. Nosé

W.E. Farrell
R.V. Lloyd
R.E. Watson Jr.
E.P. Lindell

Definition
A benign pituitary tumour producing prolactin (PRL), originating from the prolactin adenohypophysial cell.

Synonyms
Lactotroph adenoma, prolactin secreting adenoma, prolactinoma.

ICD-O code   8271/0

Epidemiology
PRL producing adenomas comprise between 11 and 26% of pituitary adenomas in surgical series, although they were the most commonly excised surgically before the introduction of dopamine agonist therapy {1889,2211}. In autopsy series, PRL producing adenoma is the most common pituitary adenoma. These tumours are usually very small. The male/female ratio in surgical series is 1:2.6 {2211} and in autopsy series 1:0.6 {1457}. In women, 76 % of PRL producing adenomas occur between 21 and 40 years; in men this age group is represented by 40% {1507}. The recurrence rate is usually under 20% {1445}. The mortality is also very low since dopamine agonists and surgical treatments stop further growth in most cases, but in a few cases PRL producing adenomas invade extensively into the surrounding tissues.

Etiology
The etiology of PRL producing adenomas is unknown. Estrogens play a major role in the development of experimental PRL producing adenomas and in pregnancy the lactotroph cells become hypertrophic and hyperplastic; moreover, pre-existing PRL producing adenomas may show an acceleration of growth during pregnancy but estrogens alone appear to be unable to induce PRL producing adenomas in humans {414,2399}. The increased growth of macroprolactinomas in contrast to the absent growth of microprolactinomas during pregnancy is rather controversial and is a much-debated issue {2331}. A PRL producing adenoma has been reported in a male-to-female transsexual patient treated with estrogen {1160}.

Localization
PRL producing microadenomas are localized in the lateral or posterior part of the anterior pituitary. Rare ectopic localizations in the suprasellar region, spinal region and sinus or the nasopharyngeal region have been described {1331}.

Clinical features
Signs and symptoms
PRL producing adenoma, the most common neoplasm of the anterior pituitary {268} is associated with hyperprolactinemia. The serum PRL levels usually parallel tumour size {1374,1613}. Pretreatment serum PRL levels in men exceed those in women at least in part because these neoplasms are usually larger in men {1374,1613}. Women usually present at a younger age and tend to have microadenomas while males have significantly larger tumours {484,1374,2424}. In one series, 74% of the tumours in males were macroadenomas compared to 40% in females {527}. Giant PRL producing adenomas and carcinomas are described almost exclusively in men {484,1746}.

PRL producing adenomas may be asymptomatic and discovered incidentally, particularly in postmenopausal females or older males. These tumours are a frequent cause of reproductive and sexual dysfunction and clinical manifestations are different depending upon gender {170,1613,2265}. In women, minor elevations in PRL levels with alterations in the secretion of gonadotropins cause early symptoms such as amenorrhea and galactorrhea. In men, the symptoms are usually reduced libido, sexual impotence and abnormal semen {170}.

Childhood pituitary adenomas are rare, comprising only 2% of combined adult and paediatric pituitary adenomas {170} and 2.7% of supratentorial tumours in childhood {1032}. PRL producing tumours are the most common pituitary adenoma in childhood and adolescence with a frequency of 41.5% and 52% in two large series {1179,1695}. PRL producing macroadenomas were found in 89% of boys versus 41% of girls {399}.

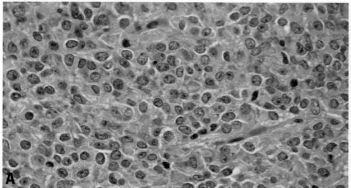
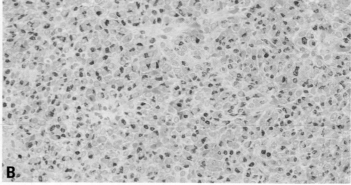

Fig. 1.07 PRL adenoma. **A** Chromophobic cells with prominent Golgi complexes. **B** PRL immunostaining (Golgi pattern).

PRL producing tumours in children are more common in females. The clinical presentation is sex and age-dependent. Growth failure, headache, and visual disturbances occur at presentation in prepubertal children. In pubertal females the usual presentation is pubertal delay, menstrual abnormalities, galactorrhea, hypogonadism, other pituitary hormone deficiencies or mass effect. Pubertal males usually present with visual impairment, headache and growth or pubertal arrest.

From a series of 123 PRL producing adenomas the mean preoperative serum PRL level in men was 2,031 ng/ml while in females it was 399 ng/ml {1374}. A single measurement greater than 250 ng/ml is diagnostic. Any sellar or parasellar process that compresses the pituitary stalk can lead to increased serum PRL, usually less than 100 ng/ml. PRL producing adenomas may also be associated with macroprolactinaemia (hyperprolactinaemia with a predominance or only big big prolactin isoform) {1547}.

Imaging

At imaging, endocrinologically active PRL producing tumours are usually microadenomas. Occasionally hormonally active macroadenomas are seen and require more extensive neuroimaging beyond the immediate sellar region. PRL producing microadenomas on pregadolinium coronal T1 MR are generally hypointense relative to the surrounding pituitary. Contrast enhancement of normal and neoplastic pituitary tissue has a dynamic relationship. Following gadolinium administration PRL producing microadenomas typically have less initial contrast enhancement than the surrounding normal pituitary when imaged in the first minute. However, with time this differential enhancement relationship may disappear, and in some cases may reverse, with retained contrast in the adenoma relative to the surrounding pituitary. Hemorrhagic and cystic changes and extension beyond the sella can be identified in macroadenomas on MRI. Adenomas are relatively soft tumours and rarely narrow the carotid arteries. In contrast to microadenomas, macroadenomas are generally characterized by robust contrast enhancement.

Macroscopy

PRL producing microadenoma may be

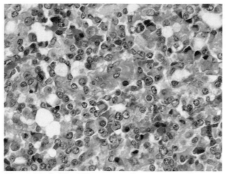

Fig. 1.08 Acidophil stem cell adenoma. Tumour cells with fibrous bodies and scattered vacuoles corresponding to giant mitochondria.

distinguished from the normal anterior lobe mostly by its soft consistency and its red tan appearance. Fibrosis and cystic changes may be present in macroadenomas.

Tumour spread and staging

The tumour starts as an intrasellar microadenoma, expanding to the capsule and to the sellar bone, which may be thinned by adenomas with enclosed growth pattern or destroyed by adenomas with invasive growth. Extrasellar extension includes (1) suprasellar growth with elevation and reduction of the sellar diaphragm, (2) rostral extension into the sphenoid sinus or nasopharynx, and (3) lateral extension into the cavernous sinus by displacement of the dura separating the sella from the sinus or by growth through natural defects in the dura (this may be seen in all adenomas) {1477A}.

Histopathology

Most PRL producing adenomas are sparsely granulated. These tumours have to be differentiated from the rare densely granulated PRL producing adenomas and also acidophil stem cell adenomas {1889,2211}.

Sparsely granulated lactotroph adenomas

These tumours show a diffuse or rarely a papillary growth pattern and are often congested. Cellular or nuclear pleomorphism is generally low, but in some cases distinct. The cells are relatively large and often elongated. The cellular membranes are indistinct. The cytoplasm is chromophobic or slightly acidophilic and PAS-negative. Calcospherites or psammoma bodies are occasionally seen. Interstitial amyloid of endocrine type is sometimes

seen in this adenoma type {2126}. PRL immunoreactivity is typically paranuclear ("Golgi pattern"), mostly strong and found in the vast majority of cells. Other pituitary hormones such as α-subunit are rarely found. The Ki-67 labeling index is usually low, but may be higher in aggressive adenomas, which correlate with increased mitotic activity.

Electron microscopy reveals large euchromatic nuclei, prominent nucleoli, an extremely developed rough endoplasmic reticulum forming concentric whorls, large Golgi areas, many immature secretory granules and sparse mature granules with diameters ranging from 150 to 300 nm {79}. Granule extrusions along the lateral cell borders into the extracellular space are found (so-called "misplaced exocytoses") {1888}.

Densely granulated lactotroph adenomas

This rare adenoma type resembles the sparsely granulated type but reveals a stronger cytoplasmic acidophilia. PRL immunoreactivity is strong and diffuse throughout the cytoplasm.

The ultrastructure shows many irregular large secretory granules, well-developed Golgi complexes and less abundant rough endoplasmic reticulum than in the sparsely granulated type {79}.

Acidophil stem cell adenoma

Some authors consider this tumour to be a variant of PRL producing adenomas although others consider this to be a subtype of GH producing adenomas (see description under GH producing adenomas).

Effect of dopamine agonists

Dopamine agonist treatment induces severe alterations in the majority of PRL producing adenomas. The cells become dramatically smaller with cytoplasmic shrinkage and increased nuclear:cytoplasmic ratios. The nuclei are hyperchromatic. In patients with longer-term treatment, adenomas develop extensive perivascular and interstitial fibrosis. Single cell necrosis is rarely found. In some cases the PRL immunoreactivity is decreased and only some cells remain immunopositive. Ultrastructurally, the volumes of rough endoplasmic reticulum and Golgi complexes are strongly reduced.

In some adenomas a variable response

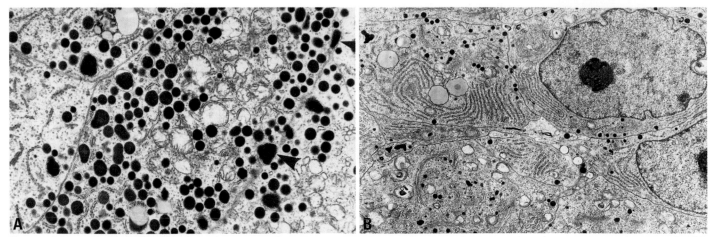

Fig. 1.09 A Mammosomatotroph adenoma showing numerous large secretory granules as well as larger than average irregular secretory granules, some of which are extruded into the extracellular space (arrowheads). **B** PRL-producing adenoma. Sparsely granulated PRL-producing adenoma illustrating its three characteristics: abundant RER, large active Golgi complex and granule extrusion.

to dopamine agonists is demonstrable: many cells shrink but others remain large and unaltered. D-2 receptor loss may be responsible for the resistance of the PRL producing cells to dopamine agonist administration. The effects of dopamine agonists appear reversible after discontinuance of treatment although some adenomas do not regrow.

Precursor lesions

Precursor lesions may be focal lactotroph hyperplasia, which can be found in some autopsy pituitaries {1888} but a clear distinction between a large hyperplastic nodule and a small PRL producing adenoma is often very difficult.

Histogenesis

The postulated cell of origin is the lactotroph or a precursor cell, since studies demonstrated bihormonal mammosomatotrophs and an embryological relationship of somatotrophs and lactotrophs, the two acidophil cell types {86}.

Somatic genetics

In common with other pituitary adenoma subtypes, PRL producing adenomas show inappropriate expression of growth regulatory molecules, their receptors, intracellular signal transduction proteins and cell cycle regulatory molecules.

Cytogenetics and CGH

Karyotyping studies, including PRL producing adenomas, have found trisomies of chromosome 12 as well as for chromosomes 5, 7, 8, 9 and 20 {628,1233}. Subsequent studies employing micro-

satellite markers and Fluorescence in situ hybridization (FISH) analysis showed trisomy of chromosome 12 in 4 of 6 PRL producing adenomas {2189}.
Comparative genomic hybridization (CGH) studies have shown chromosomal imbalances that target multiple chromosomes {604,832,1488,1824,2259}. In general, aberrations appear at higher frequency in these investigations compared to other cytogenetic techniques, are usually more frequent in functioning adenomas than their nonfunctioning counterparts. They are also more common in invasive/recurrent tumours than their noninvasive counterparts. These studies reported chromosomal imbalances in between 48% {1488} and 80% of adenomas {935}. In addition to the trisomies discussed above, the most common gains appear to be of chromosomes 4q and 5q {1824} losses on 1 and 2 {832, 1488,1824}, 11 and 13 {832,1488}.

HRAS

Mutation in the *RAS* oncogene was first described in highly aggressive PRL producing adenomas and subsequently in pituitary carcinomas or in their metastases {276,1041,1710}. There have been no other reports of molecular alterations in this adenoma subtype.

HMGA2

Recently, the *HMGA2* gene (that maps to 12q14-15) was found to be amplified in 7 of 8 PRL producing adenomas {629}. RT-PCR, Western blotting and IHC showed HMGA2 over-expression in a number of these PRL producing adenomas.

Promoter methylation

Epigenetic change, namely methylation of CpG islands (CGI) has been reported in PRL producing adenomas. To date, studies have been confined to the p16 gene (*CDKN2A*), and where expression data are included, these studies have shown an association between this epigenetic change and gene silencing {990,2000}. A further report also showed frequent methylation associated loss of p16 in adenomas that co-stained for PRL and GH {2412} and a single study has suggested that PRL producing adenomas show no epigenetic change at this locus {1882}. However, in this case this may reflect the small number of tumours investigated.

Expression profiles and proteomics

PRL producing adenomas exhibit inappropriate expression profiles for growth factors and/or their receptors where the intrinsic molecular defects have not been elucidated. In one report, it was noted that all types of pituitary adenomas, including PRL producing adenomas, express GnRH, the GnRH receptor (GnRH-R) was absent in this adenoma subtype {1926}. Alternatively spliced and truncated receptors for GHRH {842} and TRH {2437} are expressed, the former at low levels and the latter at high levels relative to full-length forms. In addition, these adenomas express TRH {1251, 1252}. TGF-β 1/2/3, EGF, VEGF and their receptors are expressed by pituitary adenomas {1006,1279,1340}. PRL receptor mRNA is found in lactotrophs as well as in PRL producing adenomas

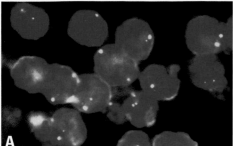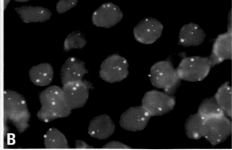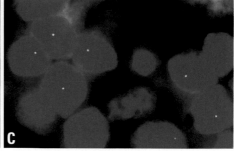

Fig. 1.10 Sporadic PRL producing pituitary adenoma. **A** FISH on paraffin section for chromosome 11 centromere (green) and MEN1 gene (BAC, red). The neoplastic cells have up to 2 signals for chromosome 11 centromere, but no more than one signal for MEN1 gene, indicating deletion of MEN1 gene. **B** FISH on paraffin section for chromosome 11 centromere (green) and MEN1 gene (BAC, red). The neoplastic cells have up to 2 signals for chromosome 11 centromere and for MEN1 gene, indicating no deletion of MEN1 gene. **C** Sporadic recurrent pituitary adenoma. FISH on paraffin section for HER2/neu (chromosome 17, green). No more than one signal per nucleus is seen, indicating monosomy of Her2/neu and absence of gene amplification.

{386,1007}. PRL producing adenomas express bFGF {596} and FGF-4 (hst) {743}. A more recent report describes a pituitary tumour derived FGF4 receptor (ptd-FGF4-R), which was constitutively active {598}. A single report has shown an inverse relationship between expression of the purine-binding factor nm23 H2 and cavernous sinus invasion in PRL producing adenoma {2183}.

The pituitary tumour-transforming gene (PTTG) is also over-expressed in PRL producing adenoma and its expression appears to correlate with invasion {2488}. Inappropriate expression of both p53 and p27 are seen in many invasive PRL producing adenomas and carcinomas {570,1006,1297,1334,1720,1781, 2222}. Reduced expression of p27 is probably a post-translation event and is thought to occur through a proteasome-ubiquitin pathway {1297}. Recently, loss of the cell cycle regulatory molecule GADD45γ as determined by RT-PCR was described in the majority of pituitary adenomas {2489}. A microarray analysis of >7000 genes showed that 47 genes were differentially expressed {585}.

Genetic susceptibility

PRL producing adenomas are usually sporadic or can be associated with MEN1, in which they are the most common pituitary tumour type {674,1422, 2310}. The primary germline mutations in MEN1 have now been identified {351}. Only a single report of isolated familial PRL producing adenomas, not a component of MEN1, has appeared in the literature {169}.

Prognosis and predictive factors

Clinical criteria for a good prognosis are the normalization of the serum PRL levels after medical or surgical therapy {2368}. Following surgery, regrowth of the adenoma is demonstrable by recurrence of hyperprolactinemia and MRI assessment of tumour mass. Macroadenomas, especially those occurring in men, show a higher recurrence rate than microadenomas {484,1693,2368}.

The role of tumour angiogenesis in predicting prognosis may prove to be important {1340}.

Markers of cell proliferation can be used for assessment of prognosis: Ki-67, c-myc protein, p53 protein {47}, and also mitotic rates can be useful but fail to distinguish clearly between benign, aggressive or malignant pituitary tumours in individual cases. Recurrences are more likely if the Ki-67 labeling index exceeds 5% and p53 protein-positive nuclei are found but clear statements for the individual patient are not possible.

Table 1.06
Comparative genomic hybridization analyses of PRL producing adenomas.

N	Abnormality	Losses	Gains	Reference
3 (Primary)	2/3	1p,2,8q,10,11,16	1q,9,12p,14,15q,22q	
3 (Recurrence)	3/3	1p,1,2,4,8q,10,11, 16	1q,4q,4,5q,5,9,12p,13q,14	{1824}
3	3/3	13q,13,Xp	3,5,6,7,8,9q,11,12,14q, 16,17q1718,19p19,20,21,22	{604}
5	1/5	–	X	{2259}
1	1/1	1p,2,10q,17p	5q	{832}
6	4/6	1,2,10,11,13,18,Y	5,7q,8,9,12,14,Xp,X	{1488}
10	8/10	1p,2q,4,5q,6q,13q,18	1p,3,5p,5q,9p.9q11,12, 14,16p,17p,19q,19,21q,22	{935}
3*	3/3	–	11	{1136}

* Interphase FISH

TSH producing adenoma

R.Y. Osamura
T. Sano
S. Ezzat
S.L. Asa

A.L. Barkan
R.E. Watson Jr.
E.P. Lindell

Definition
A benign pituitary tumour producing thyrotropin (TSH), originating from adenohypophysial cells.

ICD-O code   8272/0

Synonyms
Thyrotroph adenoma, thyrotrophic adenoma, thyrotropinoma, TSH secreting adenoma, TSHoma

Epidemiology
TSH producing adenomas are rare among the pituitary adenomas (1%) {182}. In one series the age of the 16 patients who underwent transsphenoidal surgery ranged from 23-62 years and the sex distribution was 12 women and 4 men {1927}.

Localization
Microadenomas are usually present in the mucoid wedge. However, most tumours are macroadenomas at the time of diagnosis and show no specific localization.

Clinical features
TSH producing adenomas usually secrete excess TSH and present with a goiter and hyperthyroidism (hypermetabolic state, tachycardia, tremor, proximal myopathy, neuropsychiatric abnormalities, etc.). Clinically, these patients do not differ from those with Graves disease, with the exception of absent ophthalmopathy or dermopathy. In most patients with TSH producing adenomas, the thyroid gland is nodular and this may complicate clinical distinction from multinodular thyroid disease. Because a minority of TSH producing adenomas cosecrete GH and/or PRL, patients may present primarily with acromegaly and/or amenorrhea / galactorrhea {146,147, 1927}.
The majority of lesions are macroadenomas and invasive. Misdiagnosis leads to inappropriate thyroid ablation (surgery or radioiodine); often, these tumours exhibit progressive growth and invasiveness.

Laboratory diagnosis
This is based on the finding of high (or, at least, "inappropriately normal") levels of TSH in the presence of elevated free T4 and free T3 concentrations. TSH producing adenomas frequently secrete excessive quantities of free α-subunit, and this measurement may be helpful in diagnosis. As mentioned above, elevated concentrations of GH and/or PRL suggest cosecretion by the tumour. The differential diagnosis is with pituitary resistance to thyroid hormone with clinical presentations and thyroid function tests being identical between the two entities. However, patients with TSH producing adenomas have higher α-subunit/TSH ratio. Also, TSH producing adenomas do not further increase TSH secretion after a bolus dose of TRH, whereas patients with pituitary resistance to thyroid hormone have an exaggerated TSH response. Neither group suppresses TSH secretion in response to exogenous T3. Radioactive iodine uptake is high in both entities.

Imaging
At imaging, endocrinologically active TSH producing adenomas are usually macroadenomas with extensive invasion. The rare TSH producing microadenomas on pre-gadolinium coronal T1 MR are generally hypointense relative to the surrounding pituitary.

Macroscopy
Surgical findings show unusually firm tumours that tend to be invasive and fibrotic.

Tumour and spread and staging
In a series of 16 cases, 10 showed invasion in both cavernous sinus and dura and 12 cases showed invasion in dura {1927}.

Histopathology
The tumours are composed of chromophobic cells with indistinct cell borders and varying degrees of nuclear pleomorphism. Architecturally, the tumours most commonly exhibit solid or sinusoidal patterns. Stromal fibrosis is relatively common and occasional psammoma bodies may be present. The PAS stain identifies strongly positive small cytoplasmic globules that correspond to lysosomes. The tumour cells show variable immunoreactivity for α-subunit and β-TSH. Immunohistochemistry highlights the polygonal structure of the tumour cells that usually have elongated processes. The tumour cells are also sometimes plurihormonal with reaction for GH and/or PRL by immunohistochemistry or in situ hybridisation.
Electron microscopically, the tumour cells resemble normal thyrotrophs. The polygonal cells have euchromatic nuclei and long interdigitating cytoplasmic processes that contain abundant rough endoplasmic reticulum, prominent Golgi complex and lysosomes. Secretory granules, which are spherical and range in size from 150 to 250nm tend to accumulate along the cell membrane.

Somatic genetics
TSH-releasing hormone (TRH) stimulates thyrotrophs. Untreated primary hypothyroidism is associated with hyperplasia and focal neoplastic transition {1965} suggesting that protracted TRH stimulation may lead to TSH producing adenomas. TRH is expressed in the pituitary and by different types of pituitary adenomas {2438}. TRH signalling is intact in TSH-producing pituitary adenomas as evidenced by TRH binding resulting in release of TSH {2438}. TRH gene structure and receptor mRNA expression {2437} are unaltered in thyrotroph adenomas. TRH receptor mRNA is alternatively spliced in some tumours. Deletion of exon 3 results in a truncated product that does not efficiently bind TRH. Relatively higher levels of truncated forms compared to full-length forms in some adenomas {2437} may explain paradoxical in vivo responses to TRH. There is no direct evidence for TRH involvement in pituitary tumourigenesis.
Thyroid hormones inhibit pituitary thyrotroph hormone secretion and prolifera-

tion, balancing the stimulation of hypo-thalamic TRH. Loss of negative feedback may contribute to TSH producing adeno-mas associated with primary hypothy-roidism {1965}. Thyroid hormones medi-ate their actions via nuclear thyroid hor-mone receptors (TRs) that bind specific regulatory response elements on target genes. There are two major classes of TRs, α and β, each of which undergoes alternative splicing to generate α1, α2, β1 and β2 isoforms. The β2 isoform is predominantly expressed in the hypo-thalamic-pituitary system. Screening TRα mRNA identified three novel missense mutations in the TRα region. An alterna-tively spliced variant resulting in a 135-bp deletion within the ligand-binding domain of TRβ2 was described in a TSH-producing pituitary tumour. As predicted, this tumour variant (TRβ2spl) lacks thy-roid hormone binding and displays a dominant-negative impaired negative response to ligand inhibition of TSH secretion {56}.

Genetic susceptibility
Despite the important negative feedback functions of thyroid hormones, thyroid hormone resistance, usually due to a germline mutation in the TRβ receptor, is rarely associated with pituitary tumours {1891}.
Patients with MEN 1 or Carney complex demonstrate increased susceptibility to the development of pituitary tumours including TSH producing adenomas {263,351,1094}.

Prognosis and predictive factors
Because of frequent delay in diagnosis, the tumours are frequently macroadeno-mas and tend to be invasive and aggres-sive. High Ki-67 labeling index is of sup-portive evidence for the rapid growth. Transsphenoidal surgery can achieve a good long-term outcome in about two thirds of patients with TSH producing adenomas, particularly those with

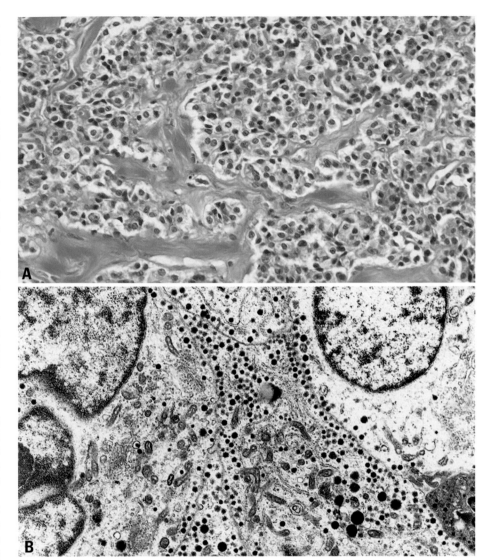

Fig. 1.11 A TSH adenoma. TSH producing adenoma with stromal fibrosis. **B** TSH-Adenoma. TSH-producing adenoma comprising angular cells with small sparse secretory granules lining up along the plasmalemma.

microadenomas. Patients with invasive or unresectable tumours need additional treatment with somatostatin analogues, radiation, and/or antithyroid therapy. Careful follow-up is necessary after sur-gery, especially in patients with a long preoperative history of hyperthyroidism.

ACTH producing adenoma

J. Trouillas
A.L. Barkan
R.E. Watson Jr.

E.P. Lindell
W.E. Farrell
R.V. Lloyd

Definition

The ACTH producing adenoma is a benign tumour, derived from corticotrophs of the anterior pituitary, that synthesize proopiomelanocortin(POMC) from which several peptides including ACTH, β-LPH and β-endorphin are cleaved.

ICD-O code   8272/0

Synonyms

Basophil adenoma, corticotroph or corticotropic adenoma, ACTH cell adenoma, ACTH secreting adenoma, ACTHoma, corticotropinoma.

Epidemiology

The incidence of Cushing disease is about 1-10 cases per million per year. ACTH producing adenomas with Cushing disease represent 10-15% of pituitary tumours {2263}. They are rare in childhood {1271} and the peak incidence is between the ages of 30 and 40 years. ACTH producing adenomas have an 8:1 female to male ratio {69}.

Etiology

Cushing disease is due to an ACTH producing adenoma, but the possibility of hyperplasia of corticotrophs, alone or associated with microadenoma, remains unclear {432,1843,2267,2467}.

Localization

ACTH producing adenomas are intrasellar tumours, with no predominant localization {125,1569}, although some studies have shown preference for the median wedge {1843,1844}.
Some suprasellar «ectopic» adenomas from the pars tuberalis {536,1014,1439} and double adenomas (ACTH producing and other tumour types especially PRL producing adenomas) have also been described {1262,2427}. The origin of some tumours from the intermediate lobe remains controversial {1473}.

Clinical features

Signs and symptoms

Pituitary ACTH-dependent disease is called Cushing disease as described by Harvey Cushing in 1932 {442}; this is in contrast to Cushing syndrome, which may have various nonpituitary aetiologies. Pituitary ACTH producing tumours retain some degree of negative feedback regulation by cortisol and this feature serves as a basis for several diagnostic tests differentiating Cushing disease from other forms of Cushing syndrome {193,1477}.
Cortisol overproduction is the underlying hormonal abnormality producing virtually the entire symptom complex of Cushing syndrome. Patients have fat deposition in the abdomen, preauricular, nuchal and supraclavicular areas and proximal muscle atrophy. Together, this results in a peculiar appearance of truncal obesity with thin extremities. Catabolic effects of excess cortisol results in thinning of the skin with plethoric facies, easy bruisability and violaceous striae particularly in the abdomen and chest. Steroid-induced osteoporosis is frequent, especially in the spine. Glucocorticoid excess results in insulin resistance and diabetes mellitus. Suppressed immune responses predispose to infections. Steroid-induced neuropsychiatric changes include depression, emotional lability, sleeplessness and poor memory. If ACTH levels are high (as in Nelson syndrome or ectopic ACTH syndrome) hyperpigmentation of skin and the mucous membranes may occur. Very high ACTH levels (macroadenomas or ectopic ACTH syndrome) may result in exceptionally high cortisol production. This may overcome the protective effect of 11-β-hydroxysteroid dehydrogenase on the mineralocorticoid receptor and result in sodium and fluid retention and hypokalemia.
The biochemical diagnosis of any form of Cushing syndrome rests of the demonstration of excessive cortisol production (best shown by high 24 hour urinary free cortisol excretion) and by loss of circadian rhythm. Simultaneous measurement of ACTH reliably distinguishes ACTH-independent Cushing syndrome in which plasma ACTH is below assay detection limit, from ACTH-dependent forms, in which ACTH may range from "normal" to grossly elevated. Plasma ACTH above 200 pg/ml is primarily seen in patients with ectopic ACTH production, although pituitary macroadenomas may also be accompanied by very high ACTH levels. Direct measurements of ACTH have largely replaced the elaborate ritual of the "low-dose/high dose" dexamethasone suppression test. In up to 20% of patients with suspected pituitary dependent

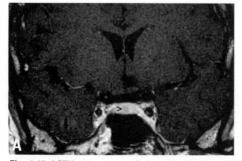 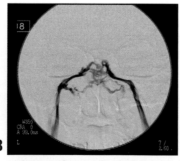

Fig. 1.12 ACTH adenomas. **A** Anterior pituitary ACTH microadenoma. Coronal T1-weighted gadolinium enhanced image demonstrates 2mm focus of decreased contrast enhancement centrally at the site of a small microadenoma (arrow head). **B** Petrosal sinus sampling. Digital subtraction venogram following injection of the distal inferior petrosal sinuses through microcatheters during petrosal sinus sampling procedure. The image demonstrates the venous drainage of the sellar and parasellar region, with opacification of the cavernous sinuses, circular sinus, clival venous plexus and inferior petrosal sinuses. ACTH concentration in blood sampled from the inferior petrosal sinuses following CRH challenge can be predictive of the lateralization of tiny pituitary microadenomas that are not demonstrable on imaging studies.

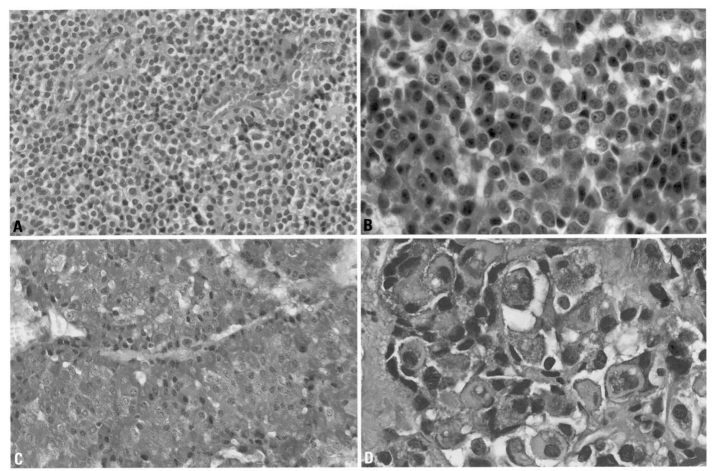

Fig. 1.13 ACTH adenoma **A** Basophilic cells in ACTH producing adenoma. **B** ACTH adenoma with Herlant tetrachrome showing basophilic adenoma cells. **C** Strong PAS positivity in a ACTH adenoma. **D** Crooke's hyaline change.

Cushing disease, no MRI abnormality is seen and the differential of occult ectopic ACTH secretion must be excluded. This should be tested with bilateral inferior petrosal sinus sampling before and after an I.V. CRH bolus. A pituitary-peripheral ACTH gradient >2 reliably establishes the diagnosis of Cushing disease, whereas a low value, especially after CRH stimulation, is diagnostic of an extrapituitary ACTH source.

Some patients with ACTH immunoreactive tumours present without evidence of hormone excess. These "silent" adenomas are usually macroadenomas that cause the symptoms of a mass lesion.

Imaging

In about 80% of patients with Cushing disease, pituitary MRI will show a microadenoma, and in another 5% a macroadenoma may be found. Some 10-20% of Cushing disease patients have no MRI abnormality (microadenomas below the MRI threshold of detection).

ACTH producing microadenomas on pre-gadolinium coronal T1 MR are generally hypointense relative to the surrounding pituitary. Contrast enhancement of normal and neoplastic pituitary tissue has a dynamic relationship. Following gadolinium administration microadenomas typically have less initial contrast enhancement than the surrounding normal pituitary when imaged in the first minute. However, with time this differential enhancement relationship may disappear, and in some cases may reverse, with retained contrast in the adenoma relative to the surrounding pituitary.

In some cases, imaging studies do not clearly demonstrate the presence of subtle ACTH producing microadenomas, despite clinical evidence of adenoma {404,518,535}.

Macroscopy

Most ACTH producing tumours are small microadenomas, measuring 4-6 mm {2127,2263}. At the time of surgery a small percentage of tumours are not identified by the pathologist even after serial sectioning. The tumours are usually red and soft and may be differentiated from the yellow tan, firm nontumourous pituitary. In some cases, the microadenoma may not be seen by the surgeon, but is identified by the pathologist. Intraoperative frozen sections or smears may help to find the tumour. Some ACTH producing adenomas invade the cavernous sinus and ACTH producing adenomas, without clinical and/or biological signs of hypercorticism {916,1333,2258}, may be discovered by the pathologist, and named "silent" ACTH producing adenoma. They are large, frequently invasive into the sphenoidal sinus and necrosed tumours. Some of them secrete high molecular weight ACTH related peptides {1805} or β-endorphin {2266}.

Histopathology

In the majority of ACTH producing adenomas, one can readily distinguish

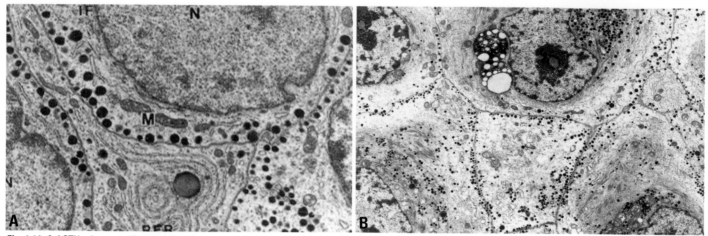

Fig. 1.14 A ACTH adenoma. Ultrastructural features. **B** Crooke cell adenoma displaying undue perinuclear accumulation of cytokeratin filaments trapping many of the secretory granules.

between the tumour and the nontumourous pituitary, although a capsule is not present. In some cases, the tumour cells may be intimately associated with the nonneoplastic pituitary. The tumours consist of monomorphic round cells, arranged diffusely with a characteristic sinusoidal pattern around the capillaries {1842}. The cells can be basophilic or amphophilic and strongly PAS-positive; some tumours, usually macroadenomas, are chomophobic and weakly PAS positive. Pleomorphism and apoptosis may be present. The nuclei are generally round and central with a conspicuous nucleolus. Mitoses are extremely rare. The non neoplastic corticotrophs often show various degrees of Crooke hyaline change due to the accumulation of cytokeratin positive intermediate filaments in the cytoplasm.

Silent ACTH producing tumours may be basophilic or chromophobic and strongly or mildly positive with the PAS stain.

In addition to the conventional ACTH producing adenomas, other variants of these tumours have been identified including *Crooke cell adenomas* and silent ACTH producing adenomas. Crooke cell adenomas consist of ACTH producing tumour cells with prominent cytoplasmic cytokeratin filaments {616}.

Immunohistochemistry

These tumours, whether functioning or clinically silent, are immunoreactive for ACTH, β-LPH and/or β-endorphin. The intensity of hormone immunoreactivity varies; chromophobic adenomas may have weak or focal positivity whereas basophilic adenomas tend to be strongly positive. Immunoreactivity for low molecular weight keratins identifies the intermediate filaments. The transcription factors neuroD1 {1665}. and Tpit {1220} are positive in ACTH producing adenomas. By in situ hybridisation, POMC mRNA can be detected {1333}.

Electron microscopy

By electron microscopy there are two variants of ACTH producing adenomas. In the vast majority of clinically functioning adenomas the cells resemble normal corticotrophs. They have moderately developed Golgi complex and rough endoplasmic reticulum. The most conspicuous feature is the presence of perinuclear bundles of 7 nm intermediate filaments of cytokeratins {859}. The secretory granules are usually numerous. They are spherical or slightly irregular ranging in size from 200 to 500 nm and tend to accumulate under the cell membrane. Silent subtype 1 adenomas, which are ACTH producing but clinically nonfunctioning, are indistinguishable from these functioning ACTH producing adenomas {916}.

Silent subtype 2 adenomas are made up of smaller than average size polyhedral cells possessing centrally placed nucleus and uncharacteristic RER and Golgi complex. There are usually sparse, irregular, drop-shaped secretory granules ranging from 150-300 nm in diameter. The tumour cells contain no cytokeratin filaments.

Somatic genetics

In one case report a *RAS* mutations was identified in a metastasis of an ACTH producing carcinoma. A single report has described a point mutation in the α-SU of protein kinase-C in an invasive ACTH producing adenoma {43}; however, this was not confirmed in a subsequent study {1970}. A novel germline mutation has been described in the glucocorticoid receptor (*GCR*) and has been implicated in the pathogenesis of Cushing disease {1042}. Somatic mutations in this receptor have been described in Nelsons syndrome, and also in cases of Cushing disease {1042A}.

Cytogenetics and CGH

Microsatellite marker analysis has shown monoallelic deletion of the glucocorticoid receptor in approximately 30% of ACTH producing adenomas, however, the functional significance is not known {936}. Interphase FISH studies have shown combined loss of chromosome 5 and 8 in 1 of 6 ACTH producing adenomas investigated and in another study loss of chromosome 11 in 3 or 4 cases {628}. CGH studies have shown chromosomal imbalances that target multiple chromosomes in pituitary tumours including ACTH producing adenomas {604,1488,2259}. In general, aberrations appear at higher frequency in this type of investigation compared to other cytogenetic techniques, are usually more frequent in functioning adenomas than their nonfunctioning counterparts, and are more common in invasive/recurrent tumours than their more benign counterparts. These studies have examined more than one adenoma subtype including ACTH producing adenomas and reported chromosomal

Table 1.07
Comparative genomic hybridization analyses of ACTH producing adenomas.

N	Abnormality	Losses	Gains	Reference
1	1/1	1q,2,4,7q,18,22	–	{604}
5	4/5	1q,2p,2q,15q,11	19p,X	{2259}
7	5/7	1p,1,2,4q,6p,6q,8p, 15,16,18q21,22	1q,5q,5,6p,7,8q,11, 12p,12q,12,13,14,X	{1488}
2*	2/2	-	11	{1136}

* Interphase FISH

imbalances in between 48% {1488} and 80% of adenomas {935}. Table 1.07 shows that multiple chromosomes are subject to both gains and losses in this adenoma subtype {1136}.

Promoter methylation.
CpG islands (CGI) methylation, associated with gene silencing, of the p16 gene (*CDKN2A*) has been shown by several groups in ACTH producing adenomas {1882,2000,2412}. Methylation of other genes found to be methylated in other pituitary adenoma subtypes (*RB1* and *DAPK*) have not been described.

Expression profiles and proteomics
ACTH producing adenomas exhibit inappropriate expression profiles for growth factors and/or their receptors where the intrinsic molecular defects have not been defined. Overexpression of the CRH receptor and of the closely related vasopressin V3 receptor have been reported {466,467,498}. ACTH producing adenomas, in common with other pituitary adenomas, express GnRH, in addition they also co-express its receptor (GnRH-R) {1926}. Single reports have described expression of receptors for GHRH {842} and for a growth hormone secretagogue {1148} in ACTH producing adenomas. Highly variable transcripts levels for EGF, VEGF and their receptors are found in the majority of ACTH producing adenomas {1279}. TGF-β-1/2/3 and the TGF-β-receptor are expressed by the majority of pituitary adenomas including ACTH producing adenomas {1006}. These adenomas also express bFGF {596}, and various isoforms of FGF receptors have been described in the majority of pituitary ade-

nomas investigated {6}. A recent report has described a pituitary tumour derived FGF4 receptor (ptd-FGF4-R) that is constitutively active, in the various hormone-secreting adenoma cell types {598}. Very recently a functional peroxisome proliferator-activated receptor-γ (PPAR-γ) that is exclusive to corticotrophs is abundantly expressed in ACTH producing adenomas {852}. A single report has shown decreased expression of the purine-binding factor nm23 H2 in ACTH producing adenomas with cavernous sinus invasion relative to other non-invasive pituitary adenoma subtypes {2183}.
ACTH producing adenomas overexpress the PTTG and expression levels correlate with invasion {2488}. A single report has described inappropriate expression of p53 in recurrent and non-invasive ACTH producing adenomas {256} while other studies suggest that immunopositivity for p53 separates non-invasive ACTH producing adenomas from invasive adenomas and carcinomas {677,1720,2222}. Loss or reduced expression of p27 appears to be a common finding in pituitary adenomas {570,1006,1297,1334, 1781}. Normal corticotrophs have low levels of p27 relative to other adenohypophysial cell types and the levels are further decreased in ACTH producing adenomas. Reduced expression is apparent as a post-translational event and is thought to occur through a proteosome-ubiquitin pathway {1297}. Loss of the cell cycle regulatory molecule GADD45γ, as determined by RT-PCR, is found in the majority of pituitary tumour subtypes investigated, including ACTH producing adenomas {2489}. A microarray analysis of >7000 genes {585}

revealed differential expression of 51 genes in ACTH producing adenomas. Expression levels for selected genes were confirmed by quantitative RT-PCR.

Genetic susceptibility
The majority of ACTH producing adenomas are sporadic; however, a small number occur with a familial aggregation as components of MEN 1 accounting for only 3.6% of cases in one series {111} and rarely affecting more than a single family member {679}. Non MEN 1 associated familial Cushing disease is an extremely rare entity and the central etiology not always certain {692,1913}.

Prognosis and predictive factors
The Ki-67 labeling index is variable {1227,2219}. The prognosis of ACTH producing adenomas is not related to the tumoural evolution but to the cardiovascular complications of the hypercorticism and to the neurosurgical difficulty in removing a very small tumour without damaging the juxtatumoural pituitary. Indeed, Cushing disease mortality has increased by a factor 3.8 {579}; the post-operative remission was achieved in around 85% of the patients {2127}. The rate of remission was significantly higher in microadenoma (92.6%) than in macroadenoma (66.7%). The recurrence rate after initially successful surgical treatment reached 15-20% at 5-6 years {2127}. Surgical failure is associated with the size and invasiveness of the adenoma {2287}. Silent ACTH producing adenomas are usually more aggressive and recur more frequently than tumours associated with hypercorticism. Histological signs of poor prognosis are being evaluated (plurihormonality, high Ki-67 labeling index, mitosis and expression of PSA-NCAM {2264}.
In some cases where patients have been treated with bilateral adrenalectomy for intractable glucocorticoid excess the ACTH producing pituitary adenoma grows at a rapid rate (Nelson syndrome) {76,677}.

Gonadotropin producing adenoma

S.L. Asa
S. Ezzat
R.E. Watson Jr.
E.P. Lindell
E. Horvath

Definition

Gonadotropin producing adenoma is a benign pituitary neoplasm composed of adenohypophysial gonadotrophs, cells that produce the gonadotropic hormones follicle-stimulating hormone (FSH) and /or luteinizing hormone (LH), or that show evidence of differentiation along the pathway of gonadotroph differentiation.

ICD-O code   8272/0

Epidemiology

Functioning gonadotropin producing adenomas with hypersecretion of gonadotropins or their subunits are more common in men {2074} and are rarely diagnosed in women, likely due to physiological elevations of gonadotropins in menopause {448}. Gonadotropin producing adenomas are more often diagnosed based on pathology, and they represent the majority of clinically nonfunctioning pituitary adenomas {79}. Accurate incidence rates are not available, since the epidemiology of pituitary adenomas is incomplete.

Localization

Gonadotropin producing adenomas are usually large macroadenomas at the time of diagnosis. They often exhibit significant suprasellar extension or parasellar invasion. They are occasionally detected as incidental findings at autopsy and these small lesions show no preferential localization within the adenohypophysis.

Clinical features

Gonadotropin producing adenomas exhibit a wide range of hormonal and proliferative behaviour. They may be small lesions with a slow rate of growth, or large, locally compressive or invasive lesions. Most are hormonally inactive and is detected either as radiographic incidental findings or because of compressive effects. According to Ebersold et al. visual disturbances, hypopituitarism, or headaches were found in 72%, 61%, or 36 % of the patients, respectively {540}. Presentation with pituitary apoplexy (acute heamorrhagic necrosis) is more common in these lesions than in other tumour types. Although not classified as malignant, since they rarely metastasize to other parts of the body, these lesions can be highly infiltrative and can cause significant morbidity due to local invasion of critical brain structures.

Biochemical diagnosis of these adenomas rests on the finding of normal or diminished non-gonadotrophin anterior pituitary hormones and/or increased concentrations of gonadotrophin subunit concentrations. Because elevated serum gonadotropin levels are typically seen in postmenopausal females, the diagnosis of gonadotroph adenomas in this population is difficult and may require the demonstration of paradoxical stimulation of FSH and/or LH, following TRH administration. Significant increases in serum β-LH in response to TRH or less commonly with FSH and LH responses are considered diagnostic of gonadotropin producing adenomas {448}.

Imaging

Other than the tendency to be invasive macroadenomas, gonadotropin producing adenomas have no specific imaging characteristics that are useful in distinguishing them from other adenomas. Critical regions to evaluate parasellar extension include the cavernous sinuses and their contents as well as the suprasellar cistern with attention to the optic chiasm. With extension into the cavernous sinus, it is important to determine the relationship with the carotid arteries, in terms of the degree of vessel encasement. Adenomas are relatively soft tumours and rarely narrow the carotid arteries.

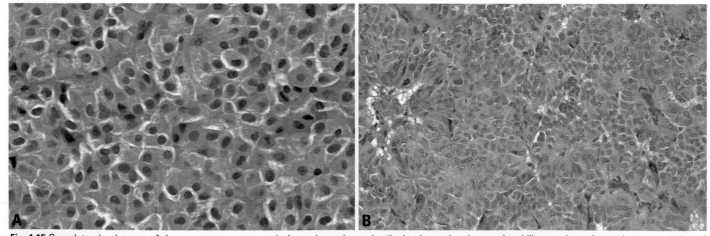

Fig. 1.15 Gonadotroph adenoma. **A** An oncocytoma composed of round to polygonal cells that have abundant eosinophilic cytoplasm due to the accumulation of numerous mitochondria. **B** A gonadotroph adenoma composed of solid nests and trabecula of cells that have variable morphology. Some are elongated, with pale acidophilic cytoplasm and these cells have distinct polarity, forming pseudorosettes around vascular channels.

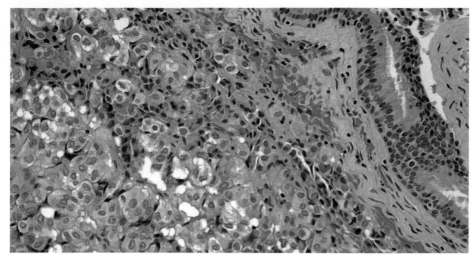

Fig. 1.16 Gonadotroph adenoma. A clinically nonfunctioning gonadotroph adenoma is usually large and invasive, as in this case where tumour is seen underlying respiratory mucosa of the sphenoid sinus.

Macroscopy

Grossly, gonadotropin producing adenomas are large and well-vascularized soft tan to brown tumours. They may exhibit areas of hemorrhage or necrosis.

Tumour spread and staging

Rarely, gonadotropin producing adenomas are diagnosed early when they are microadenomas, or macroadenomas confined to the sella. At the time of diagnosis, most gonadotropin producing adenomas are large lesions with extrasellar involvement. They range from large lesions that grow upwards and compress the optic chiasm to highly invasive lesions that infiltrate bone, cavernous sinuses and brain.

Histopathology

Several histologic patterns can be distinguished {915,919,1141,1154}. The majority of gonadotropin producing adenomas consists of uniform, tall, polar cells forming a sinusoidal pattern with characteristic pseudorosettes around vessels. Another well defined, although much less frequent, is the papillary pattern. A significant minority of tumours has a diffuse appearance. The small to middle-sized cells of some adenomas exhibit only a small degree of polarity not sufficient to generate the sinusoidal pattern described above. Adenomas comprising middle sized to large non-polar cells have either uniform spherical nuclei and moderately developed low density cytoplasm (an infrequent pattern). They may possess irregular, variable dense nuclei and large, granular, often acidophilic cytoplasm denoting oncocytic transformation, which is common in gonadotropin producing adenomas {1976,2439}. It is important to note that a combination of histologic patterns is noted in many gonadotropin producing adenomas and varying degrees of oncocytic change may be associated with all patterns. In general gonadotropin producing adenomas are chromophobe and PAS negative. However, scattered adenoma cells may contain fine, sometimes barely discernable PAS positive granules or large PAS positive globules (lysosomes).

Immunoprofile

The phenotypic variability of gonadotropin producing adenomas is fully expressed at the immunohistochemical level as well. For yet unknown reasons, only a minority of gonadotropin producing tumours exhibit generalized immunoreactivity for the two gonadotropins. The most common finding is a patchy, uneven, clonal distribution of immunoreactivities alternating with largely or entirely negative areas emphasizing the importance of adequate sampling. These tumours contain α-subunit of glycoprotein hormones, β-FSH and β-LH. There is wide variability depending on tissue fixation, antibodies and method of immunolocalization. As a rule β-FSH immunoreactivity is usually stronger and more widely distributed than that of β-LH. The immunoreactivities of the two hormones do not necessarily overlap. If present, areas of variable histologic patterns may display different patterns of immunoreactivities. Furthermore the morphology of tumour cells determines the intracellular distribution of immunopositivity; in polar cells it is the strongest within the cytoplasmic processes where most of the secretory granules reside, whereas positivity is diffuse in non-polar cells. No obvious correlation is apparent between histologic pattern and type and extent of immunoreactivities and the hormonal activity of tumours as shown by currently used hormone assays. α-SU immunoreactivity may be insignificant or absent in gonadotropin producing adenomas. These tumours are also immunoreactive for synaptophysin, chromogranin A, inhibin and activin subunits {798} and the transcription factor steroidogenic factor 1 (SF1) {80}.

Growth fraction / Ki-67 index

Gonadotropin producing adenomas have low mitotic activity and the Ki-67 labeling index is usually low (<3%).

Electron microscopy

In contrast to other pituitary adenomas, the ultrastructure of most gonadotropin producing adenomas shows no similarity to that of the normal mature human gonadotroph. The ultrastructural morphology reflects the phenotypical variations revealed by histology and immunohistochemistry. The majority of these tumours is composed of uniform, markedly polar cells with long, attenuating interwoven processes. The nuclei are uniform and largely euchromatic: the cytoplasm harbours often well developed rough endoplasmic reticulum, variably developed Golgi complex and 50-150nm spherical secretory granules most of which are distributed along the cell membranes and accumulate within cell processes leaving the nuclear pole almost completely devoid of secretory granules. These features are similar in tumours of both sexes with the notable exception of the Golgi apparatus, which displays vacuolar transformation in many adenomas of women {915,1141}. This unique anomaly is associated with poor immunoreactivity for gonadotropins, making electron microscopy mandatory for its recognition.

Another characteristic form is the infrequent tumour comprising middle sized or larger non-polar cells having centrally placed spherical, mostly euchromatic nucleus and variably developed rough endoplasmic reticulum and Golgi com-

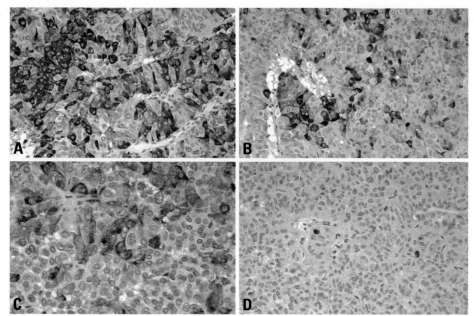

Fig. 1.17 Gonadotroph adenoma. **A** Strong reactivity for beta-FSH. **B** Staining for beta-LH in gonadotroph adenomas is usually less intense and abundant than beta-FSH. **C** Scattered strong reactivity for α-subunit of glycoprotein hormones. **D** Typical low MIB-1 labeling index.

plex. Variable numbers of cells of this type resemble mature gonadotrophs by virtue of the morphology of the secretory granules that have variable shapes and electron density and their size does not exceed 400nm.

Oncocytic transformation, i.e. the progressive accumulation of mitochondria in the cytoplasm leading to the gradual loss of the original character of the cell, is frequent.

Precursor lesions

Most gonadotropin producing adenomas are autonomous from the beginning. Associated gonadotroph hyperplasia is rare.

Histogenesis

The presursor cell of gonadotropin producing tumours may be the gonadotroph cell of the pituitary producing both FSH and LH, which may transform into a cell lacking the phenotypic markers of normal gonadotrophs but retaining its hormone production. Alternately, these tumours may arise in precursor cells subsequently differentiating into cells capable of synthesizing α and β subunits of the two gonadotropins.

Somatic genetics

Comparative genomic hybridization studies have shown gains and losses involving all chromosomes {604,832, 1824}. While some studies suggest an increased frequency of chromosomal imbalances in recurrent tumours, the regions involved differ widely between and within studies. In particular, deletions at 11q (the *MEN1* gene locus) are controversial {450,1136,1488} but losses of 13 q appear to be more consistent, suggesting that previously undescribed chromosomal regions may play a role in the tumourigenesis of pituitary tumours in general and gonadotropin producing adenomas in particular.

Members of the TGF-α family represented by at least three different forms have been implicated in pituitary gonadotrophin regulation. Inhibins and activins consist of two homo- or heterodimeric polypeptide subunits; inhibin A (a-ßA) and inhibin B (a-ßB) selectively inhibit the release of FSH from pituitary gonadotroph cells, whereas activin (ßA-ßB), activin A (ßA-ßA) and activin B (ßB-ßB) stimulate its release {38}. Activin effects are modulated by activin receptors and follistatin. Follistatin binds activin and downregulates its activity. Activin receptors are expressed in gonadotropin producing adenomas but follistatin expression is reduced or diminished {1716}, suggesting that enhanced activin signaling may also contribute to the pathogenesis of these tumours. A

truncated type I serine/threonine kinase activin receptor ActRIB (Alk4) isoform has been described exclusively in gonadotropin producing adenomas {2493}. This tumour receptor isoform fails to transduce activin-induced growth arrest signalling {2493}, underscoring the importance of the activin/follistatin balance in regulating gonadotropin producing adenoma cell growth.

Gonadal steroids participate in the negative feedback regulation of gonadotropin secretion and pituitary gonadotropin producing adenomas occasionally occur in patients with prolonged untreated primary hypogonadism {1596}. Estrogen receptor (ER) α expression correlates with production of gonadotropins {659, 2474} and splice variant of the ERα isoform is selectively expressed by gonadotropin producing adenomas {338}.

Genetic susceptibility

In spite of the important negative feedback functions of gonadal steroids in the regulation of gonadotropins, patients with androgen insensitivity due to germline mutation in the androgen receptor, have very rarely been reported to develop pituitary gonadotropin producing adenomas {2357}.

Patients with MEN 1 or Carney complex demonstrate increased susceptibility to the development of pituitary tumours including gonadotropin producing adenomas {1033,1094}.

Prognosis and predictive factors

The outcome of patients with these lesions is directly related to success of surgical excision. Transsphenoidal surgery can result in gross total removal of macroadenomas even with suprasellar extension. Transfrontal approaches may be required for some large tumours. Various forms of radiation therapy are indicated for situations where surgery is contraindicated or incomplete. Rare tumours respond to dopamine agonists {2411} or somatostatin analogues {2334}. Recurrence is common.

Null cell adenoma

T. Sano
S. Yamada
R.E. Watson Jr.

E.P. Lindell
S. Ezzat
S.L. Asa

Definition
Null cell adenomas have no hormone immunoreactivity, and no other immuno-histochemical or ultrastructural markers of specific adenohyphysial cell differenti-ation {1157}. There is controversy about the classification of tumours with only few scattered hormone immunoreactive cells.

ICD-O code   8272/0

Synonyms
Hormone immunonegative adenoma, hormonally inactive adenoma.

Epidemiology
Age and sex distribution
Null cell adenomas occur in elderly indi-viduals and are very rare in patients under 40 years of age {1420,2440}. The mean age of patients at the time of sur-gery is 6th decade in null cell adenomas, whereas it is 7th decade in oncocy-tomas, a variant of null cell adenomas {1141,2439}, with a slight male prepon-derance {1976,2440}.

Incidence and mortality
Null cell adenomas are decreasing in inci-dence due to increasing ability to classify

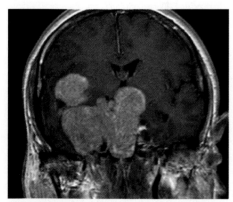

Fig. 1.18 Null cell macroadenomas. Post-gadolini-um coronal T1 weighted images show the dramat-ic growth that hormonally silent macroadenomas can achieve. Encasement of the right internal carotid artery. Note the well-defined borders and lack of low T1 signal in adjacent brain indicative of slow growth without brain edema.

adenomas with more sensitive immuno-histochemical techniques {1976, 2440}.

Localization
Almost all null cell adenomas arise in the adenohypophysis. Even if they occur ectopically, they are too large to deter-mine the exact primary site.

Clinical features
Signs and symptoms
These tumours show no clinical features of a syndrome of anterior pituitary hor-mone hypersecretion apart from mild hyperprolactinemia that is due to stalk section effect. It occurs in up to one third of non-functioning macroadenomas {1351,2468}. Other symptoms of mass effects are as in other large tumours. Moreover, they can show other less com-mon symptoms and signs depending on the extent and direction of tumour growth including cavernous sinus syndrome, cerebrospinal rhinorrhea, or various symptoms of hypothalamic disturbance {199}. In contrast, they may be inciden-tally discovered on neuroimaging without any symptoms {77}.

Imaging
Current imaging techniques are sensitive enough to demonstrate any macroade-noma showing visual impairment or hypopituitarism. MRI is currently the best tool for visualizing the pituitary gland, because of its superior spatial resolution and its ability to depict the relationship between tumour and the surrounding tis-sues. CT scans aid in demonstrating cal-cifications of the tumours. On precontrast T1-weighted images, macroadenomas are usually iso-intense, almost homoge-neous lesions, but often inhomogeneous with cystic or hemorrhagic portions {1182}. The intensity of cysts varies depending on the cyst content. Hemor-rhagic fluid appears hyper-intense on T1-weighted images, whereas non-hemor-rhagic fluid is hypo-intense. On the con-trast study, the solid portions of the tumour enhance, being usually some-what heterogeneous and less intense

than that of the normal pituitary gland. Occasionally, macroadenomas show cavernous sinus invasion or sphenoid sinus extension.

Relevant diagnostic procedures
The extent of hypopituitarism should be confirmed by measuring blood levels of anterior pituitary hormones and those secreted from the target organs (IGF-1, thyroid, adrenal, gonadal hormones) and also by assessing the data obtained by appropriate provocation tests including TRH, LHRH, insulin, GRF and CRF tests.

Macroscopy
The tumours are yellow-tan and soft. Haemorrhage and cyst formation are not infrequently observed probably because of a long history of growth.

Tumour spread and staging
Null cell adenomas often show cav-ernous sinus invasion and suprasellar extension occasionally reaching to the hypothalamus. Downward growth into the nasal cavity may also occur. Large adenomas involving the surrounding structures often recur.

Histopathology
By light microscopy, null cell adenomas are usually chromophobic, but may pres-ent a varying degree of acidophilia and are composed of round or polyhedral cells arranged in either a diffuse or pap-illary pattern of growth, often with pseudorosette formation. These tumours do not stain with periodic acid-Schiff (PAS), lead hematoxylin or other basic dyes. Nuclear pleomorphism is not marked and mitoses are rare.

Immunoprofile
Null cell adenomas are immunonegative for anterior pituitary hormones and tran-scription factors {1157}. However, some of them contain scattered cells or groups of cells that are immunopositive for one or more of anterior pituitary hormones, most commonly β-FSH and the α-SU of glycoprotein hormones, less frequently

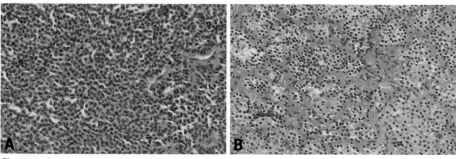

Fig. 1.19 A Null cell adenoma. Uniform adenoma cells are arranged in a diffuse and papillary pattern. **B** Oncocytic null cell adenoma. This adenoma is composed of acidophilic cells with abundant cytoplasm (oncocytes).

β-LH {1141,1932,2439}. Adenomas showing immunopositivity for either the α-SU or the β-SU are more frequent than those exhibiting immunoreactivity for both subunits. Gene expression of these hormones has been demonstrated in Northern blot methods or in situ hybridization {1976}. They also usually show immunopositivity for chromogranin A and synaptophysin.

Growth fraction / K i-67 labeling index
Null cell adenomas are slow growing tumours with less than 2% positive nuclear staining for Ki-67 antigen {1976}.

Electron microscopy
Electron microscopy demonstrates small, polyhedral cells with poorly-developed cytoplasm containing inconspicuous scattered rough endoplasmic reticulum, poorly or moderately developed Golgi complexes, numerous microtubules, and a modest number of small secretory granules measuring 100-250 nm. These granules are spherical, vary in electron density, are often haloed, and frequently line up along the cell membrane or accumulate in cell process.

Oncocytic variant
Oncocytomas are tumours composed mainly of oncocytes, cells that are characterized by an increased number and volume density of cytoplasmic mitochondria. Oncocytomas show varying degrees of acidophilia owing to uptake of the dye by accumulated mitochondria. Immunohistochemical and ultrastructural features are similar to those of null cell adenomas, except for the mitochondrial abundance.

Differential diagnosis
Based on the similarities with regard to epidemiological, clinical, biologic, prognostic, and immunohistochemical profiles, null cell adenomas, oncocytomas, and gonadotroph adenomas appear to be variants of the same entity. Other types of clinically nonfunctioning adenomas (silent GH producing adenomas, silent PRL producing adenomas, silent corticotroph adenomas, or silent subtype 3 adenomas) should be distinguished by immunohistochemical and/or electron microscopic examination, because these silent adenomas have a more rapid growth rate and demonstrate more fre-

quent recurrence than null cell adenomas.

Somatic genetics
Few studies describe cytogenetic changes in null cell adenomas. In the few published reports, the findings are even more discrepant than those described for gonadotroph adenomas. Other genetic alterations are reviewed in the introduction.

Genetic susceptibility
With very few exceptions, there is no evidence of increased development of null cell adenomas of the pituitary in patients with MEN 1 or in patients with Carney complex. On the contrary, the impression is that pituitary adenomas are much more likely to be hormonally active in the context of a background of MEN 1 {1967}.

Prognosis and predictive factors
Null cell adenomas are slow growing tumours, and therefore prognosis is good in patients with complete surgical excision. In patients with gross total resection, 6-12% radiographic recurrence rate is noted at a mean follow-up of 5-6 years after surgery {540,1302}. However, they are usually discovered in an advanced stage with supra- or extrasellar tumour extension due to hormonal silence and therefore tend to recur when surgical resection is incomplete, particularly those with significant cavernous sinus invasion.
Ki-67 labeling index, topoisomerase IIa {1890} and VEGF {1340} immunohistochemistry may prove to be additional prognostic markers.

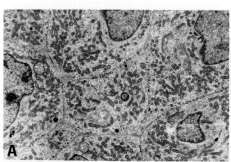
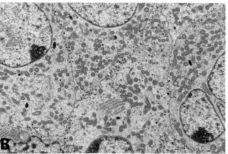

Fig. 1.20 Oncocytoma. **A** Pituitary oncocytoma displaying mitochondrial abundance, poorly developed RER and Golgi complex and small, scant secretory granules. X 5,570. **B** Oncocytoma. Charasterically numerous mitochondria are accumulated in the cytoplasm. Secretory granules are small in size and line up along the cell membrane.

Plurihormonal adenoma

E. Horvath
R.V. Lloyd
K. Kovacs
T. Sano
G. Kontogeorgos
J. Trouillas
S.L. Asa

Definition
Plurihormonal adenomas are unusual tumours that have immunoreactivities for more than one pituitary hormone which are not explained by normal cytophysiology or developmental mechanisms. They do not include the combinations of GH, PRL and TSH, or of FSH and LH.

ICD-O code
8272/0

Synonyms
Multihormonal adenoma.

Epidemiology
Age and sex distribution
These tumours are rare. Insufficient data are available to define the epidemiology, with the exception of the silent subtype 3 adenoma. These tumours occur in both sexes and show no gender-related difference in incidence. Most women are operated on between 20 and 35 years of age, while no age predilection is noted in males {916,918,1156}.

Etiology
These tumours are rare and no information is available to define the etiology.

Localization
These tumours are often macroadenomas at the time of diagnosis, since they do not give rise to characteristic clinical syndromes.

Clinical features
The clinical presentation of these lesions is highly variable and depends on the hormones produced by the adenoma. They often have symptoms of mass effects since the lesions are macroadenomas at the time of diagnosis. They often have hyperprolactinemia, that may be due to stalk effect or may be attributed to tumour production of PRL.

Imaging
No specific imaging features correlate with plurihormonality in pituitary adenomas. The silent subtype 3 adenomas are often highly invasive lesions with suprasellar and parasellar extension.

Macroscopy
The silent subtype 3 adenomas are usually macroadenomas at the time of diagnosis and are usually associated with elevated PRL blood levels which are disproportionately low for the size of the tumour. Other plurihormonal tumours have variable gross appearances.

Histopathology
These lesions tend to be chromophobic, or slightly acidophilic tumours that are usually negative with the PAS stain. Silent subtype 3 adenomas are characteristically composed of spindle shaped cells and fibrous stroma. Cellular pleomorphism and mitoses may be present.

Immunohistochemistry
The definition of a plurihormonal adenoma relies on specific immunoreactivities for unrelated hormones that are not due to antibody cross reactivities. The use of monoclonal antibodies is highly recommended, since there is frequent cross reaction between hormones of related families, and there is non specific detection of α-SU by antisera to other pituitary peptides in multiple cell types. The presence of a few scattered cells with positivity for any one hormone is insufficient evidence for true plurihormonality in a tumour; this may represent trapped non-tumourous elements.
Any combination of hormones may be found. The most common patterns include TSH, FSH and GH, or PRL and TSH. Plurihormonal adenomas rarely show immunoreactivity for ACTH and then they express α-SU {172}, β-LH {1930}, GH or PRL {1384}. Silent subtype 3 adenomas usually demonstrate reactivity for GH,PRL and TSH, as well as other hormones {916,916,918,1156}.
Pituitary cell specific transcription factors may clarify the cytologic basis of these adenomas but data are not yet available.

Electron microscopy
The only unusual plurihomonal tumour with a characteristic ultrastructure is the silent subtype 3 adenoma. This tumour type displays general ultrastuctural characteristics of well differentiated glycoprotein hormone producing adenomas. The large polar cells contain largely a euchromatic nucleus, prominent nucleolus and fragments of nuclear inclusions (spheridia). The large cytoplasm is packed with membranes of abundant RER aggregates of smooth endoplasmic reticulum and an unusually large Golgi complex. The sparse 100-200nm secretory granules tend to accumulate in cell processes.

Somatic genetics
These tumours are rare and little information is available. There is evidence of extrememly high levels of bFGF by silent subtype 3 adenomas {594,596}, that may explain the fibrosis and rapid growth.

Genetic susceptibility
These tumours are rare and no information is available.

Prognosis and predictive factors
The importance of recognizing the silent subtype 3 adenoma lies in the aggressive behaviour of these lesions. They are highly infiltrative tumours that have rapid growth and a high recurrence rate. The patients often have hyperprolactinemia and are treated with dopamine agonists; the PRL levels may fall rapidly, but the tumour continues to grow, creating a clinical conundrum.
The classification, etiology and prognosis of unusual plurihormonal tumours should evolve as more information becomes available.

Pituitary carcinoma

B.W. Scheithauer
K. Kovacs
E. Horvath
F. Roncaroli
S. Ezzat

S.L. Asa
R.V. Lloyd
V. Nosé
R.E. Watson Jr.
E.P. Lindell

Definition

The term pituitary carcinoma is restricted to a tumour of adenohypophysial cells that exhibits cerebrospinal and/or systemic metastasis.

ICD-O code   8272/3

Synonym
Adenocarcinoma of pituitary.

Epidemiology
Because of the highly restrictive definition of pituitary carcinoma, these malignancies are very rare. Pituitary carcinomas affect adults of any age; there is no significant gender bias. More than 75% are endocrinologically functional. PRL or ACTH producing tumours are the most common followed by GH and TSH producing carcinomas in this order of frequency. About half of the ACTH producing Cushing disease-associated carcinomas occur in the setting of Nelson syndrome {1720}. Accounting for 20% of all reported carcinomas as a whole, nonfunctioning examples include silent ACTH producing carcinomas {1857, 1964}, gonadotropin producing carcinomas {144,1460,1735,1856}, and carcinomas composed of null cells {1720}. Malignant transformation has also been documented in an ectopic adenoma {921}.

Etiology
The etiology of pituitary carcinomas is unknown. No predisposing genetic alterations have been identified for pituitary carcinoma. It remains to be determined whether pituitary carcinomas arise *de novo*, transform *via* genetic events from adenomas, or both. The latency period between presentation of the primary sellar tumour and metastases varies considerably (five years in PRL, and ten years in ACTH producing tumours) {1720}. Even much longer latencies support the occurrence of an adenoma-carcinoma sequence {1720}. No evidence implicates carcinogens or irradiation in the development of pituitary carcinomas.

Localization
Primary pituitary carcinomas arise from adenohypophysial cells or pre-existing adenomas and are initially located in the anterior lobe. Their growth rate varies, but many are rapidly growing invasive neoplasms, which spread to neighboring tissues and may invade the brain. Metastases occur in the craniospinal space or spread systemically to other sites, including liver, lung, bone and lymph nodes.

Epidemiology
Incidence and mortality
Primary pituitary carcinomas are very rare. More than 100 cases have been reported. They represent approximately 0.2% of all operated pituitary neoplasms. The prognosis of primary pituitary carcinomas is poor. Precise mortality figures are not available, but about 80% of patients with documented metastatic pituitary carcinoma succumb to the disease within eight years {1720}.

Clinical features
The diagnosis of carcinoma rests on the demonstration of metastatic tumour deposits. The initial clinical presentation is usually similar to that of a pituitary adenoma. Pituitary carcinomas have been associated with a number of clinical syndromes including hyperprolactinemia {2343}, Cushing disease {1150}, acromegaly {2133} and even hyperthyroidism with TSH excess {1515}. In some cases, the tumours have been unassociated with clinical or biochemical evidence of hormone excess. Rare well-differentiated gonadotropic tumours have been reported to behave in a malignant manner {144}.

Hormonal imbalance
Due to the spectrum of clinical presentations associated with pituitary carcinomas, the biochemical features are also exceedingly variable. They may follow any of the patterns of functioning pituitary tumours with hormone excess of any type, or they may be unassociated with hormone excess and may manifest with variable hypopituitarism. Measurements of pituitary hormones and the demonstration of excess and/or deficiency do not, however, permit the distinction between pituitary adenomas and carcinomas.

Mertastases
Instead the diagnosis of malignancy relies heavily on radiographic investigations to confirm the presence of metastatic tumour deposits in a patient with a known pituitary tumour. This often occurs several years after initial diagnosis. The sites of metastases include dissemination throughout the subarachnoid space {667,1150}, cervical lymph nodes {1372}, distant bony metastases excess {1515, 2343}, liver and lungs {1515,2343} and other extracranial sites. Only a few cases of hematogenous dissemination of pituitary carcinoma have been reported in

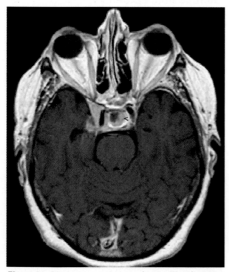

Fig. 1.21 Pituitary carcinoma (arrowhead). Axial post-gadolinium T1 weighted images demonstrate post-operative changes in the sella with invasive mass extending from the right cavernous sinus into the right temporal lobe. Note the irregular lateral border and adjacent low T1 signal in the temporal lobe, suggesting invasion of brain parenchyma and vasogenic edema. This appearance is not characteristic of indolent masses such as adenomas.

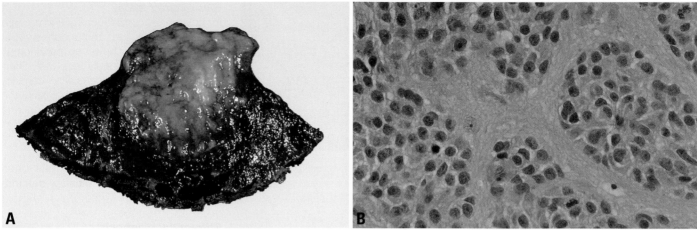

Fig. 1.22 A Metastatic pituitary ACTH carcinoma in the liver in a patient with Nelson syndrome. **B** Pituitary PRL carcinoma metastatic to the right parietal lobe of the brain with infiltration into the brain parenchyma.

the literature, primarily involving ACTH producing tumours. Recurrent ACTH producing pituitary carcinoma with cervical lymph node metastasis was described following external radiation to the pituitary fossa {2476}. Unlike other reports implicating the sustained loss of glucocorticoid negative feedback inhibition in ACTH producing carcinomas {132,1065,1358,1720}, this patient was not glucocorticoid insufficient.

Imaging
CT and MRI scans often reveal an invasive lesion extending beyond the usual confines of the sella turcica and into the parasellar structures. Cranial nerves and adjacent brain structures may be involved. Presently, there are no known imaging features unique to pituitary adenomas that are predictive of metastatic potential and behaviour.
Metastases to the brain and meninges are radiographically indistinguishable from other secondary tumours. Dura-based metastatic pituitary carcinomas may be misdiagnosed as meningiomas. In cases of pituitary carcinoma, MRI or CT imaging demonstrates foci of tumour involvement remote from the pituitary adenoma.

Macroscopy
The gross appearance of a primary pituitary carcinoma does not differ from that of an invasive macroadenoma. The essential feature of pituitary carcinoma is a) discontinuous spread in the form of single or multiple nodular subarachnoid deposits, occasionally invasive of underlying brain or overlying dura, or b) single

or multiple or systemic deposits grossly indistinguishable from metastases of carcinomas arising in other organs.

Tumour spread or staging
Most pituitary carcinomas are large and invasive of structures in the sellar region (dura, bone, cavernous sinus, cranial nerves) or of brain (hypothalamus). Spread in the central nervous sytem is by way of cerebrospinal fluid and may be cranial, spinal, or both. Systemic metastases are most often hematogenous, likely via the cavernous sinus and jugular vein, and involve primarily liver, lung, and bone {1720}. Other sites include adrenals, and even ovary or heart. In that the pituitary has no lymphatic drainage, the occasional involvement of cervical lymph nodes is presumably due to tumour invasion of the skull base and soft tissues. Whether surgery of the sellar primary facilitates metastasis is unclear, but rarely metastasis precedes sellar surgery {1720}. No formal staging scheme has been devised.

Histopathology
In that the diagnosis of pituitary carcinoma is dependent upon the demonstration of metastatic spread, there is no combination of histologic features (invasion, cellular pleomorphism, nuclear abnormalities, mitotic activity, necrosis) that is diagnostic of carcinoma. These features may be seen in varying degree in nonmetastasizing tumours (pituitary adenomas) {2219}. Mitotic activity was found in 3.9% of noninvasive adenomas, 21.4% of invasive adenomas, and 66.7% of carcinomas, but overlap was considerable.

Although it is true that mitotic activity and Ki-67 labeling index (see below) are often high in carcinomas, particularly in metastatic deposits, some carcinomas exhibit few mitoses and only low-level Ki-67 labeling index {1966,2219}. Neuronal metaplasia is rarely seen in pituitary carcinoma {1962}.

Immunohistochemistry
Similar to pituitary adenomas, primary pituitary carcinomas are invariably immunopositive for markers of neuroendocrine differentiation (synaptophysin and/or chromogranin). Staining for synaptophysin is most reliable and reproducible. Chromogranin is often positive for glycoprotein hormone-producing tumours (TSH, LH/FSH).
The diagnostic immunoprofile of primary pituitary carcinomas is based primarily upon demonstrating pituitary hormone immunoreactivity in the tumour cells. The most frequently synthesized hormones are PRL and ACTH {2219}. Tumours immunoreactive for PRL are associated with hyperprolactinemia. Tumours immunoreactive for ACTH are typically accompanied by Cushing disease {677} or Nelson syndrome {1065}; only rare examples are endocrinologically "silent," i.e., unassociated with clinical and laboratory signs of ACTH excess {1857}. Exceptionally, primary pituitary carcinomas may be immunopositive for GH-producing acromegaly {1256} or rarely gigantism {1790}. Carcinomas producing TSH {1515} and FSH/LH {144,1460} are exceptionally rare. The same is true of non-functioning tumours thought to be of null cell type {1183,1372}.

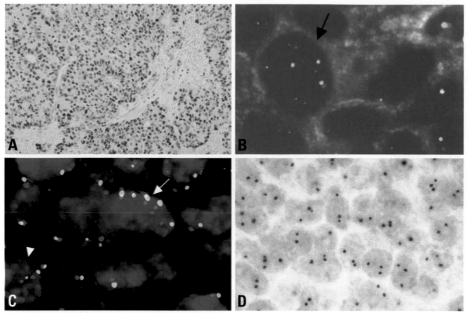

Fig. 1.23 A Pituitary carcinoma with *TP53* overexpression. **B** TSH producing pituitary carcinoma. FISH on paraffin section for Cyclin D1 (11q13). Red signal: YAC probe, centromeric to CyclinD1; green signal: BAC probe, telomeric to cyclinD1. Aneuploid chromosome numbers in occasional tumour cells (arrow). **C** PRL producing pituitary carcinoma. FISH on paraffin section for chromosome 11 centromere (green) and CyclinD1 (red). Note trisomies (arrowhead) and other aneuploid chromosome numbers in tumour cells (arrow). The immunohistochemmistry for cyclin D1 was strongly positive. **D** ACTH producing pituitary carcinoma. FISH on paraffin section for chromosome 17 centromere. There are up to three signals per nucleus, indicating trisomies.

Various other immunohistochemical studies have been applied to pituitary adenomas and carcinomas. In one study {2219}, expression of the tumour suppressor gene *TP53* was lacking in adenomas, expressed in 15% of invasive adenomas, and in 100% of all carcinomas, with higher levels being noted in metastases. Again, exceptions exist. Rare carcinomas can be p53 immuno-negative {1177}. p27, a cell cycle inhibitor is widely expressed in normal adenohypophysial cells whereas immunostaining is decreased in carcinomas {1006,1147}. In contrast, topoisomerase-2a {2317}, which plays an important role in DNA replication, and VEGF, which stimulates angiogenesis, are increased in carcinomas {1340}. It has been shown that metalloproteinases, enzymes which degrade connective tissue stroma and facilitate movement of tumour cells, are increased in rapidly growing pituitary tumours {2274}. Development of metastases, the diagnostic criterion of pituitary carcinomas obviously depends not only on the characteristics of the neoplastic cells but also upon extracellular events. Microvascular density is increased in carcinomas as compared to benign pituitary

adenomas and normal anterior pituitary {2317}. Despite these differences between adenomas and carcinomas, the various methods noted above cannot distinguish conclusively benign from malignant neoplasms. Reliable markers of malignancy remain to be elucidated. Overexpression of HER-2/neu has been reported in some pituitary carcinomas {1622}.

Markers of cell proliferation
At present, no histologic, immunochemical or ultrastructural markers have been identified which conclusively separate primary pituitary carcinoma from pituitary adenoma. Growth fraction examined by flow cytometry and the proportion of aneuploid cells are usually higher in carcinomas, however, aneuploidy may occur in benign tumours as well {1966}. Ki-67 immunostaining has been used to determine the growth fraction. One study {921} found higher mean labeling indices in carcinomas (12%) than in noninvasive adenomas (1%) or invasive adenomas (4.5%). However, it should be noted that overlaps exist and that in some carcinomas, the labeling index was in the range of benign adenomas.

Electron microscopy
In most cases, ultrastructural findings are consistent with the immunophenotype. Unlike adenomas, however, carcinomas are often ultrastructurally less well differentiated {1959}. In occasional carcinomas, it is not possible to subclassify the tumour, other than to confirm its endocrine nature.

Grading
No suitable grading system has been proposed or applied to pituitary carcinomas.

Differential diagnosis
The differential diagnosis of pituitary carcinoma necessarily focuses on its distinction from benign adenomas, other metastases, and on other neoplastic lesions occurring in the sellar region {1155}. A history of pituitary adenoma or atypical adenoma is very helpful. Application of immunohistochemistry and electron microscopy can reliably separate pituitary carcinomas from metastatic carcinoma arising from other organs. The endocrine nature of the tumour can be established with immunostains (synaptophysin, chromogranin), and the primary pituitary nature of the tumour by staining for pituitary hormones and correlating endocrine data. More conventional immunomarkers can be helpful as well. Adenohypophysial tumours may be positive for keratin and epithelial membrane antigen but lack staining for S-100 protein, carcinoembryonic antigen, vimentin, neurofilament protein, glial fibrillary acidic protein, leukocyte common antigen and immunoglobulin light chains {1340}. In a few cases, faced only with the histologic features of the primary tumour, one can perhaps suspect but cannot make a firm diagnosis of pituitary carcinoma. The histologic features (cellular pleomorphism, mitotic activity, necrosis), the immunohistochemical profile including cell proliferation markers, as well as electron microscopy cannot distinguish benign from malignant pituitary tumours. In pituitary pathology, invasion is not regarded as proof of malignancy; malignancy is documented by cerebrospinal and/or systemic metastasis.

Precursor lesions
Two variants of pituitary carcinoma are thought to occur. The most frequent

appears to involve malignant transformation of an adenoma. Histologically such tumours appear benign from the onset and, over the course of multiple surgeries for recurrence, become increasing atypical, exhibiting greater mitotic activity, Ki-67 labeling indices and *TP53* expression {1720,1962,2219}. Such "atypical adenomas" are occasionally encountered in routine practice. Just how often they will evolve into pituitary carcinomas is unclear, but it must be a rare event. The second, less common form of pituitary carcinoma is one in which histologic malignancy is apparent from the outset, there being no proof of a preexisting adenoma. To date, there is no evidence that pituitary hyperplasia, an infrequent precursor of adenoma, is implicated in the development of carcinomas.

Histogenesis

Pituitary carcinomas originate in previously normal adenohypophysial cells or in adenomas. At present, there is no evidence that pluripotential precursor cells are involved in adenoma- or carcinoma genesis.

Somatic genetics

Four pituitary carcinoma metastases (two ACTH producing and two PRL producing tumours) have been examined using CGH {1825}. Chromosomal gains were found in all samples but losses were restricted to two PRL producing carcinomas. Overall, pituitary carcinoma metastases showed an average of 8.3 chromosomal imbalances (7 gains and 1.3 losses), 10 in PRL producing carcinoma metastases (7.5 gains and 2.5 losses) and 6.5 in ACTH producing carcinomas metastases (6.5 gains and no losses). The most frequent gains were noted on chromosomes 5, 7p, and 14q. The 14q gains are extremely unusual as they have not been commonly noted in pituitary adenomas.

Examination of the clonal composition of primary, recurrent, and metastatic ACTH producing carcinoma using X-linked genes demonstrated the same allelic pattern in primary and metastatic samples. LOH analysis using 11 microsatellite allelic markers confirmed the monoclonal composition of all samples. Interestingly, however, retention of chromosomal microsatellites in the metastatic lesion that were lost in the primary and recurrent pituitary specimens suggest the possibility of divergent clonal expansion conferring different biological behaviour to metastatic compared with recurrent pituitary carcinoma {2476}.

The rarity of pituitary carcinomas does not permit valid conclusions concerning somatic defects in their pathogenesis. Point mutations in the *H-RAS* gene have been reported in metastatic deposits of several pituitary carcinomas, but not in their respective primary lesions {276,1710}. p53 immunoreactivity has been reported in pituitary carcinomas, but there is as yet no indication of whether this reflects mutation of this tumour suppressor gene {2222}.

Genetic susceptibility

There is no evidence of increased development of pituitary carcinoma in patients with MEN 1 or Carney complex. No other predisposing genetic alterations have been described for pituitary carcinoma.

Prognosis and predictive factors

In general, patients who develop malignant tumours of the anterior pituitary have a poor prognosis. The number of published cases is insufficient to draw conclusions concerning appropriate therapy. Pharmacotherapeutic agents generally reserved for the treatment of pituitary adenomas such as dopamine and somatostatin analogs are considerably less effective in controlling malignant pituitary carcinoma growth.

In three carcinomas, the Ki-67 labeling index was higher than in the benign tumours (12.8 vs 3.8%), but the reaction may be negative {1359}.

With few exceptions, the prognosis of patients with pituitary carcinoma is poor, since pituitary carcinomas are diagnosed only when tumour dissemination has occurred. The largest reported series of 15 cases {1720} found that 66% of patients died within one year of discovery of the metastases; most (75%) were systemic. The mean survival was 2 years (range 0.25-8 years). Survival was shorter in patients with systemic metastases (1 year versus 2.6 years). Occasional long-term survivors are reported {1225}.

Clinically, neuroimaging evidence of accelerating tumour growth, rapid progression of symptoms, worsening of hypopituitarism, loss of response to endocrine therapies such as dopamine agonists in the treatment of PRL producing carcinoma, and a marked increase in hormone levels are negative prognostic indicators.

Although no systematic studies of these rare tumours have correlated histopathologic features with outcome, it appears that anaplastic tumours have a less favorable prognosis {1027}.

Gangliocytoma

S.L. Asa
G. Kontogeorgos
T. Sano

K. Kovacs
R.V. Lloyd
J. Trouillas

Definition
A tumour composed of neoplastic mature ganglion cells.

ICD-O code   9492/0

Synonyms
Ganglioneuroma, hamartoma, hypothalamic hamartoma, choristoma, adenohypophysial choristoma, neuronal choristoma, pituitary adenoma with neuronal choristoma (PANCH)

Epidemiology
These are rare lesions that have no specific age or sex distribution.

Etiology
The etiology of these tumours is not known.

Localization
Gangliocytomas may arise in the pituitary or in the hypothalamus immediately adjacent to the pituitary. Other sites occur and are reviewed in the WHO Classification on Tumours of the Nervous System {1104}. This section is restricted to the unique features of these lesions that arise in the sellar region.

Clinical features
Hypothalamic and pituitary gangliocytomas may present as mass lesions, but many of these tumours are associated with pituitary adenoma and have evidence of hormone hypersecretion {1775}. The most common syndromes are acromegaly/gigantism and precocious puberty. Rare cases of hyperprolactinemia or Cushing disease have been reported {89}.

Macroscopy
These tumours have no distinguishing gross features.

Histopathology
These tumours are characterized by the presence of neuronal cells in abundant neuropil. The neurons are large, polygonal ganglion cells that are often bi- or multinucleated with characteristic prominent nucleoli. The cytoplasm harbors basophilic Nissl bodies.

Many of these tumours are intimately associated with a pituitary adenoma. In some cases, two discrete components are identified; in others, the ganglion cells are interspersed within the adenoma. The histologic features of the adenoma depend on the tumour type and are described in other sections.

Some gangliocytomas have been associated with hyperplasia of specific adenohypophysial cells while others may not show abnormalities of the hypophysial cells {91}.

Immunohistochemistry
The ganglion cells are immunoreactive for synaptophysin, chromogranin and neurofilaments, which identify the shape and axonal processes of neurons. The neuropil is strongly positive for neurofilaments. There may be positivity for S100 protein and glial fibrillary acidic protein (GFAP), the latter specifically highlighting glial elements. Ganglion cells may contain hypothalamic hormones with variable expression. They may contain GnRH, GHRH, somatostatin, TRH, CRH, and VIP. There is some correlation of hormone expression with clinical manifestations of hormone excess syndromes. Pituitary hormones may also be expressed in ganglion cells.

The associated pituitary adenomas usually have a characteristic immunoprofile. Patients with acromegaly have sparsely granulated somatotroph adenomas {91} (see above). PRL producing adenomas are sparsely granulated lactotroph adenomas and ACTH-producing adenomas have been described {1776}.

Electron microscopy
Electron microscopy highlights many important features of these tumours. They are composed of large nerve cells with well developed rough endoplasmic reticulum and elongated interdigitating cell process that contain numerous secretory granules of variable sizes. When present, the adenohypohysial cells display characteristic ultrastructural features, but there is usually evidence of synaptic process of neurons associated with the adenohypophysial cells.

Histogenesis
The exact histogenesis is not known. Some investigators propose that adenohypophysial cells can transform to neuronal cells {917,2316} implicating nerve growth factor in this process {1511}. Others argue that a primary ganglion cell tumour can induce adenohypophysial hyperplasia and adenoma by hormonal stimulation {91}. A third hypothesis is that a common tumourigenic influence induces transformation in two cell types {81}.

Prognosis and predictive factors
The prognosis depends on the size of the lesion and the clinical presentation.

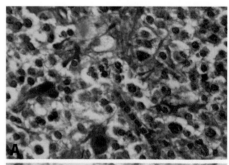
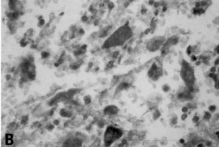

Fig. 1.24 Gangliocytoma **A** Tumour composed of anterior pituitary GH-producing cells and neuronal cells with neuropil. **B** Neurons show strong immunoreactivity for GH releasing hormone.

Mesenchymal tumours

M.B.S. Lopes
B.W. Scheithauer
W. Saeger

Definition
A variety of primary mesenchymal tumours may develop in the pituitary region. These include benign and malignant soft tissue tumours that show fibrous, fibrohistiocytic, adipose, myoid, pericytic, endothelial, chondroid or osseous differentiation.

Synonyms
The nomenclature and classification of mesenchymal tumours involving the pituitary region are those of the corresponding soft tissue tumours {638}. Detailed descriptions are provided in the WHO Classification of Tumours of Soft Tissue and Bone {638}.

Epidemiology
Age and sex distribution
Mesenchymal tumours may occur at any age. Most of the reported cases involve adults, with no obvious sex predilection. Chordomas, however, may arise in children constituting about 5% of skull base chordomas {839}.

Incidence
Primary mesenchymal tumours of the pituitary region are rare. Chordomas and chondrosarcomas collectively account for 6% of all primary skull base tumours {839} with a small number of these in the sellar region. The incidence of other benign mesenchymal tumours of the sella is uncertain due to their infrequency as separate tumour entities. Sarcomas unrelated to radiation therapy are extremely rare in this region, with only few well-documented cases {55,233, 1350}. The great majority of sarcomas reported in the area are associated with previous radiation therapy, with the lag time between irradiation and development of the sarcoma varying from 2 to 27 years {1350}. With the current recommendations for single-fraction radiosurgery in the region of the pituitary gland, for maximal protection of the optic pathways and hypothalamic area, the incidence of these highly malignant sarcomas may decrease {1246}.

Localization
Chordomas usually arise in the posterior clinoid process. The vast majority of glomangiomas are suprasellar tumours {85}. There is no preferential localization of other mesenchymal tumours in the sella turcica.

Clinical features
Signs and symptoms
Signs and clinical symptoms are nonspecific and largely depend upon the tumour size and its mass effect. Most common symptoms include visual loss and headaches, signs of hypopituitarism and/or mild hyperprolactinemia due to stalk effect. Tumours extending to the parasellar area may present with oculomotor nerve palsies. Tumours involving the clival region typically have bilateral sixth cranial nerve paresis and signs of brainstem compression {2226}.

Imaging
Descriptions of the radiologic appearance of mesenchymal tumours in the pituitary region are limited to case reports and are quite variable. These tumours usually enhance heterogeneously with gadolinium, and their signal intensity on T2-weighted image ranges from low to high. Most chordomas involving the sellar region are parasellar or suprasellar. Entirely intrasellar lesions are very rare (for review, see {2226}). Chordomas are usually hyperintense on T2-weighted MRI sequences, with various degrees of contrast enhancement. On non-contrast CT scan, calcification and sellar floor and/or clival erosion are frequently seen in chordomas {839}.

Macroscopy and histopathology
Detailed descriptions of these tumours are provided in the WHO Classification of Tumours of Soft Tissue and Bone {638}. However, due to the significance of chordomas in the routine practice, the macroscopy and histopathological features of these tumours will be herein reviewed.

Chordoma

ICD-O code   9370/3

Macroscopy
Chordomas appear myxoid or gelatinous at gross inspection with a multilocular appearance. Hemorrhages are frequent.

Histopathology
Chordomas are composed of cords of physaliferous cells with vacuoles which vary in size up to a whole-cell diameter and are PAS-positive. Between the large cells, smaller partially stellate cells are present. The broad extracellular myxoid and mucinous matrix stains strongly with Alcian blue and weakly with PAS.
Chordomas have to be distinguished from chondromas and low-grade chondrosarcomas by their typical physaliphorous cells and different immunohistochemical profile.

Immunoprofile
Chordomas express epithelial markers including epithelial membrane antigen (EMA), keratins, particularly cytokeratin 19, in addition to S-100 protein and vimentin {755}. Low-grade chondrosarcomas are immunoreactive only for S-100 and vimentin. Glycosaminoglycans

Table 1.08
Mesenchymal tumours reported in the sellar region[1]

Chondroma
Chordoma[2]
Fibroma
Glomangioma
Hemangioblastoma
Lipoma
Myxoma
Hemangiopericytoma
Rhabdomyosarcoma
Chondrosarcoma
Fibrosarcoma
Leiomyosarcoma
Osteosarcoma

[1] For review of reported cases, see {1467}
[2] For review of intrasellar chordomas, see {2226}

and collagen types do not differ significantly between these tumours. {755}.

Prognosis and predictive factors
Most of the benign soft tissue tumours of the pituitary region are controlled with surgical resection {349}. Radiation therapy is generally reserved for malignant tumours, or as palliation in invasive and/or inoperable neoplasms. Chordomas, however, tend to be more aggressive and may recur even after radical resection. Most centres recommend radiotherapy as adjuvant treatment for residual and/or recurrent tumours {839,934,1988}. Primary and post-irradiation sarcomas usually do not metastasize, but may show aggressive local behaviour with multiple recurrences and extension to adjacent structures {233, 1350,2037}. Death may result within months of the first manifestation {2037}.

Meningioma

Definition
Meningiomas are generally slow growing tumours attached to the dura mater and composed of neoplastic arachnoidal cells.

ICD-O code   9530/0

Grading
Most meningiomas are benign and graded as WHO grade I. Specific histological subtypes are associated with more aggressive behaviour and correspond to WHO grades II and III. Detailed discussion of meningiomas grading system is provided in the Tumours of the Nervous System volume {1104}.

Incidence
Meningiomas constitute approximately 15% of brain neoplasms, and about 6-10% of them occur in the sellar region {966,1785}. Meningiomas are the second most common suprasellar neoplasm in adults {1089}. Similar to tumours from other sites, meningiomas of the sellar region are tumours of adults, with a female predominance, and a peak incidence occurring during the fifth and sixth decades {1104,1785}.

Localization
Most meningiomas of the sellar region arise in the suprasellar compartment

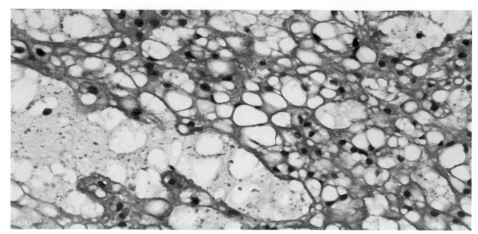
Fig. 1.25 Chordoma. Cords of tumour cells in a myxoid stroma.

from the dura of the anterior or posterior clinoidal processes, the tuberculum, the dorsum sellae or the diaphragma sellae {1920}. Truly intrasellar meningiomas are rare and originate from the inferior leaf of the diaphragma sellae {1089}.

Clinical features
Sellar meningiomas typically cause visual disturbances, mostly with reduction of visual acuity {736, 1089,1785}. Headaches may accompany the visual deficits in almost half of the patients {736,1785}. Patients with diaphragma sellae meningiomas also present with signs of hypopituitarism {1089}. Meningiomas with invasion of the cavernous sinus may manifest as third nerve palsy or as sensory loss in the trigeminal distribution {966}.

Imaging
Meningiomas are usually well-circumscribed, homogeneous isodense or hyperdense masses with diffuse enhancement on CT scan. Hyperostosis, bone erosion, and calcification may be seen {966}. Contrast enhancement is strong and uniform but not as intense as the adjacent pituitary gland and cavernous sinus, allowing most meningiomas to be distinguished from adenomas {1662}. MRI shows isointensity to gray matter on T1-weighted images. Signal on T2-weighted images is variable with about 50% being isointense and most of the remainder being hyperintense {557}. Evidence of mass effect with displacement of adjacent structures or thickening of adjacent dura may be recognized {1089}. Other features of menin-

giomas are a wide dural base of attachment and enhancement of the perilesional dura, the so-called "dura tail sign" {557}. Intrasellar meningiomas resemble pituitary adenomas by imaging, in particular the ones arising from the diaphragma sellae. Distinguishing features that might be present include the visualization of the pituitary gland, bright and homogeneous contrast enhancement, a suprasellar epicenter, and a small sellar enlargement in comparison to the size of the tumour {299}.

Macroscopy
Typically the tumours are solid and firm with whorled or lobulated appearance. Tumours with a large psammomatous component may have a gritty appearance on gross inspection. Invasion of the dura and cavernous sinus is quite common.

Histopathology
Meningiomas have a variety of histopathological appearances. The most common subtypes are the meningothelial, fibrous (fibroblastic) and transitional (mixed). Typical broad cells with meningothelial whorl formation are seen in the majority of the subtypes. Distinctive cytologic appearance of the nucleus includes well-distributed chromatin with nuclear clearing and nuclear pseudoinclusions (cytoplasmic invaginations). Other variants are listed in Table 1 and detailed in the WHO Classification of Tumours of the Nervous System {1104}. Atypical meningiomas are characterized by increased mitotic activity (4 or 5 mitotic figures per 10 high-powered fields) or

three of the following features: increased cellularity, loss of pattern or sheet-like growth, small cells with high N:C ratio, prominent nucleoli, and foci or necrosis {1104}.

Anaplastic (malignant) meningiomas are distinct from sarcomas of the meninges. Despite the high degree of nuclear and/or cellular anaplasia, increased mitotic activity (20 or more mitoses per 10 high-powered fields), and extensive necrosis, these tumours still retain histologic features of meningiomas.

Immunohistochemistry
The majority of meningiomas are immunoreactive for vimentin and EMA. EMA is particularly reactive in the "epithelial" variants such as the microcystic and the secretory subtypes. Cytokeratin and carcinoembryonic antigen (CEA) reactivity is also seen in the secretory variant. S-100 protein may be found in meningiomas with variable degree of immunopositivity. Immunoreactivity for progesterone receptor is observed in the majority of meningiomas, whereas estrogen receptor is less frequent.

Electron microscopy
Characteristic ultrastructural features of meningiomas include complex interdigitating cellular processes, abundant intermediate filaments and desmosomal junctions.

Histogenesis
Meningiomas are believed to originate from arachnoidal cells.

Genetics
Great progress has been made in the understanding of the molecular genetics of meningiomas and their frequent association with mutations in the *NF2* gene. Detailed discussion of the molecular genetics and genetic susceptibility of meningiomas is provided on the Tumours of the Nervous System volume {1104}.

Prognosis and predictive factors
The prognosis of meningiomas depends upon clinical factors, and histopathology and grading of the tumour. From the clinical point of view, the outcome of suprasellar meningiomas correlates with patient age, duration of symptoms and extent of surgical resection {602,1641}. In a large series of suprasellar menin-

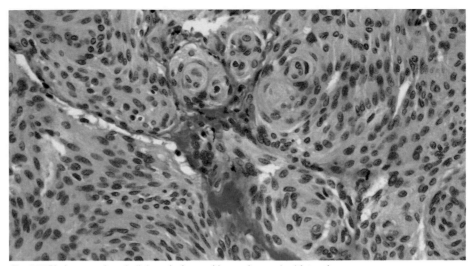
Fig. 1.26 Pituitary meningothelial meningioma with prominent whorl formation.

giomas, the outcome was more favorable in patients younger than 50 years and in those with clinical symptoms for less than 1 year {602}. Review of the literature shows a variable recurrence rate (0-62%) that appears to be highly dependent upon surgical techniques and extent of resection {602}.

The recommended grading system for meningiomas by the WHO {1104}, i.e. benign (grade I), atypical (grade II) and anaplastic (grade III) is a useful histological predictor for tumour recurrence. Additionally, histological variants with greater likelihood of recurrence and/or aggressive behaviour include the clear

cell, chordoid, rhabdoid and papillary meningiomas.

Proliferation indices have also been a valuable tool for predicting recurrence and survival in meningiomas {1729}. The Ki-67 labeling indices correlate with increased tumour anaplasia and increased risk of recurrence. Although specific labeling index values are not recognized, Ki-67 labeling indices above 5-10% suggest a greater likelihood of recurrence {1104}.

Table 1.09
Menigiomas grouped by likelihood of recurrence and grade. From WHO Classification of Tumours of the Nervous System {1104}.

Meningioma variant	ICD-O codes	WHO grading
Meningothelial	9531/0	WHO grade I
Fibrous (fibroblastic)	9532/0	
Transitional (mixed)	9537/0	
Psammomatous	9533/0	
Angiomatous	9534/0	
Microcystic	9530/0	
Secretory	9530/0	
Lymphoplasmacyte-rich	9530/0	
Metaplastic	9530/0	
Clear cell	9538/1	WHO grade II
Chordoid	9538/1	
Atypical*	9539/1	
Rhabdoid	9538/3	WHO grade III
Papillary	9538/3	
Anaplastic (malignant)*	9530/3	

* Meningiomas of any subtype may be classified as atypical or anaplastic.

Granular cell tumour

M.B.S. Lopes
B.W. Scheithauer
W. Saeger

Definition
Granular cell tumours are believed to derived from pituicytes, modified glial cells of the infundibulum and posterior pituitary gland. Granular cell tumours of this region resemble granular cell tumours elsewhere, including tongue, gastrointestinal tract and skin.

ICD-O code   9582/0

Synonyms
Choristoma, granular cell myoblastoma, granular cell pituicytoma, granular cell schwannoma, granular cell tumourettes.

Incidence
In postmortem studies granular cell tumours have been described in as high as 17% of adult autopsy cases {205}. Symptomatic cases are rare, constituting less than 0.5% of tumours involving this region in a large referral centre {2218}. Granular cell tumours arise in a wide range of age distribution. Most symptomatic tumours are diagnosed in the fourth or fifth decade of life, with a 2:1 predominance of females {1956}.

Clinical features
Most lesions are small, asymptomatic masses that are frequently diagnosed as incidental findings at autopsy.

Symptomatic granular cell tumours of the neurohypophysis are rare, with only 60 reported cases {1956, 2327}. Symptoms are related to tumour size, with signs of compression of adjacent structures including visual disturbances, headaches, hypopituitarism, and mild hyperprolactinemia due to stalk effect.

Imaging
Granular cell tumours are well-defined intra- and suprasellar lesions, homogeneously isodense on CT that strongly enhance after contrast administration {407,951}. Intra-tumoural calcification has been reported {254,1956}. MRI detection has increased the sensitivity of small lesions. The tumours are isointense to gray matter on both T1- and T2-weighted sequences and lack the normal high intensity of the neurohypophysis {407,951}. Somatostatin single-photon emission computed tomography imaging (SPECT) has been reported in one case with tumour uptake suggesting the presence of somatostatin receptors {254}.

Macroscopy
The tumours are typically firm, tan to gray and may be very vascular during surgical exploration {1956}. Most of these lesions, however, are not recognizable on gross examination.

Histopathology
Granular cell tumours are composed of large, polygonal cells, forming sheets and small lobules. The cytoplasm is eosinophilic showing distinct, fine and coarse granularity. The nuclei are round with delicate chromatin and uniform nucleoli, and tend to be located at the periphery of the cells. The cytoplasmic granules are positive for PAS-positive and diastase-resistant. Mitotic figures are absent. Perivascular lymphocytic infiltrates may be occasionally present.

Immunohistochemistry
Granular cell tumours are immunoreactive for CD68, a macrophage/lysossome marker. In addition, the majority of the cases are immunoreactive for NSE. Unlike granular cell tumour arising in the peripheral nervous system, sellar granular cell tumours are mostly negative for S-100 protein. Similarly, the tumours are only occasionally immunoreactive for glial fibrillary acidic protein (GFAP) as seen in the rare intracerebral tumours.

Electron microscopy
EM shows characteristically abundant membrane-bound, electron-dense material in the cytoplasm, consistent with lysosomes. Intermediate filaments are scarce, neurosecretory granules absent.

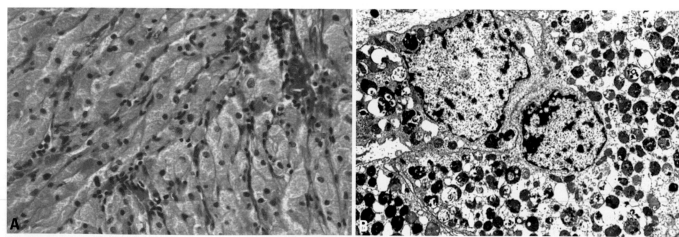

Fig. 1.27 Pituitary granular cell tumour. **A** Large, polygonal cells with granular cytoplasm are typical of granular cell tumours. **B** Electron microscopy reveals numerous lysosomes.

Histogenesis

The histogenesis of granular cell tumours is not completely understood. These tumours are believed to originate from pituicytes, modified astrocytes/glial cells of the neurohypophysis {885,1884}. Normal pituicytes were classified into five types on the basis of their ultrastructural characteristics {2182}. These authors had demonstrated that the so-called granular pituicytes of the neurohypophysis contain numerous electron-dense granules similar to those seen in granular cell tumours {2182}. Despite few reports of weak and focal GFAP immunoposivity in the tumour cells {2324}, the great majority of the granular cell tumours of the neurohypophysis lack immunoreactivity for this glial marker, questioning the definite astrocytic nature of these tumours.

Predictive factors

Granular cell tumours are generally considered to be slow-growing, benign neoplasms. However, a few cases of tumours with more aggressive behaviour have been reported {761,2327}. One particular case with infiltration of the optic chiasm demonstrated a variable Ki-67 labeling index (1-15%) in areas of the tumour and immunoreactivity for p53 {2327}. In a large review of 42 cases of symptomatic granular cell tumours {1956}, it was observed that the outcome of patients treated conservatively was poor with death within 2 to 26 months. In the same analysis, patient survival was largely increased with extended surgery or combination of surgery and radiation therapy.

Secondary tumours

K. Kovacs
E. Horvath
S. Vidal Ruibal
R.E. Watson Jr.

E.P. Lindell
S. Ezzat
S.L. Asa

Definition

Secondary tumours of the pituitary originate in extrahypophysial cells and spread to the pituitary either via the hematogenous route or by direct invasion from adjacent tissues.

Synonyms

Metastatic tumours, pituitary tumour deposits, secondary in pituitary

Epidemiology

Age and sex distribution
Secondary tumours of the pituitary are usually diagnosed in middle aged or older persons. They may occur slightly more often in women than in men. There is, however, no significant gender difference {239,878,1017,1153,1446,1458, 1851,2205}.

Incidence

Based on autopsy findings, the incidence of secondary tumours of the pituitary in cancer patients ranges between 3-23% {239,878,1017,1153,1446,1458, 1851,2205}. They occur most frequently in the terminal phase of the disease when cancer disseminates to several organs including the pituitary. Melanomas and hematologic malignancies may also involve the pituitary gland {33,754,919, 1425,2021,2028,2283}.

Etiology

The etiologic factors underlying the numerous primary tumours that affect the pituitary are reviewed in their corresponding WHO books.

Localization

Metastatic carcinomas are localized at least two times more frequently in the posterior pituitary than in the adenohypophysis. This discrepancy is due to differences in circulation. The posterior lobe has a direct blood supply from the carotid artery whereas the anterior lobe receives blood mainly from the portal vessels originating in the median eminence of the hypothalamus and reaching the anterior lobe via the pituitary stalk.

Clinical features

The most common primary sites of these lesions are breast, lung and gastrointestinal tract {339,372,387,1446,2475}. Among patients with breast carcinoma, pituitary metastases are statistically correlated with spread to other endocrine organs {163,239}, suggesting a com-

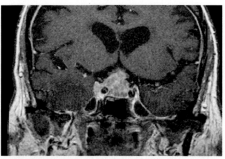

Fig. 1.28 Pituitary secondary tumours: multiple prostate cancer metastases. Coronal post-gadolinium T1 weighted image shows a heterogeneously enhancing expansile sellar mass invading the right cavernous sinus. The patient had a right oculomotor neuropathy.

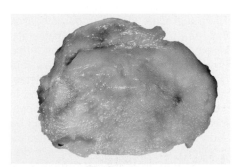

Fig. 1.29 Pituitary secondary tumours. Gross photograph of a breast carcinoma metastasis in the pituitary. The pituitary is enlarged and is almost completely replaced by carcinoma tissue.

mon mechanism that may implicate hormonal factors.

Signs and symptoms depend on the location, size and characteristics of the primary tumour, the extent of destruction of pituitary tissue and stage of the disease. Most metastases to the pituitary are unassociated with overt clinical symptomatology, mainly because the pituitary symptoms are overshadowed by non-specific manifestations of the generalized disease..Occasionally, however, patients may present with sellar tumour with no prior history of a non-endocrine malignancy {239}. The most frequently occurring endocrine abnormality is diabetes insipidus due to the destruction by metastatic deposits of the posterior lobe, pituitary stalk and/or relevant areas of the hypothalamus. Larger metastases may invade the cavernous sinus and associated structures, causing headaches, visual field defects, ophthalmoplegia, and ptosis {1054}. Only rarely is there isolated anterior pituitary involvement that can present as anterior pituitary insufficiency {239}. Pituitary metastases in some cases are associated with mild hyperprolactinemia that is explained by stalk effect.

A few examples of metastatic carcinoma involving a pituitary adenoma have been reported {992,2475}. In this situation, the metastasis can be the cause of sudden increase in size of the tumour and rapid worsening of symptoms of the mass.

Imaging

Non-symptomatic micrometastases to the pituitary are rarely subjected to dedicated sellar imaging. In the absence of known primary tumour, the finding of a pituitary mass is generally suggestive of adenoma. However, in patients with known metastatic disease, the differential of a sellar mass should include metastasis.

There are some imaging characteristics that can be suggestive of metastatic lesions as opposed to adenomas in the proper clinical context. Lesions that destroy bone are suggestive of metastases, whereas macroadenomas tend to smoothly expand and remodel bone. Invasion of the cavernous sinus can be seen with both adenomas and metastatic lesions, but when associated with cranial neuropathies is suggestive of metastatic involvement. While adenomas tend to displace the infundibular stalk, metastases can directly invade the

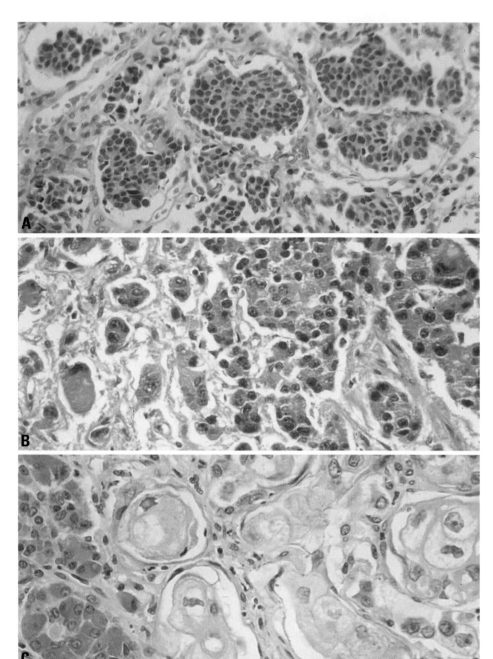

Fig. 1.30 Pituitary secondary tumours. **A** Endocrine carcinoma (carcinoid) metastasis in the anterior lobe. **B** Carcinoma of breast metastasis in the posterior lobe. Tumour cell emboli are apparent in the vessels. **C** Squamous cell carcinoma metastasis in the anterior lobe.

infundibular stalk and adjacent hypothalamus {1450}.

Relevant diagnostic procedures involve search for the primary tumour. In exceptional cases, however, no primary lesion is found and even a careful autopsy fails to reveal a primary tumour.

Diagnostic procedures

If necessary, several diagnostic procedures are available to detect abnormalities in pituitary function. Patients with dia-

betes insipidus complain of polyuria and polydipsia; the specific gravity of urine is low. Water deprivation test, blood hormone level measurements are usually not required because the diagnosis of diabetes insipidus can be established on the basis of clinical symptoms. Adenohypophysial endocrine activity can be assessed by measurement of pituitary hormone concentrations in the blood. Stimulating tests may be helpful to distinguish between lesions located in the hypothalamus versus pituitary. Reduction of adenohypophysial hormone levels may be mild, moderate or severe.

Macroscopy
Metastatic tumours can often be recognized only by routine histologic study of the pituitary. Gross examination may reveal a mass in the posterior lobe, a multinodular lesion, or the entire pituitary may be replaced. In some cases, the diagnosis is suspected because the lesion is very firm and difficult to resect surgically.

Tumour spread and staging
Tumour spreads by the hematogenous route primarily to the posterior lobe. Direct invasion from adjacent structures may also occur. Secondary tumours of the anterior lobe may also develop by direct spread from the posterior lobe via the short portal vessels or via the long portal vessels originating in the median eminence of the hypothalamus and passing through the hypophysial stalk.

Histopathology
The light microscopic findings depend on the tumour type localized as secondary deposits in the pituitary. Carcinoma of the breast, lung, colon, prostate, pancreas, thyroid usually have diagnostic morphology, however, in some cases the primary site cannot be clarified by histologic examination. Spread of melanomas and hematologic malignancies to the pituitary may also occur. Rarely cancers of various organs may metastasize to a pre-existing pituitary adenoma {8,944, 1764,1792,2475}.

Immunoprofile
The immunohistochemical characteristics are those of the primary tumour. Some tumours have characteristic immunohistochemical markers. Breast carcinomas may express estrogen receptors and progesterone receptors. Certain neoplasms of the thyroid and lung may be immunopositive for thyroid transcription factor-1 (TTF-1). Carcinomas of the prostate may be immunopositive for prostatic specific antigen (PSA). Many carcinomas are immunoreactive for keratin, EMA and CEA. Carcinomas consisting of non-endocrine cells or cells showing no endocrine differentiation are immunonegative for chromogranin and synaptophysin, the immunohistochemical markers used to verify endocrine derivation, however, metastatic endocrine carcinomas may stain for these markers.

Growth fraction / Ki-67 index
Ki-67 labeling index is usually high in metastatic carcinomas and is in the range of the primary site and other extrapituitary metastases. The diagnostic and prognostic value of other immunohistochemical markers (p27, p53, topoisomerase II, cyclo-oxygenase etc) has yet to be established.

Electron microscopy
All primary pituitary neoplasms have ultrastructural criteria of endocrine differentiation (i.e. secretory granules) and other markers specific for the adenohypophysial cell type of derivation. The ultrastructure of metastases is determined by their cytogenesis. Most are of non-endocrine origin, adenocarcinomas of non-intestinal (breast, lung), or intestinal type (colon) being most common. Small cell carcinomas (lung and other sites), melanomas and hematologic malignancies (lymphoma, plasmacytoma) occur as well.

Differential diagnosis
Histologic distinction from pituitary adenoma usually poses no major problems, with the exception of metastatic endocrine carcinomas. Many primary tumours of diverse morphologic features arise in the sella. Histologic and if necessary immunohistochemical and electron microscopic examinations can distinguish primary tumours in the sella from metastatic deposits. The identification of the primary site may not be successful in every case.

Somatic genetics
The somatic genetics of metastatic malignancies involving the pituitary are detailed in the various WHO books on these lesions.

Genetic susceptibility
No genetic susceptibility is known to predispose to pituitary metastasis. The genetic susceptibilities underlying the various primary malignancies are detailed in other WHO books on these lesions.

Prognosis and predictive factors
Since these patients have disseminated malignancy, treatment is generally of a palliative nature. Surgical decompression with or without radiotherapy can relieve symptoms {239}.
Pituitary metastases most often occur in the terminal phase of the disease, when cancer disseminates to several organs. The prognosis is poor; the majority of patients survive less than one year.

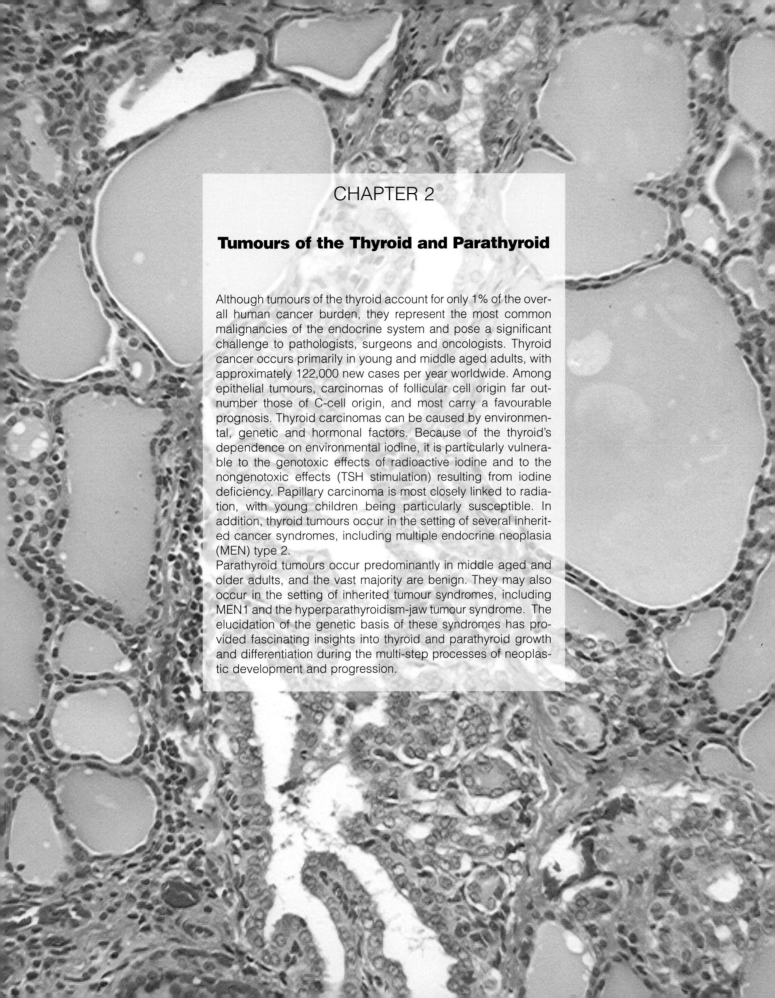

CHAPTER 2

Tumours of the Thyroid and Parathyroid

Although tumours of the thyroid account for only 1% of the over-all human cancer burden, they represent the most common malignancies of the endocrine system and pose a significant challenge to pathologists, surgeons and oncologists. Thyroid cancer occurs primarily in young and middle aged adults, with approximately 122,000 new cases per year worldwide. Among epithelial tumours, carcinomas of follicular cell origin far out-number those of C-cell origin, and most carry a favourable prognosis. Thyroid carcinomas can be caused by environmental, genetic and hormonal factors. Because of the thyroid's dependence on environmental iodine, it is particularly vulnerable to the genotoxic effects of radioactive iodine and to the nongenotoxic effects (TSH stimulation) resulting from iodine deficiency. Papillary carcinoma is most closely linked to radiation, with young children being particularly susceptible. In addition, thyroid tumours occur in the setting of several inherited cancer syndromes, including multiple endocrine neoplasia (MEN) type 2.

Parathyroid tumours occur predominantly in middle aged and older adults, and the vast majority are benign. They may also occur in the setting of inherited tumour syndromes, including MEN1 and the hyperparathyroidism-jaw tumour syndrome. The elucidation of the genetic basis of these syndromes has provided fascinating insights into thyroid and parathyroid growth and differentiation during the multi-step processes of neoplastic development and progression.

WHO histological classification of thyroid and parathyroid tumours

Thyroid carcinomas
Papillary carcinoma   8260/3
Follicular carcinoma   8330/3
Poorly differentiated carcinoma
Undifferentiated (anaplastic) carcinoma   8020/3
Squamous cell carcinoma   8070/3
Mucoepidermoid carcinoma   8430/3
Sclerosing mucoepidermoid carcinoma with eosinophilia   8430/3
Mucinous carcinoma   8480/3
Medullary carcinoma   8345/3
Mixed medullary and follicular cell carcinoma   8346/3
Spindle cell tumour with thymus-like differentiation   8588/3
Carcinoma showing thymus-like differentiation   8589/3

Thyroid adenoma and related tumours
Follicular adenoma   8330/0
Hyalinizing trabecular tumour   8336/0

Other thyroid tumours
Teratoma   9080/1
Primary lymphoma and plasmacytoma
Ectopic thymoma   8580/1
Angiosarcoma   9120/3
Smooth muscle tumours
Peripheral nerve sheath tumours
Paraganglioma   8693/1
Solitary fibrous tumour   8815/0
Follicular dendritic cell tumour   9758/3
Langerhans cell histiocytosis   9751/1
Secondary tumours

Parathyroid tumours
Parathyroid carcinoma   8140/3
Parathyroid adenoma   8140/0
Secondary tumours

---

[1] Morphology code of the International Classification of Diseases for Oncology (ICD-O) {664} and the Systematized Nomenclature of Medicine (http://snomed.org). Behaviour is coded /0 for benign tumours, /3 for malignant tumours, and /1 for borderline or uncertain behaviour.

TNM classification of thyroid carcinomas

TNM classification [1,2]
T – Primary Tumour*
TX   Primary tumour cannot be assessed
T0   No evidence of primary tumour

T1   Tumour 2cm or less in greatest dimension, limited to the thyroid
T2   Tumour more than 2 cm but not more than 4 cm in greatest dimension, limited to the thyroid
T3   Tumour more than 4 cm in greatest dimension, limited to the thyroid or any tumour with minimal extrathyroid extension (eg, extension to sternohyoid muscle or perithyroid soft tissue)
T4a   Tumour of any size extending beyond the thyroid capsule to invade subcutaneous soft tissues, larynx, trachea, esophagus, or recurrent laryngeal nerve.
T4b   Tumour invades prevertebral fascia or encases carotid artery or mediastinal vessels.

*Multifocal tumours are designated (m). The diameter of the largest determines the classification.

All anaplastic (undifferentiated) tumours are considered T4
T4a   Intrathyroid anaplastic carcinoma- surgically resectable
T4b   Extra-thyroidal anaplastic carcinoma – surgically unresectable

Regional Lymph Nodes (N)
Regional nodes are the central compartment, lateral cervical and upper mediastinal lymph node.
NX   Regional nodes cannot be assessed
N0   No regional lymph node metastasis
N1   Regional lymph node metastasis
N1a   Metastasis to level VI (pretracheal, paratracheal, and prelaryngeal/Delphian) lymph nodes
N1b   Metastasis to unilateral, bilateral or contralateral cervical or superior mediastinal lymph nodes

Distant Metastasis (M)
MX   Distant metastasis cannot be assessed
M0   No distant metastasis
M1   Distant metastasis

---

[1] {769,2078}
[2] A help desk for specific questions about the TNM classification is available at http://www.uicc.org/tnm

Thyroid and parathyroid tumours: Introduction

R.A. DeLellis
E.D. Williams

THYROID

Epidemiology

Thyroid cancer accounts for approximately 1% of all malignancies in developed countries with an estimated annual incidence of 122,000 cases worldwide {2129}. Benign thyroid tumours are common, and although cancers are relatively rare, they represent the most common malignancies of the endocrine system. Among epithelial tumours, carcinomas of follicular cell origin far outnumber those of C-cell origin. The vast majority of carcinomas of follicular cell origin are indolent malignancies with 10 year survivals in excess of 90 % {1793}. Primary lymphomas of the thyroid are uncommon while other non-epithelial malignancies are exceptionally rare.

Age and sex distribution

Thyroid cancer occurs primarily in young and middle aged adults and is rare in children. The mean age at diagnosis is the mid 40's to early 50's for the papillary type, 50's for the follicular and medullary types and 60's for the considerably less common poorly differentiated and undifferentiated types. Numerous studies have demonstrated that thyroid cancer is two to four times more frequent in females than in males, but this sex difference is far less pronounced in children and older adults. This observation suggests that a specific susceptibility gene with sex hormone receptor elements may be involved in the pathogenesis of thyroid carcinomas. Other reproductive factors, such as age at menarche, have been associated with papillary thyroid carcinoma, but these are much weaker effects {1582}.

Incidence rates

Age standardized incidence rates per 100,000 population in different parts of the world vary from 0.8 to 5.0 for males and 1.9 to 19.4 for females {2169}. Relatively low incidence rates have been reported in Denmark, the Netherlands and Slovakia while higher rates have

been noted in Sweden, France, Japan and the United States (Los Angeles). The lifetime risk of developing thyroid cancer in the U.S. is about 1:120 for females while the risk of dying from the disease is approximately 1 in 1,700 (SEER Cancer Statistics). The highest rates have been reported from Hawaii and Iceland. Studies in Hawaii have demonstrated that the incidence of thyroid cancer in all ethnic groups is higher than that in the same ethnic groups living in their respective countries of origin, particularly among Filipino females. The incidence

rates of thyroid cancer have increased in most countries since the 1970's while mortality rates due to these neoplasms have decreased. The increasing use of more sophisticated diagnostic methods with an increase in the detection of small tumours has contributed significantly to these changes.

Classification

The traditional separation of thyroid carcinoma into the major groups of papillary, follicular, medullary and undifferentiated (anaplastic) carcinoma, based on mor-

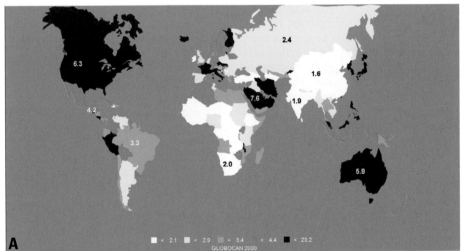

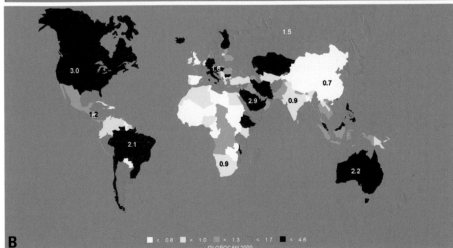

Fig. 2.001 Global incidence rates of thyroid cancer (all ages) in females (**A**) and males (**B**). Age-standardized rates (ASR, world standard population) per 100,000 population and year. From Globocan 2000 {618}.

phology and clinical features, is strongly supported by advances in molecular studies showing the involvement of distinct genes in these four groups, with little overlap. However, some areas require further clarification. For example, some tumours classified as the follicular variant of papillary carcinoma share oncogene changes with follicular tumours, and this group needs careful reassessment. The rare thyroid carcinomas that are found in a minority of patients with familial adenomatous polyposis (FAP) form a morphologically distinct group that shows a variety of patterns, including a papillary component. For convenience, the FAP associated thyroid tumours are included in the papillary group of tumours. Other rare tumour types such as squamous and mucoepidermoid carcinomas cannot be regarded as subgroups of one of the major types, and are therefore treated separately.

Poorly differentiated carcinomas may or may not show evidence of dedifferentiation from papillary or follicular carcinomas, and they are best treated as separate tumour types because of their clinical significance. Similarly, mixed medullary-follicular cell carcinomas remain of uncertain histogenesis and require separate classification.

The oncocytic thyroid tumours pose a particular problem. Traditionally, they have been regarded as belonging to the 'follicular family' of thyroid neoplasms. They are predominantly tumours with a follicular or solid architecture, and when they show a papillary architecture, they are classified as papillary carcinomas only if the nuclear features of that tumour type are present. More typical follicular tumours may show varying extents of oncocytic features, but there is a case to be made for regarding the completely oncocytic tumours as separate entities. This argument is based on evidence that they show different genetic features, that they may occur as multiple lesions with the same phenotype, and that they may be inherited, again with the same phenotype. No gene specific to oncocytic tumours has as yet been identified and sequenced. In the current classification, the tradition of regarding oncocytic tumours as variants of follicular tumours has been continued, but it remains important to identify them separately for further molecular genetic studies. This general approach applies to all subtypes of thyroid carcinoma since it is clear that hereditary non-medullary thyroid carcinoma is a term encompasing a group of syndromes with differing genetic profiles, differing clinical behaviours, and in some cases characteristic morphology.

Microcarcinomas

Any interpretation of reports of the incidence of papillary thyroid carcinoma or therapeutic success rates in its management must take into account the remarkably high prevalence of papillary microcarcinomas in thyroids removed for other reasons and in autopsy series {1738}. Patients with tumours, measuring 1 cm or less in diameter, have survival rates indistinguishable from those of the normal population {1863}. The change from nodule examination based on palpation to nodule identification based on ultrasound followed by fine needle aspiration biopsy indicates that these tumours form an increasing proportion of resected series of thyroid carcinomas. This affects the staging of papillary microcarcinomas in the most recent TNM classification of thyroid tumours.

Etiology and pathogenesis

The development of papillary thyroid carcinoma is influenced by environmental, genetic and hormonal factors and by the interactions among them. The environmental factors can be divided into genotoxic and nongenotoxic effects. Because of the thyroid's dependence on obtaining iodine from the environment, it is vulnerable to the genotoxic effects (DNA damage) of radioactive iodine and to the nongenotoxic effects (TSH stimulation) resulting from iodine deficiency. Radiation is also a causative factor for follicular adenomas and carcinomas, although follicular carcinomas occur much less frequently than papillary carcinomas, and probably have a much longer latent period.

Papillary carcinoma and the Chernobyl accident

Papillary thyroid carcinoma is most closely linked to radiation, either external radiation {1855} or internal irradiation from radioactive iodine, following exposure to radioactive fallout. Young children are particularly susceptible since thyroid growth occurs primarily in childhood and falls to low levels in adults. A striking increase in thyroid cancer in children has been reported in Belarus following the Chernobyl disaster of 1986. The worldwide incidence of thyroid cancer in children has been estimated in the order of 1 per million children per year, but in Belarus as a whole the incidence in the decade following the Chernobyl disaster reached at least 30 fold higher while in Gomel (the region closest to Chernobyl) the incidence reached about 100 fold higher {2389}.

While exposure to fallout from the atomic bomb led to whole body irradiation from neutrons and gamma rays, the Chernobyl exposure was due primarily to exposure to ^{131}I, and ^{132}I. Because of its ability to concentrate iodine, the thyroid dose from exposure to ^{131}I is, about 1000 times greater than the rest of the body. The relative risk for the development of thyroid cancer in children in Belarus under the age of 1 year at exposure reached 237 while those age 10 at exposure reached a relative risk of 6. The age related sensitivity is due to the fact that young children have a higher uptake of radioactive iodine than adults and are more likely to consume radioactive iodine in milk than older children and adults. Milk is a common source through which radioactive iodine reaches the human food chain. In addition, studies of children exposed to external radiation to the thyroid have shown that young children have an increased biological sensitivity to thyroid carcinogenesis. The role played by moderate iodine deficiency around Chernobyl is largely unknown {2389}.

Dose-response effect of radiation

In a study of 5 cohorts (atomic bomb survivors, children treated for tinea capitis, two studies of children irradiated for enlarged tonsils and infants treated for an enlarged thymus), linearity best describes the dose response even down to 0.10Gy in children less than 15 years of age {1855}. At the highest doses (>10Gy) such as those associated with cancer therapy, there is a decrease or levelling of the risk for the development of thyroid cancers which is most likely a direct consequence of cell killing.

Radiation vs. iodine deficiency

Since radiation causes double strand breaks in DNA, a necessary precursor to *RET* and *TRK* rearrangements, this may be the reason why radiation is more

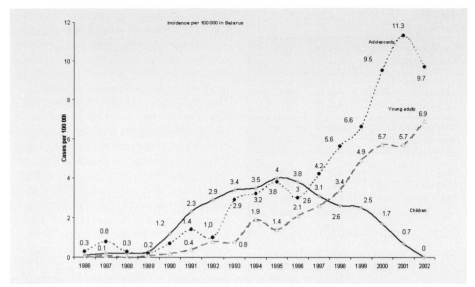

Fig. 2.002 Radiation-induced thyroid cancer. Distribution of annual rates of childhood (0-14), adolescent (15-18) and adult thyroid cancer incidence in Belarus in the population exposed to radiation from the Chernobyl accident below the age of 15. The decline in childhood incidence after 1995 is largely due to an increasing proportion of exposed children becoming adolescents; no child in 2002 had been exposed to ^{131}I from the Chernobyl accident. Courtesy of Dr. Yuri Evgenyevich.

closely associated with the development of papillary rather than follicular tumours. The etiology of follicular carcinoma is subject to the same influences described for papillary carcinoma, but with differing effects. Follicular carcinoma is particularly linked to dietary iodine deficiency {2392}, and both iodine deficiency and genetic influences could account for its link with a history of nodular goiter {1854}. The likelihood that the role of iodine is mediated through the growth stimulatory effect of high TSH levels is supported by the observation that when thyroid carcinoma occurs in dyshormonogenesis it is commonly follicular in type {411,1474}. The likelihood that progression from adenoma to carcinoma occurs is strengthened by the fact that in both dyshormonogenesis, and Cowden syndrome the defects that lead to multiple adenomas also lead to follicular carcinoma {1879}. The relative frequency of papillary carcinoma is greater in geographic regions of adequate or high dietary iodine intake compared to regions of iodine deficiency. In regions of iodine deficiency, the relative frequency of papillary carcinoma increases after iodine supplementation {825}, but it is not certain whether this is due to an absolute increase in the incidence of papillary carcinomas or a drop in the incidence of follicular carcinoma.

Lymphocytic thyroiditis
Papillary carcinoma shows a significant association with lymphocytic thyroiditis, probably both as a result of the carcinoma provoking an autoimmune response and as a possible pathogenetic mechanism {2174,2186}.

Genetic susceptibility
The familial nature of medullary carcinoma is well known, with approximately 25% of cases belonging to one or other of the recognized syndromes of MEN 2A, MEN 2B, and FMTC. Nearly all these cases show a germline mutation in the *RET* oncogene. The mutations involved and their genotype-phenotype correlations are described in the genetic section. There is a strong, but as yet unexplained familial factor in the development of papillary thyroid carcinoma. For example, in offspring of affected individuals, the rate of papillary thyroid carcinoma is 4-fold higher than in the general population {863}. Similarly, an association between papillary thyroid carcinoma, breast carcinomas and paragangliomas of the carotid body has been documented {1181,1996}. Follicular carcinoma occurs in Cowden syndrome. A histologically quite unique type of carcinoma occurs in patients with FAP, and a family with multiple oxyphil carcinomas has been reported.

Oncogenes and thyroid cancer
The past decade has witnessed significant advances in the understanding of thyroid carcinogenesis at the molecular level. *RET* and *TRK* rearrangements, which are characteristics of papillary carcinomas, are most likely related to double strand DNA breaks, often radiation induced. Recent studies have suggested that papillary carcinomas lacking these rearrangements may have *BRAF* mutations, which constitute a different route for tumorigenesis, or rearrangements in other genes involved in *RET* signaling pathways {1079,1605,2077,2389}. The majority of studies find that *RET* rearrangements and *BRAF* mutations are mutually exclusive in papillary carcinogenesis, although one considered that *BRAF* mutations may cooperate with *RET* rearrangements in the development of these tumours {2430}. Follicular neoplasms (adenomas and carcinomas) commonly demonstrate *RAS* mutations while follicular carcinomas and a minority of follicular adenomas exhibit *PAX8/PPARγ* rearrangements {1606}. Germline mutations of *RET*, on the other hand, are responsible for the development of heritable medullary carcinomas while somatic mutations are involved in the development of a subset of sporadic medullary carcinomas. The *RET* mutations associated with medullary carcinomas are point mutations or small deletions in contrast to *RET* rearrangements found in papillary carcinoma. *TP53* mutations are the most common molecular feature of undifferentiated thyroid carcinomas. A subset of poorly differentiated and undifferentiated carcinomas may also demonstrate *BRAF* mutations consistent with their origin from papillary carcinomas {1605}.

Clinical features
Ultrasound
This is particularly useful for establishing the size of a lesion and its solid or cystic nature and also for guiding the performance of fine needle aspiration biopsies (FNABs). Neither CTs nor MRIs provide higher quality images of the thyroid than ultrasound; however, CTs of the lower cervical nodes are preferable to ultrasound when tracheal or mediastinal invasion is suspected.

Nuclear scintigraphy
Scintigraphy employing technetium

pertechnetate (Tc99m) has been used extensively for the evaluation of nodular thyroid disease, particularly to determine whether the nodule has greater uptake than the normal gland ("hot"), some activity but less than that of the normal gland ("warm") or much less activity than the normal gland ("cold"). The risk of malignancy is greater in cold rather than warm or hot nodules although most cold nodules are benign and represent adenomas, cysts or focal thyroiditis. Nuclear scintigraphy is now used much less commonly than in the past because of the increased use of FNABs.

Serum TSH levels

Abnormalities in the levels of thyroid stimulating hormone (TSH) are rarely found in patients with thyroid malignancies although an elevated TSH may occur as a consequence of an associated thyroiditis, particularly in patients with lymphomas. Low TSH levels, however, may indicate the presence of a hyperfunctioning (toxic) nodule. Both papillary and follicular carcinomas may release increased amounts of thyroglobulin into the circulation; however, increased thyroglobulin levels may be found in a variety of benign conditions. Accordingly, thyroglobulin levels are not useful in the initial evaluation of patients with nodular thyroid disease. They are, however, useful in following the course of patients with recurrent and/or metastatic thyroid carcinoma particularly for patients who have undergone total or near total thyroidectomy and ^{131}I ablation for differentiated thyroid cancer {1452}.

Serum calcitonin levels

Measurements of serum calcitonin levels are used routinely in the diagnosis and follow up of cases with medullary carcinoma. They are also being performed increasingly in patients with nodular thyroid disease, and a small but significant proportion of patients with elevations have had microscopic foci of medullary carcinoma or C-cell hyperplasia detected in the resected glands {553A}. However, most investigators have found that routine measurements of calcitonin levels in patients with nodular thyroid disease are neither cost effective nor necessary unless the patient has a clinical suspicion of medullary carcinoma or abnormal results on a fine needle aspitation biopsy (FNAB).

Table 2.01
Stage Grouping.

Papillary or Follicular Carcinomas (under 45 years)			
Stage I	Any T	Any N	M0
Stage II	Any T	Any N	M1

Papillary or Follicular Carcinomas (45 years and older)			
Stage I	T1	N0	M0
Stage II	T2	N0	M0
Stage III	T3	N0	M0
	T1	N1a	M0
	T2	N1a	M0
	T3	N1a	M0
Stage IV A	T4a	N0	M0
	T4a	N1a	M0
	T1	N1b	M0
	T2	N1b	M0
	T3	N1b	M0
	T4a	N1b	M0
Stage IV B	T4b	Any N	M0
Stage IV C	Any T	Any N	M1

Medullary Carcinoma			
Stage I	T1	N0	M0
Stage II	T2	N0	M0
Stage III	T3	N0	M0
	T1	N1a	M0
	T2	N1a	M0
	T3	N1a	M0
Stage IV A	T4a	N0	M0
	T4a	N1a,b	M0
	T1	N1b	M0
	T2	N1b	M0
	T3	N1b	M0
Stage IV B	T4b	Any N	M0
Stage IV C	Any T	Any N	M1

Undifferentiated (anaplastic) carcinoma (All are considered Stage IV).			
Stage IV A	T4a	Any N	M0
Stage IV B	T4b	Any N	M0
Stage IV C	Any T	Any N	M1

Fine needle aspiration biopsy

FNAB is currently regarded as the test of choice for the diagnosis and management of thyroid nodules {167}. With the advent of FNAB, the yield of thyroid cancer at surgery has increased from 15 to 40%. Results are generally classified as satisfactory or unsatisfactory {167}. Those aspirates with insufficient cells are placed in the unsatisfactory category. Adequate samples should contain at least 6 groups of follicular cells with each group containing 15 to 20 follicular cells

present as sheets or follicular structures {701}. Satisfactory smears are subdivided into benign, malignant and indeterminate/suspicious categories. Benign aspirates include normal thyroid, multi-nodular goiter or macrofollicular adenoma. The malignant category includes papillary carcinoma, medullary carcinoma, poorly differentiated and undifferentiated carcinoma, malignant lymphoma, metastases to the thyroid and tumours of other types. The distinction between follicular adenomas and carcinomas cannot be made reliably on the basis of cytological examination, and for this reason, follicular neoplasms (including those of oncocytic type) are placed in the indeterminate/suspicious category. Other processes in the indeterminate/suspicious category include smears with features suggestive (but not diagnostic) of papillary and medullary carcinoma and cases of suspected lymphoma. In most large series of FNABs, 70% (50-90%) are benign, 4% (1-10%) are malignant, 10% (5-20%) are indeterminate/suspicious and 16% (15-20%) are unsatisfactory or non-diagnostic {701}. Surgery is recommended for lesions classified as malignant or indeterminate/suspicious while those patients with benign smears are generally followed. Rebiopsy is recommended for patients with non-diagnostic aspirates. In most series, the sensitivity of FNAB for thyroid cancer is 65-98%, the specificity is 72 to 100% and the positive predictive value is 50-96%. The false negative rate ranges from 1 to 11% while the false positive rate is 0-7%.

While a test that provided a reliable and accurate separation of follicular carcinoma from adenoma would be useful, it should be remembered that there is a strong case for removing tumours with a high risk of progression to malignancy. A method of distinguishing them from tumours with a low or absent risk of progression would be of considerable clinical value.

Staging and Prognostic factors

The TNM system is endorsed by the International Union Against Cancer (UICC) and the American Joint Commission on Cancer (AJCC). The recent TNM revision changed the definition of T1 from a tumour of 1 cm or less in diameter to a tumour of 2 cm or less, so that it is no longer consonant with the pathological definition of a microcarcinoma. Patients less than 45 years of age are classified as stage I if they have any T, any N, but no distant metastases (M0), while patients older than 45 years of age are classified as stages I to IV.

The first system proposed to define risk groups in patients with thyroid carcinoma, the EORTC (European Organization for Research and Treatment of Cancer) system, based the score determining the groups on age, sex, tumour type, extrathyroidal extension and distant metastasis. Seven other schemes have since been proposed. Three of these, which are the most frequently used, AGES (Age, Grade, Extent, Size), AMES (Age, Distant Metastasis, Extent, Size), and MACIS (Distant Metastasis, Age, Completeness of Resection, Local Invasion, Size) all rely on the same features as the EORTC, except that all three have added tumour size. Only AMES includes sex, MACIS has added incomplete resection, and only AGES uses grade {275}. A problem in using grade is that the vast majority of institutions do not grade papillary carcinomas since most are well differentiated. Interestingly none of these three schemes use nodal metastasis as a prognostic factor.

PARATHYROID

Epidemiology
Current epidemiological studies report an incidence of primary hyperparathyroidism of 17.7 cases per 1,000,000 person years in the United States (Rochester, MN) and in Western European countries {854,1557,2122}. Although studies from the Mayo Clinic have demonstrated a subsequent decline in the incidence of primary hyperparathyroidism, this trend has not been confirmed by studies from other centers {2378}.

Most of the geographic variations in the incidence of primary hyperparathyroidism may be related to variations in the utilization of routine calcium determinations. Reports from India, Saudi Arabia, Brazil, China and Vietnam indicate that many patients with primary hyperparathyroidism present with the classical phenotype and at a relatively young age. Moreover, there is a lower female predominance. This variation can be explained in part by differences in prevailing surveillance patterns and by differences in vitamin D and calcium nutrition. More severe bone disease is likely only when the secretion of parathyroid hormone is accompanied by prolonged vitamin D and calcium malnutrition. The effects of calcium and vitamin D in the diet, therefore, appear to transcend the effects of age, gender, and menopausal status in the expression of the manifestations of the disease.

Etiology and pathogenesis
Some studies have demonstrated that exposure to ionizing irradiation to the head and neck increases the risk of developing parathyroid adenomas in a dose dependent manner {911,1797}. In addition, long term stimulation of the parathyroids is associated with the development of nodules which appear to be clonal. This is seen in long standing renal failure and less commonly in celiac disease. The intense long term stimulation to parathyroid growth seen in chronic renal failure commonly leads to the development of multiple nodules in all four glands, a sequence of events reminiscent of that seen in dyshormonogenesis in the thyroid. The morphological findings in so-called 'tertiary hyperparathyroidism' may closely resemble those in primary nodular hyperparathyroidism; occasionally a dominant adenoma may develop in a background of hyperplasia.

Clinical features
Signs and symptoms
In contrast to tumours of the thyroid which typically present as mass lesions without functional abnormalities, most patients with parathyroid tumours present with evidence of parathyroid hyperfunction. Primary hyperparathyroidism is characterized by the inappropriately high level of secretion of parathyroid hormone which leads to increased renal calcium resorption, phosphaturia and increased bone resorption. The classical features of primary hyperparathyroidism, therefore, include hypercalcaemia, hypophosphatemia, hypercalciuria and progressive loss of cortical bone. This disorder predominates in women (F:M=3:1) and is recognized most commonly in the first post menopausal decade. In most series, parathyroid adenomas are responsible for hyperparathyroidism in 80-85% of cases while primary chief cell hyperplasia and parathyroid carcinoma account for 15-20% and less than 1% of cases, respectively.

Hyperparathyroidism
Once considered a rarity, primary hyperparathyroidism has emerged as the third most common endocrine disorder, following diabetes mellitus and nodular thyroid disease. This change occurred primarily as a result of the recognition of the association of primary hyperparathyroidism with renal stones in the 1930's and the introduction of the multichannel autoanalyzer in the late 1960's and early 1970's. As a result of the routine measurements of serum calcium levels, there was a dramatic increase in the proportion of patients diagnosed with asymptomatic primary hyperparathyroidism. The frequency of asymptomatic hyperparathyroidism was 0.6% between 1930 and 1965 while data from 1984-2000 indicated that of 80% of patients were asymptomatic. Concurrent with the increase in asymptomatic disease, there has been a marked decrease in the number of patients with severe metabolic complications as reflected in the skeletal system (osteitis fibrosa cystica) and kidney (nephrolithiasis), at least in the United States, Japan and Western European countries.

Diagnostic modalities
The laboratory diagnosis of primary hyperparathyroidism includes the demonstration of inappropriately high levels of parathyroid hormone. A variety of techniques, including ultrasonography, computed tomography (CT), magnetic resonance imaging (MRI) and nuclear scintigraphy, have been utilized for the localization of abnormal parathyroid tissue {683}. Technetium Tc99m sestamibi has been of particular value for the localization of parathyroid tissue. It is concentrated by thyroid and parathyroid tissue but is rapidly washed out from the thyroid while being retained by the parathyroids. Tc99m sestamibi is effective in detecting adenomas located both in their normal anatomic positions and in ectopic sites.

The sensitivity of this scanning procedure for detection of adenomas is 85 to 100% while the specificity is correspondingly high. The sensitivity for detecting hyperplastic glands is lower. While there is considerable debate on the value of this method in standard parathyroid surgical procedures, it is clear that minimally invasive parathyroid surgery necessitates a preoperative localization procedure {683,759,2088}.

Genetics and genetic susceptibility

The heritable forms of primary hyperparathyroidism occur in a number of well defined syndromes that are discussed in detail in Chapter 5. It has become evident that some of the genes involved in the development of the heritable syndromes are of equal importance in the development of sporadic parathyroid adenomas and carcinomas. Molecular studies have demonstrated that both cyclin D1 (CCND1) and the MEN1 gene play a role in the development of sporadic adenomas.

Cyclin D1 is an oncogene that encodes a key regulator of the cell cycle while MEN1 is a tumour suppressor gene that is implicated in the development of type 1 multiple endocrine neoplasia (MEN1). Other genes that have been implicated in the development of these tumours include the Ca^{2+} sensing receptor (CASR) gene and the vitamin D receptor (VDR) gene and other genes involved in their respective biochemical pathways {75,1162}. Mutations in the HRPT2 gene, the causative gene of the hyperparathyroidism-jaw tumour (HPT-JT) syndrome have also been implicated in the development of parathyroid carcinomas {927, 2026}.

Staging and prognostic factors

Because of the rarity of parathyroid carcinoma, the UICC and AJCC have not yet developed a staging system; however, Shaha and Shah have proposed a working staging system {2015}.

Conclusions

Tumours of the thyroid and of the parathyroid glands show both similarities and differences. Both are usually well differentiated, slow growing, and rarely fatal. Both can present with hyperfunction, commonly for parathyroid, rarely for thyroid. Both can be induced through a prolonged stimulus to hyperplasia and by radiation. As this brief introduction has outlined, tumours derived from thyroid follicular cells can give rise to a wide variety of distinct tumour types with differing clinical behaviours, while tumours derived from C-cells or from parathyroid cells essentially each give rise to one tumour type, with varying degrees of differentiation, growth and malignant potential. These differences could be related to the fact that C-cells and parathyroid cells are true endocrine cells, synthesizing peptide hormones and storing them as cytoplasmic granules, while follicular cells behave as modified enterocytes, secreting proteins into a lumen, resorbing proteins from that lumen, digesting them and releasing iodinated tyrosines. There are many cell types in intestinal epithelium, and it may be that follicular cells retain some of that potential diversity which is lost in the committed pure endocrine cell.

One tumour type, the mixed medullary-follicular cell carcinoma poses a particular problem because of the differing embryological origin of the two cell types A second problem is posed by the apparent dichotomy between the pathological malignancy but clinical benignity of papillary microcarcinoma. The multiplicity of tumour types derived from the follicular cell, with the main differentiated divisions of papillary, follicular, and possibly oncocytic provide a major opportunity for genotype-phenotype correlations. We know that the pathways involved appear to be distinct, and even within individual tumour types, molecular genetic studies suggest that different subpathways are involved, and they too may correlate with variations in morphology. Different morphologies are also associated with different germline defects with some, like the FAP associated tumours, showing characteristic changes.

Advances in genotype-phenotype correlation are essential if we are to understand endocrine carcinogenesis, and these advances will hopefully lead to better methods of diagnosis, and to more discriminating treatment. For this to occur we need greater understanding of morphology by molecular biologists, and greater understanding of molecular biology by morphologists. Both approaches need reproducible techniques, and both need more comparative studies of the same tumours in different centers. These studies must be carried out using a common language and framework for diagnosis. This is essential for the diagnosis that determines treatment. The pages that follow set out to provide this framework for tumours of the two endocrine glands most commonly involved by neoplastic processes, thyroid and parathyroid.

Papillary carcinoma

V.A. LiVolsi
J. Albores-Saavedra
S.L. Asa
Z.W. Baloch
M. Sobrinho-Simões
B. Wenig
R.A. DeLellis
B. Cady

E.L. Mazzaferri
I. Hay
J.A. Fagin
A.L. Weber
P. Caruso
P.E. Voutilainen
K.O. Franssila
E.D. Williams

A.B. Schneider
Y. Nikiforov
H.M. Rabes
L. Akslen
S. Ezzat
M. Santoro
C. Eng
H.R. Harach

Definition

A malignant epithelial tumour showing evidence of follicular cell differentiation and characterized by distinctive nuclear features.

ICD-O code   8260/3

Synonyms

Papillary adenocarcinoma; mixed papillary and follicular adenocarcinoma.

Epidemiology

Age and sex distribution

Although papillary carcinomas are rare before the age of 15 years, they represent the most common paediatric thyroid malignancy. Most tumours manifest in adults of 20-50 years, with a female to male ratio of 4:1. Over the age of 50 years the female predominance is less pronounced. Overall survival is excellent (greater than 90%) particularly for patients younger than 45 years.

Incidence

The incidence of papillary carcinoma has increased worldwide. For example, in the United States, 10,000 cases occurred in 1980, but 22,000 are estimated in 2004. Despite the increase in incidence, the mortality rate is declining. The prevalence of papillary carcinoma at autopsy and as an incidental finding in surgically removed glands varies between 5-35% and this variation is heavily dependent

on the sampling technique {42,657}. The incidence of clinically apparent tumours is considerably less than the autopsy data would suggest. This underscores the conundrum of understanding biological behaviour and appropriate therapy for papillary carcinoma.

Etiology

The etiology of papillary thyroid carcinoma is most closely linked to radiation exposure and is discussed in the Introduction.

Localization

Papillary carcinoma can arise in the normally situated thyroid gland and in ectopic thyroid tissue (e.g. struma ovarii).

Clinical features

Signs and symptoms

Papillary carcinoma usually presents as a thyroid mass which is typically cold on radioactive iodine scan or as cervical lymphadenopathy. In areas of iodine insufficiency, multinodular goiter remains common and papillary cancer may appear as a more distinctive nodule in the goiter. In areas with adequate iodine, papillary carcinoma usually presents as a palpable solitary nodule in a relatively normal thyroid gland. Diagnostic studies (CT, MRI, ultrasound), performed for trauma, carotid vascular disease or other indications. have revealed numer-

ous incidental, non-palpable thyroid nodules. Such preclinical nodules that prove to be thyroid cancer correspond to the prevalence of unsuspected small or microscopic foci of papillary carcinoma found as incidental lesions in thyroidectomy specimens or at autopsy. The clinical significance of incidental non-palpable papillary carcinomas is undoubtedly negligible since even large palpable papillary carcinomas in young patients have a 20-year survival in excess of 98%. These pre-clinical papillary carcinomas do not appear to alter the normal life-span.

Thyroid function tests

Thyroid carcinoma rarely interferes with the functional capacity of the thyroid gland; therefore thyroid function tests do not aid in diagnosis of thyroid carcinoma. Routine blood studies, TSH levels, or other thyroid function studies are not indicated for differential diagnosis of cancer, but should be reserved for functional evaluation.

Fine needle aspiration biopsy (FNAB)

The diagnosis of solitary thyroid nodules should begin with fine needle aspiration biopsy (FNAB) for cytologic analysis. Benign cytology may eliminate as many as 75% of patients with clinically solitary nodules from the need for further studies or surgery. Fine needle aspiration is an effective method of diagnosing papillary

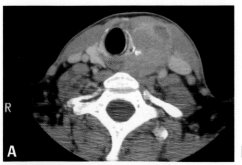 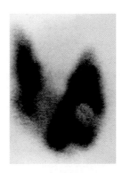 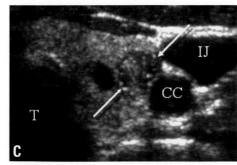

Fig. 2.003 Papillary carcinoma. **A** CT scan of a large thyroid tumour with extensive infiltration of the soft tissue of the neck. **B** I^{131} scan showing a cold nodule in the left lobe. **C** Ultrasound image showing a tumour (arrows) in the upper portion of the right thyroid lobe with internal hyperechoic foci corresponding to psammomatous calcifications in a papillary carcinoma. CC, common carotid artery; T, trachea; IJ, internal jugular vein.

carcinoma; such patients should undergo surgical treatment. Depending on the clinical context, palpable cervical lymph nodes may also be analyzed by FNAB since approximately 25% of young patients with papillary carcinoma present with palpable cervical lymph node metastases even from small or non-palpable primary papillary carcinomas.

Imaging

Other diagnostic studies include ultrasound, radio-active iodine (RAI) scans, computerized tomography (CT) scans, or magnetic resonance imaging (MRI), are discussed in the introduction. These diagnostic approaches are unnecessary in the usual patient, but in older patients with large cancers, especially when symptomatic (dysphagia, stridor, cough) or when physical examination reveals fixation or extensive involvement of local tissues, further imaging should define the extent and aid surgical management.

Macroscopy

Papillary carcinomas show a variety of gross patterns. Most lesions are grey-white firm masses, with irregular borders or even gross infiltration of the surrounding thyroid parenchyma. Some show dystrophic calcification and occasional tumours may demonstrate bone formation. The size ranges from minute (<1 mm) to several centimetres and multicentricity is common. Many tumours will show cystic change and rarely the tumour is almost entirely cystic. In some instances, the primary tumour will be solid while the nodal metastases will be cystic. Occasionally, the tumours may arise in thyroglossal duct cysts. Papillary carcinomas may show direct extension into perithyroidal fat, skeletal muscle, oesophagus, larynx and trachea.

Tumour spread and staging

Papillary carcinoma has a tendency to spread into lymphatic channels and hence regional node metastases at presentation are found in a significant proportion of cases. In addition, microscopic foci of tumour are commonly found in the thyroid, topographically separate from the main tumour mass, as a result of intraglandular lymphatic spread or, more rarely, multifocal origin. Venous invasion can also occur.

Tumour staging relies on age of patients, size of the primary tumour, extrathyroidal

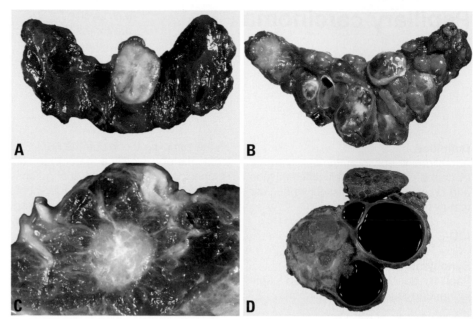

Fig. 2.004 Papillary thyroid carcinoma. **A** This encapsulated tumour arose in the isthmus. **B** The tumour is present in the upper portion of the right thyroid lobe on the background of multinodular goiter. **C** The tumour has a rounded contour. **D** The tumour has multiple foci of cystic change with haemorrhage.

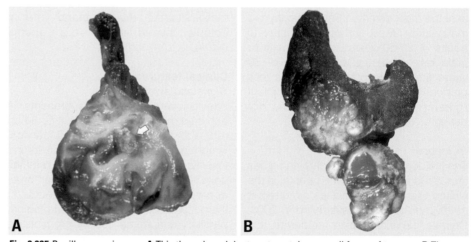

Fig. 2.005 Papillary carcinoma. **A** This thyroglossal duct cyst contains a small focus of tumour. **B** The pattern of tumour growth in the right lobe is solid while the tumour in the adjacent node is cystic.

spread and regional and distant metastases (see introduction to this chapter).

Cytopathology

Aspirates from conventional papillary carcinomas typically contain abundant cells that may be grouped in papillary tissue fragments, monolayered sheets and three dimensional clusters. The papillary fragments commonly reveal a branching pattern with a regular external contour and nuclear palisading. The tumour cells are usually cuboidal but they may also assume columnar, polygonal, spindle cell or squamous morphology. The nuclei are typically enlarged and irregular. They

contain dusty to powdery chromatin and small nucleoli which are often present adjacent to the nuclear membrane. Nuclear grooves and pseudoinclusions are common. Additional helpful features include the presence of ropy (or 'chewing gum') colloid, multinucleated giant cells, and psammoma bodies.

Histopathology

The characteristic nuclear features of papillary carcinoma include enlargement, oval shape, elongation, and overlapping. The nuclei typically show clearing, or a ground glass appearance. Irregularity of nuclear contours, including

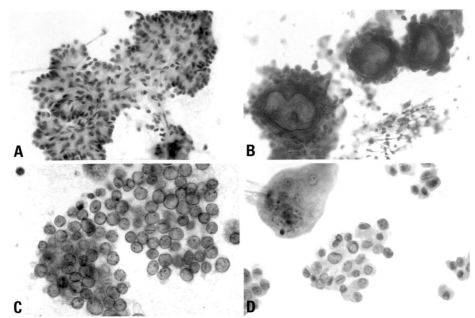

Fig. 2.006 FNAB of papillary carcinoma. A The tumour cells are arranged in a papillary fragment. B Psammoma bodies are present in the aspirate. C The nuclei have powdery chromatin, relatively thick nuclear membranes and grooves. D The tumour cell nuclei contain pseudoinclusions and a multinucleate giant cell is present in the upper left corner.

grooves and nuclear pseudoinclusions, are common. In tumours without complex papillary structures, the diagnosis of papillary carcinoma relies on these nuclear features, which should be present in a significant proportion of the neoplasm {2315}.

Papillary architecture, when present, is typically complex with branching. In occasional cases, the papillae may be markedly edematous. The papillae are covered by epithelium with disturbed polarity and pale or eosinophilic cytoplasm. Squamous metaplasia is common. Other architectural patterns often coexist with papillae and it is uncommon to find a pure papillary growth. These patterns usually include varying sized follicles; however, solid and trabecular patterns can also be seen. The tumours may be cystic and the cyst lining may show extensive squamous metaplasia. Psammoma bodies are rounded and concentrically laminated calcifications which must be distinguished from psammoma-like bodies which may be present within colloid. Psammoma bodies in papillary carcinomas are found in association with tumour cells, within lymphatic spaces or within the tumour stroma.

Intratumoural sclerosis and peritumoural lymphocytic infiltration are found frequently.

The papillae should be distinguished from papillary structures sometimes found in nodular goiter or follicular adenomas with papillae, and from the short papillary infoldings of diffuse hyperplasia. The nuclei in the latter conditions are typically round, basally situated within the cytoplasm, and most importantly, lack the features of papillary carcinoma nuclei.

Immunohistochemistry

Papillary carcinomas are reactive for cytokeratins, thyroglobulin and thyroid transcription factor–1 (TTF-1), but are negative for synaptophysin and chromogranin. A number of immunohistochemical markers have been proposed to confirm the diagnosis of papillary carcinoma. Candidate markers include S100 protein, HLA-DR, estrogen receptor, high molecular weight cytokeratins (CK), CK19, and RET. Other suggested markers of malignancy in papillary lesions include HBME-1 and galectin-3. Although galectin-3 and HBME-1 are expressed in a high proportion of papillary carcinomas, neither is specific for these tumours. CK19 has been widely applied as a marker for papillary carcinoma but also remains controversial since it is also positive in chronic lymphocytic thyroiditis and at sites of reaction, usually in response to previous aspiration biopsy. The use of RET staining to identify expression of a RET/PTC rearrangement (see somatic genetics) is dependent on the availability of reliable and sensitive antibodies {112,

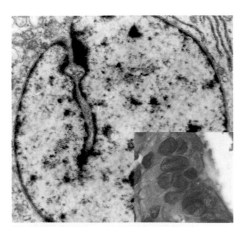

Fig. 2.007 Papillary carcinoma. EM shows highly folded nuclear membrane. Inset: inclusion-like formations and nuclear grooves.

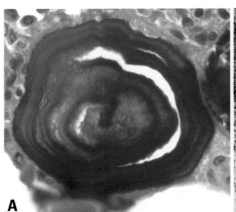
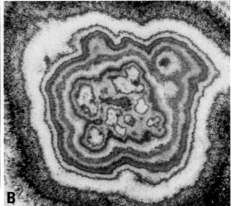

Fig. 2.008 Papillary carcinoma. A Light microscopic appearance of a psammoma body. B Electron micrograph of a psammoma body.

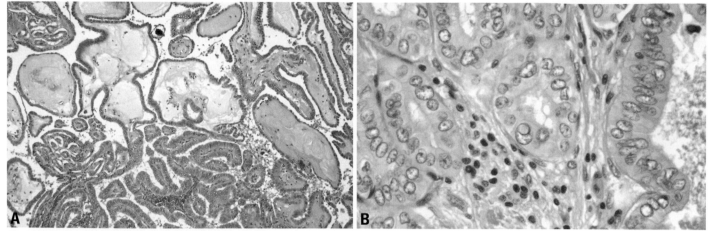

Fig. 2.009 Papillary carcinoma. **A** The papillary structures in the upper portion of the field are markedly oedematous. **B** Note the typical overlapping, grooved, ground glass nuclei with inclusion bodies.

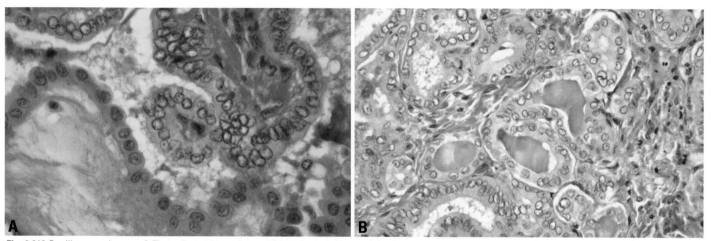

Fig. 2.010 Papillary carcinoma. **A** The cells on the surface of the oedematous papilla (left) have a metaplastic appearance with dense chromatin and are deeply eosinophilic, in contrast to the cells on the right, which have clear nuclei. **B** The colloid within the follicles is basophilic.

368,876,1073,1074,1335,1495,1794, 2158,2434}.

Tumours with metastases typically show loss of p27 or upregulation of cyclin D1 while non-metastatic papillary carcinomas are positive for p27 and negative for cyclin D1 {1667,1750}.

Metastatic papillary carcinomas of thyroid origin are positive for TTF-1 and thyroglobulin while pulmonary primaries may be positive for TTF-1 but are negative for thyroglobulin. Papillary carcinomas from sites other than the lung and thyroid are typically negative for both TTF-1 and thyroglobulin.

Histopathological variants

Some papillary carcinomas show special features, i.e., combinations of certain growth patterns, cell types and stromal reactions. Tumours should be dominated by a certain feature in order to qualify as a specific histological variant.

Follicular variant

Grossly, many of these tumours resemble encapsulated follicular neoplasms. They are composed of small to medium sized, irregularly shaped follicles with virtually no papillary structures. A variable amount of colloid, which may appear hypereosinophilic and scalloped, is seen in the follicles. The majority of cells lining the follicles contain large clear nuclei with grooves and nuclear pseudoinclusion. Where a small minority of cells in a follicular nodule show these features the clinical significance is uncertain. The term "well differentiated tumour of uncertain malignant potential" has been suggested for tumours of this type {2391} but the use of this nomenclature has not as yet been generally accepted. Intrafollicular multinucleate giant cells may be frequent in this variant while stromal sclerosis and psammoma bodies are seen occasionally. Approximately one third of

the tumours are encapsulated. Despite complete encapsulation, lymph node and rarely, hematogenous metastasis can occur; however, the prognosis of these tumours is similar to that of usual papillary carcinoma {2496}. An exception is the rare diffuse or multinodular follicular variant, which has an aggressive clinical course {114,978,2241}.

Fine needle aspiration biopsy shows non-cohesive cells, sometimes arranged in follicles are found in a background usually containing little colloid. The nuclear changes typical of papillary carcinoma allow this variant of PTC to be distinguished from the other follicular patterned lesions. However, in the follicular variant, the number of intranuclear inclusions is less than that seen in conventional PTC.

Macrofollicular variant

The macrofollicular variant of papillary

carcinoma is probably the rarest form. It is composed predominantly or exclusively of macrofollicles (>50 % of a cross sectional area), and is often confused with colloid or hyperplastic nodules or macrofollicular adenoma since most of the tumours are encapsulated. Moreover, many of the macrofollicles are lined by cells with hyperchromatic nuclei and the colloid often shows peripheral vacuolization. However, some follicles are lined by cells with large clear nuclei with grooves and pseudoinclusions characteristic of papillary carcinoma. This variant is characterized by a low incidence of lymph node metastasis {27,599,1696}. However, when metastases do occur, they often maintain the macrofollicular architecture seen in the primary tumours.

Oncocytic variant

Oncocytic papillary carcinomas are characterized grossly by a distinct mahogany brown appearance and may have a papillary or follicular architecture. Occasional tumours of oncocytic type may appear grey-white. Papillary tumours are characterized by complex branching papillae in which oncocytic cells cover thin fibrovascular stromal cores {178,873,886,1363,2086}. The "Warthin-like" tumour has abundant chronic inflammatory cells and is frequently associated with Hashimoto thyroiditis {67}. Tumours with follicular architecture may be macro- or micro-follicular with variable colloid storage {369}. The tumours may be well delineated and even encapsulated, but careful evaluation usually identifies at least some degree of infiltration of the surrounding capsule. Some lesions are frankly and widely invasive. The diagnosis of the oncocytic variant is based on the nuclear features of these lesions which are identical to those seen in papillary carcino-

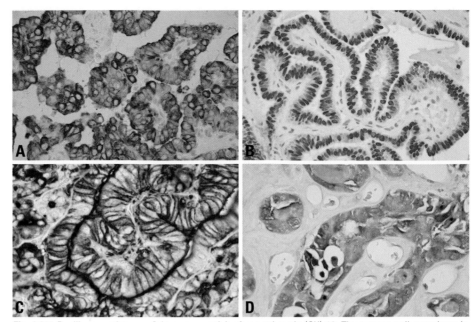

Fig. 2.011 Papillary carcinoma. **A** Immunoreactivity for cytokeratin (CK)-19. The tumour cell cytoplasm is strongly reactive. **B** Immunoreactivity for TTF-1. Each of the nuclei is positively stained. **C** Papillary carcinoma immunostained for HBME-1. Positive staining is present primarily within the plasma membranes of the tumour cells. **D** Galectin-3 staining is confined to the cytoplasm of tumour cells.

mas of conventional type. The oncocytic cells are usually polygonal but may be columnar; they have abundant granular eosinophilic cytoplasm.

On FNAB, large cells arranged in irregular clusters or papillary aggregates are found. The nuclei are clear and have grooves and pseudoinclusions. Follicular carcinomas of oncocytic type generally lack these nuclear features.

Clear cell variant

Both conventional papillary carcinomas and the follicular variants may be composed predominantly of clear cells. Often a papillary architecture predominates but some tumours may have a follicular growth pattern. In some of these tumours an admixture of oncocytic and clear cells is seen. The nuclear features are those of

conventional papillary carcinoma. Moreover, some cells have partially clear and partially oncocytic cytoplasm. Both intra- and extra-cellular alcian blue-positive mucin is occasionally seen. Recognition of these types of papillary carcinoma in metastatic sites may be problematic, especially without immunostains for thyroglobulin and TTF-1 {302,389}.

Diffuse sclerosing variant

This tumour tends to occur in young patients {300} and is characterized by diffuse involvement of one or both thyroid lobes, usually without forming a dominant mass. In most tumours, small papillary structures are seen within dilated lymphovascular spaces. They are characterized by extensive squamous metaplasia,

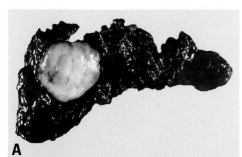
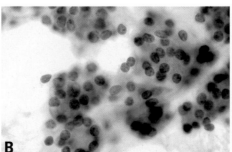
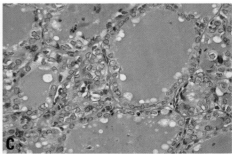

Fig. 2.012 Follicular variant of papillary carcinoma. **A** This tumour is encapsulated and grossly resembles a follicular adenoma. **B** FNAB demonstrating nuclear crowding with powdery chromatin and grooves. **C** The nuclei are enlarged, irregularly shaped and clear in the corresponding histological section.

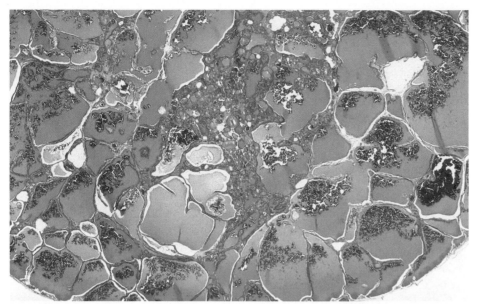

Fig. 2.013 Papillary carcinoma, macrofollicular variant. The tumour is composed predominantly of macro-follicles.

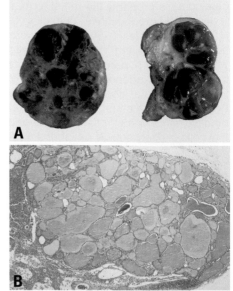

Fig. 2.014 A Papillary carcinoma. This nodal metastasis contains large colloid filled follicles resembling colloid goiter. **B** Lymph node metastasis of a macrofollicular papillary carcinoma, surrounded by a thin rim of lymph nodal tissue.

numerous psammoma bodies, dense lymphocytic infiltration and stromal fibrosis. When a dominant nodule is present, the neoplastic cells appear similar to those of conventional papillary carcinoma or they may have a clear glycogen-rich cytoplasm. In dominant nodules, the tumour occasionally shows a predominantly follicular pattern. The nontumourous thyroid often shows chronic lymphocytic thyroiditis and many patients have serologic evidence of autoimmune thyroid disease. There may be prominent regional node metastases; lung metastases are also common at presentation (about 25% of patients).

Tall cell variant
This rare variant of papillary carcinoma is uncommon. It is composed predominantly of cells whose heights are at least three times their widths. This form of papillary carcinoma has been poorly defined because the height of the neoplastic cells is quite variable and depends upon the plane of section and, also, because a significant proportion of tall cells is seen in different types of papillary carcinoma. A combination of papillary, trabecular or cord-like patterns predominate in most tumours while follicular structures are rare. The neoplastic cells have abundant eosinophilic cytoplasm and nuclei similar to those of conventional papillary carcinoma although nuclear grooves and nuclear pseudoinclusion tend to be more abundant. Necrosis, mitotic activity and extrathyroidal extension by the tumour are common. These tumours occur in older patients, often males, and tend to show a more aggressive clinical behavior than usual papillary carcinoma {1663}.

Columnar cell variant
This rare variant is composed of pseudostratified columnar cells some of which may contain supranuclear and subnuclear cytoplasmic vacuoles reminiscent of those of early secretory endometrium. Hyperchromatic nuclei predominate while the characteristic large clear nuclei of conventional papillary carcinoma are only focally present in some tumours. A variable proportion of papillary, follicular, trabecular and solid patterns is seen in most tumours. The follicles may appear elongated and empty resembling tubular glands. When these structures predominate in metastatic deposits the tumour may be confused with metastatic adenocarcinoma from the gastrointestinal tract or lung. The neoplastic cells show variable thyroglobulin immunoreactivity and are typically positive for TTF1. These tumours more often have advanced local growth and

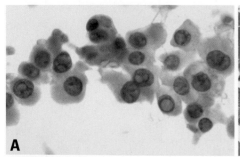
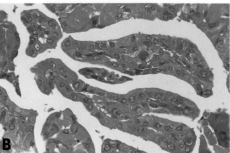
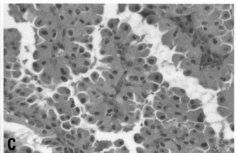

Fig. 2.015 Papillary carcinoma, oncocytic variant. **A** FNAB: the nuclei contain prominent pseudoinclusions (Courtesy of G. Guiter, M.D.). **B** The papillae are covered by tumour cells with deeply eosinophilic cytoplasm. **C** Tumour nuclei show apical polarization and the cytoplasm is deeply eosinophilic.

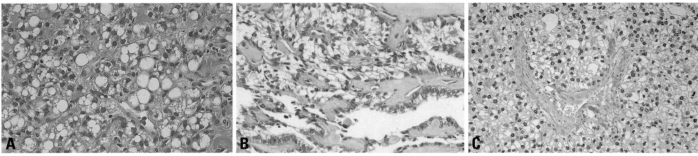

Fig. 2.016 Papillary carcinoma, clear cell variant. **A** The tumour cells have abundant clear/vacuolated cytoplasm. **B** The cytoplasm of the tumour cells is extensively vacuolated. **C** Nuclear immunoreactivity for TTF-1 confirms the thyroid origin of this clear cell tumour.

extrathyroidal extension and tend to show a more aggressive clinical behavior than conventional papillary carcinomas {2377}. Nonetheless, those tumours that are partially or completely encapsulated appear to have a lower metastatic potential than those tumours that are non-encapsulated or partially encapsulated.

Solid variant

These tumours are dominated by solid sheets of tumour cells with typical nuclear features of papillary carcinoma. Vascular invasion and extrathyroidal extension are found in about one-third of cases. These tumours are more common in children, including those who have been exposed to radiation. If a solid growth is combined with marked nuclear pleomorphism and tumour cell necrosis,

a poorly differentiated carcinoma should be considered.

Cribriform carcinoma

In some schemes, cribriform carcinoma is considered a variant of papillary thyroid carcinoma while in other classifications, it is considered a distinct entity. It is characterized by focal papillary architecture, cribriform features, solid and spindle cell areas as well as squamoid morules. This tumour typically occurs in patients with FAP or Gardner syndrome. In this setting tumours are usually multifocal and predominate in young women. A solitary sporadic counterpart rarely occurs {282}. Focally, the nuclei are clear and show grooves. Most nuclei, however, appear hyperchromatic. Most tumours are thyroglobulin positive only focally. {830,1727}

Papillary carcinoma with fasciitis-like stroma

Rare examples of papillary carcinoma with peculiar fibrous stromal reactions (fasciitis-like, fibromatosis-like) have been described {1568}. No particular adverse prognostic significance to these changes has been identified.

Papillary carcinoma with focal insular component

A small proportion of papillary carcinomas may show a focal insular component, and trabecular/solid growth patterns may be present. The cells of the insular, solid and trabecular components are similar to those of conventional papillary carcinoma. The neoplastic cells are immunoreactive for thyroglobulin and TTF1. The clinical significance of a focal

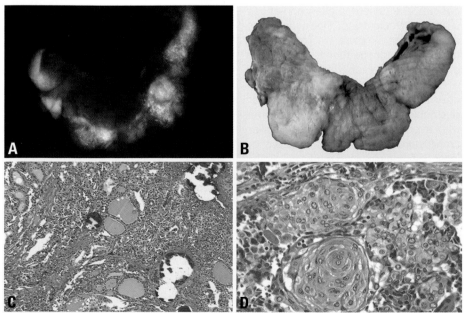

Fig. 2.017 Papillary carcinoma, diffuse sclerosing variant. **A** Radiograph demonstrating extensive areas of calcification. **B** This tumour extensively involves both lobes. **A, B** from {23A}. **C** Lymphocytic thyroiditis and multiple intravascular psammoma bodies are common. **D** Note the prominent squamous metaplasia.

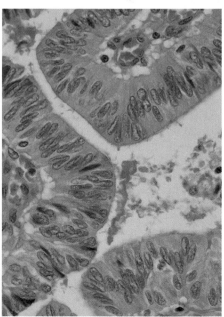

Fig. 2.018 Papillary carcinoma, tall cell type. In this focus, the tumour cells are at least 3 times taller than they are wide.

insular pattern is not known {28,94}.

Papillary carcinoma with squamous cell or mucoepidermoid carcinoma

Papillary carcinoma rarely coexists with squamous cell carcinoma. The papillary carcinoma that is frequently the tall cell variant merges imperceptibly with the squamous cell carcinoma. This combined carcinoma should not be confused with papillary carcinoma with squamous metaplasia because the former follows an aggressive clinical course and the latter behaves as conventional papillary thyroid carcinoma. Papillary carcinoma can also be admixed with mucoepidermoid carcinoma that is usually not associated with eosinophilia or Hashimoto thyroiditis {115}.

Papillary carcinoma with spindle and giant cell carcinoma

Rarely papillary carcinomas may have a minor or focal undifferentiated component. If the undifferentiated or spindle cell component predominates, the tumours should be classified as undifferentiated carcinomas. Since the natural history of focal undifferentiated carcinoma is unknown, it should be designated as papillary carcinoma with focal spindle and giant cell component {303} (See undifferentiated carcinoma below).

Combined papillary and medullary carcinoma

In this form of combined thyroid carcinoma, the papillary carcinoma usually represents a minor component (<25%) of the tumour.(See section on mixed medullary and follicular tumours) Although the medullary and papillary carcinoma components are intimately admixed, each component can be identified by its nuclear features. The cells with large clear nuclei are immunoreactive for thyroglobulin and negative for calcitonin, whereas the round or ovoid cells with coarsely granular chromatin are immunoreactive for calcitonin and negative for thyroglobulin; both components are positive for TTF1 {26}.

Papillary microcarcinomas

The term microcarcinoma should be used for a papillary carcinoma, which is found incidentally, and which measures 1 cm or less in diameter {1738}. It is the most common form of papillary carcinoma. In Finland, for example, it was found in over

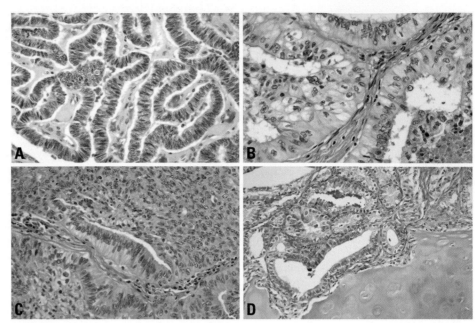

Fig. 2.019 Papillary carcinoma, columnar cell variant. **A** The tumour cell nuclei have an elongate shape and demonstrate pronounced pseudostratification. **B** This lesion exhibits prominent subnuclear vacuoles. A focus of necrosis is present in the right lower portion of the field. **C** Subnuclear vacuolization is seen along with a solid growth pattern. **D** The tumour is invading the tracheal cartilage.

one third of the autopsies and it has been reported in up to 24% of surgical thyroidectomies performed for disorders unrelated to papillary carcinoma {630}. Because of its small size, it is frequently overlooked on gross examination. In children these tumours can behave more aggressively, and rarely in adults they may present with cervical nodal metastasis. Commonly located near the thyroid capsule, the tumour is often non-encapsulated and sclerosing. However, encapsulated variants exist. The smallest tumours (<1 mm) frequently show a follicular pattern and lack stromal sclerosis, whereas, larger microcarcinomas (average size 2 mm) show a prominent desmoplastic stroma. Microcarcinomas with a predominant or a pure papillary architecture are the largest tumours but least common (mean, 5 mm).

Terminology. In some schemes, papillary carcinomas measuring less than 1 cm in diameter, are considered a variant of papillary carcinoma {630,826,2443}. These tumours have been referred to by a number of terms including occult, latent or small papillary carcinoma, non-encapsulated thyroid tumour and occult sclerosing carcinoma. The term "papillary microtumour" has been proposed for this group of neoplasms, but specifically excludes tumours in patients less than 19 years of age and tumours presenting

with metastases {1863}.

Metastatic spread. Occasionally, a papillary carcinoma of 1 cm or less in diameter represents the primary tumour for a large cervical lymph node metastasis. These rare lesions have distinct immunohistochemical features, with loss of p27 {1074} and upregulation of cyclin D1 {1073}, reflecting a different biology compared with the very common incidental microcarcinomas.

Grading

Tumour grading in papillary carcinoma is of little value since more than 95% of cases are well differentiated using standard grading criteria {1316}. However, certain features such as tumour necrosis, vascular invasion, numerous mitoses and marked nuclear atypia have been associated with a less favourable prognosis {23}.

Precursor lesions

There is no known precursor lesion of papillary thyroid carcinoma.

Histogenesis

The cell of origin of papillary carcinoma is the follicular cell.

Somatic genetics

RET/PTC rearrangements

Chromosomal rearrangements of receptor tyrosine kinase genes (*RET* and *TRK*)

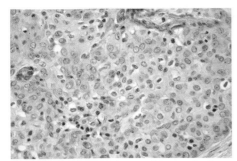

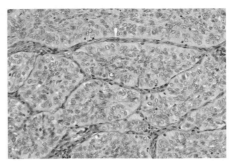

Fig. 2.020 Papillary carcinoma with a predominant solid growth pattern.

Fig. 2.021 Papillary carcinoma, with focal insular growth pattern.

represent the most common structural genetic alterations in papillary thyroid carcinoma. Rearrangements involving the *RET* gene, called *RET/PTC*, are found with highly variable frequency (0-80%) in different studies and geographic regions. The average incidence of *RET/PTC* is 20-30% in sporadic adult papillary carcinomas {224,1933}, and is higher in tumours from children and young adults (45-60%) {222,617}, and in populations subjected to either accidental or therapeutic irradiation (50-80%) {234,1784}. *RET/PTC* fusion after irradiation is thought to be mediated by spatial proximity of the participating chromosomal loci in the nucleus {1607} and by short-sequence homology in DNA at the breakpoints {1117,1602}.

Several types of *RET/PTC* exist, all formed by fusion of the tyrosine kinase domain of *RET* on 10q11.2 with the 5' terminal sequences of different genes located on

chromosome 10q or on other chromosomes. *RET/PTC1* {774} is typically the most common, followed by *RET/PTC3* {221,1936}, whereas *RET/PTC2* {223} and novel types {419, 1115, 1116,1118, 1574,1908} account for less than 5% of all rearrangements. The exception is a population of papillary carcinomas in children that developed less than 10 years after accidental exposure to radiation, where *RET/PTC3* was the dominant type and novel types of *RET/PTC* constituted up to 12% of all rearrangements {1784}. All types of *RET/PTC* have in common a replacement of the extracellular ligand-binding domain of *RET* by *RET*–fused genes which typically exhibit expression in the thyroid and dimerization potential. This leads to ligand-independent activation of the RET kinase, clonal expansion and neoplastic transformation of thyroid follicular cells {1004,1766,1935}. *RET*-

fused genes may have an impact on tumour phenotype: *RET/PTC1* is more common in papillary microcarcinomas and tumours with classic papillary architecture {2158,2319}, whereas *RET/PTC3* predominates in the solid and tall cell variants {128,1603}.

Oncocytic papillary carcinomas have *RET/PTC* rearrangements {369,373} with similar frequency as non-oncocytic papillary carcinomas.

TRK rearrangements

Chromosomal rearrangements involving the *TRK* gene are found in approximately 10% of papillary carcinomas {224,1563}. They result from the fusion of the tyrosine kinase domain of *TRK* on chromosome 1q22 to the 5' terminal sequence of the tropomyosin (*TPM3*) {1418,1787} or TPR {766} genes also located on 1q, or of the *TFG* gene on chromosome 3 {765}. All types of *TRK* rearrangement occur with approximately similar frequency {224,1563}, whereas *TRK-TPM3* predominates in radiation associated papillary thyroid carcinomas {154}.

RAS mutations

Activating point mutations of one of three *RAS* proto-oncogenes occur in less than 10% of papillary carcinomas {597,819, 1579}, with *N-RAS* codon 61 being the most frequently affected hot spot in this type of tumour. In one series, however, ras mutations were found in 43% of cases of the follicular variant {2494}.

BRAF mutations

Point mutation of the *BRAF* gene at nucleotide position 1796, a thymine-to-adenine transversion, has been identified in a high proportion of papillary carcinomas (up to 70%) {1079,2077,1605}. This mutation was not detected in other types of thyroid neoplasms. There was no overlap between papillary carcinoma with mutated *RET/PTC*, *BRAF*, or *RAS*, all of which encode proteins that act along the same intracellular signaling pathway leading to the activation of the MAPK cascade. The studies of Xu et al, demonstrated that a substantial proportion of *BRAF* positive tumours also harbour *RET* rearrangements suggesting that mutated *BRAF* may cooperate with *RET/PTC* to induce the development of papillary carcinoma {2433}.

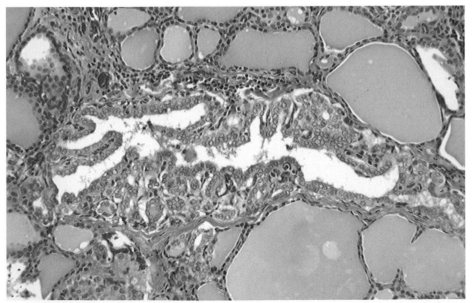

Fig. 2.022 Papillary microcarcinoma. This tumour has a papillary architecture and shows typical nuclear clearing.

Table 2.02
Characteristics of different types of *RET/PTC* rearrangement in papillary thyroid carcinoma.

Type of RET/PTC	Gene fused with RET	Mechanism of rearrangement	Prevalence among all RET/PTC	Association with radiation exposure
RET/PTC1	H4 (D10S170)	inv(10)(q11.2;q21)	60-70%	some
RET/PTC2	RIa	t(10;17)(q11.2;q23)	<10%	some
RET/PTC3 (and RET/PTC4)	ELE1 (RFG, ARA70)	inv(10)(q11.2)	20-30%	strong
RET/PTC5	GOLGA5	t(10;14) (q11.2;q?)	rare	yes
RET/PTC6	HTIF1	t(7;10)(q32;q11.2)	rare	yes
RET/PTC7	RFG7	t(1;10)(p13;q11.2)	rare	yes
RET/ELKS	ELKS	t(10;12)(q11.2;p13)	rare	no
RET/KTN1	KTN1	t(10;14)(q11.2;q22.1)	rare	yes
RET/RFG8	RFG8	t(10;18)(q11.2;q21-22)	rare	yes
RET/PCM-1	PCM-1	t(8;10)(p21-22;q11.2)	rare	yes

β-Catenin

Frequent somatic mutations of the *CTNNB1* gene encoding β-catenin {2430}, and the rare case of somatic APC mutation {285A} have been observed in the FAP associated cribriform variant, but not in conventional papillary carcinoma.

Genetic susceptibility

The genetic significance of the diagnosis of papillary thyroid carcinoma (PTC) includes association with familial adenomatous polyposis coli (FAP), Cowden syndrome, and the syndromes referred to as familial site-specific papillary thy- roid carcinoma, and perhaps Carney complex. The great majority of epithelial thyroid carcinomas seen in Cowden syndrome, however, are follicular thyroid carcinomas. Occasionally, PTCs are seen in this syndrome, but are typically the follicular variant. For patient care, and hence purposes of differential diagnosis, it is important to separate the morphology of tumours associated with FAP from conventional papillary carcinoma. For details see Chapter 5.

Prognosis and predictive factors

Papillary carcinoma prognosis is excellent; 10-year survival is over 90% and for young patients is over 98%. The relative proportion of papillary and follicular areas does not correlate with prognosis, but vascular invasion and nuclear atypia may be adverse prognostic signs {1316}. Principal clinical features correlating with prognosis depend on risk group definition, which is defined primarily by age, but also by size, extrathyroidal extension, completeness of surgery, and distant metastases (see introduction). The adverse prognostic effects of older age are accentuated by frequent larger tumour size and extraglandular extension of the tumours. The tall cell and columnar cell variants have a less favourable prognosis than conventional papillary carcinomas.

Follicular carcinoma

M. Sobrinho Simões
S.L. Asa
T.G. Kroll
Y. Nikiforov
R. DeLellis
P. Farid
Y. Kitamura

S.U. Noguchi
C. Eng
H.R. Harach
E.D. Williams
A.B. Schneider
J.A. Fagin
R.A. Ghossein

E.L. Mazzaferri
R.V. Lloyd
V. LiVolsi
J.K.C. Chan
Z. Baloch
O.H. Clark

Definition

A malignant epithelial tumour showing evidence of follicular cell differentiation and lacking the diagnostic nuclear features of papillary carcinoma.

ICD-O code   8330/3

Synonyms

Follicular adenocarcinoma; oncocytic carcinoma; Hurthle cell carcinoma.

Epidemiology

Follicular carcinoma accounts for 10-15% of clinically evident thyroid malignancies. It is more common in women, and tends to occur in patients in the fifth decade. The peak incidence of oncocytic follicular carcinomas is approximately 10 years later than follicular carcinomas of conventional type. At variance with papillary carcinoma, follicular carcinoma rarely occurs in children. A single case of a follicular carcinoma in a newborn has been reported to date {1474}. The incidence of follicular carcinoma is higher in iodine-deficient areas. Dietary iodine supplementation has been associated with an increase in the relative frequency of papillary carcinoma and a decrease in the relative frequency of follicular carcinoma. The frequency of follicular carcinoma has also decreased recently, due to the exclusion from this category of the follicular variant of papillary carcinoma.

Etiology

Both iodine deficiency and irradiation

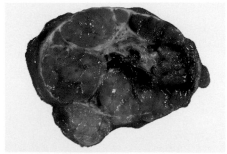

Fig. 2.023 Follicular carcinoma, widely invasive type. The entire lobe is replaced with tumour.

have been implicated in the development of follicular carcinoma, as discussed in the introduction.

Localization

Follicular carcinoma can arise in the normally situated thyroid gland and in ectopic thyroid tissue (e.g. struma ovarii).

Clinical features

Follicular carcinomas most commonly present as asymptomatic intrathyroidal mass lesions, and are often larger than papillary carcinomas at presentation. The frequency of ipsilateral lymphadenopathy is considerably less than that observed in patients with papillary carcinoma and has been reported to be less than 5% in most series. Similar to papillary carcinomas, follicular carcinomas are typically cold on scintigraphic scan. Hoarseness, dysphagia and dyspnea are rare at presentation and may occur in those patients with widely invasive follicular carcinomas. Distant metastases have been reported in up to 20% of patients at presentation with the most common sites of involvement being lungs and bone.

Oncocytic follicular carcinomas have a similar clinical presentation. A somewhat higher proportion of patients with these tumours have ipsilateral nodal involvement. In addition, oncocytic follicular carcinomas have a greater propensity to recur in the neck and are more likely to cause death by local invasion than follicular carcinomas of conventional type. In the series from Memorial Sloan Kettering, there were no significant differences in the frequency of distant metastases in patients with follicular carcinomas of conventional and oncocytic types. However, the cumulative incidence of metastases was somewhat higher in oncocytic (33%) than in non-oncocytic (22%) follicular carcinomas.

Macroscopy

Follicular carcinomas are usually encapsulated round to ovoid solid tumours generally measuring more than 1 cm in

diameter. On cross section, they have bulging surfaces and vary in color from gray-tan to brown. Minimally invasive tumours are indistinguishable grossly from follicular adenomas except for the fact that follicular carcinomas tend to have thicker and more irregular capsules. Widely invasive follicular carcinomas may demonstrate extensive permeation of the capsule. In some instances, however, widely invasive tumours may lack any evidence of encapsulation. Rarely, widespread vascular invasion may lead to permeation of thyroid veins and even the superior vena cava.

Tumour spread and staging

Multifocality is uncommon, as is recurrence in the residual thyroid after partial thyroidectomy. Regional lymph node metastases from follicular carcinomas are uncommon. The most common sites

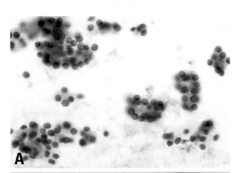

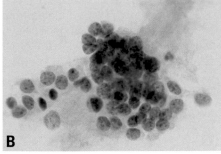

Fig. 2.024 FNA of follicular carcinoma. **A** Groups of follicular cells arranged in a microfollicular pattern. Malignancy was established by demonstrating capsular and vascular invasion in the resected thyroid gland. **B** Moderately pleomorphic tumour cells. Aspirate prepared from a recurrent mass that developed after a thyroidectomy for follicular carcinoma.

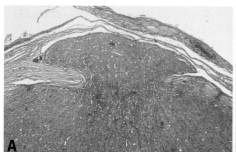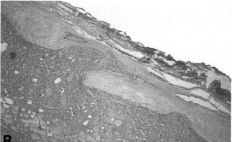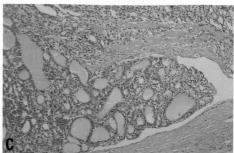

Fig. 2.025 Follicular carcinoma, minimally invasive type. **A** Tumour demonstrates complete penetration of the capsule and has a mushroom-like configuration. **B** This tumour demonstrates both minimal capsular and vascular invasion. **C** Focal invasion of a capsular vessel.

of distant metastases are lung and bone. Staging of follicular caracinomas is discussed in the introduction.

Cytopathology

Aspirates from follicular carcinomas are generally hypercellular with a dispersed microfollicular arrangement of tumour cells and scant colloid. Microfollicles consist of groups of follicular cells with 6 to 12 nuclei forming a small ring-like structure. The presence of nuclear atypia does not correlate with malignancy since some follicular carcinomas may have bland cytological characteristics while some adenomas may demonstrate considerable nuclear atypia. The diagnosis of malignancy depends on the demonstration of capsular or vascular invasion which is demonstrable only in histological preparations.

Histopathology

Follicular carcinomas are invasive neoplasms of follicular cells that lack the typical nuclear features of PTC. The diagnosis and classification of these neoplasms is one of the most contentious issues in thyroid pathology. Follicular carcinomas show variable morphology ranging from well formed colloid-containing follicles to solid or trabecular growth patterns.

Poorly formed follicles or atypical patterns (eg cribriform) may occur and coexistence of multiple architectural types is common. However, neither architectural nor cytological atypical features, by themselves, are reliable criteria of malignancy since these changes may be present in benign lesions, including nodular (adenomatous) goiters and adenomas.

Invasiveness

Classically, follicular carcinomas have been divided according to their degree of invasiveness into two major categories. Minimally invasive follicular carcinomas have limited capsular and/or vascular invasion. Widely invasive follicular carcinomas have widespread infiltration of adjacent thyroid tissue and/or blood vessels.

Capsular invasion is defined by tumour penetration through the tumour capsule unassociated with the site of a previous fine needle aspiration biopsy.

Vascular invasion is defined by the presence of intravascular tumour cells either covered by endothelium or associated with thrombus. In order to qualify as vascular invasion, involved vessels must be within or beyond the tumour capsule. Foci of vascular invasion should be distinguished from subendothelial collec-

tions of tumour cells, retraction artifacts surrounding entrapped groups of tumour cells within the capsule, artifactual dislodgement of tumour cells that may be present within vascular spaces and foci of intravascular endothelial proliferation. Artifactually dislodged tumour cells within vessels often have an irregular configuration and are not attached to the vessel walls while the spaces around areas of retraction are not covered by endothelial cells. The cells in foci of intravascular endothelial proliferation typically have a spindled appearance and are positive for vascular markers, including CD31 and CD34.

The probability of aggressive behaviour increases with the extent of vascular invasion. Tumours that show only minimal capsular invasion carry minimal risk of recurrence or metastases while the risk of recurrence of metastases in tumours with minimal vascular invasion is low. The risk of metastatic disease in those tumours with widespread vascular invasion, on the other hand, is substantial.

Terminology

In most classifications, the term *minimally invasive follicular carcinoma* is used for tumours that demonstrate focal capsular and/or vascular invasion. In some

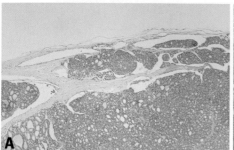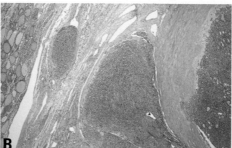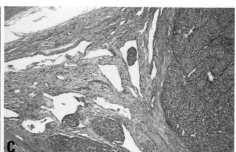

Fig. 2.026 Follicular carcinoma, widely invasive type. **A** There are multifocal areas of invasion of capsular vessels. **B** The tumour has extended beyond the capsule and is present within a vascular space. **C** Multiple foci of vascular invasion are present.

schemes, however, thus term has been assigned to tumours that show only capsular invasion. The term "grossly encapsulated angioinvasive follicular carcinoma" has been suggested for those tumours that demonstrate vascular invasion. {1070,1318}

Immunohistochemistry
The tumours show thyroglobulin, TTF1 and low molecular weight cytokeratin immunoreactivity. In some follicular carcinomas, as in rare follicular adenomas and nodular goiters, there is focal immunoreactivity for cytokeratin 19 and for some native and sialylated Lewis blood antigens in contrast to the widespread immunostaining observed in papillary carcinomas {45,46,640,641}. Galectin-3, HBME-1, CD15 and CD44v6 have also been reported in these tumours {126,1495}.
Follicular carcinomas usually display membranous immunoreactivity for E-cadherin and beta-catenin, as do normal thyroid, benign follicular lesions and the follicular variant of papillary carcinoma {1846,1848,2075}. There is a subgroup of widely invasive follicular carcinomas that demonstrates E-cadherin downregulation {1050}.
In general, follicular carcinomas have a Bcl-2 positive, TP53 negative phenotype and display low levels of cyclin D1, high levels of p27 and low proliferation rates {511,576,2184}. Most follicular carcinomas, like most follicular adenomas and papillary carcinomas, are telomerase negative; the percentage of follicular carcinomas exhibiting telomerase expression is nevertheless higher than that of follicular adenomas or papillary carcinomas {1441}.

Histopathological variants
Oncocytic variant
Oncocytic follicular carcinomas are malignant neoplasms of follicular cell origin composed exclusively or predominantly (greater than 75%) of oncocytic cells. Although these tumours have been categorized as a separate entity in other classifications, they are included as a variant of follicular carcinoma in this classification. Other terms for these tumours include oxyphil and Hurthle cell carcinoma. The oncocytic variant of follicular carcinoma represents 3-4% of thyroid malignancies {472,939,940}. The median age at diagnosis is 61 years and the

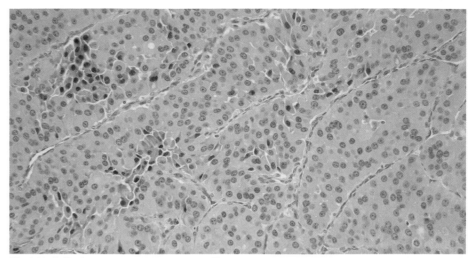

Fig. 2.027 Follicular carcinoma, oncocytic type. This tumour demonstrates a trabecular growth pattern.

female to male ratio is 6.5:3.5 {939}. There is no evidence at present to suggest that the etiology of the oncocytic follicular carcinomas differs from that of follicular carcinomas of conventional type although some studies have suggested a primary role of mitochondrial abnormalities in the genesis of these tumours {1447,2477}.
Patients with oncocytic follicular carcinomas most commonly present with a painless thyroid nodule. The carcinomas tend to be larger than adenomas of the oncocytic type and they tend to occur in older patients. In contrast to follicular carcinomas of conventional type which typically present as unifocal masses with nodal metastases in less than 5% of cases, the oncocytic variants are associated with nodal metastases in approximately 30% of cases. Occasional patients may present with distant metastases involving lung and bone.
Oncocytic follicular carcinomas are char-

acterized by a distinct mahogany brown appearance. They have a tendency to undergo infarction usually after fine needle aspiration biopsy. Associated changes include haemorrhage, cyst formation or areas of scarring; however, similar changes may also occur spontaneously. Minimally invasive tumours are indistinguishable grossly, except for their mahogany brown color, from minimally invasive follicular carcinomas of conventional type. Widely invasive tumours have irregular boarders and may form distinct satellite nodules that result in a multinodular appearance.
Oncocytic follicular carcinomas have a variety of architectural patterns ranging from well formed follicles to solid and/or trabecular growth patterns {1315}. The solid and trabecular forms of these tumours tend to have scant or absent colloid. The nuclei tend to be hyperchromatic and pleomorphic and generally have prominent eosinophilic nucleoli

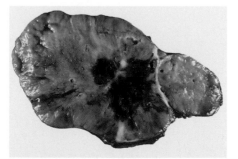

Fig. 2.028 Follicular carcinoma, oncocytic type. Note the mahagony brown appearance with central haemorrhages and focal scarring. The capsule is largely preserved. On the right a satellite nodule.

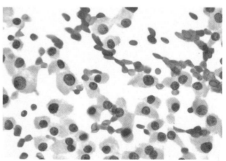

Fig. 2.029 FNA of oncocytic carcinoma. Loosely cohesive cells with round nuclei and moderate amounts of cytoplasm. Malignancy indicated by capsular and vascular invasion.

{1315}. When colloid is present, there is a tendency for it to be basophilic with frequent concentric rims of calcification, resembling psammoma bodies. The cytoplasm of the tumour cells is deeply eosinophilic and granular. Clear cell change may be prominent in some tumours. The diagnosis of oncocytic follicular carcinoma depends on the demonstration of capsular and/or vascular invasion. The tumours are classified into minimally and widely invasive types, as described for follicular carcinomas of conventional type.

Oncocytic follicular carcinomas are typically positive for thyroglobulin and TTF-1 and usually exhibit a cytokeratin 7 positive and cytokeratin 20 negative phenotype {155,1646}. Ultrastructurally, the cells are filled with mitochondria with an increase in the number, size and pleomorphism of intramitochondrial dense bodies. Swelling of the mitochondria may lead to a disappearance of the cristae.

FNAB. Aspirates from oncocytic follicular carcinomas are generally impossible to distinguish from oncocytic adenomas. Aspirates are usually hypercellular and consist of oncocytes with absent or scanty colloid. In contrast to cases of Hashimoto's thyroiditis, oncocytic carcinomas lack an associated lymphoplasmacytic infiltrate. Renshaw has suggested that an oncocytic lesion should be considered particularly suspicious for malignancy in the presence of: (1) small cell dysplasia; (2) large cell dysplasia; (3) crowding with the formation of syncytia; (4) dyshesion {1812,1813}. Additional studies will be required to assess the value of these parameters in the diagnosis of oncocytic lesions.

Clear cell variant

Follicular carcinomas may be composed predominantly of clear cells that contain glycogen, mucin, lipid or dilated mitochondria. It should be noted that clear cell change may be particularly prominent in oncocytic neoplasms. Signet-ring follicular cells can also be a minor or a major component of follicular carcinomas.

Differential diagnosis

Minimally invasive follicular carcinomas may be difficult to distinguish from follicular adenomas and nodular (adenomatous) goiters due to the limited evidence of unequivocal invasion. The possibility of designating tumours where it is not possible to be certain about the presence or absence of invasion as 'follicular tumours of uncertain malignant potential' has been suggested {2391}. If used at all, this term should be restricted to adequately sampled tumours with real uncertainty about whether the criteria for invasion have been fulfilled. It should not be used as an excuse for inadequate study of the lesion.

Various cell cycle related proteins have been used to distinguish oncocytic follicular adenomas and carcinomas {373, 412,572,912}. Only Ki-67 has been shown to be a robust marker that correlates with the diagnosis of carcinoma, particularly the widely invasive type {572,912}. However, Ki-67 positivity is not an independent prognostic factor because of its strong correlation with the presence of extrathyroidal extension and vascular/lymphatic invasion {912}.

Follicular carcinoma can be difficult to

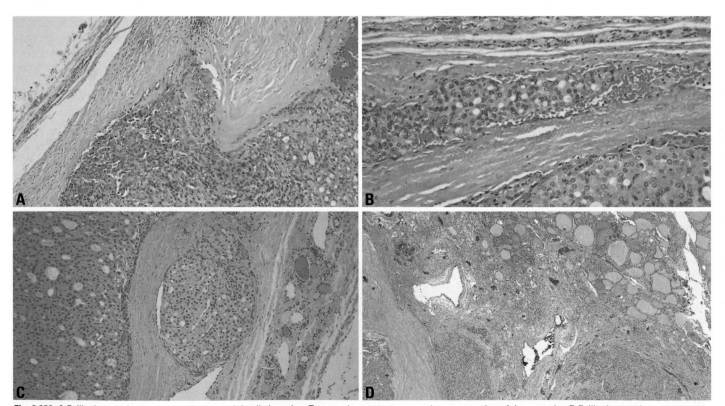

Fig. 2.030 A Follicular carcinoma, oncocytic type, minimally invasive. Tumour demonstrates complete penetration of the capsule. **B** Follicular carcinoma, oncocytic type, minimally invasive. There is a focus of vascular invasion within the capsule. **C** Follicular carcinoma, oncocytic type, minimally invasive. This tumour shows a single focus of vascular invasion within the capsule. **D** Follicular carcinoma, oncocytic type, widely invasive. The adjacent thyroid parenchyma is extensively invaded by tumour.

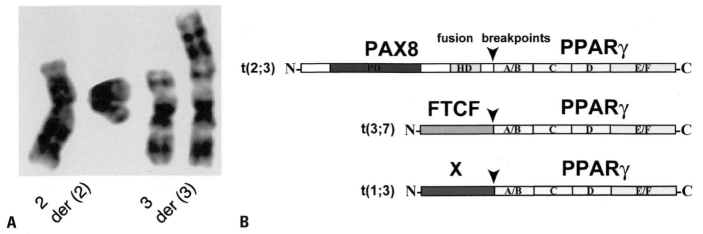

Fig. 2.031 Follicular carcinoma. **A** t (2;3) (q13; p25) rearrangement harboring the *PAX8-PPARγ* gene fusion in a follicular carcinoma (der, derivate chromosome). **B** Schematic representation of distinct PPARγ fusion proteins produced by different *PPARγ* rearrangements.

distinguish from the follicular variant of papillary carcinoma. In a small number of apparent follicular tumours with definite capsular or vascular invasion a minority of nuclei may show changes suggestive of a papillary carcinoma. In this situation a diagnosis of 'well differentiated carcinoma not otherwise specified' may be appropriate {2391}. The distinction is clinically immaterial since the treatment is similar and depends upon the extent of invasion.

Widely invasive follicular carcinomas are occasionally difficult to separate from poorly differentiated carcinomas {2083}. The features of the latter tumours are discussed in a subsequent section.

Oncocytic follicular carcinomas can be confused with oncocytic medullary carcinomas. The latter lesions usually have a nesting or insular architecture and the cells are polygonal rather than having the spindle-shaped morphology of the classical medullary carcinoma. The nuclei of medullary carcinomas resemble neuroendocrine nuclei (round to oval with

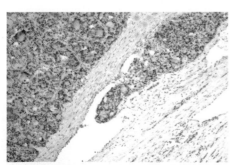

Fig. 2.032 Follicular carcinoma. Nuclear overexpression of PPARγ, detected by immunohistochemistry in a follicular carcinoma.

salt and pepper chromatin). The diagnosis of medullary carcinoma is confirmed by identifying chromogranin, calcitonin and CEA immunoreactivity and by demonstrating a lack of thyroglobulin staining in tumour cells {361}.

Immunostains may be required to rule out non-thyroid oncocytic tumours, such as oncocytic parathyroid neoplasms. In contrast to parathyroid tumours, oncocytic follicular carcinomas are typically positive for thyroglobulin and TTF-1. Parathyroid tumours, on the other hand, are typically positive for parathyroid hormone and chromogranin while oncocytic follicular carcinomas are negative for these markers.

Clear cell follicular carcinomas must be distinguished from clear cell adenoma, parathyroid adenoma or carcinoma and metastatic clear cell carcinomas, particularly of renal origin.

Precursor lesions
No definite precursor lesions are known. Follicular carcinomas may arise from follicular adenomas.

Histogenesis
The cell of origin is the follicular epithelial cell.

Somatic genetics
Chromosomal imbalance
Allelic imbalance, comparative genomic hybridization, and cytogenetic studies have suggested involvement of chromosomes 2 {2273}, 3p {764,874,1098,1859, 2001,2273,2353}, 6 {1860,2215}, 7q {1098,1860,1861,2215,2268,2487}, 8 {1860,1861}, 9 {2001,2215}, 10q {2453,

2484}, 11 {1098,1440}, 13q {1098,2001}, 17p {764} and 22 {662,861,1098} in follicular carcinomas. These studies have included both conventional and oncocytic follicular carcinomas.

Oncocytic neoplasms show frequent chromosomal DNA imbalance, with numerical chromosomal alterations being the dominant feature {2185}. Somatic mutations and sequence variants of mitochondrial DNA (mtDNA) have been identified in oncocytic thyroid carcinomas {1447,2452}. Similar changes have been found in the non-tumourous thyroid tissue of patients with oncocytic neoplasms {1447}, suggesting that certain polymorphisms predispose to this cytologic alteration.

PPARγ rearrangemets
Rearrangements of the peroxisome proliferator-activated receptor gamma (*PPARγ*) gene are found in 25-50% of follicular carcinomas {534,655,1171, 1411,1604}. *PPARγ* rearrangements produce various PPARγ fusion proteins {999,1171,1364,1366}, the most common of which (PAX8-PPARγ) can deregulate ligand-inducible transcription by PPARγ {1171}, inhibit apoptosis, and promote proliferation and anchorage-independent growth of thyroid follicular cells {1415,1767}. *PPARγ* rearrangements have been found most consistently in low stage follicular carcinomas with vascular invasion {655,1606} and in some locally aggressive and metastatic follicular carcinomas {534,1859}. *PPARγ* gene rearrangements have been identified at apparent lower frequency in adenomas {655,1171,1411,1604,1606,1767}.

Point mutations

Mutations of the *RAS* genes {1274,1275, 1398,1578,1606,2038,2157} are found in 20-50% of follicular carcinomas.

Activating mutations in codon 61 of the *N*- and *H-RAS* genes are the most common. *RAS* mutation and *PPARγ* rearrangement appear to define independent pathways in follicular carcinogenesis {1606}.

Mutation and down-regulation of the *TP53* {511,601,976}, *PTEN* {447,661,720, 802}, tumour suppressor genes and of β-catenin {689,690} gene may facilitate progression from well-differentiated to poorly differentiated follicular carcinoma in some cases.

Genetic susceptibility

The genetic differential diagnosis of follicular thyroid carcinoma includes Cowden syndrome, and perhaps Werner syndrome and Carney complex. For details of the hereditary aspects of thyroid carcinomas, please refer to the chapters dedicated to the hereditary endocrine cancers, chapter 5 (Inherited Tumour Syndromes).

Prognosis and predictive factors

Although there are numerous data on the risk group assessment of differentiated thyroid carcinomas, there are relatively few studies that specifically focus on the prognosis of follicular carciomas {762,1793}. In general, minimally invasive follicular carcinomas have a very low long term mortality in the range of 3 to 5% with survival curves approaching those of a normal population matched for age and sex. Widely invasive carcinomas, on the other hand, have a long term mortality of approximately 50% and the probability of metastatic disease is considerably higher than that seen in association with minimally invasive tumours. These generalizations apply both to conventional follicular carcinomas and follicular carcinomas of oncocytic type.

Table 2.03
Risk group analisis for follicular carcinomas. From Shah et al. {1793}

Factor	Low	Intermediate	Intermediate	High
Age (yr)	<45	>45	≥45	≥45
T	T1/T2	T3/T4 and/or	T1/T2	T3/T4 and/or T1/T2
M	M0	M1 and/or	M0	M1 and/or M0
Type	Non-oncocytic	Oncocytic and/or	Non-oncocytic	Oncocytic and/or non-oncocytic
Grade	Low	High	Low	High

The results of earlier studies had suggested that all oncocytic tumours were potentially malignant {2234}; however, more recent studies have shown that histologic features, similar to those used for conventional follicular carcinomas, can be used to predict biological behavior {297,301,572}. Interestingly, cases showing some but not all of the features of malignancy such as questionable capsular and vascular invasion, ("indeterminant" malignant potential) have behaved in a clinically benign fashion {301,572}.

Generally, oncocytic carcinomas behave more aggressively than follicular carcinomas of conventional type, with higher frequencies of extrathyroidal invasion, local recurrence and nodal metastases. However, this view is not universally accepted. For example, Evans and Vassilopoulou-Sellin {590} have demonstrated that when cases of conventional follicular carcinoma and oncocytic follicular carcinoma are stratified according to the extent of invasion, there are no statistically significant differences in the rates of local recurence, frequency of nodal or distant metastases or patient survivals {590}.

In a series of more than 200 patients with follicular carcinomas of both conventional and oncocytic types, 10 year survivals for low, intermediate and high risk groups were 98%, 88% and 56%, respectively {1793,2014}. Twenty-year survivals for the same group were 97%, 87% and 49%. Risk group analysis in this series was based on age, tumour size, local extension, histological findings (presence or absence of oncocytic change and grade) and presence or absence of distant metastases. Adverse prognostic factors included age greater than 45 years (p <0.001), oncocytic tumour type (p= 0.05), extrathyroidal extension, tumour size in excess of 4 cm, and the presence of distant metastases (p <0.01). Gender, multifocality and lymph node metastases, on the other hand, had no significant impact on prognosis.

Risk group analysis

Although flow cytometric anaysis of DNA content and nuclear DNA ploidy are not useful in the distinction of benign and malignant oncocytic tumours, this type of analysis is useful in the prognostic assessment of oncocytic carcinomas {247,1469}. Fluorescence in situ hybridization studies have suggested that loss of chromosome 22 may have prognostic value in oncocytic carcinomas {571}.

Poorly differentiated carcinoma

M. Sobrinho Simões
J. Albores-Saavedra
G. Tallini
M. Santoro
M. Volante
S. Pilotti

M.L. Carcangiu
M. Papotti
X. Matias-Guiu
G.E. Guiter
M. Zakowski
A. Sakamoto

Definition

Follicular-cell neoplasms that show limited evidence of structural follicular cell differentiation and occupy both morphologically and behaviourally an intermediate position between differentiated (follicular and papillary carcinomas) and undifferentiated (anaplastic) carcinomas.

Synonyms

Poorly differentiated follicular carcinoma; solid type of follicular carcinoma {651, 2083}; poorly differentiated papillary carcinoma; grade III papillary carcinoma {2083,2271,2419}; trabecular carcinoma {273,1362}; "insular carcinoma" {304}; poorly differentiated carcinoma with a primiordial cell component {1682}.

Epidemiology

Poorly differentiated carcinoma remains a controversial entity. It is therefore difficult to evaluate whether the different prevalence rates among different geographic regions reflect true etiological differences or mere variations in diagnostic criteria. For example, this etitity accounts for 4-7% of all the clinically evident thyroid carcinomas in Italy and in some Latin American countries {304, 2080} compared to much lower rates in United States. The disease is more common in women and in patients older than 50 {304,2083}.

Etiology

The etiology is unknown. While some of these tumours appear to arise from pre-existing papillary and follicular thyroid carcinomas, others most likely arise de novo {1744}.

Clinical features

Most poorly differentiated carcinomas appear as solitary large thyroid masses, cold by scintigraphy, with or without concurrent enlarged regional lymph nodes. Frequently, there is a history of recent growth in a long-standing uninodular or multinodular thyroid. Conversely, poorly differentiated carcinomas may occasionally present as rapidly growing masses. In addition to nodal metastases, lung and bone metastases are also relatively frequent at the time of diagnosis.

Macroscopy

Most of the tumours are over 3 cm in diameter at the time of diagnosis and are solid and gray-white with frequent foci of necrosis. Most tumours have pushing borders and, rarely, a thick capsule. In many cases there is also invasive, peritumoural growth that occasionally leads to satellite nodules within the thyroid parenchyma. Extrathyroidal extension is less commonly present than in undifferentiated carcinomas.

Tumour spread and staging

In addition to direct local invasion, poorly differentiated carcinomas most commonly spread to regional lymph nodes and have a propensity to metastasise to liver and bone. Staging is discussed in the introduction.

Cytopathology

The cytologic features of poorly differentiated carcinoma include high cellularity with numerous dyscohesive, small to intermediate sized cells, some microfollicles and scant colloid. The nuclei are deceptively bland with fine chromatin and small nucleoli. In general atypia is mild, nuclear pleomorphism being unusual. Necrosis and mitoses are relatively common. A definitive diagnosis of poorly differentiated carcinoma, howev-

er, can be made only at the histological level {787,1594,1739}.

Histopathology

The histopathologic appearance of poorly differentiated thyroid carcinoma is variable {273,304,1324,1362,1682,1901}. Three different histologic patterns are recognized: insular, trabecular and solid {1682,2081}. The diagnosis relies on the identification of these patterns in the majority of the tumour together with an infiltrative pattern of growth, necrosis, and obvious vascular invasion. Discrepancies do exist with regard to the significance of a minor poorly-differentiated component in an otherwise well differentiated carcinoma {94,1612,1942}, but one study has shown that the presence of more than 10% of such patterns is associated with extrathyroidal invasion, lymph node and distant metastases at diagnosis {1612}. Some tumours display clear and/or oncocytic cells {1686,2007}. Rarely these tumours may contain cells with rhabdoid features {31}.

The insular pattern is characterized by well-defined nests of tumour cells surrounded by thin fibrovascular septa, which are frequently separated from tumour cells by artefactual clefts {304}. The nests are predominantly solid, but may contain small follicles. Tumour cells are generally small and uniform and contain round hyperchromatic or vesicular nuclei with indistinct nucleoli. Mitotic figures are common. Occasionally, a

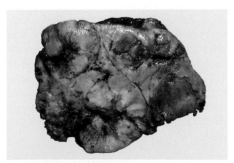

Fig. 2.033 Poorly differentiated thyroid carcinoma. This tumour has replaced the entire lobe.

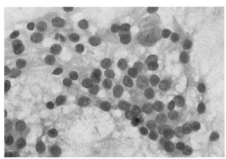

Fig. 2.034 FNA of insular carcinoma. The cells are loosely cohesive with round densely staining nuclei.

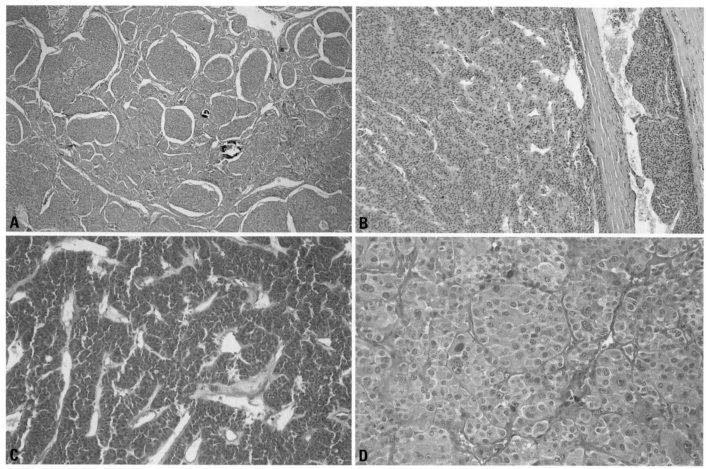

Fig. 2.035 Poorly differentiated carcinoma. **A** This tumour demonstrates a prominent insular growth pattern. **B** This tumour has a trabecular architecture and is associated with vascular invasion. **C** The tumour has a trabecular arrangement. **D** Insular growth pattern.

peritheliomatous growth pattern is seen coexisting with necrosis and/or fibrosis. The trabecular pattern is characterized by cells arranged in cords or ribbons, while the solid pattern exhibits large sheets of tumour cells that occasionally may show small abortive follicles or some colloid droplets. In most cases of poorly differentiated carcinoma, regardless of the predominant pattern of growth, there are nuclei that superficially resemble those of papillary carcinoma {2083}.

Poorly differentiated carcinomas may contain a minor component showing features of papillary or follicular carcinoma {304,2082}. Other cases may show focal nuclear pleomorphism, resembling an undifferentiated carcinoma although the significance of this finding is uncertain. Examples showing transition from a poorly differentiated component to areas of undifferentiated carcinoma have been described {1435}. The presence of the undifferentiated component should be reported because some of these tumours

have behaved as undifferentiated carcinomas.

Immunohistochemistry
Poorly differentiated carcinomas typically show immunoreactivity for thyroglobulin and TTF1, although the thyroglobulin positivity may be restricted to isolated tumour cells or poorly developed follicles {304,1651,1652,1682,1739}. Focal TP53 nuclear positivity {503,1743} and increased Ki-67 (MIB-1) index {2184} are also common features. Most poorly differentiated carcinomas show absence of E-cadherin membranous expression in contrast to normal thyroid and well-differentiated thyroid carcinomas {1846}. Immunohistochemistry with markers relevant for the analysis of thyroid follicular cell replication and death demonstrates that the proliferation, survival and cell cycle regulation patterns observed in poorly differentiated thyroid carcinomas have features which are intermediate between those of well- and undifferentiat-

ed tumours {503,576, 1399,1743,2184}.

Differential diagnosis
This includes medullary carcinoma, follicular carcinoma, and the solid variant of papillary carcinoma. Metastatic tumours to the thyroid, especially carcinoids, may also enter into the differential diagnosis {1432}. Demonstration of positive immunostaining for thyroglobulin is useful in the distinction of these tumours from medullary and metastatic carcinomas. Rarely, poorly differentiated carcinomas may coexpress calcitonin and other neuro-endocrine markers in scattered cells {279,673,1324,2081,2083}. Thyroid papillary carcinoma with solid areas usually occurs in young patients and exhibits typical nuclear features with ground-glass appearance and grooves {978}.

Precursor lesions and Histogenesis
Poorly differentiated carcinomas can occur either de novo or from preexisting

well-differentiated carcinomas, which are regarded as precursor lesions {304}. The ultrastructural, lectin histochemical and morphometric study of poorly differentiated carcinomas has shown their closer relationship to follicular than to papillary carcinoma {2083}. This does not challenge, however, the fact that some poorly differentiated carcinomas derive from preexisting papillary carcinomas {304, 2082}.

Somatic genetics
Complex clonal alterations are common in the few cases of poorly differentiated thyroid carcinomas that have been analyzed by conventional cytogenetics {874}. The proportion of unbalanced DNA profiles detected by CGH in poorly differentiated thyroid cancer is 80%, similar to that detected in undifferentiated thyroid cancer, with a median number of chromosomal gains or losses (5.5 per case) which is midway between that observed in well differentiated (1 per case) and undifferentiated (10 per case) tumours {2422}. Specific types of chromosomal alterations such as +1p34-36, +17q25, +20q, -1p11-31, -6q21, -13q21-31 are associated with the transition from well differentiated carcinoma to poorly differentiated carcinomas {2422}. These alterations are common to both poorly differentiated and undifferentiated carcinomas while additional specific changes are observed in undifferentiated thyroid cancer {2422}.

Molecular genetic alterations
Poorly differentiated thyroid carcinomas have a frequency of genetic alterations

Table 2.04

Expression profile of common immunohistochemical markers relevant for thyroid follicular cell proliferation (Ki-67/MIB1), survival (BCL2) and regulation of the cell cycle (CYCLIN D1 and P27)

	Ki-67/MIB1	BCL2	CYCLIN D1	P27
Normal thyroid follicular cells	Very low (positive cells <5%)	Positive	Negative	Positive
Well differentiated thyroid carcinoma	Low (often <10% positive cells)	Positive	Low	High*
Poorly differentiated thyroid carcinoma	Intermediate (usually 10-30% positive cells)	Usually positive	Intermediate	Intermediate
Undifferentiated (anaplastic) thyroid carcinoma	High (often >30% positive cells)	Negative	High	Low

*Some groups found low levels of expression in papillary carcinoma.

intermediate between well-differentiated and undifferentiated carcinomas. Analysis of TP53 exons 5-9 shows mutations in 20-30% of poorly differentiated carcinomas and there is a broad correlation between mutations and TP53 immunohistochemical reactivity {504, 511}. Aberrant TP53 immunoreactivity is detectable in 40-50% of poorly differentiated carcinomas, a prevalence that is not very different from that observed in undifferentiated carcinomas (50-80%) {503, 1743,2076}. H-, K- or N-RAS mutations occur in approximately 50% of poorly differentiated thyroid carcinomas {129,691, 1398,1544,1744}. Although RAS mutations are also present in well differentiated carcinomas, multiple activating mutations are restricted to poorly and undifferentiated tumours with undifferentiated carcinomas showing the highest degree

of RAS mutation heterogeneity {691}. WNT activation, as indicated by stabilizing mutations and/or aberrant nuclear localization of β-catenin, has recently been identified in poorly differentiated thyroid carcinomas {689,1846}. A small number of poorly differentiated thyroid carcinomas express rearranged tyrosine kinase genes such as RET/PTC or NTRK1 {224,1937}; however, there is no evidence that these tumours are associated with unfavourable clinicopathologic features or decreased survival {224, 1937}.

Prognosis and predictive factors
The mean five-year survival rate is about 50% in most series {304,1612,1682, 2080,2083}. The majority of patients die in the first three years after diagnosis and few patients survive >5 years. Death is

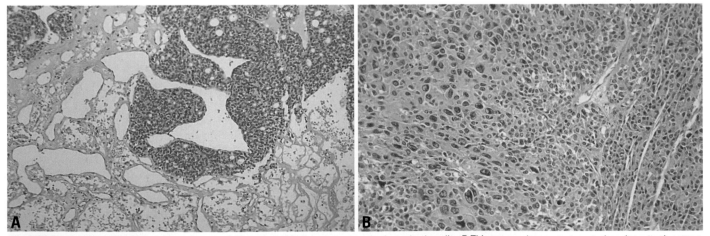

Fig. 2.036 Poorly differentiated thyroid carcinoma. **A** There is peritheliomatous growth of neoplastic cells. **B** This tumour demonstrates a trabecular growth pattern (right) with areas of transformation to undifferentiated carcinoma (left).

usually caused by regional and distant metastases rather than by local invasion. The prognosis of patients with poorly differentiated carcinoma depends primarily on the TNM staging, completeness of surgery and responsiveness to radioactive iodine therapy. The prognostic significance of the prominence of necrotic foci, histologic pattern (insular, solid or trabecular), extent of vascular invasion and degree of aneuploidy remains controversial {1612,1682,1901,2083}. There is no sufficient evidence that any molecular genetic alteration plays a significant role in prognosis.

Table 2.05
Molecular alterations relevant for thyroid tumour progression in poorly differentiated thyroid tumours compared with well- and undifferentiated (anaplastic) thyroid cancers.

	TP53 [a]	H-, K-, N- RAS [a]	WNT / β-catenin [b]
Well differentiated thyroid carcinoma	Absent	10-20%	Absent
Poorly differentiated thyroid carcinoma	20-30%	50%	0-30%
Undifferentiated (anaplastic) thyroid carcinoma	70-80%	50%	80%

a) Mutations detected by PCR/SSCP and sequencing.
b) CTNNB1 exon 3 mutations which prevent β-catenin degradation detected by PCR/SSCP and sequencing, and/or aberrant nuclear localization of β-catenin.

Undifferentiated (anaplastic) carcinoma

N. Ordonez
Z. Baloch
X. Matias-Guiu
H. Evans
N.R. Farid
J.A. Fagin
Y. Kitamura

G. Tallini
C. Eng
P.I. Haigh
W.C. Faquin
I. Sugitani
D. Giuffrida
S. Boerner

Definition
Undifferentiated thyroid carcinomas (UTC) are highly malignant tumours that histologically appear wholly or partially composed of undifferentiated cells that exhibit immunohistochemical or ultrastructural features indicative of epithelial differentiation.

ICD-O code   8020/3

Synonyms
Spindle and giant cell carcinoma, sarcomatoid carcinoma, pleomorphic carcinoma, dedifferentiated carcinoma, metaplastic carcinoma, carcinosarcoma.

Epidemiology
UTC occurs mainly in the elderly. Only 25% of patients are younger than 60 years at diagnosis. The sex distribution shows that females are affected more frequently than males, with a female-to-male ratio of 1.5:1.
The incidence of UTC is approximately one or two cases/million annually, but this varies geographically, with a higher incidence in Europe than in the USA. A higher incidence has also been reported in endemic goiter regions. Although UTC accounts for less than 5% of clinically recognized malignant thyroid neoplasms, more than half of the 1200 deaths attributable to thyroid cancer annually in the USA result from UTC. Mortality rate is over 90%, with a mean survival of 6 months after diagnosis {725, 1040}.

Etiology
Most cases of UTC show evidence of a pre-existing differentiated or poorly differentiated thyroid carcinoma.

Clinical features
Almost all patients with UTC present with a rapidly expanding neck mass. The most frequent and important signs and symptoms are hoarseness (80%), followed by dysphagia (60%), vocal cord paralysis (50%), cervical pain (30%) and dyspnea (20%). The tumours may be fixed and hard (75%), and may present as a single (60%) or multiple nodules (40%) with bilateral involvement in 25% of cases. Surrounding structures are frequently invaded: muscles (65%), trachea (50%), oesophagus (45%), laryngeal nerve (30%) and larynx (15%). Cervical adenopathy is present in more than 40% of patients. At least 40% of patients have distant metastases at the time of diagnosis, 50% involving the lungs, 15% the bones and 10% the brain {1464}. Cardiac metastases have also been described {726}.

Macroscopy
The tumours are large, fleshy, and white-tan in colour, often exhibiting areas of necrosis and haemorrhage. They are typically infiltrative and in most instances replace most of the gland parenchyma with invasion into the surrounding soft tissue and adjacent structures including lymph nodes, larynx, pharynx, trachea, and oesophagus.

Tumour spread and staging
Undifferentiated carcinomas typically spread beyond the thyroid by direct local extension. Metastases to regional nodes are also common but their presence is often overshadowed by the presence of extensive soft tissue invasion. Distant metastases may be present in any site.
All undifferentiated carcinomas are considered to be T4 tumours. (see Introduction)

Cytopathology
Aspirates from undifferentiated carcinoma are typically highly cellular. The cells are present singly or in clusters and there is marked nuclear pleomorphism. The cell types include squamoid, giant cell and spindle cell. The nuclei are bizarre and single or multiple. They reveal coarsely clumped chromatin and single or multiple prominent nucleoli. Mitotic figures may be numerous. Occasional osteoclast-like giant cells can be seen. The background smear reveals necrotic debris often with accompanying polymorphonuclear leukocytes. Because of the presence of the latter cells care must be taken to distinguish these cases from acute thyroiditis.

Histopathology
Histologically, the majority of UTCs are widely invasive tumours composed of an admixture of spindle cells, pleomorphic giant cells and epithelioid cells. There is considerable variation in both the percentage and distribution of these cellular elements from case to case. The spindle cells can be slender or plump, and the giant cells may contain single or multiple, bizarre nuclei. About 20-30% of the cases can present frankly epithelioid areas, sometimes exhibiting squamoid features. In most cases, mitotic figures are a frequent finding. Extensive coagulative necrosis with irregular borders and palisading is often seen. Infiltration of vascular walls often accompanied by obliteration of the vascular lumina is common. Occasional osteoclast-like giant cells are common. A prominent

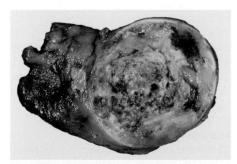

Fig. 2.037 Undifferentiated carcinoma. This tumour has a fleshy cut surface with areas of haemorrhage and necrosis.

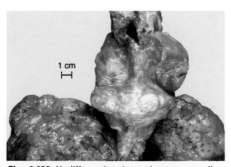

Fig. 2.038 Undifferentiated carcinoma spreading into both thyroid lobes, adjacent soft tissue, larynx and trachea. Note bilateral lung metastases.

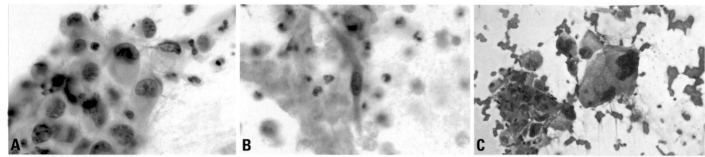

Fig. 2.039 FNA of undifferentiated carcinoma. **A** The tumour is present in sheets and is composed of cells with pleomorphic nuclei and prominent nucleoli. **B** A keratinized spindle shaped cell is present in the center of the field. **C** Markedly atypical cells are present.

neutrophilic infiltrate can be seen in some cases.

Tumours composed predominantly or exclusively of spindle cells often present a sarcomatoid appearance. When the tumour cells are arranged in fascicles, they can resemble either fibrosarcoma or leiomyosarcoma; whereas, when they are arranged in a storiform pattern, they can mimic malignant fibrous histiocytoma. Tumours can be composed predominantly of large anaplastic cells containing a single or multiple, hyperchromatic, eccentric nuclei, and dense, eosinophilic cytoplasm. Some tumours may be highly vascularized and the neoplastic cells can be arranged in a hemangiopericytic-like pattern or may form irregular anastomosing tumour cell-lined clefts mimicking an angiosarcoma.

Immunohistochemistry
Among the epithelial markers investigated, cytokeratin is the most frequently expressed in UTC (40-100% of the cases) {303,1320,1494,1653}. This wide range is due mainly to differences in the epitope retrieval procedures and the antibody used. In two large studies using the AE1/AE3 cytokeratin antibody "cocktail", cytokeratin expression was demon-

strated in about 80% of the cases {1653, 2308}. Epithelial membrane antigen is less commonly expressed (30-50%) {1494}. CEA expression is uncommon (less than 10% of the cases) and usually occurs in those cases having squamoid features {303,1653}. Thyroglobulin is almost invariably negative and, when present, is usually the result of diffusion from entrapped non-neoplastic thyroid or from residual well-differentiated neoplastic components. TTF-1 is rarely expressed in UTC's. Typically, undifferentiated carcinomas are strongly positive for TP53.

Immunohistochemistry can be very useful in distinguishing UTC from other tumours that may present a similar morphology. Desmin, myogenin and Myo-D1 can assist in distinguishing UTC from rhabdomyosarcomas; smooth-muscle actin and desmin from leiomyosarcomas; factor VIII-related antigen, CD31 and CD34 from angiosarcomas; S-100 protein, HMB-45, and Melan A from melanomas; and CD45 from large cell lymphomas.

Electron microscopy
EM can demonstrate the presence of epithelial type cell junctions and tonofila-

ments, but in some cases, these structures may be difficult to find or may be absent.

Variants
Several histologic variants of UTC have been recognized, all of which are uncommon. The osteoclastic variant is characterized by the presence of a large number of multinucleated, non-neoplastic, osteoclast-like giant cells that, because they strongly express CD68, are believed to be histiocytes {675, 1653}. Neoplastic bone or cartilage characterize the carcinosarcoma variant {513}. Two additional variants have recently been described: the paucicellular anaplastic carcinoma and the lymphoepithelioma-like carcinoma variants. The paucicellular variant is characterized by a hypocellular proliferation of mildly atypical spindle tumour cells embedded in a dense fibrous stroma that resembles Riedel thyroiditis {291,2349}. The lymphoepithelioma-like variant histologically resembles nasopharyngeal lymphoepithelioma but it has not been found to be associated with EBV infection {510}.

Precursor lesions
When an UTC is well-sampled, it is possible to find well differentiated or poorly differentiated thyroid carcinoma, in a significant proportion of the cases {1213, 1341,2108}. This finding supports the belief that UTC arises from the transformation (dedifferentiation) of a pre-existing better differentiated carcinoma. Some cases may, however, arise de novo.

Histogenesis
Current evidence indicates that undifferentiated thyroid carcinomas originate from follicular cells.

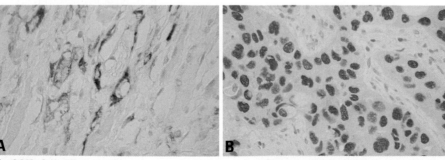

Fig. 2.040 **A** Undifferentiated carcinoma, paucicellular variant. Tumour cells are highlighted by the presence of immunoreactivity for cytokeratins. **B** Undifferentiated carcinoma immunostained for TP53. Positive staining is confined to the nuclei.

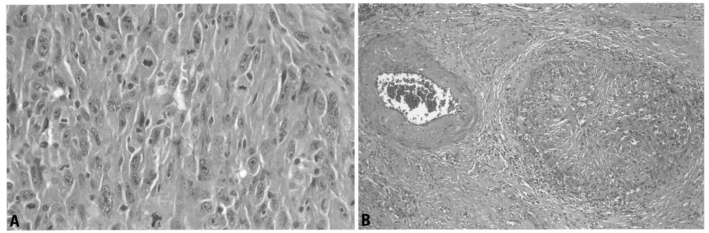

Fig. 2.041 Undifferentiated carcinoma. **A** Spindle cells with numerous atypical mitoses. **B** This tumour contains foci of vascular invasion.

Somatic genetics

Chromosomal imbalances

UTC is characterized by complex chromosomal alterations {1969} and CGH demonstrates DNA imbalance at a variety of chromosomal loci {2422}. Thus, the median chromosomal loss or gain in UTC is 10/case, compared to 5.5 and 1 in poorly differentiated thyroid carcinoma (PDTC) and well differentiated thyroid carcinoma (WDTC), respectively {2422}. Allelic losses have been described at 1q, 1p, 5, 8, 9p,11,17p,19p,22q and 16p and 18q {1018,1099,1102,2387,2422}. Specific loss or gain of chromosomal material, e.g. 3p13-14+, 5q11-31-, 11q13+, losses and gain at 8p and 8q may be associated with the transition from PDTC to UTC {1018,1099,1102, 2387}. Studies of coexisting well differentiated and undifferentiated thyroid carcinomas with a molecular genotyping

panel of tumour suppressor genes implicated in the thyroid carcinogenesis have demostrated that most cases have a core of conserved mutations in the two components. The undifferentiated component typically demonstrate increased mutation rates, consistent with the theory of multistep carcinogenesis {942,943}.

Molecular genetic alterations

Multiple molecular genetic and expression studies have been performed in UTC, many involving small sample sizes. The increased replicative potential is reflected by alterations in components involved in cell cycle control such as over-expression of cyclin D1, decreased expression of p27, and inactivation of *PTEN* and *p16* {720}. The most consistent finding is the strong association of UTC with *TP53* mutations. {511, 601,606,976,2016}. β-catenin (*CTNNB1*)

mutations have also been described {690}.

Genetic susceptibility

The genetic differential diagnosis for undifferentiated thyroid carcinoma could include all inherited cancer syndromes with non-medullary thyroid cancer, Cowden syndrome, Carney complex, familial adenomatous polyposis, familial site-specific non-medullary thyroid carcinoma and Werner syndrome. For details on inherited thyroid cancers, see Chapter 5.

Prognosis and predictive factors

Undifferentiated thyroid carcinoma is a highly aggressive malignant neoplasm typified by rapidly progressive local disease. The overall five-year survival ranges from 0-14%, and the median survival is 2.5-6 months {800,1341,1464,

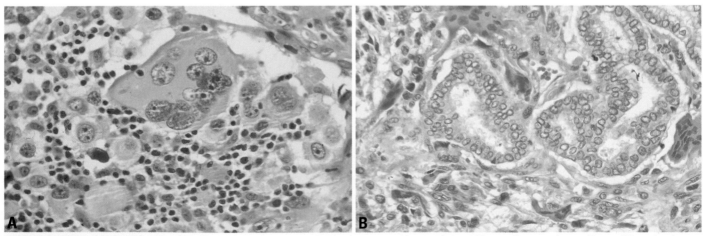

Fig. 2.042 Undifferentiated carcinoma. **A** Markedly atypical giant cells. **B** This tumour arose in association with a papillary carcinoma. The undifferentiated component has spindle cell features.

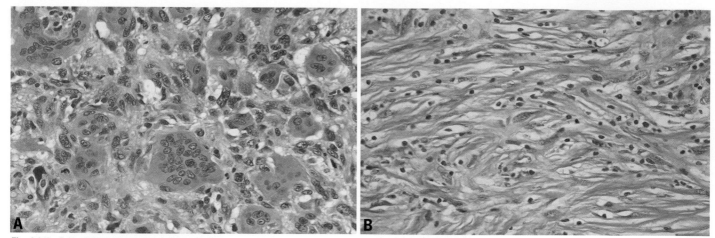

Fig. 2.043 A Undifferentiated carcinoma. Numerous osteoclast-like giant cells are present. **B** Undifferentiated carcinoma, paucicellular variant. The tumour is densely fibrotic with relatively sparse cellularity.

2160,2336}. Prognostic factors are related primarily to the extent of disease at presentation. Rare cases exhibiting a better prognosis usually include localized tumours less than 5 cm, particularly small foci that are only identified microscopically {36,486,2160}. Undifferentiated thyroid cancer may be associated with adjacent well-differentiated thyroid cancer, but the prognosis depends on the size of the undifferentiated component and the efficacy of eradicative surgery {800,2308}. Those patients with tumours that are amenable to complete surgical resection combined with preoperative or postoperative adjuvant doxorubicin-based chemotherapy and irradiation may have prolonged survival {800,1609,1737,2160,2336}. Predictive factors associated with histomorphologic and genetic features of the tumour have not been identified.

Squamous cell carcinoma

K.Y. Lam
A. Sakamoto

Definition
Squamous cell carcinoma of the thyroid is a malignant epithelial tumour composed entirely of cells with squamous cell differentiation.

ICD-O code
8070/3

Synonym
Epidermoid carcinoma

Epidemiology
These tumours account for up to 1% of thyroid malignancies {591,739,1215, 2040}. Squamous cell carcinoma of the thyroid is a disease of the elderly and more commonly occurs in women, with a female to male ratio of 2:1 {1215}.

Clinical features
The clinical features do not differ from those of undifferentiated carcinoma of thyroid. Squamous cell carcinoma of thyroid grows rapidly, and often presents with pressure symptoms resulting from tracheal or oesophageal compression {1215}. A long-standing history of thyroid disease is noted in some cases {410}. Hashimoto thyroiditis has been reported in some patients with squamous cell carcinoma {356}. Rarely, patients with squamous cell carcinoma develop a paraneoplastic syndrome, with hypercalcaemia and leukocytosis {1826,1897}.
Imaging studies are important for the exclusion of primaries from other sites and delineation of the extent of the disease. Laryngoscopy, bronchoscopy, oesophagoscopy examination and chest X-ray are recommended to exclude the origin of squamous cell carcinoma from other sites.

Macroscopy
Squamous cell carcinoma is typically a large tumour involving one or both lobes of the thyroid gland {2061}. Satellite tumour nodules are often noted. The tumour frequently has a firm consistency and a greyish-white colour with areas of necrosis.

Tumour spread and staging
The most common route of spread is local extension into adjacent structures. Nevertheless, distant metastases do occur in approximately 20% of the cases, and nodal metastases are common {410, 1215,1779}. The staging of squamous cell carcinoma is identical to that of undifferentiated carcinoma.

Cytopathology
Fine needle aspiration biopsy is useful to establish the diagnosis {1178}. The cytological features are identical to squamous cell carcinomas arising in other sites.

Histopathology
By definition, squamous cell carcinoma of thyroid should be comprised entirely of tumour cells with squamous differentiation. Undifferentiated carcinoma or papillary carcinoma may show areas of squamous differentiation {1213,2492}. However, there should be no evidence of other types of thyroid carcinoma in close proximity to the carcinoma if a tumour is classified as squamous cell carcinoma of the thyroid. Squamous cell carcinoma of thyroid often shows extensive infiltration of perithyroidal soft tissue, prominent vascular invasion and perineural invasion.
The most important differential diagnoses include squamous differentiation in undifferentiated carcinoma, extension or metastases from squamous cell carcinoma of other sites, squamous metaplasia associated with nodular goiter, lymphocytic thyroiditis and carcinoma showing thymus-like differentiation (CASTLE).

Immunoprofile and growth faction
Squamous cell carcinomas of the thyroid are strongly positive for CK19 but negative for CK1, CK4, CK10/13 and CK20 {1215,1218}. Focal positivity for CK7 and CK18 may be present in some tumours. Occacional cases have been reported as positive for thyroglobulin, but these most likely represent non-specific absorption from adjacent cells; epithelial membrane antigen has also been reported to be positive {2492}. In addition, the tumour often shows a high proliferative index {1103}.

Grading
The tumours are graded as are squamous carcinomas in other anatomic locations. Approximately half of the squamous cell carcinomas of the thyroid gland are poorly-differentiated {410, 1215}.

Somatic genetics
Expression of abnormal TP53 has been noted in approximately 50% of squamous cell carcinomas of thyroid and loss of p21 expression is apparent in all tumours {1204,1206,1213,1215}.

Prognosis and predictive factors
The prognosis in most cases is similar to that of undifferentiated carcinoma {410, 1215}.

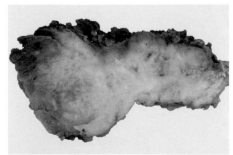
Fig. 2.044 Squamous cell carcinoma. This tumour has replaced an entire lobe of the thyroid.

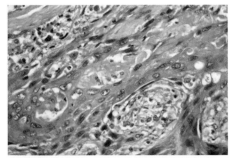
Fig. 2.045 Squamous cell carcinoma. Fascicles of keratinized cells were present throughout the tumour.

Mucoepidermoid carcinoma

J.Cameselle-Teijeiro
B. Wenig
M. Sobrinho Simões
J Albores-Saavedra

Definition
A malignant epithelial neoplasm showing a combination of epidermoid and mucinous components.

ICD-O code
8430/3

Epidemiology
Mucoepidermoid carcinoma (MEC) comprises about 0.5% of all thyroid malignancies {653} and shares most of the epidemiological features of papillary carcinoma {1847}. This tumour affects women more frequently than men (2:1), and has a bimodal age distribution.

Etiology
An association between radiation exposure to the neck during childhood has been documented in two cases {218, 2376}.

Clinical features
Most patients are euthyroid and present with a firm, "cold", painless mass in the neck. Extra-thyroidal extension is observed in about 20% of the cases {115,653,1916,2376}. Symptoms of oesophageal, tracheal, or recurrent laryngeal nerve compression are occasionally observed {115,653,1916,2376}.

Macroscopy
MEC show considerable size variations and may measure up to 10 cm. The tumours are rubbery to firm and the cut surfaces show a tan-brown to yellowish-white, well circumscribed but non-encapsulated mass, sometimes showing mucoid and/or cystic spaces. Necrosis and infiltration of the thyroid capsule and surrounding tissues are also found in occasional cases {73,283}.

Tumour spread and staging
Cervical lymph node metastases occur in a significant proportion of patients while lung and bone metastases have been reported in a few cases {115,653, 1916,2376}. Staging is discussed in the introduction.

Cytopathology
Cytologic smears from MECs show epidermoid cells and mucus-secreting cells with vacuolated cytoplasm often containing mucinous material, and/or signet-ring features {218,284,286,2306}. Cellular sheets showing a microcystic-like pattern containing hyaline bodies and/or amorphous material are also found {284}.

Histopathology
The histopathological features of mucoepidermoid carcinoma of the thyroid are similar although not identical to mucoepidermoid carcinomas of the salivary glands. In the thyroid, MEC is characterized by anastomosing compact clusters of epidermoid cells and mucocytes surrounded by fibrous stroma. The cuboidal or goblet-like mucous cells line ducts or glandular spaces. Extracellular mucin is also observed {2376}. Sometimes, intermixed in squamous sheets, are cells with abundant foamy cytoplasm often with hyaline colloid-like PAS positive intracellular droplets (hyaline body). Cystic spaces containing mucinous material or keratinized debris may be prominent. In some areas a cribriform-like pattern with elongated lumens and papillary infoldings is seen. Ciliated epithelium is also present in some cases {2376}. The tumour cells have medium-sized nuclei with rather pale chromatin resembling those of papillary carcinoma. The most frequent nuclear features include grooves and pseudoinclusions {218,2192}. Mitotic figures are rarely seen. Small foci of necrosis are seen occasionally in some tumour islands {653}. Foci of papillary carcinoma have been found in about 50% of the cases {115,1916}.

Mucinous material is PAS positive and diastase resistant. Positivity is also seen with with Mayer's mucicarmine, alcian-blue at pH 2.5, and the high-iron-diamine-alcian-blue method {1916}. The thyroid gland adjacent to the tumour is usually infiltrated focally by lymphoid tissue with or without germinal centres (lymphocytic thyroiditis), but oncocytic metaplasia is rare {1053}.

Immunohistochemistry
Tumour cells are positive for low and high molecular weight cytokeratins and usually for polyclonal CEA. Most MECs are focally positive for thyroglobulin and TTF-1 and negative for calcitonin {115,283, 653,1506,1916,2376}. P-cadherin expression is found in most MEC {1847}.

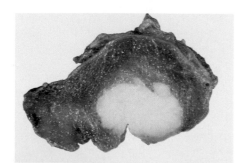

Fig. 2.046 Mucoepidermoid carcinoma. This tumour is sharply circumscribed but not encapsulated.

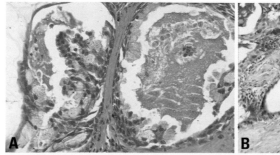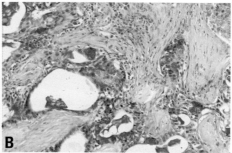

Fig. 2.047 A Mucoepidermoid carcinoma containing cystic foci with prominent mucous cells. B This tumour contains cystic foci with prominent mucous cells. Mucicarmine stain.

Histogenesis

MEC is most likely derived from meta-plastic follicular thyroid epithelium. In support of this hypothesis is the occurrence of MEC in the background of lymphocytic thyroiditis in which squamous metaplasia is common. Solid cell nests (SCN) also have been considered as the progenitor for thyroid MECs {1770}. However, the presence of keratinization, intercellular bridges and thyroglobulin reactivity with absent calcitonin are supportive of a follicular cell origin rather than origin from SCNs.

Prognosis and predictive factors

Thyroid MECs are low grade malignant tumours with an indolent biological behaviour and excellent long term prognosis. Transformation to undifferentiated carcinoma has been reported rarely {283,2306}. Extrathyroidal invasion and regional nodal metastases may occur but distant metastases are rare. Death due to tumour has occurred in about 20% of patients, especially in elderly patients {115,283,653,1916,2306}.

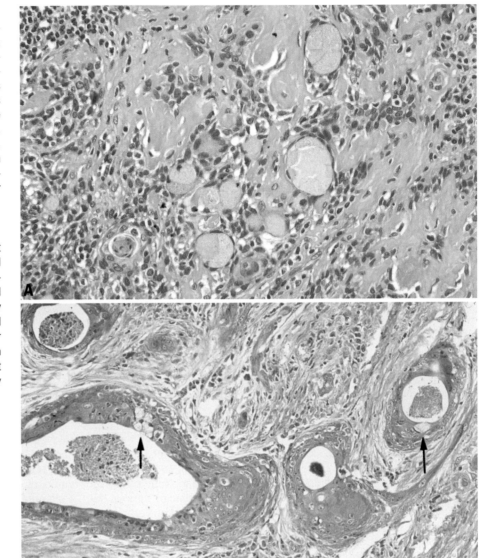

Fig. 2.048 **A** Mucoepidermoid carcinoma with extensive fibrosis. Mucocytes show compression of the nucleus by globules of mucin. **B** Admixture of squamous cells and mucous cells (arrows).

Sclerosing mucoepidermoid carcinoma with eosinophilia

J.K.C. Chan
V. LiVolsi
L. Bondeson

J. Albores-Saavedra
K. Geisinger
M. Sobrinho Simões

Definition
Sclerosing mucoepidermoid carcinoma with eosinophilia is a rare malignant neoplasm showing epidermoid and glandular differentiation, accompanied by prominent sclerosis and by eosinophilic and lymphocytic infiltration.

ICD-O code   8430/3
(mucoepidermoid carcinoma)

Epidemiology
The tumour occurs in adults and affects women almost exclusively {115,216,334, 341,384,695,2054,2099,2376}.

Etiology
Thyroiditis, in particular fibrosing Hashimoto thyroiditis has been reported in association with this tumour type.

Clinical features
Most patients present with a slowly growing thyroid mass. However some patients give a history of recent rapid enlargement and rarely, patients may present with symptoms resulting from extrathyroidal extension of the tumour, such as hoarseness, dyspnoea or vocal cord paralysis. These tumours are always "cold/hypofunctioning" on radionuclide scan.

Macroscopy
The tumours often show ill-defined borders, although occasionally they may be well-circumscribed. The cut surfaces are usually firm, white to yellow, and solid; rare tumours may demonstrate areas of cystic change. The maximum size ranges from 1.2-13 cm.

Tumour spread and staging
In about half of the cases, there is involvement of the perithyroidal soft tissues. Approximately one-third of patients show regional lymph node metastasis at presentation. Lung and bone metastasis can also occur {216,341,695,2054}.

Histopathology
Sclerosing mucoepidermoid carcinoma with eosinophilia is characterized by a sclerotic stroma richly infiltrated by eosinophils, lymphocytes and plasma cells. The tumour cells form anastomosing cords and nests and are polygonal, with only mild to moderate nuclear pleomorphism and distinct nucleoli. Interspersed with the epidermoid nests are mucous secreting cells and small pools of mucin. A pseudo-angiomatous appearance may be present due to loss of cohesion of tumour cells. Perineural invasion and obliteration of blood vessels are common. Rarely the tumour is associated with conventional papillary thyroid carcinoma. The background thyroid almost always shows Hashimoto thyroiditis or lymphocytic thyroiditis, often with fibrosis and areas of squamous metaplasia.

Immunohistochemistry
The tumour is immunoreactive for cytokeratin, negative for calcitonin, and is usually negative for thyroglobulin. Approximately half of the cases are positive for TTF1. Some tumour cells, especially the mucin-containing cells, may express carcinoembryonic antigen.

Differential diagnosis
This includes undifferentiated or squamous carcinomas of the thyroid on one hand, and benign squamous metaplasia on the other. Undifferentiated or squamous cell thyroid carcinoma usually exhibits more sheet-like growth, frank nuclear atypia, prominent necrosis and sparse or absent eosinophils. Benign squamous metaplasia of thyroid follicular epithelium does not exhibit invasive growth or eosinophilic infiltration.

Histogenesis
The tumour probably arises from follicular epithelium-derived metaplastic squamous nests that occur in a setting of Hashimoto or lymphocytic thyroiditis {341,2054,2376}.

Prognosis and predictive factors
Based on the limited follow-up information available, about half of the patients have been disease-free on follow-up of 3 months to 9 years, and about half have shown local-regional or distant spread. Predictive factors are not known.

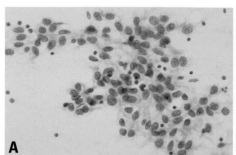 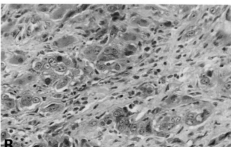 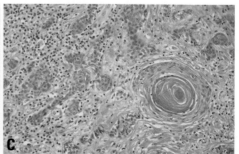

Fig. 2.049 Sclerosing mucoepidermoid carcinoma with eosinophilia. **A** FNAB demonstrating bland-looking epithelial cells. **B** Infiltration of skeletal muscle, associated with marked eosinophilia. **C** This tumour contains a well formed squamous pearl.

Mucinous carcinoma

M. Sobrinho Simões
J. Cameselle-Teijeiro
H.R. Harach

Definition
Mucinous carcinoma of the thyroid is characterized by clusters of neoplastic cells surrounded by extensive extracellular mucin deposition.

ICD-O code   8480/3

Epidemiology
Mucinous carcinoma of the thyroid is very rare with only a few cases reported and virtually nothing is known about its epidemiology {436,497,2085,2087}.

Clinical features
The tumours present as a rapid or slow growing, occasionally painful, "cold" thyroid nodules with or without palpable regional lymph nodes.

Macroscopy
The reported tumours have presented as well- or poorly-circumscribed grey-brown gelatinous nodules ranging up to several centimetres in diameter {436,497,2085, 2087}.

Histopathology
The hallmark of mucinous carcinoma is the presence of abundant mucoid lakes around strands or clusters of tumour cells that usually show large regular nuclei and prominent nucleoli. Focal squamous differentiation may occur. Mitoses, necrosis, and capsular or vascular invasion have been reported. The mucosubstance is of the sulfated type as shown by the "iron" diamine method, and

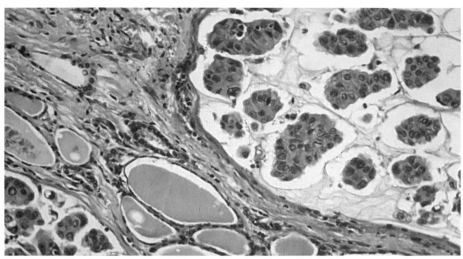

Fig. 2.050 Mucinous carcinoma. Neoplastic cells are present in pools of mucin.

stains positively with mucicarmine, Alcian blue and PAS before and after diastase digestion {436,2087}. The cells are typically positive for cytokeratins Ultrastructurally, the neoplastic cells are scattered in a granular extracellular matrix and generally show abundant intracytoplasmic mucin droplets, a prominent Golgi apparatus, and lumina lined by microvilli with glycocalix but lacking rootlets {436,2085,2087}.

Immunohistochemistry
The tumours usually show focal thyroglobulin, TTF1, low molecular weight cytokeratins and MUC2 immunoreactivity and are negative for calcitonin and CGRP {436,2085,2087}.

Differential diagnosis
Mucinous carcinoma of the thyroid should be distinguished from other thyroid primaries that may produce mucins, mostly intracellular, including follicular adenoma, and papillary, follicular, medullary and mucoepidermoid carcinomas (see respective sections in this chapter). Metastatic carcinoma from lung, breast, colon or other organs must always be considered as differential diagnosis when dealing with a thyroid tumour with a large mucinous compo-

nent. Follicular and papillary carcinomas displaying focal mucin production should not be regarded as mucinous carcinoma.

Histogenesis
The histogenesis of mucinous carcinoma of the thyroid suggests a dual cell origin {283,1809,2393}. The main cellular components, mucinous and thyroglobulin-immunoreactive cells, have been described in ultimobranchial bodies {2393} and related lateral thyroid lobe tissue constituents like solid cell nests, mixed follicles and thyroid follicles with acid mucin {820,821}.

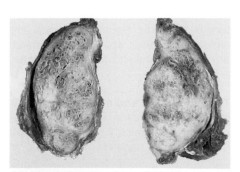

Fig. 2.051 Mucinous carcinoma: Cut sections demonstrate a gelatinous appearance.

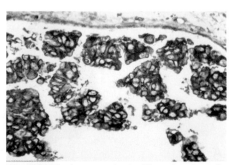

Fig. 2.052 Mucinous carcinoma. Thyroglobulin stain shows neoplastic cells within pools of mucin.

Medullary thyroid carcinoma

X. Matias-Guiu
R. DeLellis
J.F. Moley
R.F. Gagel
J. Albores-Saavedra

G. Bussolati
K. Kaserer
E.D. Williams
Z. Baloch

Definition
A malignant tumour of the thyroid gland showing C-cell differentiation.

ICD-O code   8345/3

Synonyms
Solid carcinoma; solid carcinoma with amyloid stroma; C-cell carcinoma; compact cell carcinoma; neuroendocrine carcinoma of the thyroid.

Epidemiology
Medullary thyroid carcinoma (MTC) comprises 5 to 10% of all thyroid malignancies. Up to 25% of these tumours are heritable, caused by gain of function germline mutations in the *RET* proto-oncogene [multiple endocrine neoplasia (MEN) type 2A and 2B and familial MTC (FMTC)] with an autosomal dominant mode of inheritance. In sporadic cases, the mean age at presentation is 50 years with a slight female predominance. Tumours occurring in patients with MEN 2B present in infancy or early childhood while MEN2A associated tumours occur in late adolescence or early adulthood. Medullary carcinomas in patients with FMTC manifest at a mean age of 50 years. Sporadic forms of MTC occur with similar frequency in different parts of the world.

Etiology
The etiology of sporadic MTC is unknown. In rare instances, these tumours may arise in the setting of Hashimoto disease, but this association is probably coincidental. Limited data suggest that chronic hypercalcemia may be associated with an increased incidence of these tumours {1321}. The incidence of MTC is not increased in patients with a history of irradiation to the head and neck; however, rats treated with low doses of ^{131}I have an increased incidence of these tumours {2239,2261}.

Localization
Medullary carcinoma typically is located in the middle third of the lobe, which corresponds to the area where C cells predominate normally.

Clinical features
Most patients with sporadic MTC present with a painless thyroid nodule that is "cold" on scintigraphic scan. Up to 50% of patients may present with nodal metastases and up to 15% may have distant metastases. Extensive local growth may be associated with upper airway obstruction and dysphagia. Virtually all MTCs produce calcitonin and serum levels of the hormone are typically increased. Large tumour volume is often associated with diarrhea and flushing in part due to the high calcitonin levels. Since the tumour cells may produce a number of other peptide products and amines, paraneoplastic syndromes due to the release of these substances may occur. For example, Cushing syndrome due to the paraneoplastic production of adrenocorticotropin has been well documented in some patients with MTC.

Table 2.06
Variants of medullary thyroid carcinoma (MTC)

1 Papillary or pseudopapillary, characterized by the presence of true papillae or artefactual pseudopapillae, caused by tissue fragmentation {1023,1915}.
2 Glandular (tubular or follicular) {829,1915}.
3 Giant cell {1483}.
4 Spindle cell {1684}.
5 Small cell {584} and Neuroblastoma-like {823}.
6 Paraganglioma-like {953}.
7 Oncocytic cell {509,822}.
8 Clear cell {1228}.
9 Angiosarcoma-like {1685}.
10 Squamous cell {509}.
11 Melanin-producing {1405}.
12 Amphicrine {741}.

Over the past 5 years, there has been an increase in the reported frequency of medullary microcarcinomas (less than 1 cm in diameter). Most of these tumours have been incidental findings, or were discovered by elevated serum calcitonin levels in patients with nodular thyroid disease {796}. In one study of 1385 patients with nodular thyroidal disease, the prevalence of MTC was 0.57% of all thyroid nodules and 15.7% of all carcinomas that were found incidentally in these patients {1670}.

Macroscopy
The tumours are firm, white-grey to tan in colour, gritty in consistency, and are well circumscribed, but not encapsulated. They vary in size from less than 1 cm ("microcarcinomas") to several centimeters in diameter. Sporadic tumours are typically unilateral, while familial tumours are characteristically multiple and bilateral.

Tumour spread and staging
Medullary carcinoma tends to metastasize early, particularly to cervical lymph nodes. Distant metastases are found at operation in approximately 20% of patients who present with palpable MTC [176]. Hematogenous MTC metastases

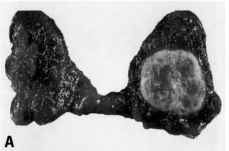
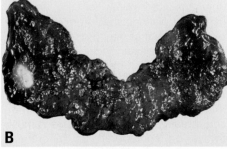

Fig. 2.053 Medullary thyroid carcinoma **A** This sporadic tumour involves a single lobe. **B** Medullary microcarcinoma.

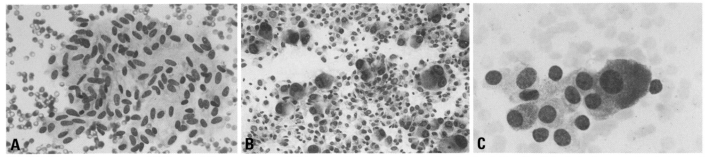

Fig. 2.054 Fine needle aspirates (FNA) of medullary carcinoma. **A** This tumour is composed predominantly of spindle cells. **B** Aspirate demonstrating features of the giant cell (pleomorphic) variant. **C** Tumour cells contain metachromatic cytoplasmic granules, as demonstrated with the May-Grunwald Giemsa stain.

often occur in the liver, lungs, and bone; occasionally they are found in the brain, soft tissues outside the neck, and bone marrow. Occult distant metastases are most likely the cause of most cases of persistent hypercalcitoninemia after thyroidectomy and lymph node dissection. Microcarcinomas may also be associated with metastases. The staging of medullary carcinoma is discussed in the introduction to this chapter.

Cytopathology

Aspirates from medullary carcinomas are typically hypercellular with non-cohesive or loosely cohesive cells. The cells are variable in shape with polygonal, bipolar or spindle shapes. The nuclei are typically hyperchromatic with coarsely granular chromatin and moderate degrees of pleomorphism. Multinucleate tumour giant cells are common. The nuclei are often eccentric thereby imparting a plasmacytoid appearance to the cells. Cytoplasmic granules can be particularly prominent in Romanowsky stained

preparations. Amyloid deposits may be found in 50-70% of aspirates. In Papanicolaou stained preparations, the amyloid deposits appear deep green. With Congo red stains, the amyloid deposits exhibit a typical apple green birefringence.

Histopathology

The histopathologic appearance of medullary thyroid carcinoma is quite variable {29,850,914,1684,2285}. The characteristic features are sheets, nests or trabeculae of polygonal, round or spindle cells, separated by varying amounts of fibrovascular stroma, giving rise to a more or less lobular (organoid) or trabecular arrangement {29,1684,2285}. Some tumours may have a histological pattern reminiscent of carcinoid {824}. The epithelial nests vary in size and configuration. Tumour cells contain round to oval, regular nuclei with coarse chromatin. Nucleoli are usually not prominent (except in the oncocytic variant), and mitotic figures are usually scant.

Occasionally, nuclei are enlarged, pleomorphic and hyperchromatic or even multiple, however, medullary carcinomas with these features do not carry the ominous prognosis of undifferentiated carcinoma. The cytoplasm is granular, eosinophilic to amphophilic, and has ill-defined margins. Occasionally, tumour cells exhibit a prominent plasmacytoid appearance. Non-cohesive growth is common. Necrosis and haemorrhage are infrequent and restricted to large tumours. Mucin production has been described in a high proportion of cases, but it is usually present in limited amounts {1417,2472}. Small psammoma-like concretions may also be seen. Lymphatic permeation by tumour cells is also common.

S-100 protein positive sustentacular cells can occur at the periphery of the tumour cell nests, and are said to be more common in heritable tumours {1433}. Although true encapsulated medullary carcinomas do exist {528,1023}, tumour cells usually infiltrate the surrounding

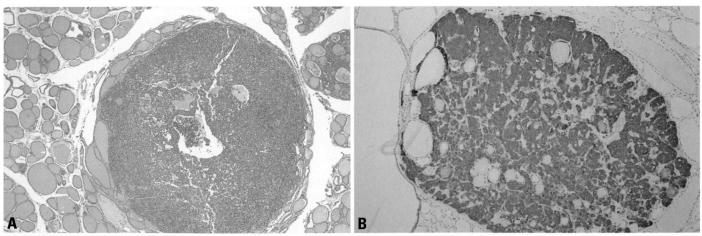

Fig. 2.055 A Microscopic medullary thyroid carcinoma. The tumour nodule is sharply circumscribed. **B** This microscopic medullary carcinoma is positively stained for calcitonin.

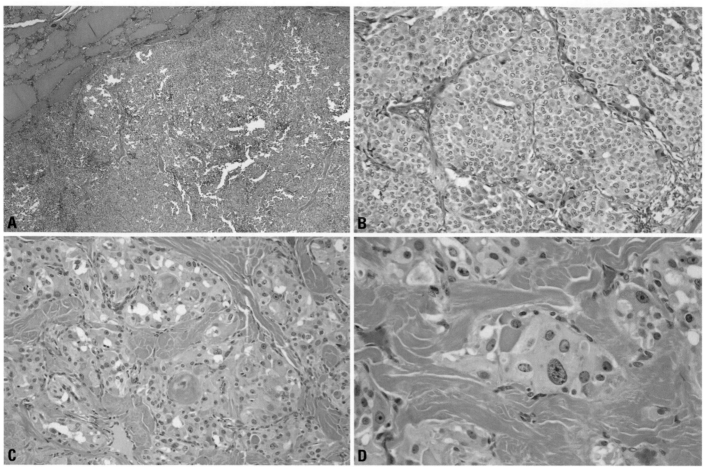

Fig. 2.056 Medullary carcinoma. **A** Predominantly solid growth pattern. The interface between tumour and the adjacent thyroid is irregular. **B** Insular pattern of growth. **C** This tumour is intersected by fibrous tissue and amyloid deposits. **D** Occasional cells with enlarged hyperchromatic nuclei are present in this area.

thyroid tissue, often entrapping normal thyroid follicles. The appearance of the tumour stroma is also variable {29,850, 914,1684,2285}. In some cases it is highly vascular and frequently contains abundant hyalinized collagen. Congo red positive stromal deposits of amyloid can be identified in 80% of cases. They are occasionally associated with a foreign-body type giant-cell reaction and calcification.

Immunohistochemistry

Medullary carcinoma is usually positive with argyrophilic stains. The tumour cells are immunoreactive for calcitonin in the vast majority of cases, with in-situ hybridization techniques revealing calcitonin mRNA in the remaining cases. Carcinoembryonic antigen is expressed in most cases {481,1338}. Tumour cells are typically positive for a variety of generic neuroendocrine markers such as chromogranin A and synaptophysin.

There is also positivity for TTF-1 and low-molecular-weight keratins. Tumour cells may also contain a great variety of neuroendocrine substances including: somatostatin, proopiomelanocortin-derived peptides (some of which are associated with Cushing syndrome), bombesin/gastrin-releasing peptide family members, neurotensin, histaminase, serotonin, catecholamines. About 30% of tumours exhibit aneuploidy by flow or static cytometry. In some studies, aneuploidy and high growth fractions have been associated with worse prognosis {175,1981}. MIB-1 (Ki-67) index is usually low {2351}.

Electron microscopy

Ultrastructurally, the tumour cells contain two main types of secretory granules: type I granule is about 280 nm, and type II granules are more electron dense membrane bound, with a mean diameter of 130 nm {909,2084}.

Differential diagnosis

The diagnosis of medullary carcinoma should be considered in any thyroid tumour showing unusual features. Histopathologic differential diagnosis of medullary carcinoma includes thyroid paraganglioma, hyalinizing trabecular tumour, follicular carcinomas with trabecular growth patterns, poorly-differentiated carcinomas with solid, trabecular or insular patterns, oncocytic tumours, intrathyroidal parathyroid tumours, and the rare thyroid metastases from neuroendocrine carcinomas from other organs {1432}. On the other hand, medullary carcinomas metastatic to lymph nodes without a proven primary thyroid tumour can be confused with metastatic melanoma or metastatic neuroendocrine carcinoma of other organs. The characteristic cytomorphology of tumour cells, the presence of delicate fibrovascular septa, absence of extensive necrosis, and positive immunostaining for calcitonin, CEA and low-molecular-weight keratins are helpful in the diagnosis of medullary carcinoma.

Precursor lesions

C-cell hyperplasia is the precursor of heritable medullary carcinoma {2407}, as discussed in Chapter 5 on inherited tumour syndromes. However, the term C-cell hyperplasia refers to two different pathologic conditions with different neoplastic potential {32,1317,1728}, "neoplastic" and "reactive". "Neoplastic" C-cell hyperplasia can usually be seen on H&E sections, while the "reactive" type usually requires immunohistochemistry for its identification {1728}.

"Neoplastic" C-cell hyperplasia (so-called C-cell carcinoma in situ, or medullary carcinoma in situ) is the precursor lesion of heritable medullary thyroid carcinoma, associated with germline mutations in the *RET* protooncogene. Neoplastic C-cell hyperplasia usually occurs in the thyroid tissue of the upper two thirds of the lateral lobes, adjacent to invasive medullary carcinomas of heritable type, and also in prophylactic thyroidectomy specimens in asymptomatic carriers of *RET* germline mutations {1309}. In such cases, C-cell hyperplasia (focal, diffuse, or nodular) is characterized by groups of intrafollicular atypical C-cells, which may encircle the follicles, and lead to partial or complete obliteration of the follicular spaces {479}. There is a progressive increase of the proliferation index accompanied by an increase of molecular alterations and monoclonality, leading to invasive medullary carcinoma {496,1434}.

The role of C-cell hyperplasia in the development of sporadic medullary carcinoma remains unknown, although it has been reported in association with apparent sporadic tumours {1043}.

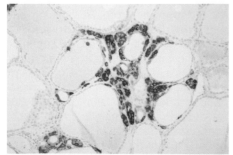

Fig. 2.057 C-Cell hyperplasia in a patient with MEN2A. Immunostain for calcitonin.

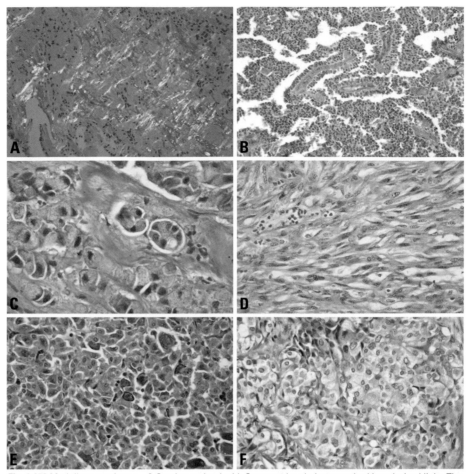

Fig. 2.058 Medullary carcinoma. **A** Section stained with Congo red and photographed in polarized light. The amyloid deposits show green birefringence. **B** Pseudopapillary pattern. **C** This lesion is composed of vacuolated amphicrine cells. **D** Spindle cell growth pattern. **E** Melanotic variant containing scattered cells with melanin pigment. **F** This tumour has a focally solid growth pattern.

Differential diagnosis of "neoplastic" C-cell hyperplasia includes intraglandular spread of medullary carcinoma, solid cell nests and palpation thyroiditis. Distinction of C-cell hyperplasia from microinvasive medullary carcinoma may be very difficult in individual cases. The presence of fibrosis around tumour cell nests and demonstration of defects in the follicular basement membrane by immunohistochemistry or electron microscopy may be helpful {1461}. Hyperplastic C cells usually show greater reactivity for calcitonin than the cells of invasive medullary carcinoma.

Outside of the setting of heritable medullary thyroid carcinoma, an increase in the size and numbers of C-cells has been described in association with a great variety of pathophysiologic conditions including ageing, hyperparathyroidism, hypergastrinemia, lymphocytic thyroiditis, adjacent to follicular tumours. The malignant potential of this second type of C-cell hyperplasia (also designated as "reactive", "secondary" or "physiologic") has not been fully demonstrated, although there are examples of C-cell hyperplasia secondary to hyperparathyroidism that have been associated with sporadic medullary carcinomas {1321}. "Reactive" C-cell hyperplasia is characterized by an increased number of normal-appearing C-cells (at least more than 50 C-cells per low power field in areas of high C cell concentration) {32}. Exceptionally, "reactive" C-cell hyperplasia shows focal obliteration of follicles. Adequate sampling of the normal thyroid is needed before C-cell hyperplasia can be excluded.

Histogenesis

In 1966, Williams suggested that medullary carcinoma derived from the C-

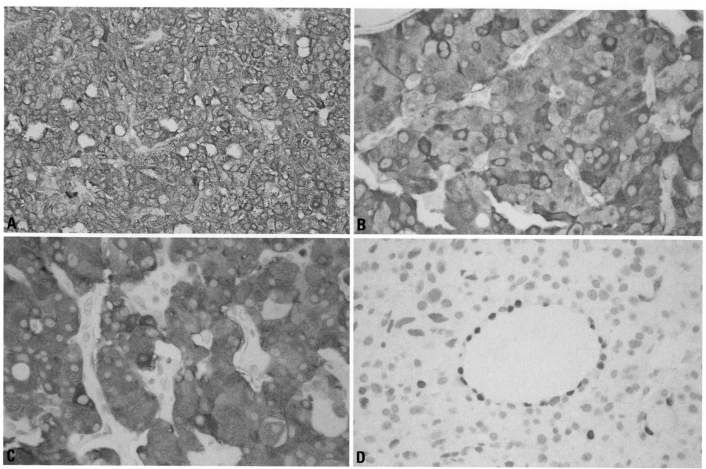

Fig. 2.059 Medullary thyroid carcinoma **A** Immunostain for calcitonin. The tumour cells are uniformly reactive. **B** Chromogranin immunostain. All of the cells are positively stained. **C** All tumour cells are immunoreactive for synaptophysin. **D** An entrapped follicle demonstrates strong TTF-1 immunoreactivity; in the surrounding medullary carcinoma only scattered cells are strongly stained.

cell {2390}, and Meyer and Abdel-Bari, and Bussolati and coworkers, demonstrated calcitonin production in tumour cells {271,1489}. In 1973, Wolfe described C cell hyperplasia in the vicinity of familial MTC, and identified it as the precursor of heritable medullary carcinoma {2407}. C cells are derived from the neural crest via the ultimobranchial body. However, demonstration of C-cells in patients with Di George anomaly has raised the possibility that a small subset of C-cells is of endodermal derivation {267}.

Somatic genetics
Despite more than a decade of somatic genetic studies, little is known about the etiology of sporadic MTC. Allelotyping studies have demonstrated loss of heterozygosity of markers at 1p (42%), 3p (30%), 3q (38%), 11p (11%), 13q (10%), 17p (8%), and 22q (29%), which have been corroborated by CGH studies as

well {1413,1556}. Somatic *RET* mutations, most commonly the M918T mutation, have been shown to occur in 20-80% of sporadic MTC, depending on the series and mutation detection technologies {559}. This large range of somatic M918T mutation frequencies is likely due to subpopulations within each MTC that variably harbour this mutation {566}. This heterogeneity suggests either that the codon 918 mutation can arise as an event in progression within a metastatic clone or within a single tumour, or that MTC can be of polyclonal origin. One CGH study reports on the increased number of CGH-detectable chromosomal aberrations in M918T somatic mutation positive MTC compared to those without this mutation {663}.

Genetic susceptibility
There is only a single differential diagnosis to consider for heritable forms of medullary thyroid carcinoma, multiple

endocrine neoplasia type 2 (MEN 2), which comprises MEN 2A, MEN 2B and familial medullary thyroid carcinoma (see Chapter 5). There have been two reports from a single center that suggest that up to a third of patients who are apparently sporadic, defined as lacking germline *RET* mutations, had tumours with histological features similar to those of hereditary MTC, ie, C-cell hyperplasia and even multifocal disease {1043,1044}. However, the first report appeared in 1998 and most clinical *RET* testing pre-1998 was limited to exons 10 and 11. Indeed, current clinical *RET* testing across different centers in the world do not necessarily test all the necessary 'hotspot' codons. Germline *RET* mutations in codon 768, 790, 791, and 804 have been subsequently identified to predispose to familial MTC and low penetrance (mild disease, later onset, no family history) disease, and hence associated with apparently sporadic MTC

{559,719}. It is, therefore, plausible that these apparently sporadic tumours showing C-cell hyperplasia and other features of heritable disease actually have germline *RET* mutations in these low penetrance and perhaps other as yet unidentified codons. When a series of 10 individuals who were sent in as sporadic (no germline mutations) and subjected to comprehensive mutation analysis of *RET*, 7 were found to harbour germline mutations in one of exons 10, 11, 13, or 14, which were previously undetected by the first centre (C. Eng, unpublished data).

Prognosis and predictive factors

United States SEER data of 499 cases of medullary carcinoma showed 5 and 10-year survivals of 83.2% and 73.7%, respectively {185}. Older age, male gender and extent of local tumour invasion were associated with substantially reduced survival {185}. In addition, Voutilainen and coworkers demonstrated that the presence of distant metastases was an independent predictor of poor prognosis {2335}.

Micromedullary carcinoma

The 10-year survival rate for patients with sporadic micromedullary carcinomas is better than that observed in patients with tumours greater than 1 cm (p = 0.04). Normal postoperative calcitonin levels were observed in 71.1% of patients with microcarcinomas treated by total thyroidectomy as compared to 33.6% in patients with larger tumours {168}.

Prognosis in familial cases

In a series of 104 cases reported by Kebebew et al. {1060}, more than 90% of patients with familial tumours diagnosed by biochemical or molecular studies were disease-free at last follow-up as compared to those patients who were not screened (P<0.001). Moreover, screened patients had a lower incidence of lymph node metastases (P<0.05). Thyroidectomy in MEN 2A patients less than 5 years of age resulted in a significant reduction in the number of cases of medullary carcinoma with or without metastases when compared to patients whose thyroidectomies were performed between the ages of 6 and 20 {2167}. Interestingly, metastatic, persistent or recurrent disease occurred more commonly in MEN 2A patients with codon 634 mutations than in those with mutations affecting other codons.

Widespread metastases have been associated with systemic symptoms of diarrhea, bone pain or flushing, and approximately one third of these patients died within 5 years. In the series reported by Kebebew et al, overall cause specific mortality at 5 and 10 years was 10.7% and 13.5%, respectively {1060}. In univariate analyses, age, gender, TNM stage, sporadic vs hereditary status, distant metastases and extent of thyroidectomy were significant prognostic factors. However, only age and stage were significant variables in multivariate analyses {1060}. These observations underscore the fact that screening and early treatment by thyroidectomy, with central lymph node dissection, are associated with a rate of cure approaching 100%. Patients with persistent hypercalcitoninemia without clinical or radiological evidence of residual tumour after apparent curative surgery may enjoy long-term survival in the presence of occult medullary thyroid carcinoma.

Type of RET mutation

Whether somatic *RET* M918T mutation in sporadic MTC is associated with metastatic outcome remains controversial. A few studies suggest that this genotype-prognosis association exists {1971}. However, these studies relied on examining for this mutation in both primary MTC and metastatic deposits. Because of this experimental design and biased ascertainment, these studies selected for the presence of metastatic disease and M918T. However, well-controlled and designed studies did not show the association between somatic M918T and outcome {559,1413}.

Medical management is currently based on the known patterns of germline RET mutations in heritable medullary thyroid cancer, as discussed in Chapter 5. Children with MEN 2B usually present at an earlier age than children with MEN 2A and have a higher risk for aggressive forms of medullary carcinoma {241}.

Histopathological criteria

The main histopathological parameters that have been suggested to have a relationship to survival are necrosis and squamous metaplasia {646}. The presence of less than 50% of calcitonin immunoreactive cells and the finding of immunoreactive CEA in the absence of calcitonin have also been considered to represent a poor prognostic feature {646,1484}.

Mixed medullary and follicular cell carcinoma

M. Papotti
G. Bussolati
P. Komminoth
X. Matias-Guiu
M. Volante

Definition
Mixed medullary and follicular cell carcinomas (MMFCC) are tumours showing the morphological features of both, medullary carcinoma with immunoreactive calcitonin and follicular (or papillary) carcinomas with immunoreactive thyroglobulin {856}.

ICD-O code   8346/3

Synonyms
Mixed follicular and C-cell carcinoma; mixed medullary and papillary carcinoma; composite carcinoma; biphasic carcinoma; simultaneous carcinoma; compound medullary-follicular carcinoma; concurrent medullary-follicular carcinoma; stem cell carcinoma; differentiated carcinoma, intermediate type

Epidemiology
MMFCC are very rare tumours and most have been described in single case reports. The largest series includes 11 cases collected in two Institutions over a period of more than 20 years {1683}. After reviewing all medullary carcinomas, 3-5% of cases displayed mixed features, having a follicular or papillary carcinoma component both in primary tumours and metastases {1683}. These numbers reflect the extreme rarity of this condition, with percentages averaging less than 0.15% of all thyroid tumours {1045,1683}. The mean age of 36 reported cases {1688} was 48 years, not differing from

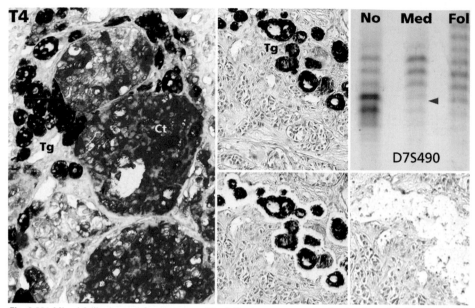

Fig. 2.061 Mixed follicular and C-cell tumour. The follicular component stains for thyroglobulin (black), the C-cell (medullary) component for calcitonin (red). Following laser capture microdissection, LOH at D76S490 is detected in the medullary (Med) but not in the follicular component (Fol), as compared to the corresponding normal tissue (No).

conventional medullary carcinoma, with a 1.3:1 male to female ratio. Patients usually present with a "cold" thyroid nodule. Occasional examples of MMFCC have been shown to occur in kindreds with inherited medullary thyroid carcinoma caused by a germline *RET* mutation.

Clinical features
Most patients with MMFCC present with a thyroid mass which is usually cold on scintigraphic scan and solid on ultrasonography.

Macroscopy
Macroscopic features of MMFCC overlap those of conventional medullary and follicular-derived neoplastic counterparts. Most tumours are solid, whitish, firm, non-capsulated lesions with a mean diameter of 3.7 cm {1688}.

Tumour spread and staging
Most reported cases had lymph node involvement, at the time of diagnosis or in the course of disease progression {1688}. Distant metastases were present

in 26% of these, occurring in the lung, liver, mediastinum or bone. Metastases may exhibit a predominant medullary, or follicular cell component, but can also show a combination of both. According to tumour diameter, the majority of cases were classified as pT2.

Histopathology
MMFCC is an extremely heterogeneous group of tumours. The vast majority present as a predominant medullary carcinoma admixed with follicular-derived structures in variable proportions. The medullary component, which generally comprises the majority of the tumour, shows no specific features.
Concerning the follicular population, the majority of MMFCC are composed of single follicles admixed in an otherwise classical medullary carcinoma. Because non-neoplastic follicles may be observed in classical MCT due to entrapment, strict criteria should be applied for those tumours not showing both components in the metastases. In these cases, the diagnosis of MMFCC should only be consid-

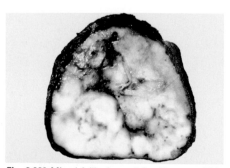

Fig. 2.060 Mixed follicular and C-cell tumour. This tumour has a solid appearance and is not encapsulated.

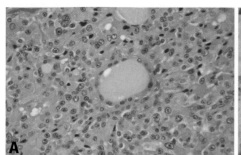 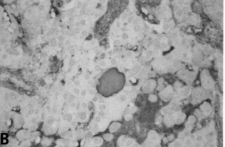 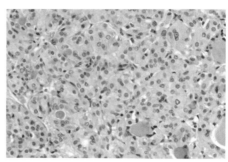

Fig. 2.062 A Medullary thyroid carcinoma. An entrapped normal thyroid follicle is present in the center of the field. **B** Medullary thyroid carcinoma immunostained for thyroglobulin. Entrapped thyroglobulin deposits are positively stained while the tumour cells are non-reactive

Fig. 2.063 Mixed medullary and follicular carcinoma.

ered when the follicular-cell component is either that of papillary carcinoma or consists of thyroglobulin positive follicles showing neoplastic features, often deep within the tumour. The cells that line the follicles are enlarged and have hyperchromatic nuclei, larger than those of peritumoural follicular cells.

Other morphological patterns of growth in the follicular cell component include conventional papillary carcinoma, both classic and follicular variants, associated with medullary carcinoma {26,745,1247, 1429,1699}. The mixed medullary and papillary carcinoma can be recognized with conventional stains due to the distinctive nuclear features of papillary carcinoma. The lymph node metastases may have a similar pattern of growth.

In addition, virtually all other types of follicular-derived carcinomas have been identified in MMFCC, including oxyphilic carcinoma {1683}, poorly differentiated solid/trabecular carcinoma {2194} and foci of anaplastic carcinoma {1692}.

Histogenesis
Several hypotheses have been postulated to explain the histogenesis of MMFCC {1428}. On the one hand, the clonal origin from a common stem cell, capable of differentiating towards both follicular and C cell lineages, has been proposed by some authors {1325}, supported by the evidence of co-expression of calcitonin and thyroglobulin protein and mRNA in the same cells {910,1614,1683}. The demonstration of C-cells in the thyroid of patients with DiGeorge syndrome, has provided support for the hypothesis that a subset of C-cells may be of endodermal derivation; and these cells could give rise to mixed medullary and follicular tumours {267}. Other authors have favoured the hypothesis of a collision phenomenon {66,1429,1699}. Genetic analysis of individual tumour cells or clusters taken from the two tumour components by means of laser-based microdissection {2329} revealed different molecular abnormalities, suggesting an origin from different cell clones. It was suggested that in some cases follicular structures may be hyperplastic or adenomatous (rather than malignant), sequestrated by the medullary carcinoma counterpart, (so-called "hostage" theory) {2329}.

Somatic genetics
Very few cases of MMFCC reported in the literature have been analysed for specific genetic alterations. Somatic point mutations of the *RET* proto-onco-

gene show a similar range to those found in sporadic medullary thyroid carcinoma {1657,2329}. No specific molecular alterations have been recognized in the follicular derived neoplastic component.

Genetic susceptibility
The majority of MMFCCs are sporadic tumours, but six reported cases were associated with MEN2 syndrome {1152, 1519,1614,1683}

Prognosis and predictive factors
Since the predominant component of this tumour is medullary carcinoma the prognosis is similar to that of medullary thyroid carcinoma. The follicular component has been shown to concentrate radioactive iodine {803,1688,1692}.

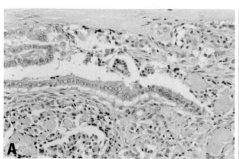 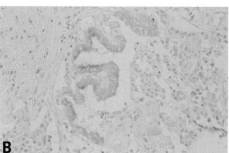 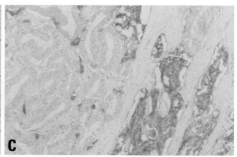

Fig. 2.064 A Conventional papillary carcinoma associated with medullary carcinoma. **B** Thyroglobulin stain. **C** Calcitonin stain.

Spindle cell tumour with thymus-like differentiation

W. Cheuk
J. K.C. Chan
D.M. Dorfman
T. Giordano

Definition
Spindle cell tumour with thymus-like differentiation (SETTLE) is a rare, malignant tumour of the thyroid characterized by a lobulated architecture and biphasic cellular composition featuring spindle shaped epithelial cells that merge into glandular structures.

ICD-O code
8588/3

Synonyms
Thyroid spindle cell tumour with mucinous cysts; malignant teratoma; and thyroid thymoma in childhood {828,1088, 1281,1559,2369}.

Epidemiology
SETTLE usually affects children, adolescents and young adults, with a mean age of 19 years (range 4-59), and a male predominance (M:F=1.5:1) {237,521,904, 981,1952,2118}.

Clinical features
The most common presentation is a painless thyroid mass present for a variable duration. Less common presentations include rapidly enlarging neck mass, local tenderness, tracheal compression, and diffuse thyroid enlargement mimicking thyroiditis {365,1107}. The tumour appears "cold" on thyroid scan, and displays heterogeneous solid and cystic densities on CT scan. Thyroid function tests are not affected.

Macroscopy
The tumour is grossly encapsulated, partially circumscribed, or infiltrative with a mean size of approximately 3 cm. The cut surface is firm, greyish-white to tan, and vaguely lobulated. Small cysts may be present.

Tumour spread and staging
SETTLE is typically associated with delayed blood-borne metastasis. Sites of metastasis, in descending order, are the lungs, lymph nodes, kidney and soft tissues. Metastasis usually occurs many years after diagnosis {344}, although regional metastasis at presentation can sometimes be present {365,1107}.

Histopathology
SETTLE is a highly cellular tumour with a lobulated pattern imparted by fibrous septa. Most cases are biphasic, but occasional cases may be composed exclusively of spindle cells or glandular structures, the so-called monophasic variant {365}. Compact interlacing to reticulated fascicles of spindle cells merge imperceptibly with tubulopapillary glands. The spindle cells possess elongated nuclei with fine chromatin and inconspicuous nucleoli, and scanty cytoplasm. Mitotic figures are rare in most cases, but occasional cases may show high mitotic activity and focal necrosis {1091}. The glandular component usually takes the form of tubules, papillae, cords, small pale-staining islands, and epithelium-lined cystic spaces. The glandular cells are cuboidal to columnar, and are sometimes mucinous or ciliated. Their nuclei are similar to those of the spindle cells except for an oval or round contour. Exceptionally, there can be focal squamous metaplasia {2429}. Lymphocytes are typically scanty. Vascular invasion may be present.

Immunohistochemistry
Both the spindle and glandular cells express cytokeratins. Rarely, the spindle cells may demonstrate myoepithelial differentiation {2156,2429}. The tumour cells are negative for thyroglobulin, calcitonin, CEA, S-100 protein and CD5. Ultrastructurally, the epithelial nature of the spindle cells is evidenced by presence of tonofilaments, desmosomes and basal lamina.

Differential diagnosis
SETTLE must be distinguished from sarcomatoid undifferentiated carcinoma.

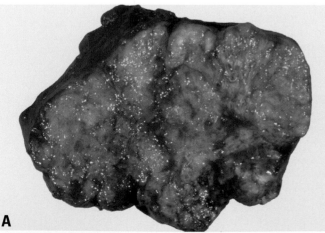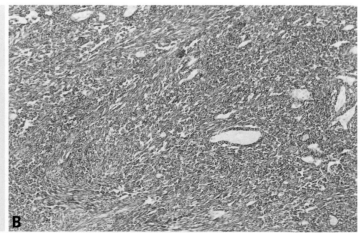

Fig. 2.065 A SETTLE. The cut surface shows a fleshy tumour with invasion of the entire thyroid gland. **B** Pan-cytokeratin (MNF-116) immunohistochemistry shows diffuse strong staining of spindle cells as well as glandular structures.

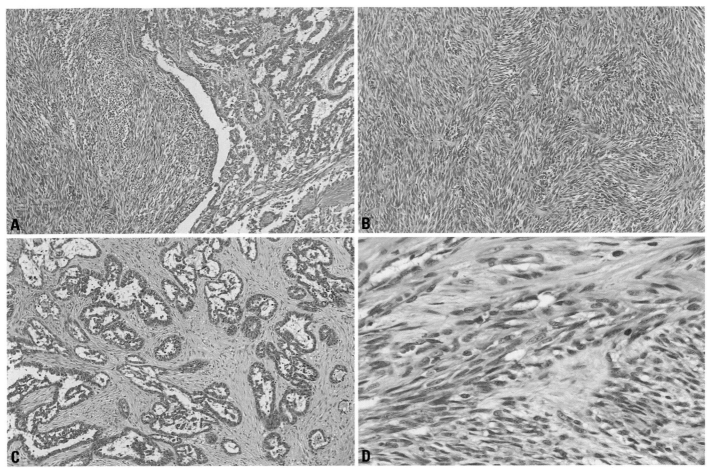

Fig. 2.066 SETTLE of the thyroid gland. **A** A biphasic growth pattern is evident, with spindle cells on the left merging into well formed tubulopapillary structures on the right. **B** This tumour is composed of interlacing bundles of spindle cells. **C** Tumour with a monophasic appearance dominated by epithelial cells forming glandular structures. **D** Tumour cell nuclei show mild variation in size and shape.

Ectopic thymoma can be distinguished from SETTLE by the jigsaw puzzle-like lobulation, a rich infiltrate of TdT-positive immature T cells, and the presence of interdigitating cell processes on electron microscopy. SETTLE is difficult to distinguish from synovial sarcoma, although the presence of t (X;18) translocation with *SYT/SSX* gene fusion may be of assistance in this distinction.

Somatic genetics
Study on one case has revealed somatic mutations in the *K-RAS* gene, but no mutations in the *TP53* gene {2429}.

Prognosis and predictive factors
SETTLE is a slow growing tumour, but the overall metastatic rate is over 60% with long-term follow-up {366}. Metastatic disease, nevertheless, can still be compatible with long survival after treatment.

Carcinoma showing thymus-like differentiation

W. Cheuk
J. K.C. Chan
D.M. Dorfman
T. Giordano

Definition
Carcinoma showing thymus-like differentiation (CASTLE) is a carcinoma of the thyroid gland with architectural resemblance to thymic epithelial tumours.

ICD-O code   8593/3

Synonyms
Lymphoepithelioma-like carcinoma of the thyroid gland {2030}; intrathyroid epithelial thymoma {1517}; primary thyroid thymoma {82}.

Localization
The great majority of cases occur in the thyroid gland, most commonly the lower poles, but rare cases may arise in the perithyroid soft tissues of the neck.

Epidemiology
CASTLE is a very rare tumour that affects middle-aged adults with a slight female predominance (M:F=1:1.3).

Clinical features
Patients frequently present with a painless mass in the thyroid, followed by symptoms related to tracheal compression and hoarseness. Enlarged metastatic nodes may be found at initial presentation in approximately 30% of patients {344}. The tumour appears as a "cold nodule" on thyroid scan. On ultrasound, the tumour appears hypoechoic, lobulated and heterogeneous. On CT scan, the tumour displays soft tissue density with slight contrast enhancement.

Macroscopy
Grossly, the tumour is fleshy and grey-tan. The interface of the tumour with the thyroid is smooth and well-demarcated.

Tumour spread and staging
CASTLE is locally invasive with early regional lymph node metastasis.

Histopathology
The tumour invades the thyroid in broad fronts. It grows in the form of variably sized smooth-contoured islands and cords, and occasionally jagged islands, accompanied by a moderately cellular desmoplastic stroma. The architecture thus shows a superficial resemblance to the lobulation seen in thymomas and thymic carcinomas. Tumour islands are commonly penetrated by delicate vessels. In contrast to perivascular spaces seen in thymomas, the vessels are surrounded by fibrous stroma often containing plasma cells. The tumour is characterized by squamoid or syncytial-appearing cells with lightly eosinophilic cytoplasm. Nuclei are oval, pale to vesicular, and have small distinct nucleoli. The nuclear atypia is mild to moderate, and the mitotic count averages one to two per 10 HPFs. In some cases, the tumour cells appear spindle shaped or display variable degrees of squamous differentiation in the form of distinct cell borders, intercellular bridges and even focal keratinization. The tumour islands and stroma are infiltrated by variable numbers of small lymphocytes and plasma cells.

Immunohistochemistry
The immunophenotype of CASTLE is identical to that of thymic carcinoma. {171,522,523}. There is no known association with EBV {2030}.

Differential diagnosis
It is important to distinguish CASTLE from undifferentiated thyroid carcinoma, squamous cell carcinoma of the thyroid and metastatic lymphoepithelioma-like carcinoma. In contrast to CASTLE, undifferentiated carcinomas often exhibit frankly invasive or permeative growth, generally more marked cytologic atypia, readily identified mitotic figures and coagulative necrosis. Positive immunostaining for CD5 would support a diagnosis of CASTLE over these tumour types. Follicular dendritic cell sarcoma can also show lobulation and perivascular

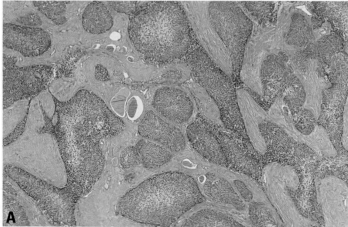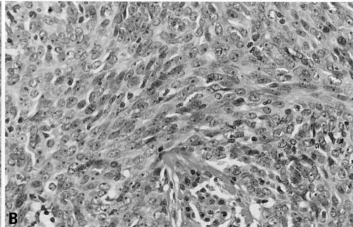

Fig. 2.067 CASTLE of the thyroid gland. **A** Broad anastomosing islands of tumour cells separated by a desmoplastic stroma. **B** Focally, CASTLE may show a spindle cell appearance. Note the pale nuclei and small, distinct nucleoli.

spaces, mimicking CASTLE, but lacks immunoreactivity for cytokeratin and expresses follicular dendritic cell markers {375}.

Histogenesis
CASTLE probably arises from thymic remnants in the thyroid glands, as evidenced by presence of ectopic thymic tissue in the vicinity of the tumour in some cases and CD5 immunoreactivity {1024}.

Prognosis and predictive factors
CASTLE generally pursues a protracted clinical course, although occasional cases may pursue a rapidly fatal course {1518}. There are currently no reliable clinical or histologic factors that can predict the clinical course of the tumour.

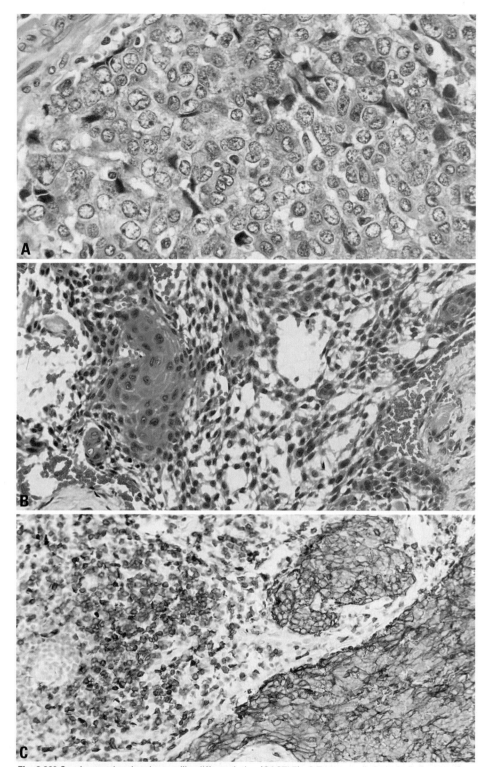

Fig. 2.068 Carcinoma showing thymus-like differentiation (CASTLE). **A** Tumour cells have indistinct borders and moderately atypical nuclei. A few admixed lymphocytes and plasma cells are also present. **B** Occasionally, tumour cells show definite squamous differentiation. **C** Immunostaining for CD5 shows tumour cells exhibiting cell membrane staining (right field). The intermingled T lymphocytes serve as internal positive control.

Follicular adenoma

J.K.C. Chan
M. Hirokawa
H. Evans
E.D. Williams
Y. Osamura
B. Cady

M. Sobrinho-Simões
M. Derwahl
R. Paschke
G. Belge
J. Oriola
H. Studer

C. Eng
S.L. Asa
R.V. Lloyd
Z. Baloch
R. Ghossein
E. Mazzaferri
J.A. Fagin

Definition
A benign, encapsulated tumour of the thyroid showing evidence of follicular cell differentiation.

ICD-O code   8330/0

Epidemiology
The epidemiology of follicular adenoma is difficult to analyse because of the lack of consistent criteria for distinguishing hyperplastic nodules and adenomas. Many do not make the diagnosis of adenoma in a multinodular gland, preferring to regard all of the lesions as nodules providing there is no evidence of malignancy. In a large, pooled analysis of the relationship between benign thyroid disease and the development of thyroid cancer, nodules and adenomas were treated together {647}. The biological basis for separating nodules from adenomas is dependent on their clonality {2228} and up to 60% of lesions in multinodular goiter have been shown to be monoclonal {68,383,835,1169}.
Solitary cold thyroid nodules occur in 4–7% of adults in an iodine sufficient area {1108}; in iodine deficient areas, the incidence of nodules, usually multiple, is related to the level of dietary iodine intake, and can rise to 50% of the population. Females are more commonly affected than males. The rate of progression to malignancy is similar for both solitary cold nodules and multinodular goiter, but although males are less frequent-ly affected, the risk of progression to malignancy in males is relatively greater {157,1454}. Changing incidence of the occurrence of adenoma is related to changes in iodine intake, and in radiation exposure of differing populations.

Etiology
The etiological factors involved in follicular adenomas are largely shared with follicular carcinoma. The association with radiation is better documented than that for follicular carcinoma, and radiation induced adenomas show a very long mean latent period {2047}. Adenomas are common in iodine deficient areas, usually as part of a nodular goiter. They can also occur as part of nodular goiters in Cowden syndrome, and in dyshormonogenesis.

Localization
Follicular adenoma can arise in the normal thyroid gland and in ectopic thyroid tissues (e.g. struma ovarii).

Clinical features
While small follicular adenomas are usually asymptomatic, they may be detected by the patient or may be palpable on careful physical examination. Spontaneous haemorrhage into an adenoma occasionally results in an acute episode of pain and enlargement.

Diagnostic modalities
Follicular adenomas are frequently dis-covered by ultrasound studies. Most follicular adenomas are relatively small, while follicular carcinomas tend to be larger.
Radioactive iodine scans of follicular adenomas generally show hypofunction, while ultrasound demonstrates a solitary solid nodule. These lesions are generally well demarcated by imaging studies. A minority of adenomas are "hot" on scan and are associated with hyperthyroidism.

Macroscopy
Follicular adenoma is usually a solitary, round or oval, nodule surrounded by a thin capsule. The cut surfaces show grey-white, tan or brown fleshy tumour. Generally, those tumours with a grey-white colour have a solid or trabecular growth pattern while tan to brown tumours show evidence of follicle formation with colloid deposition. Secondary changes such as haemorrhage and cystic degeneration may be present. The tumour usually measures 1-3 cm, but can be much larger. Occasionally, follicular adenomas can arise in a background of nodular hyperplasia, and the tumour is distinguishable from the background nodules (colloid or hyperplastic) by the encapsulation and the fleshy appearance.

Tumour spread and staging
Transection of this benign tumour at surgery may rarely be linked to recurrence or implantation in the operative field.

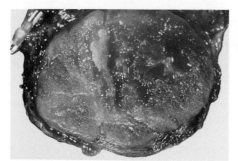
Fig. 2.069 Follicular adenoma. This encapsulated tumour has a bulging cut surface.

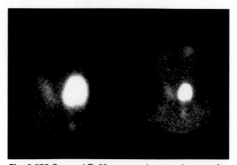
Fig. 2.070 Coronal Tc99m pertechnetate image of a hyperfunctioning thyroid adenoma / nodule.

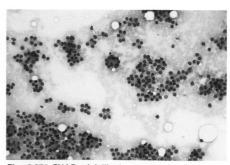
Fig. 2.071 FNAB of follicular adenoma, showing a microfollicular pattern. Histologic examination of the excised lesion confirmed the diagnosis of adenoma.

Cytopathology

Aspirates of follicular adenomas are usually cellular with numerous follicular cells and little or no colloid. Most often, the follicular cells are both dissociated and arranged in syncytial fragments and exhibit a microfollicular pattern. Microfollicles consist of groups of 6-12 nuclei in a small ring sometimes with a central dot of colloid. Macrofollicular adenomas demonstrate abundant colloid with follicular cells arranged in monolayer sheets. This appearance is very similar to that observed in adenomatoid nodules. The distinction of follicular adenomas and carcinomas is not possible in cytologic preparations.

Histopathology

Follicular adenoma is typically enclosed in a fibrous capsule of variable thickness. By definition, capsular or vascular invasion are absent. The architectural pattern and cytologic features are different from those of the surrounding thyroid tissue. The tumour can show a variety of architectural features, most commonly follicular or trabecular. The tumour cells are cuboidal, columnar or polygonal, and often have uniform, dark, round nuclei, although occasional enlarged hyperchromatic nuclei can be present. In the central portion of the tumour, where fixation is often delayed, the nuclei may appear "blown up", large and pale, but fall short of the cytologic criteria for the diagnosis of papillary carcinoma. Mitotic figures are rare. There is usually only scanty stroma, which is richly vascularized by delicate capillaries that may not be obvious in conventional histologic sections. Focal myxoid change may be seen in the subcapsular region. Secondary changes such as stromal oedema, fibrosis, hyalinization, haemorrhage, calcification, cartilaginous metaplasia, cyst formation, and infarction can supervene.

Growth patterns

Follicular adenomas have been referred to as "normofollicular", "macrofollicular" and "microfollicular", reflecting the size of the follicles comprising the tumour. Since a single tumour may show more than one of these architectural patterns, it can be difficult to apply these descriptive designations. Rarely, papillae can be present focally.

Immunohistochemistry

Follicular adenomas are immunoreactive for cytokeratins, thyroglobulin and TTF1, but not CK 19 {1795}, calcitonin or pan-neuroendocrine markers.

Differential diagnosis

The distinction between follicular adenoma and adenomatoid nodule (cellular colloid nodule) is sometimes rather arbitrary. In general, adenomatoid nodules are multiple, lack a well-defined fibrous capsule, and are composed of follicles morphologically similar to those in the surrounding thyroid tissue. The only histologic features which reliably distinguish a follicular carcinoma from a follicular adenoma are the presence of vascular or capsular invasion, underscoring the importance of adequate sampling of any suspicious tumour to search for such features. Capsular invasion should be distinguished from sites of prior fine needle aspiration biopsies which most commonly appear as linear tracts at right angles

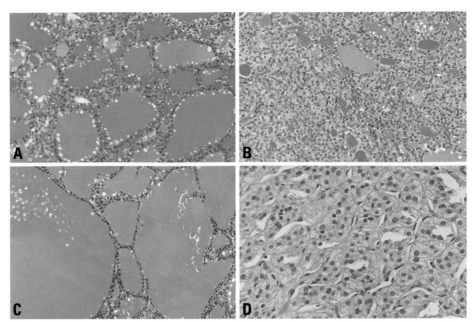

Fig. 2.072 Follicular adenoma of the thyroid. **A** Normofollicular variant, comprising follicles with size similar to that of normal thyroid follicles. **B** Predominant microfollicular architecture. **C** Macrofollicular variant, comprising large follicles distended with colloid, mimicking colloid nodule. **D** Trabecular growth pattern. Tumour cells have finely vacuolated cytoplasm due to the accumulation of liquid deposits.

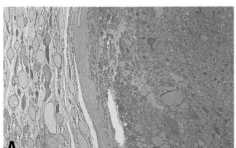
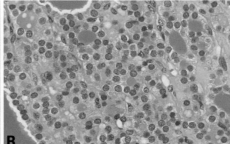
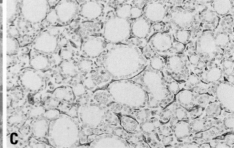

Fig. 2.073 Follicular adenoma. **A** The tumour is completely surrounded by a thin fibrous capsule. **B** Predominant microfollicular pattern; nuclei are round, uniform and non-overlapping. **C** The inconspicuous capillaries between the follicles are highlighted by immunostaining for CD34.

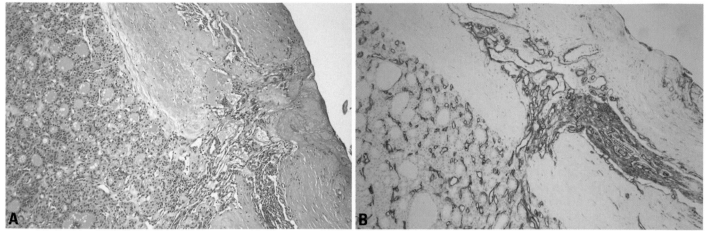

Fig. 2.074 A Follicular adenoma resected following a fine needle aspiration biopsy. There is a capsular defect and the capsular vessels show a marked degree of endothelial cell proliferation. **B** Same case as **A**, immunostained for CD34. The cells within the capsule and capsular vessels are CD34 positive, establishing their endothelial origin.

to the capsule. Vascular endothelial proliferation should be distinguished from sites of vascular invasion, and this can be facilitated by the use of endothelial markers. As a group, the fibrous capsule is often thicker in follicular carcinoma compared with follicular adenoma. Medullary carcinoma should be excluded when a tumour presumed to represent follicular adenoma shows unusual histologic features, such as prominent fibrovascular septa, solid growth, or spindle cells. Parathyroid adenoma arising within the thyroid gland can mimic follicular adenoma of the microfollicular, clear cell or oncocytic type. The cytology (such as presence of water-clear cells) should provide an important clue to the correct diagnosis, which can be further confirmed by positive immunostaining for parathyroid hormone and chromogranin.

Variants

Many histologic variants of follicular adenoma have been recognized. Hyalinizing trabecular tumour is dealt with separately on page 104.

Oncocytic adenoma

These solitary, well-delineated and encapsulated tumours are characterized by a distinct mahogany brown appearance, often with central areas of scarring. They are particularly prone to developing infarction after FNAB but this phenomenon may also occur spontaneously. The tumours are composed of cells with abundant granular eosinophilic cytoplasm and large open nuclei with prominent nucleoli, although rarely the nuclei can be hyperchromatic. Like other follicular adenomas of thyroid, oncocytic follicular adenomas have a variety of architectural patterns ranging from well-formed follicles to solid and/or trabecular growth. Colloid often appears dense and may form structures mimicking psamomma bodies. Focally one can see the formation of papillary structures. Occasionally, there is an almost exclusive papillary architecture. Oncocytic papillary

carcinoma must be excluded and this distinction relies on establishing lack of nuclear criteria for the diagnosis of papillary carcinoma {369}. The distinction from oncocytic follicular carcinoma is based on lack of capsular or vascular invasion {1315}. Adenomatoid oncocytic nodules often occur in association with Hashimoto thyroiditis and are difficult to distinguish from true adenomas. Multiple oncocytic adenomas can occur, particularly in young female patients and are associated with a risk of progression to carcinoma {1052}.

The overall cytological features of oncocytic adenomas are generally similar to follicular adenomas of usual type. The individual cells, however, are large with abundant granular eosiniphilic cytoplasm and large nuclei with prominent nucleoli. They may show prominent anisokaryosis.

Follicular adenoma with papillary hyperplasia

Also known as papillary variant of follicu-

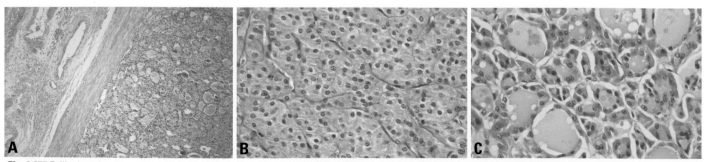

Fig. 2.075 Follicular adenoma, oncocytic type. **A** The tumour is surrounded by a fibrous capsule. Follicular cells have a micro-to-normo- follicular architectural pattern. **B** The tumour cells are arranged in a trabecular pattern. **C** The component cells have deeply eosinophilic, granular cytoplasm.

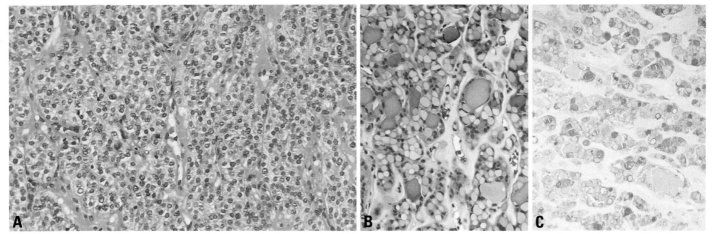

Fig. 2.076 Follicular adenoma of the thyroid. **A** Trabecular/embryonal variant. This tumour shows a solid growth and prominent fibrovascular septa. Medullary carcinoma should be ruled out by the appropriate immunohistochemical tests. **B** Signet ring type. The tumour cells contain large intracellular vacuoles that displace the nuclei to the periphery of the cells. **C** The intracytoplasmic vacuoles are positive for thyroglobulin.

lar adenoma, this subtype is usually encapsulated and partially cystic. It comprises broad or delicate branching papillae as well as follicles, lined by columnar cells with uniform, round and hyperchromatic nuclei, regularly aligned at the base. By definition, nuclear features of papillary thyroid carcinoma should be absent. This tumour occurs predominantly in children and adolescents and may be multiple {588,1386}.

Fetal adenoma
This variant is characterized by a microfollicular/trabecular structure in an oedematous stroma, particularly in the center of the tumour. More than 50% of these tumours are aneuploid {330}.

Signet-ring cell follicular adenoma
This lesion is characterized by signet ring tumour cells with a discrete cytoplasmic vacuole displacing the nucleus to the periphery {40,703,1482,1829}. The vacuoles are immunoreactive for thyroglobulin, and often stain for mucosub-

stances. Ultrastructurally, they represent intracellular lumens lined by microvilli.

Mucinous follicular adenoma
A variant characterized by accumulation of abundant extracellular mucin, often accompanied by a microcystic, reticular or multicystic growth pattern {485}. Typical features of follicular neoplasm are often evident in some areas of the tumour. In addition, there can be signet ring cell change.

Lipoadenoma
This is a follicular adenoma with mature adipose cells interspersed throughout the tumour {895,1200}.

Clear cell follicular adenoma
Ther term refers to the cytoplasmic clearing of the tumour cells which can result from ballooning of mitochondria, accumulation of lipid or glycogen, or deposition of intracellular thyroglobulin {302, 1980,1982,2257}. As in clear cell follicular carcinoma, immunoreactivity for thy-

roglobulin and TTF1 are useful in separating this entity from metastatic renal cell carcinoma.

Toxic (hyperfunctioning) adenoma
This is a follicular adenoma associated with symptoms of hyperthyroidism due to autonomous production of thyroxine. Histologically, the follicles are lined by tall cells, often showing papillary projections within the lumina, similar to the follicles seen in Graves disease. The tumour appears as a "hot" nodule on radioactive iodine scan.

Atypical adenoma
The term "atypical adenoma" has been variably used to refer to follicular neoplasms exhibiting high cellularity, nuclear atypia, or unusual histologic patterns (such as spindle cell fascicles), but lacking vascular and capsular invasion on thorough sampling. Despite the histologically worrisome appearance, this tumour pursues a benign course {851,1229, 1230}. Use of this term is discouraged.

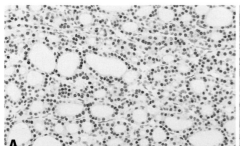 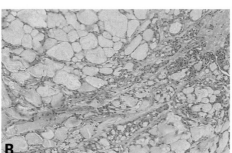 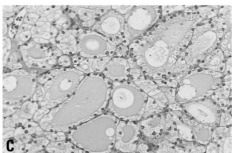

Fig. 2.077 **A** Follicular adenoma of the thyroid. The follicular cells show nuclear labeling for thyroid transcription factor-1 (TTF-1). **B** Mucinous follicular adenoma. Note the presence of abundant extracellular, lightly basophilic mucin. A reticulated pattern is produced. **C** Follicular adenoma with clear cell features.

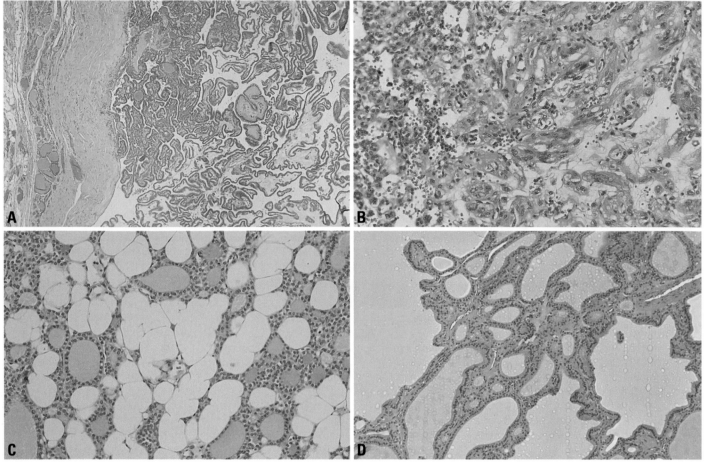

Fig. 2.078 A Follicular adenoma. This encapsulated tumour demonstrates papillary hyperplasia. Some of the papillae show marked stromal edema. **B** Atypical follicular adenoma. This richly vascular tumour is composed predominantly of spindle shaped cells. **C** This adenoma contains stromal fat cells. **D** Toxic adenoma of the thyroid. Many follicles show papillary infoldings, reminiscent of Graves disease.

Follicular adenoma with bizarre nuclei
A variant characterized by the presence of isolated or small groups of monstrous tumour cells with enlarged hyperchromatic nuclei within an otherwise typical follicular adenoma {1862}.

The use of the term *"well differentiated tumour of uncertain malignant potential"* has been suggested for tumours with questionable capsular or vascular invasion {2391}. However, the use of this nomenclature has not been generally accepted. If used at all, this term should be restricted to adequately sampled tumours with real uncertainty about whether the criteria for invasion have been fulfilled {2391}.

Somatic genetics
Cytogenetics and LOH
Clonal cytogenetic aberrations have been detected in about 45% of thyroid adenomas. Trisomy 7 alone or with other

trisomies are the most frequent type of aberrations. Among the structural aberrations translocations involving the long arm of chromosome 19 (19q13) and of the short arm of chromosome 2 (2p21) predominate {159}. Interestingly, both breakpoints have been cloned recently and candidate genes have been identified {158,1839,1840}. An additional small subgroup of thyroid adenomas is characterized by deletions of chromosome 13. There are multiple allelotyping studies in follicular adenomas and a variable range of frequencies of deletions have been found scattered across the genome, especially chromosomes 3p, 10, 13 and 19.

Molecular genetics
The molecular alterations that confer a growth advantage to the adenoma cells are largely unknown {2153}. Mutations of *RAS* genes have been detected in follicular adenomas {1579}, in multinodular

goiters, but not in toxic adenomas {1170}. For the subgroup of hyperfunctioning adenomas and thyroid nodules, mutations in the TSH receptor gene and the gene encoding the α-subunit of stimulatory GTP-binding protein have been described {488,1168}.

The *oncocytic variant* shows frequent chromosomal DNA imbalance, with numerical chromosomal alterations being the dominant feature {2185}. Somatic mutations and sequence variants of mitochondrial DNA (mtDNA) are found in benign as well as malignant oncocytic tumours and even in non-tumourous tissues adjacent to oncocytic neoplasms {1447,2452}. It has been suggested that polymorphisms and large deletions in mtDNA predispose to this cytologic alteration {1447}. Some cases may show *PPARγ* rearrangements.

Genetic susceptibility

The genetic differential diagnosis for follicular adenoma includes Cowden syndrome and Carney complex, the details of which are discussed in Chapter 5 (Inherited Tumour Syndromes).

Prognostic and predictive factors

Provided the adenoma is completely removed, there is no further risk.

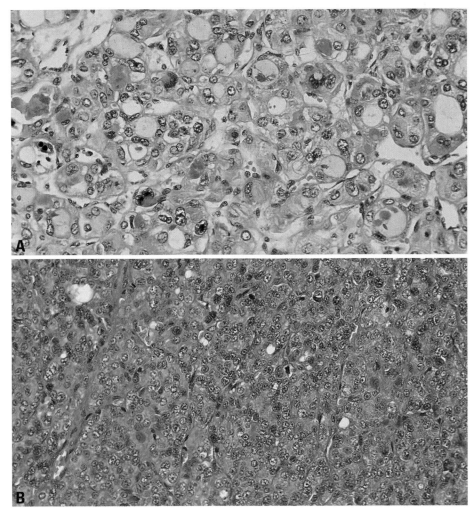

Fig. 2.079 **A** So-called atypical adenoma of the thyroid. Note the significant cytologic atypia. **B** Atypical follicular adenoma. This encapsulated tumour demonstrates high cellularity with generalized, mild nuclear atypia.

Hyalinizing trabecular tumour

J.A. Carney
M. Volante
M. Papotti
S. Asa

Definition
Hyalinizing trabecular tumour (HTT) is a rare tumour of follicular cell origin with a trabecular pattern of growth and marked intratrabecular hyalinization.

ICD-O code 8336/0

Synonyms
Hyalinizing trabecular adenoma, para-ganglioma-like adenoma; hyaline cell tumour with massive accumulation of cytoplasmic microfilaments; hyalinizing trabecular adenoma-like lesion; papillary carcinoma; hyalinizing trabecular variant.

Epidemiology
The tumour is unusual under the age of 30 years and is about equally distributed in the fourth through the seventh decades with a mean age of 47 years. There is a marked female predilection.

Etiology
The etiology of HTT is unknown. The nuclear features of the tumour suggest that it may be related to papillary carcinoma of the thyroid and *RET/PTC* rearrangements described in two studies {367,1687} have bolstered this suggestion. The tumour commonly arises in a background of chronic lymphocytic thyroiditis; it may occur in association with conventional papillary carcinoma or as a component of a multinodular goiter {247, 346}. Several cases have occurred following radiation exposure.

Clinical features
The tumour usually presents as a single asymptomatic mass, detected on examination or, less commonly, by the patient who feels or sees a mass in the neck. A few patients have a diffuse or multinodular thyroid enlargement. Ultrasonography and scintigraphy reveal solid "cold" nodules, with heterogeneity and sometimes hyperechoic spots in the former.

Macroscopy
HTT is usually a single, solid, encapsulated or circumscribed neoplasm of medium size, measuring 2.5 cm or less in diameter. The cut surface is homogeneous, delicately lobulated, with a yellow tinge and occasionally marked with off-white flecks and streaks, and gaping vessels. Gross calcification is rare. Some tumours are microscopic.

Cytopathology
Fine needle aspiration biopsy is often interpreted as papillary carcinoma because of the nuclear features in the tumour. It is less commonly interpreted as medullary carcinoma, the significance of the elongated shape of the tumour cells and the hyaline material being misinterpreted {20,204,247,1322}. Lumpy stromal deposits of basement membrane material constitute an important diagnostic clue {215}.

Histopathology
HTT is a solid epithelial neoplasm that is circumscribed and may be surrounded by a thin capsule. It features a trabecular-alveolar growth pattern of medium to large-sized cells with finely granular, acidophilic, amphophilic or clear cytoplasm, intratrabecular hyaline (PAS-positive basement membrane material), polygonal and fusiform cells, nuclei with prominent grooves and cytoplasmic pseudoinclusions, and small nucleoli, occasional mitoses, round paranuclear cytoplasmic bodies with a slight yellow tinge, and occasional mitotic figures {315,1877}. Calcospherites (psammoma bodies) may be present. The cells are arranged in sinuous or straight trabeculae supported by a delicate fibrovascular stroma. The PAS-positive hyaline material resembles amyloid but amyloid stains are negative. Colloid is scant or absent. The amount of fibrous stroma ranges from minimal to modest. Care must be exercised to distinguish the trabecular-associated hyalinization of the hyalinizing trabecular tumour from the usual often perivascular stromal hyalinization that is a common feature of other thyroid tumours.

Immunohistochemistry
The tumours are thyroglobulin and TTF-1 positive and calcitonin-negative {315}. The majority of tumours have a distinctive cell membrane staining pattern with MIB-1 {891} Discrepant results have been obtained with high molecular weight cytokeratin {892} and cytokeratin 19

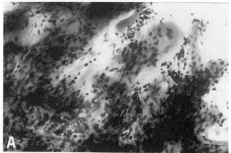
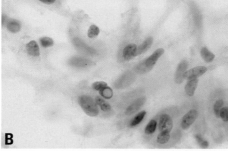

Fig. 2.080 Fine needle aspirate (FNA) of hyalinizing trabecular tumour. **A** Elongated cells associated with abundant hyaline stromal material. **B** A nuclear pseudoinclusion is present.

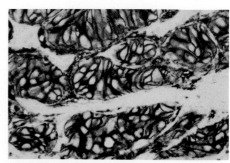

Fig. 2.081 Hyalinizing trabecular tumour with plasma membranes strongly immunoreactive for MIB-1.

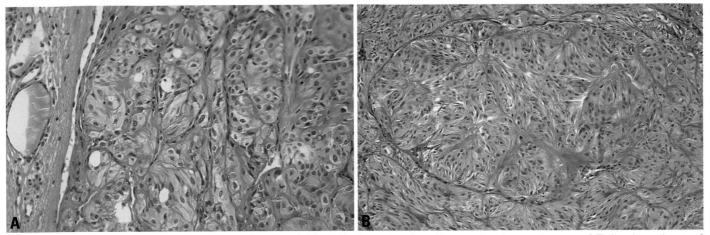

Fig. 2.082 Hyalinizing trabecular tumour. **A** This tumour is surrounded by a thin fibrous capsule and has a trabecular growth pattern. **B** Trabeculae and nests of spindle cells with a prominent hyaline stroma.

{641,892}. Galectin-3 immunoreactivity is expressed in many HTTs {678}.

Electron microscopy

HTT features a population of polymorphic cells, accumulation of extracellular basement membrane material, intracellular intermediate filaments, and lysosomes with "finger-print" pattern {315, 1877,1918}.

Histogenesis

The recognition of *RET/PTC* rearrangements in some of the tumours suggests a relationship with papillary thyroid carcinoma {367,1687}.

Somatic genetics

A close relationship between HTT and papillary thyroid carcinoma (PTC), suggested by peculiar morphological and cytological features, seems to be confirmed by genetic analysis. In fact, two groups of investigators independently reported the presence of *RET/PTC* somatic translocations in HTT, in a per-

centage of cases ranging from 21% (3/14 cases) {1687} to 62% (5/8 cases) {367}. All the positive cases harboured the *RET/PTC1* fusion gene. *H-*, *N-* and *K-RAS* gene mutations were absent in three cases investigated {296}. TP53 protein over-expression was not identified in two cases investigated by immunohistochemistry {1025}.

Genetic susceptibility

There is a single report of HTT in a patient with familial polyposis {1524}, but a causal association remains to be proven.

Prognosis and predictive factors

The great majority of the lesions have behaved as benign neoplasms and should be treated as such. Occasional tumours associated with lymph node metastases have been reported but the precise classification of these cases is controversial {1456,1917}. In view of these observations and the molecular biological evidence of a close relation-

ship to papillary carcinoma, the term "hyalinizing trabecular tumour" is preferred to "hyalinizing trabecular adenoma".

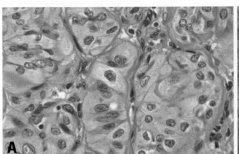
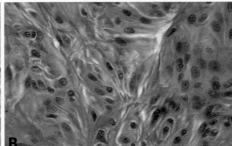
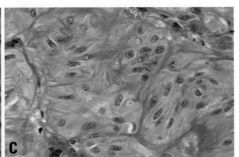

Fig. 2.083 Hyalinizing trabecular tumour. **A** Trabecular growth pattern. Granules are present within the cytoplasm. **B** The nucleus in the center of the field contains a prominent pseudoinclusion. **C** The nuclei are elongated and contain prominent grooves.

Teratoma

L.D.R. Thompson
R.D. Craver

Definition
A neoplasm displaying mature or immature tissues from ectoderm, endoderm, and mesoderm. Tumours of the cervical region are regarded as thyroid teratomas if: (1) the tumour occupies a portion of the thyroid gland; (2) there is direct continuity or close anatomic relationship with the thyroid; and/or (3) a cervical teratoma is accompanied by total absence of the thyroid gland.

ICD-O code   9080/1

Synonyms
Choristoma; hamartoma; heterotopia; epignathus; dermoid.

Epidemiology
There are approximately 300 cases of thyroid teratomas reported, representing less than 0.1% of all benign or malignant primary thyroid gland neoplasms {782, 1012,2199,2230,2486}.The tumours can occur at any age, but the peak is in the newborn {782,1012,2199,2230,2486}. Two distinct groups can be created by separating the neonates and infants from the children and adults: >90% of the tumours in the neonatal group are benign while 50% or more in the adult group are malignant. There is no gender predilection, although malignant teratomas may-occur more frequently in men {2230}.

Localization
Primary thyroid teratomas must involve

Table 2.07
Summary of clinical and pathological features of thymic teratomas. Compiled from publications with >3 cases {110,134,180,405,440}.

Histology	All	Mature	Immature	Malignant
Cases analyzed*	101	56	27	18
Females	55	27	17	12
Males	44	27	11	6
Age range, all	Newborn – 85.0 yrs	Newborn – 72.0 yrs	Newborn – 6.0 yrs	Newborn – 85.0 yrs
Average age, all	9.8 yrs	6.3 yrs	Newborn	31.2 yrs
Neonates and infants	75	44	26	5
Children and adults	26	12	1	13
Tumour size, average (cm)	6.5	5.9	6.2	8.7

*Parameter was not always stated in the report, and therefore the numbers do not necessarily equal the total values in the columns.

the thyroid gland or be in direct continuity with it. Teratomas of the mediastinum and posterior neck are considered separate entities. It is axiomatic that thyroid gland tissue can be present in a teratoma, but a thyroid teratoma is recognized by the presence of thyroid tissue identified at the periphery of the main tumour mass.

Clinical features
Patients present with a mass in the neck, often reaching a significant size. Other congenital anomalies may be present in neonatal patients. In addition, patients may experience dyspnoea and/or stridor. The duration of symptoms ranges from days to years. Tumours associated with symptoms other than a mass (i.e., stridor, hoarseness) are on average larger than those without these symptoms {782, 1012,2199,2230,2486}.

Radiographic images obtained in-utero may identify the thyroid mass. A multicystic mass of the thyroid gland, which may compress the airway, is most frequently identified {257,2230,2279}.

Macroscopy
Average tumour size is 6 cm. The tumours are usually multiloculated, with the cystic spaces containing white-tan creamy material, mucoid material, or dark brown haemorrhagic fluid admixed with necrotic debris. Material resembling brain tissue is frequently noted. Islands of bone and cartilage may also be present {782,1012,2199,2230,2486}.

Tumour spread and staging
Benign (mature or immature) teratomas may cause compression atrophy or in-utero, maldevelopment of the organs of the neck. However, malignant teratomas may invade by direct extension into the surrounding tissues. Local recurrence associated with metastatic disease to the regional lymph nodes, followed by metastatic disease to the lungs is the usual course of the malignant tumours. Staging is not usually applied since the local effect is more prognostically significant than other features {257,427,501, 1261,2230,2279}.

Cytopathology
FNAB will demonstrate various cellular components, often misinterpreted as contamination or a "missed" lesion. In

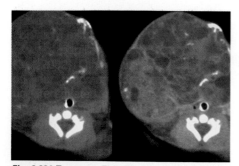

Fig. 2.084 Teratoma. This CT scan demonstrates a large multicystic neoplasm in the anterior neck that completely replaces the thyroid.

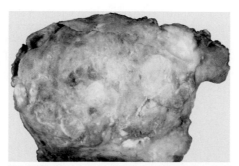

Fig. 2.085 Mature thyroid teratoma. The tumour has a multinodular appearance and completely replaces the thyroid gland.

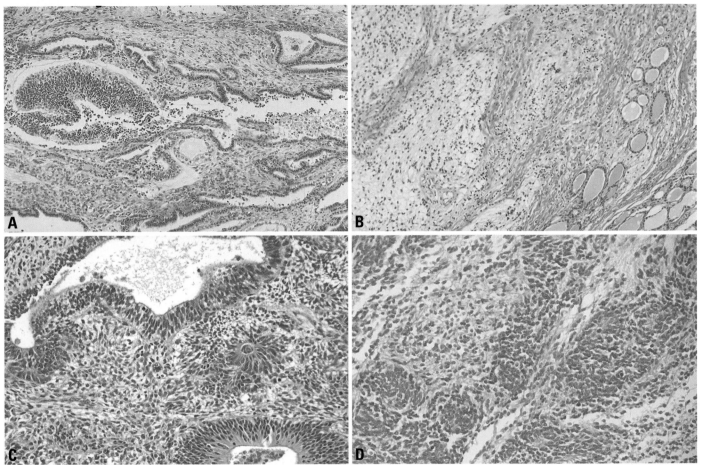

Fig. 2.086 Teratomas. **A** This tumour includes retinal anlage epithelium in addition to epithelial and mesenchymal elements. **B** Benign teratoma. Thyroid follicular epithelium (right corner) is present adjacent to areas of benign neural tissue. **C** Benign immature (grade 2) teratoma, with immature neuroectodermal tissue arranged in Flexner-Wintersteiner rosettes. **D** Malignant teratoma (grade 3). Focus of immature neuroectodermal cells with occasional pseudorosettes.

malignant teratomas, the FNAB smears will show a "neuroepithelial" small-round-blue cell appearance when taken from the immature/malignant neural elements. These cells are frequently interpreted as "malignant cells" {257,2230,2279}.

Histopathology
Characteristically, these tumours display a wide array of tissue types and growth patterns, as seen in other teratomas. Small cystic spaces may be lined by squamous, pseudostratified ciliated columnar, cuboidal, glandular, or transitional epithelia. Neuroblasic elements often arranged in sheets or rosette-like structures are characterized by small to medium-sized cells with dense hyperchromatic nuclei and mitoses. The maturation of the neural-type tissue determines the grade: completely mature (Grade 0), predominantly mature (Grades 1 and 2), and exclusively imma-

ture (Grade 3 or malignant). Cartilage, bone, striated skeletal muscle, smooth muscle, adipose tissue, and loose myxoid to fibrous embryonic mesenchymal connective tissue are admixed with the neural and epithelial elements {257,427, 501,1261,2230,2279}.

Immunohistochemistry
Immunohistochemistry for S-100 protein, glial fibrillary acidic protein, neuron specific enolase, neurofilament and myo-D1 may be of value for the characterization of the various immature elements {1261, 2230}.

Differential diagnosis
Entities to be considered in the differential diagnosis clinically in the neonate, include cystic lymphangioma (cystic hygroma), thyroglossal ductal cyst, and branchial cleft cyst, all of which are easily recognizable at the microscopic level.

Histologically, immature and malignant teratomas largely comprised of neural tissue need to be distinguished from extraskeletal Ewing sarcoma/primitive neuroectodermal tumour, small cell carcinoma, malignant lymphoma, and other malignant small cell tumours {22}. The diagnosis of teratoma under these circumstances is largely dependent on the identification of other tissue elements, the immature/malignant neural tissues, and a confirmatory immunohistochemical panel {22,427,2230,2279}.

Grading
Benign, immature, and malignant teratomas are graded based on the presence of immature neuroectodermal tissues. Mature teratomas contain only mature elements (Grade 0). Benign, immature teratomas with a limited degree of immaturity (embryonal-type tissue in only 1 low-power field, Grade 1) while also

encompassing tumours with >1 but <4 low-power fields of immature foci (Grade 2). Malignant tumours contain >4 low-power fields of immature tissue, along with mitoses and cellular atypia (Grade 3) {2230}. The presence of embryonal carcinoma or yolk sac tumour would place a teratoma into the malignant category (Grade 3) by definition {782,1012,2199, 2230,2486}.

Histogenesis
Teratomas are thought to arise from misplaced embryonic germ cells.

Prognosis and predictive factors
The outcome for thyroid teratomas is dependent largely on the age of the patient, the size of the tumour at the time of presentation, and the presence and proportion of immature elements. Among

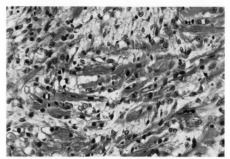
Fig. 2.087 Malignant teratoma (grade 3). This tumour has areas of rhabdomyosarcomatous differentiation.

neonates and infants, there is a preponderance of immature (Grade 1 or 2 immaturity) over mature teratomas and a near absence of malignant behaviour. Conversely, among children and adults there is a preponderance of malignant teratomas (Grade 3), with recurrence and dissemination occurring in up to 30% of cases. Thyroid teratomas in infants can cause significant morbidity, despite their favourable histology because of respiratory distress or the presence of associated malformation of vital structures in the neck {1145,2230}.

Primary lymphoma and plasmacytoma

S. Abbondanzo
K. Aozasa
S. Boerner
L.D.R. Thompson

Lymphoma

Definition
Primary lymphoma arising within the thyroid.

ICD-O code   [type specific]

Synonyms
The recent WHO classification of tumours of haematopoietic and lymphoid tissues is now generally accepted {989}.

Epidemiology
Primary thyroid gland lymphomas are uncommon and have been estimated to represent approximately 5% of all thyroid tumours {2117} and 2.5-7% of all extranodal lymphomas {65,654, 884,1706}. They occur predominantly in older individuals (mean age, 65 years) with a female to male ratio of 3-7:1.

Etiology
Most cases of extranodal marginal zone B cell lymphoma of the thyroid gland are associated with chronic lymphocytic thyroiditis {487}. It has been postulated that lymphomas arise in the setting of acquired mucosa-associated lymphoid tissue (MALT) as a result of an autoimmune or inflammatory process. Patients with Hashimoto thyroiditis have a strikingly higher incidence of thyroid lymphoma when compared to sex and age-matched healthy individuals.

Localization
Primary thyroid lymphomas should be distinguished from lymphomas which arise elsewhere in the neck or mediastinum with secondary involvement of the thyroid gland. However, in patients with very large tumours, this distinction may be impossible. Hodgkin lymphoma involving the thyroid is almost always by direct extension from a lymph node or thymic mass.

Clinical features
Presenting symptoms include pain, dyspnoea, dysphagia, hoarseness, choking, coughing and hemoptysis. Because of the association with Hashimoto's thyroiditis, patients may present with hypothyroidism. Patients may rarely present with hyperthyroidism {1921}. Areas of lymphomatous involvement are usually "cold" with ^{131}I scan {60,61,487,702, 1706,1752,2065}.

Macroscopy
There is a wide variation in tumour size, ranging up to 20 cm in maximum dimension. Tumours may involve one or both lobes of the thyroid gland and have variable features, including a soft or firm consistency, lobulation, multinodularity or diffuse effacement of the normal thyroid architecture, with solid and cystic areas. The cut surfaces are smooth or slightly bulging, pale tan, white-grey or red with a "fish-flesh" appearance. There may be a uniformly homogeneous or mottled appearance. Foci of haemorrhage or necrosis may be noted in large tumours. Extension into adjacent adipose tissue or skeletal muscle is common.

Tumour spread and staging
The majority of patients with thyroid lymphoma present with Stage IE (extranodal) or IIE disease. In disseminated cases, the most frequently involved sites are cervical or perithyroidal lymph nodes, followed by mediastinal and abdominal lymph nodes. Other sites of involvement include bone marrow, gastrointestinal tract, lung, bladder and liver. Patients who present with diffuse large B-cell lymphoma of the thyroid are much more likely to have Stage IIIE or IVE disease {487}.

Cytopathology
Aspirates from large cell lymphomas are typically hypercellular with non-cohesive cells showing cytological features similar to those of large cell lymphomas in other sites. Marginal zone lymphomas typically contain admixtures of small atypical lymphocytes, centrocytes, monocytoid B-cells, immunoblasts and plasma cells. Because of this admixture of cell types, the distinction of a marginal zone lymphoma from a reactive process may be impossible in cytological preparations, and molecular studies are usually required to establish or definitive diagnosis.

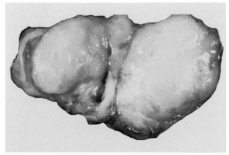

Fig. 2.088 Malignant lymphoma with a characteristic fish-flesh appearance.

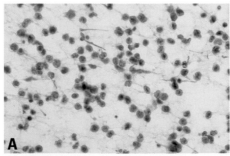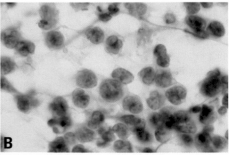

Fig. 2.089 FNA of large cell lymphoma. **A** The tumor cells are loosely cohesive. **B** The cells have large vesicular nuclei and prominent nucleoli.

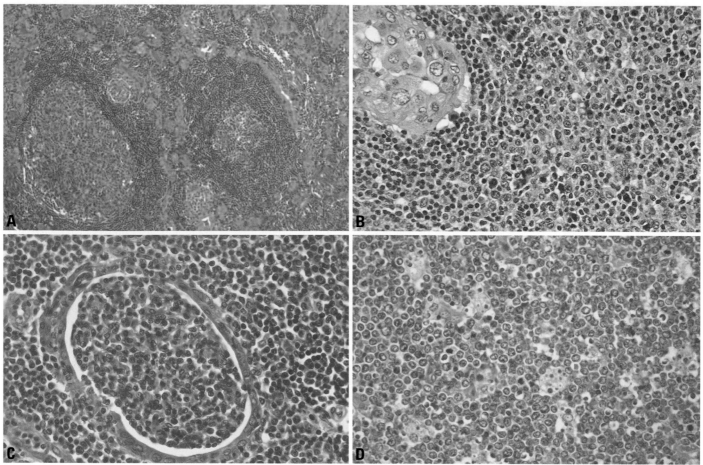

Fig. 2.090 **A** Lymphocytic thyroiditis, characterized by the presence of well formed follicles. **B** This marginal zone lymphoma is composed of monocytoid B-cells, centrocyte-like cells and immunoblasts. A focus of papillary carcinoma is present on the left. **C** Neoplastic lymphocytes are present within this thyroid follicle. **D** Malignant lymphoma. This high grade lymphoma has a 'Burkitt-like' pattern. Numerous tingible body macrophages are present.

Histopathology

The lymphomas of the thyroid include extranodal marginal zone B-cell lymphoma (EMZBCL), and diffuse large B-cell lymphoma (DLBCL) with areas of transition between the two types. Other types of lymphoma, specifically follicular lymphoma, have been described, but are rare {2225}. Lymphomas of the thyroid gland occur in the setting of chronic lymphocytic thyroiditis in almost all cases. In cases of EMZBCL, there is a vaguely nodular to diffuse heterogeneous B-cell infiltrate that is comprised of atypical small lymphocytes, centrocyte-like (cleaved) cells, monocytoid B-cells, scattered large immunoblasts and plasma cells. Reactive germinal centres, which often exhibit colonization by neoplastic cells, are invariably present. Lymphoepithelial lesions, which represent infiltration of thyroid follicles by neoplastic B cells, are frequent features. In thyroid EMZBCL, the lymphoepithelial lesions may have a distinctive appearance as rounded balls or masses, filling and distending the lumen of the thyroid follicle ("MALT balls"). Immunostains for cytokeratins are particularly helpful in demonstrating the infiltration of follicles by the lymphoma cells. Plasma cells and plasmacytoid cells with Dutcher bodies or cytoplasmic immunoglobulin are also seen. Perithyroidal extension may be present in approximately half of the cases. There may be single or multifocal foci of large cell transformation adjacent to the low-grade component. Areas of diffuse large B-cell lymphoma (DLBCL) may occur in the absence of any recognizable low-grade areas. The large cells demonstrate a spectrum of cytologic features that resemble centroblasts, immunoblasts, monocytoid B cells and plasmacytoid cells. Some thyroid lymphomas may represent Burkitt-like tumours with brisk mitotic activity, apoptosis and a starry sky pattern. Atrophy of residual thyroid parenchyma and fibrosis are often noted. The adjacent uninvolved thyroid parenchyma may contain adenomatoid nodules, adenomas or foci of carcinoma {63,360}.

Immunohistochemistry

The B cell immunophenotype of EMZBCL and DLBCL are confirmed by immunoreactivity for CD20 and/or CD79a. Bcl-2 reactivity in the neoplastic, colonizing B cells (but not in the residual, reactive germinal centre cells) is also characteristic. Immunoglobulin light chain restriction for either may be demonstrated, especially in the plasma cell or plasmacytoid component. Co-expression of CD43 with CD20 may be seen in a small percentage of EMZBCL. An antibody to cytokeratin may be useful to highlight the epithelial remnants in the lymphoepithelial lesions.

Differential diagnosis

The distinction between EMZBCL and

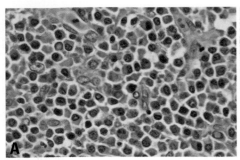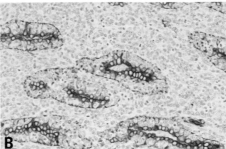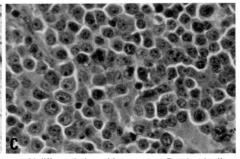

Fig. 2.091 Malignant lymphoma of the thyroid gland. **A** This marginal zone lymphoma shows extensive plasmacytoid differentiation with numerous Dutcher bodies. **B** Malignant lymphoma immunostained for cytokeratin. There is extensive infiltration of the residual thyroid follicles by tumour cells. **C** Plasmacytoid cells are present in this diffuse large cel lymphoma.

lymphocytic thyroiditis may be difficult at times. Although histologic evaluation remains the gold standard for diagnosis, immunohistochemical, flow cytometric or molecular genetic analyses may be required {2177,2178,2444}. Extranodal marginal zone lymphoma with prominent nodularity may simulate a follicular lymphoma (FL). It is necessary, therefore, to distinguish the reactive, colonized germinal centres in EMZBCL from the neoplastic germinal centres in FL. The majority of cases of FL will show immunoreactivity for bcl-2 and will express the germinal centre cell markers CD10 and bcl-6. Diffuse large B cell lymphoma may be indistinguishable from carcinoma (primary undifferentiated carcinoma of thyroid origin), metastatic carcinoma, melanoma or myeloid sarcoma by histology alone. An antibody-screening panel, including CD45RB, CD20, cytokeratin, S-100 protein, HMB-45 and myelomonocytic markers is essential to make the correct diagnosis.

Precursor lesions
Chronic lymphocytic thyroiditis is almost certainly a prerequisite for the development of lymphoma in the thyroid gland. The few cases that do not have docu-

mented lymphocytic thyroiditis may have been inadequately sampled or may have had complete obliteration of the thyroid architecture by the lymphomatous infiltrate. Atrophy of the residual thyroid parenchyma and fibrosis support the chronicity of the underlying process that is associated with the subsequent development of lymphoma.

Postulated cell of origin
The cell of origin of EMZBCL is the post germinal center marginal zone B-cell while peripheral B-cells of either germinal center or post germinal center origin are thought to give rise to diffuse large B-cell lymphomas (DLBCL)

Somatic genetics
The cytogenetic and molecular genetic features of extranodal marginal zone B-cell lymphoma (EMZBCL), of the thyroid gland have not been as extensively reported as those arising in other sites {1120}. Clonal rearrangement of the heavy chain variable region {1514} and Fas gene mutations have been reported in thyroid lymphomas {2175}, as well as monoclonal rearrangements of the immunoglobulin heavy chain gene {2177,2178,2444}.

Prognosis and predictive factors
The prognosis of thyroid MALT type lymphomas is very favorable in general, although it is dependent on clinical stage and histology. Tumours that are localized (Stage IE) at the time of presentation and demonstrate purely low grade histology have an excellent prognosis. Patients whose tumours have either a large cell component or are composed of large B-cells, have a significantly poorer prognosis. Prognostic features associated with a poor prognosis include perithyroidal extension, vascular invasion, high mitotic rate and apoptosis {64,487,884,2401}.

Plasmacytoma

Plasmacytomas are rare in the thyroid, and it has been suggested that these lesions may represent a MALT type lymphoma with prominent plasma cell differentiation. Complete correlation of clinical, laboratory, radiologic and pathologic features, is therefore, important to document the localized or systemic nature of the neoplasm and to determine the treatment options.

Ectopic thymoma

J. K.C. Chan
W. Cheuk
D.M. Dorfman
T. Giordano

Definition
An organotypic thymic epithelial tumour occurring within the thyroid.

ICD-O code
8580/1

Epidemiology
Ectopic thymoma only rarely occurs within the thyroid gland {344,1187,1288, 1419,1635,1841}. Most patients are middle-aged, with a strong female predominance.

Clinical features
Patients typically present with a neck mass of a few months to several years in duration, with or without compressive symptoms. Paraneoplastic syndromes such as myasthenia gravis, have not been reported to date. Thyroid scan reveals a "cold" nodule, and thyroid function tests are normal.

Macroscopy
Almost all reported cases of ectopic thymoma in the thyroid have been non-invasive. The cut surface shows lobulated yellowish-tan tumour tissue interspersed with whitish fibrous septa {344}.

Tumour spread and staging
Ectopic thymoma of the thyroid gland is predominantly a localized tumour.

Histopathology
Ectopic thymoma displays the same repertoire of histologic subtypes as found in mediastinal thymoma. Residual ectopic thymus tissue may be identified in the periphery in some cases {1841}. Epithelium-rich thymomas have to be distinguished from undifferentiated carcinoma and squamous cell carcinomas, while lymphocyte-rich tumours may be potentially mistaken for lymphoma.

Somatic genetics
Not known for ectopic thymoma of the thyroid. Epstein-Barr virus (EBV) is negative {1187}.

Histogenesis
Thyroid thymoma is believed to arise from thymic remnants entrapped in the thyroid gland {1841}. The thymic and third branchial pouch remnants have been postulated to give rise to a spectrum of neoplasms that retain the potential for thymic differentiation to variable extent {344}, including four clinicopathologically distinct entities: ectopic thymoma, ectopic hamartomatous thymoma, spindle cell tumour with thymus-like differentiation (SETTLE) and carcinoma showing thymus-like differentiation (CASTLE). All except ectopic hamartomatous thymoma can occur in the thyroid gland.

Prognosis and prognostic factors
Thyroid thymoma usually does not recur after surgical excision. To date, only one reported case of thyroid thymoma has been complicated by cervical lymph node metastasis, which occurred one year after diagnosis {1187}. There are no established prognostic factors.

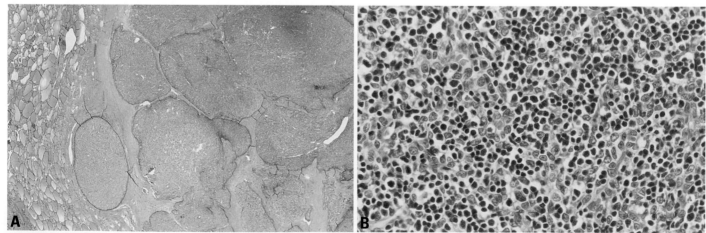

Fig. 2.092 Ectopic thymoma. **A** The tumour is composed of sheets of tumour cells in a jigsaw puzzle-like arrangement. **B** There is an intimate admixture of neoplastic epithelial cells and small lymphocytes.

Angiosarcoma

V. Eusebi

Definition
A malignant tumour, primary in the thyroid showing evidence of endothelial cell differentiation.

ICD-O code   9120/3

Synonyms
Malignant hemangioendothelioma

Epidemiology
Angiosarcomas of thyroid were originally reported in Alpine countries of central Europe, and were linked to dietary iodine deficiency. In Switzerland they accounted for 4.3% of all thyroid tumours during the period 1962-1973 {855}. This view has been challenged by cases occurring in flatland areas or seaside regions, suggesting that other as yet unknown factors may be involved in the pathogenesis of these tumours. The fact that angiosarcomas are not exclusive to mountainous areas is shown by cases reported in Hong Kong {348}, Northern France {1780}, the United Kingdom {152} and the United States {583}. In one Italian Institute of Pathology that reviews cases from non-mountainous areas, the percentage of angiosarcomas was 2.3% of all malignant thyroid tumours (excluding lymphomas) between 1990-1994 {1387}. Thyroid angiosarcomas manifest as a "cold" nodule in elderly patients with a mean age in the 7th decade {1387,1689} and a female to male ratio of 4.5:1 {1689}. Thyroid angiosarcomas develop

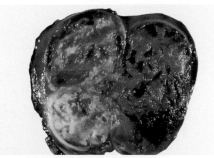

Fig. 2.093 Angiosarcoma. The tumour is surrounded by fibrous pseudocapsule. The central portion of the tumour is hemorrhagic and necrotic.

most often in longstanding nodular goiters which may, when cystic, be misdiagnosed by FNAB {1387}.

Etiology
Iodine deficiency has been suggested as a possible etiological factor.

Clinical features
With the exception of occasional cases that manifest first with signs of metastasis, the tumour presents with pain or pressure symptoms {1222} or with a rapidly growing painless nodule {2193}.

Macroscopy
Tumours often appear circumscribed but are invariably invasive. The cut surface is variegated, with cystic and solid areas. Haemorrhage is usually present within cysts and the solid areas are often necrotic. The size ranges from 3-10 cm {1387,2193}. Occasional cases are extensively invasive with direct involvement of the tracheal wall and surrounding tissues {583}.

Cytopathology
FNAB smears consisting of necrotic material with occasional large neoplastic cells with abundant cytoplasm and round central nuclei are seen. Care must be taken to exclude metastases and undifferentiated thyroid carcinomas.

Histopathology
Thyroid angiosarcomas are similar to those of corresponding tumours in soft tissues. Solid areas show extensive necrosis surrounded by a rim of neoplastic tissue. Anastomosing channels with papillary fronds lined by endothelial cells are regularly found. Solid areas are frequent and simulate undifferentiated and poorly differentiated carcinomas. Thyroid angiosarcomas are frequently epithelioid. The neoplastic cells have abundant eosinophilic cytoplasm with round, vesicular nuclei with well defined nuclear membranes and prominent, eosinophilic nucleoli. Occasional binucleated forms are present, but multinucleated giant

cells are very rare. Numerous mitoses.

Immunohistochemistry
Thyroid angiosarcomas are positive for Factor VIIIR-Ag, Ulex Europeus, CD34, and CD31 {542,583,1387,1733,2193}, and are variably positive for low molecular weight keratins {583,1387}. Angiosarcomas analyzed for thyroglobulin mRNA expression by in situ hybridization have been negative {1689}.

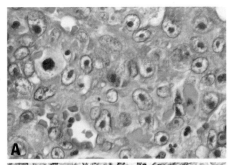
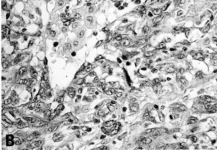
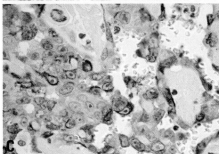

Fig. 2.094 Angiosarcoma of the thyroid gland. **A** The tumour cells have large vesicular nuclei with prominent eosinophilic nucleoli. **B** Many tumour cells are positively stained for CD31. **C** Angiosarcoma immunostained for cytokeratins (CAM 5.2). There are numerous positive cells.

Electron microscopy

Ultrastructurally, single membrane-bound rod-shaped cytoplasmic structures, reminiscent of Weibel-Palade bodies, have been identified {583,1387, 2193}. Occasional intracytoplasmic lumina may also be seen.

Differential diagnosis

This includes undifferentiated, poorly differentiated and metastatic carcinoma as well as endothelial hyperplasia in nodular goiters which has undergone degenerative changes {1938}.

Histogenesis

A debate on the nature of this type of thyroid tumour has been going on for more than two decades. Some pathologists have been sceptical of the existence of this neoplasm, believing that most of the cases reported as angiosarcoma were in reality anaplastic carcinomas with angiomatoid features {1503}. At present we feel that this view is no longer tenable since the histological, immunohistochemical, ultrastructural and molecular evidence is overwhelmingly in favour of the endothelial nature of these tumours.

The hypothesis that there are malignant tumours exhibiting dual differentiation toward endothelial and epithelial cells has been proposed {542,1502}. We feel that this occurrence is difficult to discard; nevertheless, this phenomenon must be very rare and it is not present in most of the cases reported in the literature and/or seen by us.

Prognosis and predictive factors

Most patients die from tumour in less than six months {548,1198} regardless of the treatment, with a few surviving up to 5 years {583,1198,1222,1387}. Entirely intrathyroid tumours generally have a longer survival than those with extrathyroidal extension.

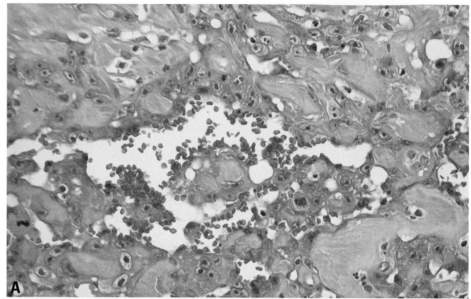
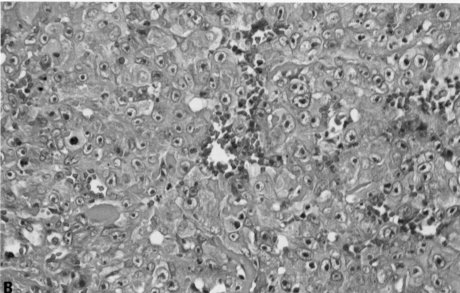

Fig. 2.095 Angiosarcoma. **A** Papillary fronds of tumour are present within the vascular lumina. **B** This area of tumour is composed of solid cells sheets with large vesicular nuclei containing prominent central nucleoli. A few dilated vascular channels are also present.

Smooth muscle tumours

L.D.R. Thompson

Definition
A benign or malignant tumour derived from or showing evidence of differentiation towards smooth muscle.

ICD-O code
Leiomyoma	8890/0
Leiomyosarcoma	8890/3

Epidemiology
Primary smooth muscle tumours of the thyroid gland are exceedingly rare {57,187,362, 1056,2272}.

Etiology
There is no known etiology, although a single case of an Epstein-Barr virus-associated thyroid smooth muscle tumour has been reported in a child with a congenital immunodeficiency disease {2232,2272}.

Localization
The smooth muscle-walled vessels at the periphery of the gland (thyroid gland capsule) may account for the frequent peripheral localization of the tumour {2232}.

Clinical features
In contrast to their benign counterparts, primary thyroid leiomyosarcomas tend to occur in older patients, with both demonstrating a roughly equal gender predilection. Patients have non-specific signs and symptoms. Radiographic studies, specifically CT, will help to identify the extent of disease {2180,2232}.

Macroscopy
The tumours range in size up to 12 cm in greatest dimension, while leiomyomas tend to be smaller {57,187,362,1056, 2180,2232}.

Tumour spread and staging
Staging is not usually applied since the local effect is more prognostically significant than other features.

Histopathology
The tumour cells are arranged in bundles or fascicles of smooth muscle fibers, intersecting in an orderly fashion. The tumour cells are spindled, with blunt ended cigar-shaped, slightly hyperchromatic nuclei occupying a central location within the cytoplasm. Occasional cytoplasmic vacuoles can be seen adjacent to the nucleus. In malignant cases, capsular invasion, vascular invasion, haemorrhage, necrosis, nuclear pleomorphism and increased mitotic figures (including atypical forms) can be seen. Entrapment of normal thyroid follicles is seen frequently at the periphery of the tumour.

Immunohistochemistry
The tumour cells are immunoreactive for vimentin, smooth muscle actin, muscle specific actin, and desmin and non-reactive for thyroglobulin, cytokeratin, chromogranin, and calcitonin {362,1056, 2232}.

Differrential diagnosis
This includes solitary fibrous tumour, SETTLE, thyroid undifferentiated carcinoma, and other sarcomas {303,1493,1653, 2232}. Undifferentiated thyroid carcinoma usually occurs in older patients who have a long-standing history of a pre-existing thyroid lesion with recent rapid enlargement. This tumour does not express desmin or actins {1056,1258, 1493,1653,2232}.

Histogenesis
The neoplasms probably arise from the smooth muscle-walled vessels in the capsule of the thyroid gland {1056,2232}.

Prognosis and predictive factors
Leiomyomas are curable by excision whereas leiomyosarcomas are associated with a poor clinical outcome.

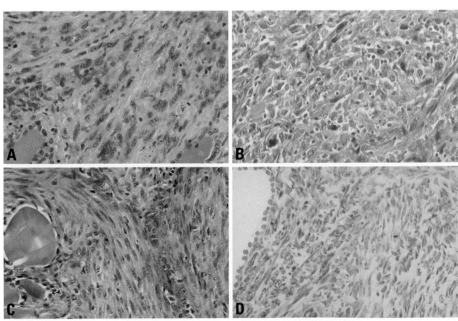

Fig. 2.096 Leiomyosarcoma. **A** The tumour is composed of spindle shaped cells with hyperchromatic nuclei. Normal follicles are present in the lower portion of the field. **B** The tumour cells exhibit considerable nuclear pleomorphism. **C** Spindle shaped tumour cells infiltrate the adjacent thyroid parenchyma. **D** Leiomyosarcoma immunostained for smooth muscle actin. The tumour cells are positively stained while the adjacent follicle (left) is negative.

Peripheral nerve sheath tumours

L.D.R. Thompson

Definition
A benign (schwannoma) or malignant neoplasm (malignant peripheral nerve sheath tumour, MPNST) arising from peripheral nerves or displaying differentiation towards Schwann or perineurial cells.

ICD-O code
Schwannoma	9560/0
MPNST	9540/3

Epidemiology
Neurogenic tumours of the thyroid gland are exceedingly rare but have been reported in all ages without a known gender predilection {24,57,793,2159,2231}.

Localization
Association with medium to large nerves at the periphery of the gland (thyroid gland capsule) has been shown {2231}.

Clinical features
Patients present with non-specific signs and symptoms. CT images show an inhomogeneous, low-density mass, showing compression of the upper airway, infiltration into the soft tissues or destruction of the thyroid gland in MPNST {24,2159,2231}.

Macroscopy
The tumours range in size up to 7 cm in greatest dimension. The tumours are tan to white and glistening with a "neural" appearance {24,57,793,2159,2231}.

Tumour spread and staging
Staging is not usually applied since the local effect is more prognostically significant than other features.

Histopathology
Schwannomas and MPNSTs are identical in appearance to those occuring in other anatomic sites {24,57,793,2159, 2231}. The tumour cells are immunoreactive with S100 protein and vimentin, while non-reactive for thyroglobulin, TTF-1, cytokeratin, chromogranin, smooth muscle actin, muscle specific actin, and

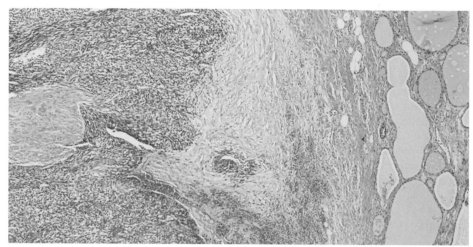

Fig. 2.097 Malignant peripheral nerve sheath tumour (MPNST). The tumour infiltrates the adjacent thyroid tissue.

desmin {24,57,2159,2231}. Cytological features are similar to schwannoma and MPNST in other sites {996,2231}.

Benign PNSTs are usually sufficiently well developed to be accurately diagnosed on hematoxylin and eosin stained slides alone. However, MPNSTs mimic undifferentiated thyroid carcinoma and other sarcomas, whether primary or secondary. Therefore, a primary MPNST of the thyroid should only be diagnosed when there is no direct extension from a perithyroidal neoplasm, there is complete absence of all epithelial and thyroid differentiation and there is definite evidence of specific Schwann cell derivation histologically, immunophenotypically and/or ultrastructurally {24,36,303,2159, 2231,2231}.

Histogenesis
The postulated origin includes the sympathetic and parasympathetic innervation of the thyroid (cervical plexus) or the sensory nerves {531,2231}.

Prognosis and predictive factors
Schwannomas are curable by surgical excision whereas primary MPNST of the thyroid is associated with a poor clinical outcome {24,2231}.

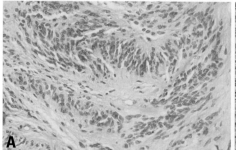
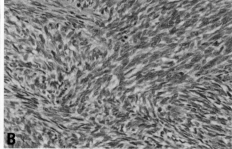

Fig. 2.098 A Schwannoma. This tumour demonstrates a typical Verocay body. B Malignant peripheral nerve sheath tumour (MPNST). Spindle shaped tumour cells are arranged in a fascicular pattern.

Paraganglioma

R. A. DeLellis

Definition
An intrathyroidal neuroendocrine tumour of paraganglionic origin.

ICD-O code   8693/1

Epidemiology
Thyroid paragangliomas are rare tumours, with approximately 15 well documented cases reported in the literature {1201}. All cases have occurred in females with a mean age of 48 years (range 9-73 years).

Clinical
Most patients present with an asymptomatic neck mass.

Macroscopy
Intrathyroidal paraganglioma is typically circumscribed or encapsulated and is gray-tan to brown in color. The mean tumour size is 3 cm (range, 1.5-10 cm).

Tumour spread and Staging
While most paragangliomas are confined to the thyroid, occasional tumours may extend into the trachea or larynx. One case extended into the mediastinum. There have been no cases with documented metastatic spread.

Cytopathology
The cytopathological features of a single case of thyroid paraganglioma have been reported {2326}. Aspirates showed single cells and loose clusters of large cells with ovoid nuclei, focally discrete nucleoli, moderate anisocytosis and anisonucleosis. A few cells with irregular nuclei and coarse chromatin were also present.

Histopathology
Thyroid paragangliomas are similar to parasympathetic paragangliomas at other sites. The tumours typically show a lobular or nesting (Zellballen) growth pattern with occasional areas of anastomosing cell cords or diffuse sheet like patterns of growth. Lobules and nests are separated by fibrovascular connective tissue. Tumours are composed of a mixture of chief cells and sustentacular cells. The chief cells are polygonal, with finely granular amphophilic cytoplasm. The nuclei are round to ovoid with finely granular chromatin and generally small nucleoli. Occasional cells with enlarged hyperchromatic nuclei may be present. A second population of elongated sustentacular cells with deeply eosinophilic cytoplasm is present at the periphery of the nests or intermingled with the chief cells. The mitotic rate is low.

Immunohistochemistry
The chief cells are typically positive for neuron specific enolase, synaptophysin and chromogranin, while stains for cytokeratins, EMA, thyroglobulin, calcitonin, calcitonin gene related peptide, serotonin and vimentin are negative. Sustentacular cells are positive for S-100 .protein.

Differential diagnosis
The differential diagnosis includes medullary thyroid carcinoma, hyalinizing trabecular tumour and metastatic carcinoid tumour. Medullary thyroid carcinomas, in contrast to paragangliomas, are positive for cytokeratins, calcitonin, calcitonin gene related peptide and carcinoembryonic antigen. Most medullary carcinomas are positive for amyloid while paragangliomas of the thyroid are negative. Hyalinizing trabecular tumours are positive for thyroglobulin and have distinctive nuclear features which permit their distinction from paragangliomas. Metastatic carcinoids involving the thyroid are cytokeratin positive and typically demonstrate a prominent interstitial growth pattern, multiple tumour foci within the gland and folliculotropism {1201}.

Histogenesis
Thyroid paragangliomas most likely arise from the inferior laryngeal paraganglia which rarely may be found within the thyroid gland.

Prognosis and predictive factors
In all reported cases, thyroid paragangliomas have behaved as benign neoplasms.

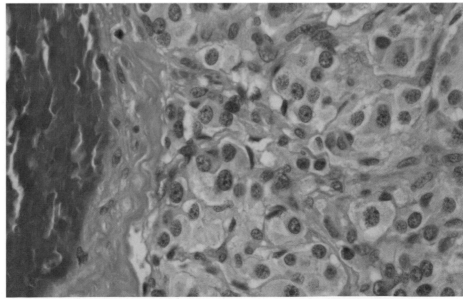

Fig. 2.099 Paraganglioma. Note the typical arrangement of tumour cells in nests (Zellballen) with chief cells and sustentacular cells.

Solitary fibrous tumour

M. Sobrinho Simões
J. Cameselle-Teijeiro

Definition
Thyroid solitary fibrous tumour (SFT) is an uncommon mesenchymal tumour indistinguishable from pleural and other extrapleural SFTs.

ICD-O code   8815/0

Synonyms
Fibroma, fibrosarcoma. Use of these terms is no longer recommended {638}.

Epidemiology
SFT of the thyroid gland is an uncommon neoplasm observed in middle-aged adults, with a slight predominance of females {253,285,288,489,1076,1850, 2168}.

Clinical features
Most patients are clinically euthyroid and present with an asymptomatic, slowly growing mass in the neck. The tumour is cold on scintigraphy, and ultrasonography reveals usually a solid, circumscribed well encapsulated nodule.

Macroscopy
SFT occurs anywhere in the thyroid gland, as well as in the perithyroid soft tissues, mimicking an epithelial thyroid tumour {2321}. Most thyroid SFTs present as well circumscribed or encapsulated masses, measuring between 2 and 8 cm (mean, 4.7 cm). On section, they have a firm, solid, grey-white to brown appearance; cystic changes are occasionally observed {1076,1850,2168}.

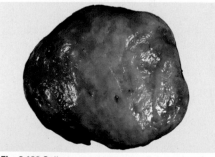

Fig. 2.100 Solitary fibrous tumour, demarcated from the adjacent thyroid tissue.

Histopathology
Thyroid solitary fibrous tumours display a variegated, wavy, storiform, hemangiopericytic- or desmoid-like arrangement of spindle cells, with occasional cysts. The spindle cells may infiltrate the thyroid parenchyma. A highly characteristic feature of SFT is a mixture of hypocellular (collagen-rich) and hypercellular areas, as well as branching hemangiopericytoma-like vessels. Myxoid change, extravasated erythrocytes, and interstitial chronic inflammatory cells, mainly mast cells, can be seen. The tumour cells have little cytoplasm with indistinct borders and vesicular nuclei with finely, regularly dispersed chromatin. Nuclear atypia is rare {1850,2168}. Tumour cellularity is usually low or moderate, mitotic figures are absent or rare. The adipocytic variant contains several mature lipomatous areas with a lobular or cord-like pattern poorly delimited from the surrounding proliferative spindle cells {285,2168}.

Immunohistochemistry
Solitary fibrous tumours (SFTs) of the thyroid gland are characteristically immunoreactive for vimentin, CD34, CD99 and for BCL2 {285,287,288,489,1076,1850, 2168}. In the adipocytic variant, positivity for factor XIIIa, progesterone and estrogen receptors is found, with immunoreactivity for S100 protein in the lipomatous foci {285}.

Differential diagnosis
The differential diagnosis of STF includes hemangiopericytoma and other spindle cell mesenchymal tumours, post-fine-needle aspiration spindle cell nodules, undifferentiated carcinoma (paucicellular variant) and medullary carcinoma {116,285,638,2198}.

Histogenesis
The precursor cell of SFT may be a vimentin+/CD34+ primitive mesenchymal cell capable of fibroblastic, myofibroblastic, adipose, and/or hemangiopericytic differentiation {285,2168}.

Cytogenetics and somatic genetics
No specific data on SFT of the thyroid are available.

Prognosis and predictive factors
Recurrence or distant metastasis from thyroid SFT have not been reported but there are too few documented cases to allow a definitive conclusion {253,285, 288,489,1076,1850,2168}.

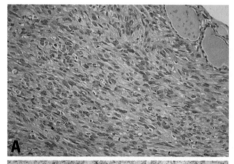
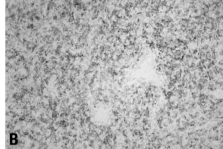
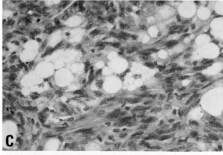

Fig. 2.101 Solitary fibrous tumour of the thyroid. A This tumour is composed of spindle cells and should be distinguished from leiomyosarcoma. B Tumour cells are strongly positive for bcl-2. C This tumour contains scattered adipocytes.

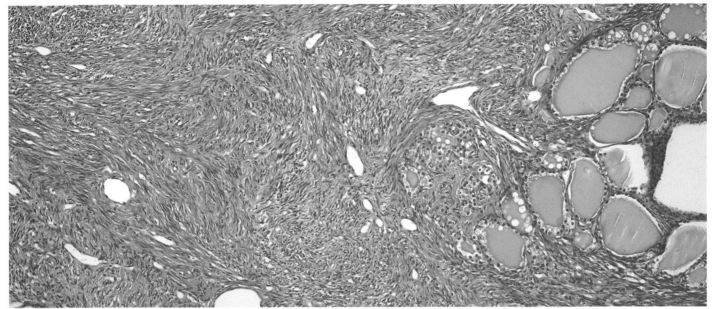

Fig. 2.102 Solitary fibrous tumour of the thyroid with an infiltrative growth pattern.

Rosai-Dorfman disease

L.D.R. Thompson
L.B. Kahn

Definition
A rare histiocytic syndrome of unknown etiology, characterized by histiocytic and lymphocytic infiltration of the thyroid gland.

Synonym
Sinus histiocytosis with massive lymphadenopathy.

Epidemiology
There are only exceedingly rare, isolated case reports in the literature of primary thyroid involvement by Rosai-Dorfman disease {395,1232,1768,2187}.

Clinical features
Only adult women have been reported to develop this disorder. Non-specific findings are usually noted, although the mass may masquerade as undifferentiated carcinoma {395,1232,1768,2187}.

Histopathology
The characteristic histiocyte-like cells are arranged in nodules and show emperipolesis of lymphoid cells {395, 1232,1768,2187}. A background of lymphocytic thyroiditis is usually seen, with clinical evidence of Hashimoto thyroiditis.

Prognosis and predictive factors
In general, isolated thyroid involvement has not progressed to systemic disease and the patients enjoy an excellent outcome {395,490,1232,1768,2187}.

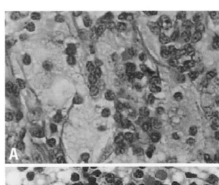
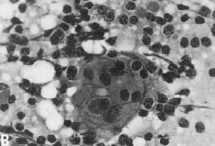

Fig. 2.103 Rosai-Dorfman disease of a thyroid isthmic lymph node. **A** Large histiocytic cells with engulfed lymphocytes. **B** FNAB showing a large histiocyte with foamy cytoplasm containing intact lymphocytes. From R.S. Cocker et al. {395}.

Follicular dendritic cell tumour

R.A. DeLellis

Definition
Thyroid follicular dendritic cell tumour is a rare neoplasm composed of cells showing morphologic and phenotypic features of follicular dendritic cells {989}.

ICD-O code
9758/3

Synonyms
Reticulum cell sarcoma/tumour; dendritic reticulum cell sarcoma/tumour.

Sites of involvement
The tumour most commonly arises in cervical lymph nodes, but other lymph node compartments may also be involved {188,989,2300}. The tumours also may arise in a variety of extranodal sites, including the thyroid {681}.

Epidemiology
Primary follicular dendritic cell tumours are exceptionally rare in the thyroid, and the few reported cases have occured in adults. In approximately 10-20% of extrathyroidal cases the tumour has occured in association with Castleman disease, usually of the hyarline vascular type {989}.

Clinical features
Most patients present with a painless, slowly growing mass. In the case reported by Galati et al, the patient presented with a mass in the neck, in association with a lesion in the thyroid {681}.

Etiology
Cases of follicular dendritic tumour with features of inflammatory pseudotumour have been associated with Epstein-Barr virus infection when they are inflammatory cell rich and located in the spleen or liver. The relationship to EBV is unknown {70,2004}.

Macroscopy
Tumours usually present as well circumscribed masses that are tan-grey on gross section. Foci of necrosis and haemorrhage may be present, particularly in large tumours.

Microscopy
The tumour cells range from spindle shaped to epithelioid with moderate amounts of eosinophilic cytoplasm with indistinct cell borders {342,1718}. The rounded to spindle shaped nuclei are vesicular and contain small but distinct nucleoli. Mitotic rate varies from 0 to10 per 10 high power files although the rate may be considerably higher in some cases. Occasional multinucleate giant cells resembling Warthin-Finkeldy cells may be present. Variable numbers of small lymphocytes may also be present. In some cases, the tumours may resemble inflammatory pseudotumours.

Immunohistochemistry
The tumour cells are typically positive for CD21, CD23, and CD35 {1593}. They are often positive for vimentin and epithelial membrane antigen but stains for cytokeratins (AE1/AE3, CAM5.2) are negative {681}. They are variably positive for S100 protein and CD68. Stains for CD45 and CD20 may be positive focally. The surrounding small lymphocytes reveal a mixed T-cell and B-cell phenotype.

Histogenesis
The normal cellular counterpart of the tumour is the follicular dendritic cell.

Prognosis and predictive factors
Because of the rarity of thyroid primaries, little is known about the prognosis of this tumour. In the case reported by Galati, 4 of 17 cervical lymph nodes resected at the time of thyroidectomy contained metastases {681}. The treatment includes complete surgical excision with or without adjuvant chemotherapy or radiotherapy.

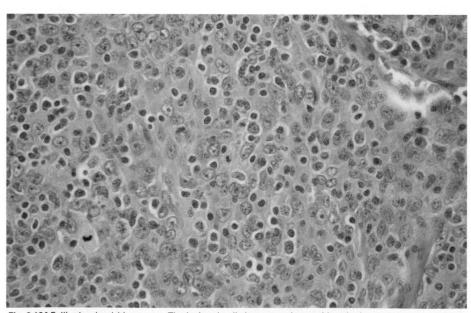

Fig. 2.104 Follicular dendritic tumour. The lesional cells have round to ovoid vesicular nuclei with prominent nucleoli. Small lymphocytes are dispersed between the tumour cells.

Langerhans cell histiocytosis

L.D.R. Thompson

Definition
A type of histiocytosis characterized by the proliferation of dendritic Langerhans cells with varying numbers of mature eosinophils.

ICD-O code 9751/1

Synonyms Histiocytosis X; Hand-Schüller-Christian syndrome; Letterer-Siwe disease.

Epidemiology
The incidence of this disorder when isolated to the thyroid gland is very low {153,493,553,740,1097,2352,2449}. Patients may present at any age although most patients have been less than 20 years of age. There is no gender predilection.

Etiology
Although the etiology remains unknown, considerations include a neoplastic process {2397}, a possible viral origin {1257,1455}, or an abnormal proliferative process {1385}.

Localization
A sub-capsular and septal location within the thyroid is frequent.

Clinical features
The clinical presentation depends upon the degree of thyroid involvement. Thyroid enlargement, when present, may be associated with a number of features, particularly in patients with systemic involvement. Radioactive ^{131}I studies demonstrate a "cold" nodule of variable size depending upon the extent of the disease {1444,1896,1899,2233}.

Macroscopy
The nodules of Langerhans cell histiocytosis are grossly indistinguishable from other thyroid nodules. Most lesions are small although complete replacement of the thyroid can occur in diffuse disease.

Tumour spread and staging
Although not universally accepted, the classification established by the Writing Group of the Histiocyte Society is used. Local disease involves a single location and is confined to the organ/location of the initial biopsy and is the sole manifestation of the disorder. Systemic disease involves more than one anatomic site, typically the bone, skin, liver, lymph nodes, lungs, central nervous system (including the pituitary gland), spleen, and gastro-intestinal tract {71,137,381, 2423}.

Cytopathology
FNAB smears will demonstrate scant amounts of colloid in a haemorrhagic background with a high cellularity; thyroid follicular epithelial cells are rare. There are large collections of eosinophils, lymphocytes, and isolated discrete, large mononucleated or multinucleated Langerhans cells with prominent nuclear folds (grooves) and abundant foamy cytoplasm {493,553}.

Histopathology
Langerhans cell histiocytosis can be either diffuse or focal. The Langerhans' histiocyte is characterized by an enlarged cell containing delicate appearing pale or eosinophilic cytoplasm surrounding a vesicular nucleus with an indented, notched, lobated, folded, grooved, vesicular or "coffee-bean" shaped appearance. An increased number of eosinophils, concentrated in collections around areas of necrosis, are seen frequently. Lymphocytic thyroiditis appears to be a common background disorder {1305,1424,1899,2233}.
Ultrastructurally, the histiocyte contains a variable number of invaginations of the plasma membrane, arranged in a pentilaminar pattern, referred to as Birbeck or Langerhans granules {37,2423}.
Langerhans cells are immunoreactive for S-100 protein, CD1a, and occasionally CD68 {1658,2233,2423}. The macrophage antigens generally demonstrate a concentration in the perinuclear space and Golgi region {1880, 2233}.

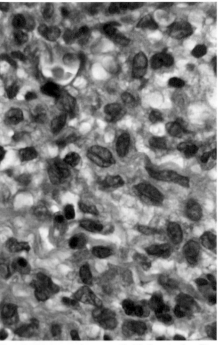

Fig. 2.105 Langerhans cell histiocytosis. The Langerhans histiocytes have prominent nuclear folds. Numerous histiocytes are also present.

The *differential diagnosis* includes a number of histiocytic disorders, as well as papillary or undifferentiated thyroid carcinoma {1097,1305,1658,1745,2352}. However, the characteristic nuclear features of the histiocytes are usually sufficient to make an accurate diagnosis.

Histogenesis
The Langerhans histiocyte is the putative cell of origin, believed to be a modified histiocyte derived from the dendritic system {1745,2423}.

Prognosis and predictive factors
Recognition of these lesions should prompt correlation with the patient's clinical history and the exclusion of systemic disease, since the prognosis is closely related to the presence or absence of involvement of other organs {1197}. Patients with localized thyroid disease usually do not develop subsequent systemic disease {1592,2233}.

Secondary tumours of the thyroid

R. DeLellis

Definition

Tumours that occur in the thyroid as a result of direct extension of malignancies from contiguous structures or as a result of hematogenous/lymphatic spread from distant sites.

Epidemiology

Metastases to the thyroid gland are found at autopsy in up to 25% of patients with disseminated malignancies. In clinical series, the frequency of secondary involvement of the thyroid is considerably lower.

Etiology

The thyroid gland is a richly vascularized structure, and as such, would be expected to harbour metastases with a relatively high frequency {1577,2395}. Several studies have suggested that abnormal glands (nodular goiter, adenomas, thyroiditis) are more likely to harbour metastatic disease than completely normal glands. In the series of cases reported by Heffess et al., 42% of the glands with metastases showed other abnormalities {857}. Metastases involving pre-existing thyroid carcinomas have also been documented {113}.

Localization

Metastases may occur in any portion of the thyroid gland. Tumours arising in the pharynx, larynx, trachea, oesophagus, cervical lymph nodes, soft tissue and mediastinum involve the thyroid by direct extension.

Clinical features

Patients usually present with a mass lesion involving the thyroid, hoarseness (due to compression of the recurrent laryngeal nerve), dyspnoea, dysphagia and neck pain. In one series of renal cell carcinomas metastatic to the thyroid, 80% of the cases involved a single lobe and presented as a solitary mass {857}. In this series, sixty-four percent had a prior history of renal cell carcinoma and the mean time to the appearance of a thyroid mass following nephrectomy was

9.4 years (range 2 to 21.9 years). In 36% of patients, the thyroid metastasis was the initial presentation of the tumour. Rarely, metastases to the thyroid may be associated with transient hyperthyroidism, presumably due to destruction of thyroid parenchyma and release of thyroid hormones.

Macroscopy

In autopsy series, metastases to the thyroid are most often multifocal and are variable in size. In clinical series they are more commonly solitary and may measure up to 15 cm in diameter. In cases in which there is direct extension of tumour from an adjacent site, the tumour tends to be large with involvement of a single lobe of the gland initially.

Origin of metastases

In the clinical series reported by Nakhjavani et al {1577}, the most common primary sites were kidney (33%), lung (16%), uterus (7%), and melanoma (5%) Breast, lung and skin (melanoma) have been the most common sites of origin of metastases in autopsy series. In one study from Hong Kong {1208}, the majority of the tumours secondarily involving the thyroid gland were carcinomas, and of these cases, lung was the most common (43%), followed by breast (8.8%) and stomach (7.7%). Lymphomas and leukemias accounted for 15% of cases. Rare sources of primary tumours included nasopharyngeal carcinoma, choriocarcinoma, malignant phyllodes tumour and osteosarcoma.

Cytology

Fine needle aspiration biopsy is a useful approach for the diagnosis of secondary tumours of the thyroid {2071}. A source of difficulty is the distinction of metastatic disease from poorly differentiated or undifferentiated thyroid carcinomas.

Histopathology

Most tumours involving the thyroid by direct extension are squamous cell carcinomas or malignant lymphomas. In the

majority of these cases, direct involvement of the gland by contiguous neoplasms is apparent on clinical grounds. Because of the rarity of primary squamous cell carcinomas of the thyroid, the possibility of secondary involvement of the gland by a contiguous or metastatic squamous cell carcinoma should always be considered.

Metastatic tumours generally retain the histologic features of the primary tumours but are frequently less differentiated. The distinction of metastatic renal cell carcinoma from follicular tumours showing clear cell change may be particularly difficult. Features favoring a diagnosis of metastatic renal cell carcinoma include prominent vascularity, glandular lumina filled with red blood cells and clear cytoplasm. The identification of metastatic renal cell carcinoma is aided by the absence of thyroglobulin in the neoplastic cells and the presence of CD10. It should be noted, however, that interstitial deposits of thyroglobulin may be present in metastases involving the thyroid gland and in some instances, thyroglobulin may diffuse into the tumour cell cytoplasm. Stains for TTF-1 are more reliable in this situation since a positive reaction is manifested by nuclear rather than cytoplasmic staining. A subset of secondary tumours from the lung would also be TTF-1 positive.

Metastatic neuroendocrine and carcinoid tumours may be particularly difficult to distinguish from medullary thyroid carcinomas. The diagnosis of metastatic neuroendocrine tumours should be suspected in the presence of a predominantly interstitial pattern of spread, the occurrence of multiple tumour foci, folliculotropism, rosette formations with lumens and cuticular borders and lack of immunoreactivity for calcitonin and CEA {1432}.

Prognosis

Although solitary thyroid prognosis of patients with metastases to the thyroid gland is generally poor, surgical resec-

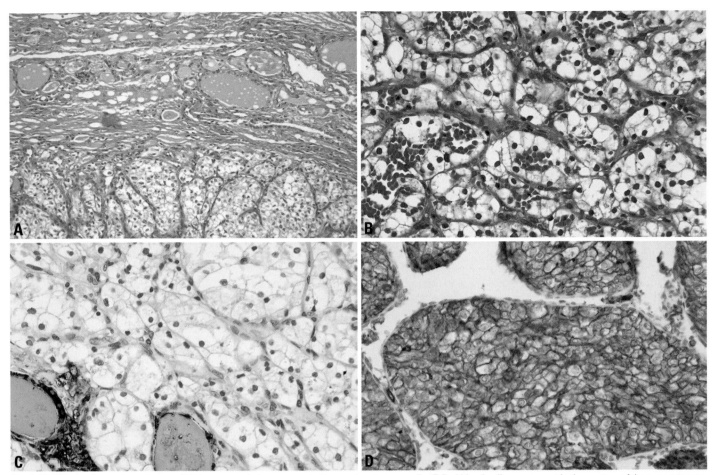

Fig. 2.106 Metastatic renal carcinoma. **A** This metastasis is composed of large, clear tumour cells. **B** Red blood cells are present in the centers of the tumour nests. **C** Metastatic renal cell carcinoma is negative for thyroglobulin while the entrapped follicles are positively stained. **D** Intense CD10 staining is present in the plasma membranes of tumour cells (same case as **A**).

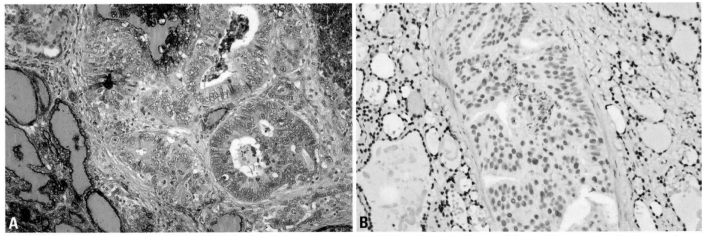

Fig. 2.107 **A** Colonic adenocarcinoma metastatic to the thyroid gland. The normal thyroid tissue is positive for thyroglobulin while the metastatic adenocarcinoma is negative. **B** A metastatic focus of breast carcinoma within a vascular channel in the thyroid gland does not react with TTF-1, while the surrounding thyroid parenchymal cell nuclei are immunoreactive.

tion of solitary thyroid metastatic disease is recommended. This approach may lead to prolonged survival, particularly in patients with renal cell carcinoma.

Parathyroid carcinoma

L. Bondeson
L. Grimelius
R.A. DeLellis
R. Lloyd
G. Akerstrom

C. Larsson
A. Arnold
C. Eng
E. Shane
J.P. Bilezekian

Definition
A malignant neoplasm derived from parathyroid parenchymal cells.

ICD-O code   8140/3

Epidemiology
Parathyroid carcinoma is a rare disease accounting for less than 1% of all patients with primary hyperparathyroidism in Western countries. The corresponding figure reported from Japan is 5% {2019}. In contrast to the marked female predominance among patients with parathyroid adenomas, the gender distribution is about equal in patients with parathyroid carcinoma, which occurs in all ages from early childhood {807}.

Etiology
The etiology of parathyroid carcinoma is unknown but some cases are associated with various types of hereditary predisposition, particularly the hyperparathyroidism-jaw tumour syndrome (see Chapter 5). Case reports indicate that secondary parathyroid hyperplasia and neck irradiation are possible risk factors {997,2019}.

Localization
Parathyroid carcinoma may occur in any site in which parathyroid tissue may be found.

Clinical features
The clinical manisfestations of parathyroid carcinoma are due primarily to the effects of excessive parathyroid hormone (PTH) secretion. However, several features are more common in association with parathyroid carcinomas than adenomas {413,801,941,1631,1925,2019,2020, 2428}. These include severe hypercalcemia often associated with typical symptoms (fatigue, weakness, weight loss, anorexia, nausea, vomiting, polyuria, polydipsia), extremely high PTH levels and frankly elevated serum alkaline phosphatase activity. A palpable neck mass, reported in up to 75% of patients with parathyroid carcinoma, is distinctly unusual in parathyroid adenomas {1283}. Recurrent laryngeal nerve palsy in a patient with primary hyperparathyroidism should raise the possibility of parathyroid carcinoma.

The classical target organs of PTH, kidney and skeleton, are affected with greater frequency and severity in patients with parathyroid carcinomas than in those with adenoma {801,2019, 2020}. Nephrolithiasis, nephrocalcinosis, and renal insufficiency are frequent presentations of parathyroid carcinoma. Clinical and radiological signs of PTH related bone disease are considerably more common in patients with parathyroid carcinoma. Concomitant bone and stone disease are frequent in association with parathyroid carcinoma and are now distinctly unusual in patients with parathyroid adenomas.

Macroscopy
Parathyroid carcinomas can be indistinguishable grossly from adenomas. Usually, however, the malignant tumours present as larger masses that are often adherent to adjacent structures. The presence of adhesions is suspicious but not diagnostic for malignancy since periglandular fibrosis occasionally is related to scarring after haemorrhage in a benign parathyroid lesion. In contrast to the soft tan appearance of adenomas, carcinomas are more firm and gray-white with occasional foci of necrosis. Frozen section is of little value in distinguishing benign from malignant disease, and inci-

sional biopsy should be strongly discouraged in order to prevent seeding of tumour cells, which may cause implants and recurrent hyperparathyroidism both in benign and in malignant cases.

Tumour spread and staging
Spread of parathyroid carcinoma is most commonly heralded by the presence of recurrent local disease in the soft tissues of the neck. Metastases most often develop in cervical and mediastinal lymph nodes, lungs, bone, and liver. In most series, the lungs are the most common sites of distant spread. Bone metastases must be distinguished from benign "brown tumours" caused by severe hyperparathyroidism {789}. Ossifying fibromas, a component of the hereditary hyperparathyroidism-jaw tumour syndrome may also mimic bone metastases. The average time between initial surgery and recurrent disease is 2-3 years {1925}, but disease-free intervals as long as 20 years have been reported. Neither tumour size nor lymph node status have been found to be significant prognostic factors according to the National Cancer Center data base report {941}.

Cytopathology
Fine needle aspiration is useful for the identification of parathyroid tissue {217} particularly in lesions with an aberrant location, including metastases, but it is not a method suited for distinction between benign and malignant primary tumours.

Histopathology
Histologic evidence of parathyroid carcinoma is often equivocal, and a definitive diagnosis should be restricted to lesions displaying vascular invasion, perineural space invasion, capsular penetration with growth into adjacent tissues, and/or metastases. The specific criteria for the identification of vascular invasion are essentially identical to those used in assessing this feature in thyroid follicular carcinomas. Importantly, vascular inva-

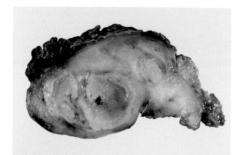

Fig. 2.108 Macroscopic appearance of a carcinoma of the parathyroid gland. From V.A. LiVolsi and S. Asa {1319}.

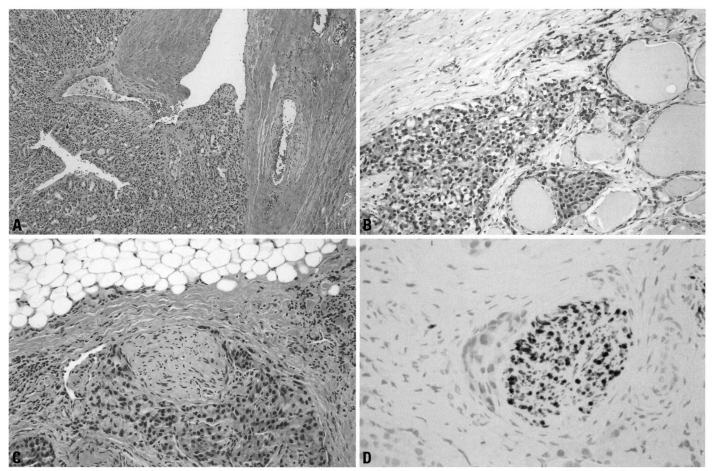

Fig. 2.109 Parathyroid carcinoma. **A** This tumour has invaded a large vascular channel. **B** This oncocytic tumour invades the thyroid gland. **C** Extensive perineural space invasion is present. **D** A nerve, highlighted with positive staining for S-100 protein, is surrounded by tumour.

sion should be present in the tumour capsule or in the surrounding soft tissue rather than within the tumour. Non-penetrating capsular invasion is an unreliable sign of malignancy that is difficult or impossible to distinguish from entrapment of epithelial remnants in areas of fibrosis secondary to degenerative changes in benign lesions. Local recurrences are highly suspicious for malignancy, but seeding from an intraoperatively ruptured adenoma or hyperplastic gland occasionally causes implants mimicking malignant growth {19}. Likewise, intentionally autotransplanted hyperplastic parathyroid tissue may give rise to clinically benign lesions with a seemingly invasive growth pattern involving fat and muscle. It should also be mentioned that benign parathyroid lesions located within the thyroid gland often lack a well-defined capsule and may show pseudoinvasive growth patterns.

Band-forming fibrosis is a common but inconstant and non-pathognomonic fea-

ture of parathyroid carcinoma {219, 1957}. Scarring from haemorrhage or infarction in benign parathyroid lesions may give rise to similar patterns of fibrosis. In addition, perinodular fibrosis is quite common in parathyroid hyperplasia associated with tertiary hyperparathyroidism. Hemosiderin deposits occur in malignant as well as benign parathyroid lesions and cannot be used as a distinguishing feature.

Similar to parathyroid adenomas, most parathyroid carcinomas display a solid growth pattern with tumour cells arranged in diffuse masses or closely packed nests. Trabecular growth, also shown by some adenomas and hyperplastic glands, occurs in a minority of cases. Follicular and acinar patterns are uncommon but do not exclude malignancy {219}. Rarely, tumours may demonstrate rosettes. Spindle cell growth is a rare feature without a clear-cut association with malignancy in parathyroid lesions {39,219,589}.

Carcinomas composed of chief cells predominate but oncocytic tumours occur in the same proportion as seen among parathyroid adenomas {214,219,2414}. Mixtures of these cell types are not uncommon, and cases containing clear cells are also encountered. Oncocytic carcinomas do not differ from chief cell carcinomas with respect to clinical behaviour {573}.

Mitotic activity
The mitotic activity in parathyroid carcinoma is extremely variable and shows broad overlap with adenoma and hyperplasia. In some clinically aggressive carcinomas mitotic figures are difficult to detect while a minority shows mitoses in numbers well above those recorded in adenomas {214,219,589,1957,2073}. Furthermore, tertiary hyperplasia may show focal mitotic activity in each of four glands with mitotic rates higher than those in most carcinomas. The presence of scattered foci of coagulative necroses

plus macronucleoli and mitotic activity in excess of five mitoses per 50 high power microscopic fields constitutes a triad indicating high risk of clinically malignant behaviour {219}.

Parathyroid carcinoma vs. adenoma
Paralelling the data regarding mitoses, the proliferation marker Ki-67 is of limited diagnostic value due to the overlap of labelling indices shown by benign and malignant parathyroid lesions {573,575, 607,1330}. An index greater than 5% should lead to a closer and prolonged follow-up of the patient due to an increased risk of malignancy and recurrent disease {607,1330}. DNA quantitation cannot be used as a diagnostic tool since adenomas may show aneuploid patterns {1395} and clinically aggressive carcinomas quite often are euploid {1925}. On an individual basis, there is no consistent difference between these two tumour categories with respect to immunoreactivity for p53, bcl-2, p27, cyclin D1, or retinoblastoma gene expression {573, 575,607,1058,1330,1567,2301,2303}. Based on tissue microarray analyses, however, Stojadinovic and coworkers have reported that 76% of adenomas have a p27(+) bcl-2(+), Ki-67(-), mdm-2(+) phenotype while no carcinomas exhibited this phenotypic profile {2136}.
If a non-functioning (non-hypercalcaemic) parathyroid carcinoma is suspected, immunostaining of PTH is a potential diagnostic adjunct {1655}. A parathyroid tumour lacking unequivocal evidence of invason but showing some other feature(s) suspicious for malignancy is referred to as atypical adenoma.
Some parathyroid carcinomas have such a bland appearance that they differ from benign lesions only by their invasiveness. Two thirds of carcinomas, however,

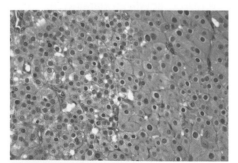

Fig. 2.110 Parathyroid carcinoma, composed of an admixture of chief cells (left) and oncocytes (right).

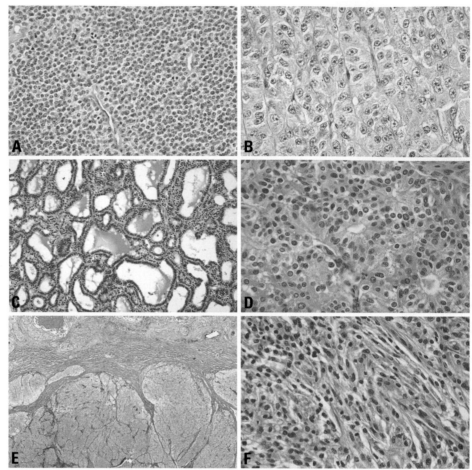

Fig. 2.111 Growth patterns of parathyroid carcinoma. **A** This carcinoma is cytologically bland but was associated with metastases. **B** Trabecular growth pattern and markedly enlarged nuclei with prominent nucleoli. **C** Predominant follicular growth pattern. **D** This tumour has a rosette-like pattern. **E** Band-forming fibrosis is a common but neither a constant nor pathognomonic feature of parathyroid carcinoma. **F** Predominant spindle cell growth pattern.

show conspicuous atypia. General nuclear enlargement and macronucleoli are the most important diagnostic clues {219,986,2070}. Nuclear pleomorphism is common but is also a fairly frequent finding in adenomas {217,219,478}.

Grading
There is no generally accepted system for grading of parathyroid carcinomas.

Precursor lesions
Rare cases of parathyroid carcinoma in patients with secondary hyperparathyroidism indicate that hyperplasia occasionally may precede the development of malignancy {2019}. Seemingly adenomatous remnants have been observed in a few cases of parathyroid carcinoma {589} but this finding is uncommon {1957}, and genetic studies support the hypothesis that most parathyroid carci-

nomas arise *de novo* rather than from pre-existing adenomas {1188}.

Somatic genetics
While distant metastases and extensive local invasion are specific features of parathyroid malignancies, other histopathological features of carcinoma can overlap with those of adenomas. Molecular and genetic differences between these entities, therefore, carry potential diagnostic and therapeutic importance.
CGH and molecular genetic studies have uncovered certain recurrent clonal alterations that suggest the involvement and location of genes that contribute to parathyroid malignancies. *Cyclin D1*, a parathyroid adenoma oncogene, appears to be overexpressed in many parathyroid cancers but sample sizes have been limited {2303}. Recurrent loss-

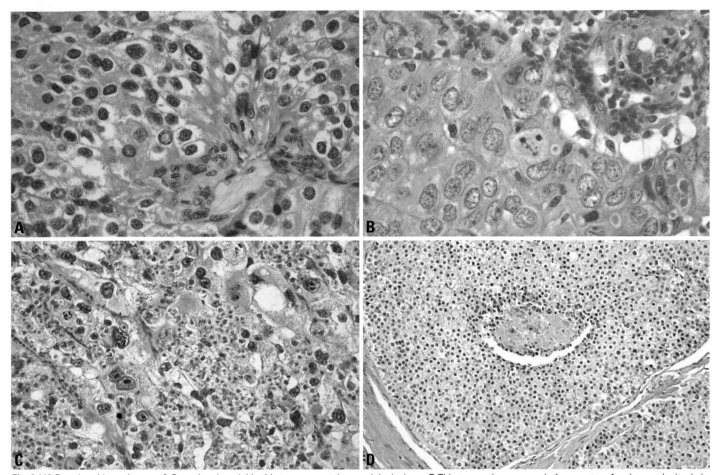

Fig. 2.112 Parathyroid carcinoma. **A** Occasional nuclei in this tumour contain pseudoinclusions. **B** This tumour is composed of oncocytes. An abnormal mitosis is present in the center of the field. **C** This locally recurrent carcinoma shows marked nuclear atypia. **D** Focal necrosis is a common feature of some carcinomas.

es of chromosome 13q in parathyroid carcinomas have been reported both by CGH {1188} and molecular allelotyping {438} and decreased Rb protein expression has been reported {438}. Importantly, several genomic regions frequently lost in parathyroid adenomas, including 11q (the location of the *MEN1* gene), are rarely, if ever, lost in carcinomas, suggesting that parathyroid carcinomas do not arise from pre-existing adenomas {1188}.

HRPT2
Recent studies have suggested that mutations of *HRPT2* are an important contributor to the pathogenesis of parathyroid carcinoma. Inactivating germ-line mutations of this tumour suppressor gene, located on1q25, cause the hyperparathyroidism-jaw tumour syndrome, a rare form of hyperparathyroidism with an increased prevalence of parathyroid malignancies, as well as a small subset of cases of familial isolated hyperparathyroidism {319,927,2320}. Sporadic parathyroid carcinomas can frequently arise as a consequence of acquired inactivation of *HRPT2*. Specifically, the two available studies have shown one or two inactivating mutations in parathyroid carcinomas from 10/15 and 4/4 cases studied {927,2026}. In contrast, only 2/47 sporadic adenomas with cystic features and 0/25 unselected adenomas showed *HRPT2* mutations {319,927}. Furthermore, certain patients with sporadic parathyroid carcinoma can carry germline mutations in *HRPT2* and may represent new probands of HPT-JT or a phenotypic variant, mandating special considerations for their clinical management and genetic screening {2026}.

Genetic susceptibility
Parathyroid carcinoma has yet to be a proven component tumour of MEN 1, but have been reported to be a component of hyperthyroidism-jaw tumour syndrome (see Chapter 5).

Prognosis and predictive factors
The average time between surgery and the first recurrence is approximately three years although intervals of up to 20 years have been reported {1925,2019}. In the United States, a 10-year survival rate of approximately 50% has been reported {941}. Patients treated with extensive surgery had a longer survival and a longer relapse-free period {1925}. Recurrence rates from 30-67% and 5-year survival between 40 and 86% have been reported {941,2019,2428}. Most patients developing metastases eventually die from the effects of excessive PTH secretion. Localization studies should be performed in patients with parathyroid carcinoma with recurrent hypercalcemia {670,1010,1630}.

Parathyroid adenoma

L. Grimelius
R.A. DeLellis
L Bondeson
G. Akerstrom
A. Arnold

K.O. Franssila
G.N. Hendy
D. Dupuy
C. Eng

Definition

A benign neoplasm composed of chief cells, oncocytic cells, transitional oncocytic cells, or a mixture of these cell types.

ICD-O code   8140/0

Epidemiology

The incidence of primary hyperparathyroidism increased dramatically in the past three decades, primarily as a result of the introduction of the multichannel autoanalyzer in clinical laboratories. The true incidence of this disorder has been difficult to determine but data from the Mayo Clinic and European centers indicate an incidence of 17.7 cases per 100,000 person / year {854,1557,2122}. The prevalence has been reported to be as high as 1:100 but a figure of 1:1000 is probably closer to the true prevalence of the disease. More recent studies from the Mayo Clinic have demonstrated a 3-fold decline in the incidence of primary hyperparathyroidism; however, other centers have not been able to document a similar trend {2378}.

Age and sex distribution

Primary hyperparathyroidism due to adenomas occurs in all age groups but the peak incidence occurs between 50 and 60 years of age, with a female to male ratio of approximately 3:1. This finding may be related to the fact that the disease may appear concurrent with a fall in estrogen levels since estrogens may oppose some of the skeletal actions of parathyroid hormone.

Etiology

Factors that predispose to the development of parathyroid adenomas are poorly understood although prior irradiation to the head and neck has been implicated in the development of some of these tumours {398,2250}. Hyperparathyroidism following radioactive iodine treatment occurs rarely {213}. Long term growth stimulation leads to multiple nodule formation; occasionally a dominant nodule may show features of an adenoma. Heritable factors may also play a role in the development of these tumours and are discussed in a subsequent section.

Localization

The vast majority of adenomas involve a single parathyroid gland, the remaining glands being normal. Exceptionally, two adenomas may occur {2309}. Parathyroid adenomas may also occur within the thyroid, the retroesophageal space and the mediastinum. Rarely, they may arise from ectopic or supernumerary parathyroid tissue present within the pericardium, vagus nerve or soft tissue adjacent to the angle of the jaw {347,520}. Preoperative identification of adenomas has been discussed in the Introduction.

Clinical features

Primary hyperparathyroidism is characterized by the excessive and incompletely regulated secretion of parathyroid hormone, leading to the mobilization of calcium from bone, enhanced renal resorption of calcium, phosphaturia and increased calcium resorption from the gastrointestional tract. Affected patients typically demonstrate hypercalcemia and hypophosphataemia.

Plasma calcium levels

Prior to the introduction of the multichannel autoanalyzer in the late 1960´s allowing liberal serum calcium determination, most patients with primary hyperparathyroidism presented with classical symptoms of nephrolithiasis or bone disease. In current series, most patients are recognized by routine serum calcium measurements and have vague symptoms of fatigue, weakness and psychiatric disturbance with mild depressive symptoms, or appear asymptomatic. Nephrolithiasis still occurs especially in younger patients. Reduction of bone mineral and bone density is common, but overt bone disease is encountered only in occasional patients with severe hypercalcaemia, and raised alkaline phosphatases. Some patients with severe hypercalcaemia may have polydipsia, polyuria, constipation and musculoskeletal pain. Few patients have pancreatitis, possibly related to hyperparathyroidism. Surgery is recommended in patients with overt symptoms of renal stones or nephrocalcinosis, evident bone disease or fractures, or a rare neuromuscular syndrome with marked muscular

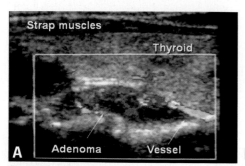
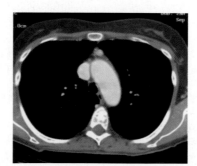
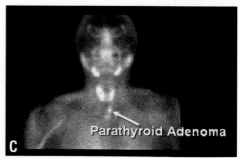

Fig. 2.113 A Sagittal color Doppler image of a posterior parathyroid adenoma with a typical hypervascular flow pattern. **B** Axial image of contrast enhanced CT image of chest. A parathyroid adenoma is present anterior to the heart. **C** Anterior 2 hour delayed planar image from a technetium 99m labeled sestamibi scan shows a region of uptake in the left inferior cervical region below the thyroid gland, consistent with a parathyroid adenoma.

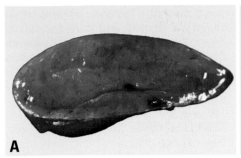 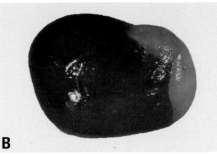 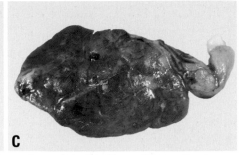

Fig. 2.114 Parathyroid adenoma. **A** This encapsulated tumour is tan in color. **B** This tumour has a yellowish cap of normal glandular tissue. **C** Oncocytic adenoma with remnant yellowish normal tissue at the vascular pole.

weakness. Neuropsychiatric symptoms are considered strong indication by many and can be markedly relieved by surgery, but benefit from parathyroid operation may be difficult to predict in individual patients.

In asymptomatic patients, surgery is recommended if serum calcium, adjusted for current albumin concentration, is greater than 1 mg/dl (0.25 mM) above the normal reference, e.g. > 11.4 mg/dl (reference < 2.60 mM), or if creatinin clearence is reduced by 30 %, 24-h urinary calcium is greater than 400 mg, bone mineral density at any site is more than 2.5 SD below peak bone mass (t-score >-2.5). Surgery is always recommended in patients younger than 50 years {3} and those who cannot follow a medical surveillance program.

Approximately 25% of asymptomatic patients who did not undergo parathyroidectomy show evidence of disease progression {2053}. An increased mortality rate, primarily due to cardiovascular disease, has been noted in patients with chronic hypercalcemia {1678}.

Macroscopy

The typical adenoma is tan to reddish-brown in colour, soft and homogeneous in consistency, with a smooth surface and a thin capsule. Tumour weight varies from 0.06 to 300 g. In current series, most adenomas weigh between 0.2 and 1 g. Microadenomas may be so small that they may be missed on surgical exploration and frozen section examination {328,1298,1796}. Adenomas may be round, ellipsoid, bean- or kidney-shaped, or flattened and elongated. Ocasional tumours may be bi- or multilobar {328, 841}. The edges are usually rounded as a result of the expanding parenchymal tissue. Adenomas, especially larger ones, may display fibrosis, haemosiderin deposits, cystic degeneration and calcifications {328,841,1756}. Macroscopic cysts may occur, but are not common {2039}.

A yellowish-brown rim of glandular normal tissue is seen in about 50-60% of the adenomas, most often adjacent to the vascular hilus of the gland. It usually represents a remnant of the original parathyroid gland.

Cytopathology

Smears from aspirated parathyroid tissue may show follicular, papillary and lymphoid patterns. Follicular elements may contain colloid-like substances and may resemble a thyroid neoplasm. Other phenomena shared with thyroid lesions are oncocytic metaplasia and nuclear pseudoinclusions (as seen in papillary carcinomas). Fluid aspirated from secondary cystic lesions in large parathyroid adenomas has the same appearance as fluid in cystic goiter, but the origin can be established by measuring the fluid's content of parathyroid hormone. Smears from parathyroid lesions containing clear cells may be mistaken for metastatic hypernephroma. Other pitfalls that may lead to overdiagnosis of malignancy include the marked nuclear pleomorphism occasionally seen in parathyroid adenomas {217}.

Histopathology

Parathyroid adenomas are benign encapsulated neoplasms usually involving a single gland; however some ade-

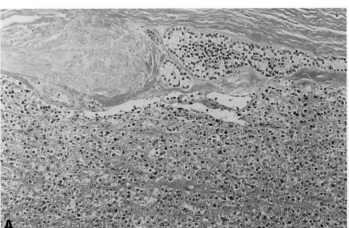 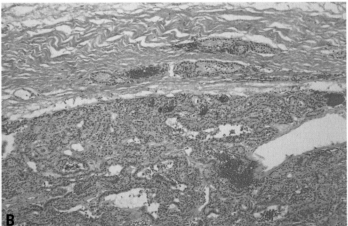

Fig. 2.115 Parathyroid adenoma. **A** This tumour is composed predominantly of transitional oncocytic cells and has a broad capsular zone containing remnants of normal parathyroid tissue. **B** A small rim of normal parathyroid is present adjacent to this adenoma.

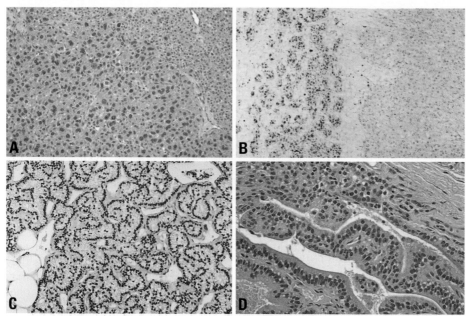

Fig. 2.116 Parathyroid adenoma **A** This tumour contains a focus of cells with enlarged hyperchromatic nuclei. **B** In this oil red O stain, the tumour (right) is almost devoid of neutral lipid deposits while the adjacent normal gland is strongly positive. **C** Predominant glandular (trabecular) growth pattern. **D** Pseudopapillary growth pattern.

nomas may lack a well defined connective tissue capsule. Chief cells predominate in most adenomas {195,841}, but a mixture of oncocytic and transitional oncocytic cells is common, and the latter cells may be either diffusely scattered among chief cells or aggregated into nests.

Chief cells
The chief cells of adenomas are generally larger than corresponding cells in the adjacent rim of normal glandular tissue and in associated normal parathyroid glands. {118,1327} The cytoplasm is either faintly eosinophilic ("dark") or vacuolated ("light"); the light cells are rich in glycogen. The oncocytic cells display a finely granular eosinophilic cytoplasm. The chief cells may be devoid of fat or may contain finely dispersed fat. In contrast, chief cells in the peripheral glandular rim or in associated parathyroid glands, contain one or a few lipid droplets, with a diameter of 2-7 µm. This difference in lipid content is valid only for the chief cells {1326,1875}.

The neoplastic chief cell nuclei, which are usually round and chromatin dense, occasionally with a small nucleolus, may vary in size. In some adenomas obvious nuclear pleomorphism occurs, with giant hyperchromatic and occasional multilobar nuclei. These cells are either diffuse-

ly spread throughout the tumour or occur in clusters {841}. In the absence of other features of malignancy, pleomorphic nuclei should not be regarded as a criterion of malignancy. Mitotic activity may occur in adenomas, but usually in a low frequency; Snover and Foucar {2073} found no mitoses or less than 1 per 10 high-power fields (HPF) in 15 of 17 adenomas, and more than 1 mitosis in two cases. San-Juan et al. {1923} reported a similar mitotic frequency.

Growth patterns
The parenchymal cell arrangement varies from solid sheets to a nodular, trabecular, follicular and/or acinar pattern, but there may also be a rosette-like, papillary or pseudopapillary pattern {657, 1895}. Often a mixture of different arrangements is seen. In cases with a more solid sheet-like pattern the chief cells may display a palisaded arrangement around blood vessels. Small cysts lined by parenchymal cells may be present and cystic degeneration may occur in some adenomas, particularly larger ones. Entrapped neoplastic cells occurring in the fibrotic cyst walls may arouse suspicion of infiltrative growth. Some of the adenomas reported in patients with the hyperparathyroidism-jaw tumour syndrome are cystic {319}. The lumina of follicular or acinar glandular structures con-

tain eosinophilic material, which is occasionally laminated and may sometimes be focally calcified,resembling psammoma bodies {478}. Congo red staining has shown that some of the intrafollicular material displays green birefringence typical of amyloid {54,1268}.

Fat cells are usually absent or sparse in adenomas. When fat cells are present, they may be diffusely distributed or may occur in small groups, particularly in peripheral parts of the adenomas. Rarely the fat cells have a frequency and distribution pattern reminiscent of a normal gland.

The *stroma* of adenomas is generally sparse but richly vascularised. Stromal oedema, fibrotic areas and bands with or without haemosiderin deposits, and chronic inflammation may also be seen, particularly in larger adenomas. Calcifications and even bone formation may also occur in fibrotic areas and in the sclerotically thickened capsules {1756}.

Massive *infarction* of adenomas, spontaneous or following FNA, may be associated with hypercalcaemic crisis.

Immunohistochemistry
The chief cells show positive immunostaining for parathyroid hormone and chromogranin A. These cells also display an argyrophil reaction {1731}. The chief cells contain the low molecular weight cytokeratins 8 (52kD), 18 (45kD) and 19 (20 kD) {1492}. TTF1 is negative.

The proliferation marker Ki67/MIB-1 may be of some diagnostic help in the distinction of parathyroid adenomas and carcinomas. The Ki67 index is generally lower for adenomas than for carcinomas, but overlapping occurs, which limits its diagnostic value {607,1330}, as discussed in the section on parathyroid carcinomas. An index higher than 5% should, however, raise the possibility of malignant behaviour and motivate a closer and prolonged follow-up of the patient {1330}.

Markers involved in the cell growth, such as p53, bcl-2, p27Kipl, cyclin D1 and retinoblastoma protein, have shown no consistent differences in expression between adenomas and carcinomas {575,607,1058,1330,1567,2301,2303}.

Flow DNA cytometry is of limited diagnostic and prognostic value in the individual case, since both adenomas and carcinomas may exhibit euploid and aneuploid patterns {1395,1925}, and clinically aggressive carcinomas quite often are euploid {1925}.

Electron microscopy
Ultrastructurally, the chief cells of adenomas often show signs of increased endocrine activity compared with the chief cells in the rim of "normal" glandular tissue adjacent to the adenoma and in associated parathyroid glands. Signs of increased activity are reflected by increased endoplasmic reticulum, large Golgi regions, paucity of secretory granules and small amounts of cytoplasmic fat. Oncocytic cells contain abundant mitochondria, while the Golgi apparatus and endoplasmatic reticulum are less prominent than those in chief cells. These cells mostly contain few secretory granules {388,1463,1608,1876}.

Associated parathyroid glands
The rim of uninvolved glandular tissue adjacent to the adenomas is generally located close to the vascular hilus, often, but not always, separated from this by the adenoma capsule. This remnant of glandular tissue is more difficult to detect with increasing adenoma size {328}. Chief cells usually predominate in the remnant, and fat cells are usually abundant but may also be few or even absent. A diagnosis of adenoma, however, cannot be based on the demonstration of such a remnant alone, since a similar appearance may be seen in glands of nodular chief cell hyperplasia.

The parathyroid glands associated with adenomas may show atrophic or normal macroscopical and microscopical features. In elderly persons oncocytic nodules may be seen in glands without signs of hyperparathyroidism {1323}; in young and middle-aged persons, however, oncocytic nodules may represent an abnormal finding.

Histological variants
Oncocytic adenoma
A minority of adenomas causing hyperparathyroidism are composed largely or exclusively of oncocytic cells {149,1463, 1654,1763}. These tumours are usually red-brown on cross-section. Non-functioning oncocytic adenomas may be found incidentally at neck exploration or autopsy. The oncocytic cells may be arranged in solid sheets, trabeculae, anastomosing cords or a mixture of these

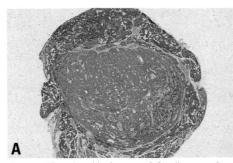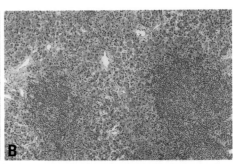

Fig. 2.117 Parathyroid adenoma. **A** Small oncocytic adenoma surrounded by a rim of normocellular parathyroid tissue. **B** This tumour is composed of oncocytic cells and contains aggregates of small lymphocytes. The patient had a history of psoriatic arthritis.

patterns. The nuclei are typically round and chromatin dense, but nuclear pleomorphism sometimes occurs. In addition, oncocytic adenomas may also contain prominent nucleoli.

Water-clear adenoma
Rarely, water-clear adenomas have been reported, including double adenomas {1173,1513}. Most of the neoplasms with clear-like cells probably represent chief cells with multiple vesicles and an abundant content of glycogen {1608}.

Lipoadenoma
Lipoadenomas are rare tumours that contain abundant mature adipose tissue and/or myxoid stroma with only scattered nests, cords and/or delicate anastomosing trabeculae of chief cells predominantly. They are encapsulated, soft, often lobulated on cross-section, yellow-tan in colour and can attain a considerable size {694,780,834,1632,2278,2410}. The chief cells contain a reduced amount of fat {2278}. These lesions have also been referred to as hamartomas {1632}. Ectopic lipoadenomas have also been reported {834,2410}.

Atypical adenoma
There are tumours without unequivocal signs of capsular or vascular invasion, but with other features similar to those of parathyroid carcinomas, including broad fibrous bands with or without haemosiderin deposits, mitoses, and neoplastic cell groups in a thickened fibrous capsule. These tumours, which may be adherent to the adjacent thyroid or surrounding soft tissues, are considered of uncertain malignant potential, and are therefore referred to as atypical adenomas {219,1283}. However, follow-up of these cases has demonstrated a benign outcome in most, following local excision {1282}. By using standard DNA fluorometric methods, these workers demonstrated 12 cases of atypical adenomas, 10 of which had a non-aneuploid pattern and 2 of which had an aneuploid pattern. The 2 patients with aneuploid adenomas developed recurrent disease while the remaining 10 did not with an average follow-up of 25 months. These findings suggest that patients with lesions diagnosed as atypical adenomas with an aneuploid DNA pattern by static DNA fluorometric methods should be

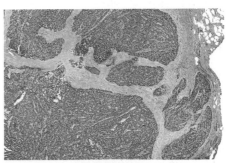

Fig. 2.118 Parathyroid lipoadenoma. The stroma contains adipose tissue with myxoid change and clusters of lymphocytes.

Fig. 2.119 Atypical parathyroid adenoma, composed of nodules of neoplastic chief cells separated by broad bands of fibrous tissue. There was infiltration into the adjacent soft tissue or vessels.

closely followed to rule out recurrence or metastasis {1283}.

Differential diagnosis

Chief cell hyperplasia
When two or more glands are enlarged and abnormal, primary chief cell hyperplasia should be considered in the differential. This indicates that the pathologist must examine an associated gland or at least have information from the surgeon on PTH levels or on the size and colour of the glands left in situ. Tiny glandular biopsies from normal associated glands are difficult to interpret since the distribution of parenchymal and fat cells are often irregular. Before operation, renal failure, a cause of diffuse and nodular hyperplasia, should be excluded.

Parathyroid glands in primary chief cell hyperplasia may have a microscopical appearance similar to that of adenomas, and microadenomas may be difficult to differentiate from hyperplastic nodules. Slight nuclear pleomorphism may be seen in hyperplasias, but if it is more pronounced, a diagnosis of adenoma must be considered. Overall, the adenoma and hyperplasia diagnoses are to a great extent based on the macro- and/or microscopical findings in the remaining associated glands. Fat staining of cryostat sections may help to discriminate between normal and slightly hyperplastic glands {212}.

The development of highly sensitive pre-operative techniques for the localization of parathyroid adenomas and the use of intraoperative parathyroid hormone assays has had a profound impact on the treatment of patients with primary hyperparathyroidism {683,759,1035,1624}. An intraoperative decline of parathyroid hormone to normal levels at 10 minutes and greater than 50% of the initial baseline value suggests surgical cure {2088}. These intraoperative analyses have lent considerable credibility to minimal access surgery with uniglandular removal.

Adenoma vs. carcinoma
Parathyroid adenomas may be difficult to distinguish from carcinomas. The features that permit this distinction is discussed in the previous section.

Parathyroid vs. thyroid lesion
The glandular pattern in an adenoma may be so prominent that difficulties may arise in discriminating between parathyroid adenoma and a thyroid follicular nodule or neoplasm. The rim of normal parathyroid tissue seen in some adenomas can be of diagnostic help for the diagnosis of adenoma. Parathyroid glands and adenomas can lie within the thyroid capsule and give the impression of representing a thyroid nodule or thyroid neoplasm. Moreover, parathyroid adenomas with a papillary pattern can be mistaken for papillary carcinoma. Immunohistochemical staining for parathyroid hormone, TTF1 or thyroglobulin are helpful in this discrimination. Thyroid follicular colloid usually contains birefringent oxalate crystals, which are rarely seen in parathyroid tissue. Accordingly, polarised light microscopy may be of diagnostic help in identifying thyroid tissue {974}. In situ hybridisation with probes for parathyroid hormone mRNA is another way to identify parathyroid cells {1066,2138}. Metastases from medullary thyroid carcinoma may occasionally be difficult to distinguish from abnormal parathyroid tissue. Immunostaining with calcitonin antibodies is of diagnostic help in identifying medullary thyroid carcinoma.

Precursor lesions
Histological studies in an autopsy series have suggested that adenomas may arise in nodular hyperplasia, as a result of a growth advantage in individual nodules. In the multiple endocrine neoplasia (MEN) type 1 syndrome, multiple adenomas occur in a background of polyclonal hyperplasia {18}.

Somatic genetics
Cyclin D1/PRAD1 was identified as an oncogene activated by clonal DNA rearrangement in parathyroid adenomas {75,865,1545}, and is overexpressed by rearrangement or alternative mechanisms in up to 40% of sporadic adenomas {75,865}. Overexpression of cyclin D1, a central regulator of the cell cycle, has been confirmed to cause parathyroid neoplasia and biochemical hyperparathyroidism, including an altered PTH-calcium setpoint, in transgenic mice {961}. The 11q13-based *MEN1* tumour suppressor gene, in which germline mutations cause MEN 1 {351}, has incurred biallelic somatic mutation and/or deletion in 12-19% of sporadic adenomas {305,609,869,1491}. A mouse model of *MEN1* deficiency causes a phenotype that includes parathyroid hypercellularity {425}. The *in vivo* oncosuppressor function of the *MEN1* gene product menin may involve transcriptional regulation through interaction with JunD {12}, modulation of the TGFβ pathway through interaction with Smad3 {1021}, or other actions. *HRPT2* on 1q, the cause of the rare familial hyperparathyroidism-jaw tumour syndrome, has been reported to bear somatic inactivating mutations in 4% of sporadic adenomas but the function of its tumour suppressor protein product, parafibromin, is unknown {319}. Several candidate genes, including *CASR*, *VDR*, *SMAD3*, and *RET* are not somatically mutated in parathyroid adenomas {75,335,865,922,2025}. Molecular allelotyping and CGH have identified subchromosomal losses or gains in adenomas but most, excepting losses on 1p/q, 6q, 11 (focused on 11q23 in addition to 11q13/*MEN1*), 13q, and 15q, have not been validated across studies or with more than one method {14,75,608,1225}.

Genetic susceptibility
The genetic differential diagnosis includes MEN 1, MEN 2 and hyperparathyroidism-jaw tumour syndrome. See Chapter 5.

Prognosis and predictive factors
Typically, parathyroid adenomas are well circumscribed and are relatively easy to excise. There may occasionally be a risk for incomplete excision of bilobar or multilobar adenomas. Disruption of the adenoma capsule during surgery may cause implantation of adenomatous parathyroid tissue and can give rise to persistent or recurrent hyperparathyroidism (parathyromatosis) {19,645}. Occasionally, hyperparathyroidism may persist after surgical excision owing to the presence of a second adenoma or other causes.

Atypical adenomas are tumours of uncertain malignant potential and patients with these tumours should be followed for persistent hyperparathyroidism and signs of local recurrence and/or metastases.

Secondary tumours of the parathyroid

R.A. DeLellis

Definition

Tumours involving the parathyroid that arise as a result of direct extension from contiguous structures or as a result of hematogenous /lymphatic spread from a distant site.

Clinical features

Most patients with secondary tumours of the parathyroid are asymptomatic. However, some patients may present with evidence of a mass lesion involving the neck. Depending on the extent of the tumour, there may be hoarseness, dysphagia and neck pain. Hypoparathyroidism resulting from tumourous involvement of the parathyroid is exceptionally rare {920}.

Origin of metastases

The most common sites of origin of tumours involving the parathyroid glands include breast, skin (melanoma), lung, kidney and soft tissue.

Macroscopy

Metastases to the parathyroid glands may be inapparent by gross examination

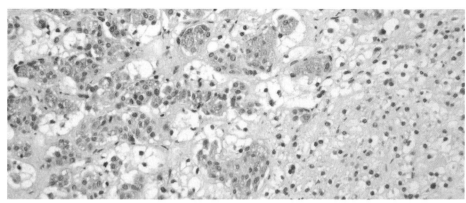

Fig. 2.120 Metastatic carcinoma. This metastatic breast carcinoma stains positively for mucin (mucicarmine stain) while the adjacent parathyroid adenoma is negative.

or may lead to enlargement of one or more glands {470}. In cases in which there is direct extension of tumour from an adjacent site, the primary tumour tends to be large with involvement of multiple parathyroid glands.

Histopathology

Most tumours involving the parathyroid glands by direct extension are thyroid carcinomas, squamous cell carcinomas, malignant lymphomas or soft tissue

tumours. Metastatic tumours generally retain the cytohistological features of the primary tumours.

Prognosis and predictive factors

Prognosis is dependant on the nature of the primary malignancy.

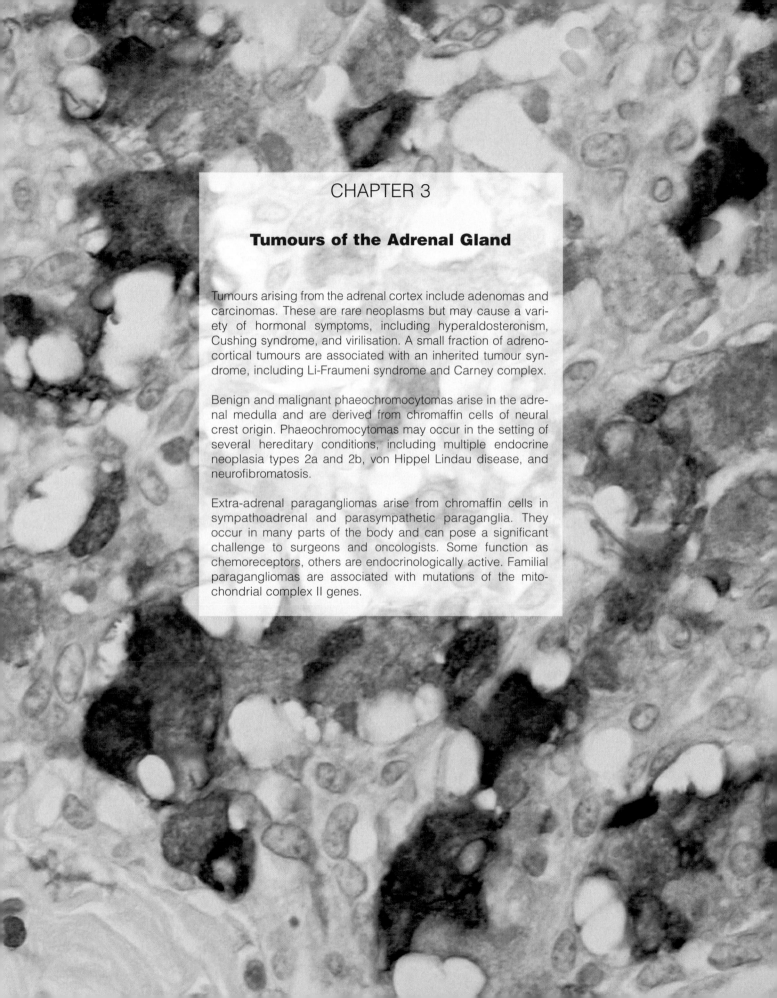

CHAPTER 3

Tumours of the Adrenal Gland

Tumours arising from the adrenal cortex include adenomas and carcinomas. These are rare neoplasms but may cause a variety of hormonal symptoms, including hyperaldosteronism, Cushing syndrome, and virilisation. A small fraction of adrenocortical tumours are associated with an inherited tumour syndrome, including Li-Fraumeni syndrome and Carney complex.

Benign and malignant phaeochromocytomas arise in the adrenal medulla and are derived from chromaffin cells of neural crest origin. Phaeochromocytomas may occur in the setting of several hereditary conditions, including multiple endocrine neoplasia types 2a and 2b, von Hippel Lindau disease, and neurofibromatosis.

Extra-adrenal paragangliomas arise from chromaffin cells in sympathoadrenal and parasympathetic paraganglia. They occur in many parts of the body and can pose a significant challenge to surgeons and oncologists. Some function as chemoreceptors, others are endocrinologically active. Familial paragangliomas are associated with mutations of the mitochondrial complex II genes.

WHO histological classification of tumours of the adrenal gland

Adrenal cortical tumours
Adrenal cortical carcinoma   8370/3
Adrenal cortical adenoma   8370/0

Adrenal medullary tumours
Malignant phaeochromocytoma   8700/3
Benign phaeochromocytoma   8700/0
Composite phaeochromocytoma / paraganglioma

Extra-adrenal paraganglioma   8693/1
    Carotid body   8692/1
    Jugulotympanic   8690/1
    Vagal   8693/1
    Laryngeal   8693/1
    Aortico-pulmonary   8691/1
    Gangliocytic   8683/0
    Cauda equina   8693/1
    Orbital Nasopharyngeal   8693/1
    Extra-adrenal sympathetic paraganglioma   8693/1
    Superior and inferior para-aortic paraganglioma   8693/1

Urinary bladder   8693/1
Intrathoracic and cervical paravertebral   8693/1

Other adrenal tumours
Adenomatoid tumour   9054/0
Sex-cord stromal tumour   8590/1
Soft tissue and germ cell tumours
    Myelolipoma   8870/0
    Teratoma   9080/1
    Schwannoma   9560/0
    Ganglioneuroma   9490/0
    Angiosarcoma   9120/3

Secondary tumours

---

[1] Morphology code of the International Classification of Diseases for Oncology (ICD-O) {664} and the Systematized Nomenclature of Medicine (http://snomed.org). Behaviour is coded /0 for benign tumours, /3 for malignant tumours, and /1 for borderline or uncertain behaviour.

TNM classification of adrenal cortical carcinoma

TNM classification [1,2]

T – Primary Tumour
TX   Primary tumour cannot be assessed
T0   No evidence of primary tumour
T1   Tumour ≤5 cm, localized
T2   Tumour >5 cm, localized
T3   Tumour any size, locally invasive but not involving adjacent organs
T4   Tumour any size, involving adjacent organs

N – Regional lymph nodes
NX   Regional lymph nodes cannot be assessed.
N0   No regional lymph node metastasis
N1   Regional lymph node metastasis

M –   Distant metastasis
MX   Distant metastasis cannot be assessed.
M0   No distant metastasis
M1   Distant metastasis

Stage Grouping

Stage	T	N	M
Stage I	T1	N0	M0
Stage II	T2	N0	M0
Stage III	T1 or T2	N1	M0
	T3	N0	M0
Stage IV	T3	N1	M0
	T4	N0	M0
	Any T	Any N	M1

---

[1] {2402}
[2] A help desk for specific questions about the TNM classification is available at http://www.uicc.org/tnm

Adrenal tumours: Introduction

R.V. Lloyd
A.S. Tischler
N. Kimura
A.M. McNicol
W.F. Young Jr.

Adrenal tumours

Most primary tumours of the adrenal glands consist of two distinct types of neoplasms. Those arising from the adrenal cortex include adenomas and carcinomas while tumours arising from the medulla represent neural crest-derived chromaffin cell tumours or phaeochromocytomas. Paragangliomas are closely related to adrenal phaeochromocytomas and are extra-adrenal in location. Some of these tumours are also referred to as extra-adrenal phaeochromocytomas, and chemodectomas.

Adrenal cortical adenomas

The prevalence of adrenal cortical adenomas greater than 1 cm in diameter in autopsy series has ranged from 1.5% to 7% {2132}. With the use of high resolution imaging such as CT and MRI, incidentally discovered adrenal masses (incidentalomas) have become a common finding and are uncovered in up to 4% of patients imaged for nonadrenal disorders {1109}. Incidentalomas are uncommon in patients below the age of 30, and they increase in frequency with age. They occur equally in males and females, and in more than 85% of cases, they represent nonfunctioning adenomas {2132}. In up to 20% of cases, they may cause abnormal hormone secretion without obvious clinical manifestations {1870}. Nonfunctioning incidentalomas less than 5 cm are likely to be benign, but larger tumours may be malignant.

The most frequent endocrine abnormalities associated with adenomas are primary hyperaldosteronism followed by Cushing syndrome, virilisation, and rarely feminisation {1194,2097,2132}.

Variants. In addition to the classical adrenal cortical adenomas, a few variants may be seen: Pigmented "black" adenomas - These benign tumours have abundant intracytoplasmic lipofuscin, and the tumours appear dark brown to black and may be functional and associated with Cushing syndrome. There is no clinical significance associated with the excessive pigment.

Oncocytic adrenal cortical adenoma. These tumours have cells with abundant compact eosinophilic cytoplasm that is finely granular. They are usually nonfunctional, and ultrastructural features include abundant mitochondria and a paucity of lipid droplets.

Myxoid variant of adrenal cortical adenomas {250}. These tumours have abundant extracellular mucin and may show pseudoacinar formation.

Adrenal cortical carcinomas

These are rare tumours with an incidence of one per million population per year. Women are more often affected than men (2.5:1), and the mean age of onset is 40-50 years; but men tend to be older at presentation {2132}. About 80% of the tumours are functional most commonly secreting glucocorticoids (45%), glucocorticoids and androgens (45%), or androgens alone (10%). Less than 1% of all cases secrete aldosterone {1067,2132}. There is usually no significant racial predilection, but a recent epidemiologic study showed a trend of increased rates among blacks {417}.

Unusual variants of adrenal cortical carcinomas include:

Oncocytic adrenal cortical carcinomas - These are mitochondria-rich tumours that are usually nonfunctional. Although many oncocytic adrenal cortical tumours are benign, some can be malignant {1194}.

Myxoid variant of adrenal cortical carcinoma - These have similar features as the myxoid variant of adenomas with obvious malignant features as well {250}.

Adrenal carcinosarcoma - These are very rare malignancies with features of adrenal cortical carcinomas and sarcomas such as rhabdomyosarcomas {122}, but they may also have osteogenic or chondroid differentiation {476,634}.

Paediatric adrenal cortical neoplasms

These tumours are usually functional in paediatric patients. Children often show signs and symptoms of endocrine abnormalities. In one series, there were only 17 of 200 nonfunctional cortical tumours {1581}. Most present with virilisation followed by Cushing syndrome along with a mixed endocrine syndrome including virilisation {1194}. Pure Cushing syndrome is uncommon in this population. Feminisation is unusual, as is primary hyperaldosteronism {1194}.

There is usually a female predominance with an average age of 4.6 years, and half the patients are diagnosed in the first four years of life {1581}.

Etiology of adrenal cortical neoplasms

Some hereditary syndromes have been associated with adrenal cortical tumours {1804,1806}, including Li-Fraumeni syndrome, Beckwith-Wiedemann syndrome,

Table 3.01
Functional classification of adrenal cortical tumours.

1. Endocrine hyperfunction (hypercorticalism)   Hypercortisolism (Cushing syndrome)   Hyperaldosteronism (Conn syndrome)   Virilisation   Feminisation   Mixed endocrine syndrome
2. Non functional or nonhyperfunctional
3. Functional status unknown

Table 3.02
Oncogenes, tumour suppression genes and growth factors implicated in adrenal cortical tumourigenesis.

Oncogenes   G protein (Gas) {1373}   *RAS* {2450}   Calcium-dependent protein kinase C activity {1242}   ACTH receptor deletions {1808}
Tumour suppressor genes   *TP53* {1636}   *MEN1* {1986,1987}   *P57Kip2* {1312}   *H19* {1312}
Growth factors   IGF II overexpression {712,713,958}

Table 3.03
Functional classification of tumours of intra-adrenal (phaeochromocytomas) and extra-adrenal (paraganglioma) tumours.

1. Functional disturbance
Hyperfunction
Hypertension
Watery diarrhoea, hypokalaemia,
achlorhydria syndrome
Cushing syndrome
Others, including acromegaly
2. No functional disturbance
3. Functional status unknown

Table 3.04
Genetic alterations in familial phaeochromocytomas and paragangliomas.

MEN2A	(10q11.2)
MEN2B	(10q11.2)
Von Hippel-Lindau (*VHL*)	(3p25.3)
NF1	(17q11.2)
SDHD, SDHB, SDHC	(11q23, 1p36, 1q21)
References {16,568,795,1123,1131,1587,1599}	

and Carney complex (*see* Chapter 5). These account for only a small percentage of adrenal cortical neoplasms, since most of these tumours are sporadic. Various oncogenes, tumour suppressor genes and growth factors have been implicated in the pathogenesis of adrenal cortical tumours. The exact role of these genes in tumour development and progression remains to be elucidated.

Phaeochromocytoma and paragangliomas

Phaeochromocytomas and paragangliomas are tumours of neural crest origin arising from chromaffin cells {1194,2097}. The incidence of phaeochromocytoma was calculated to be 0.8 per 100,000 person-years {502, 1377,2381}. Paraganglia are specialized neural crest-derived cells that are dispersed in many parts of the body {660,2097}. These paraganglionic cells are usually divided into sympathoadrenal and parasympathetic paraganglia. The sympathoadrenal paraganglia are more or less symmetrically distributed along the paravertebral axis from high in the neck near the superior cervical ganglion to the abdomen and pelvis. There are also small paraganglia associated with organs such as the urinary bladder and prostate gland. The greatest concentration of chromaffin cells are in the adrenal medulla and function to make more rapid adjustments to environmental changes ("fight or flight") mediated by norepinephrine and epinephrine.

Paraganglia of the head and neck region and middle mediastinum are closely aligned with the parasympathetic nervous system and have a special relationship with the branchial arches such as the carotid body paraganglia {2097}. Some of these paraganglia such as the carotid body function as chemoreceptors by detecting changes in PaO_2, $PaCO_2$, and pH leading to reflex alterations in breathing and cardiovascular functions. Individuals living at high altitudes such as the Peruvian Andes often have AN increased incidence of paraganglionic hyperplasia, including carotid body paraganglionic hyperplasia, and neoplasia.

In general, sympathoadrenal paraganglia are often functionally active and secrete catecholamines. With rare exceptions, the paraganglia of the head and neck are endocrinologically silent. Some tumours arising from the aorticopulmonary paraganglia can actively secrete catecholamines.

Malignant phaeochromocytomas and paragangliomas

Malignant tumours constitute 3% to 13% of all cases {1194,2132}. The five-year survival is 23% to 44% compared to 97% for benign phaeochromocytomas. Malignancy is defined strictly by metastatic disease to sites where chromaffin tissues are usually not present. Metastatic sites include lungs, bones, liver, and lymph nodes. Malignant tumours may also recur locally. Intra-abdominal extra-adrenal paragangliomas probably have the highest rate of malignancy among these tumours {1194}. Malignant tumours are larger, have a higher mitotic count, and have extensive local or vascular invasion. They also express fewer peptides on immunohistochemical studies compared to benign tumours.

Benign phaeochromocytomas

These tumours are usually unilateral and solitary within the adrenal. Familial tumours may be bilateral and multicentric. In the familial setting of multiple endocrine neoplasia types 2A and 2B, there is usually medullary hyperplasia preceding the development of phaeochromocytomas. Historically, the chromaffin reaction was used to identify these tumours. In this reaction, a section of tumour is immersed in a dichromate-containing fixative, and this results in a tan-brown reaction product. Most tumours are functional and they may produce ectopic hormones.

Benign paragangliomas

These extra-adrenal paragangliomas and chemodectomas constitute 10% or less of total phaeochromocytomas/paragangliomas. In the series of Fries and Chamberlin, 205 extra-adrenal tumours were examined; 3% were cervical, 12% were intrathoracic, and 85% were intra-abdominal. Of the intra-abdominal tumours, 45% were in the superior para-aortic location, 30% in the inferior para-aortic location, and 10% were in the urinary bladder {660}. In the series of 107 phaeochromocytomas and paragangliomas reported by Melicow, 98% of the tumours were intra-adrenal and intra-abdominal, while only 2% were cervical or intrathoracic, and less than 1% of these arose in the urinary bladder {1478}.

Genetic susceptibility

Various hereditary conditions have been linked to familial phaeochromocytomas including multiple endocrine neoplasia types 2a and 2b, von Hippel Lindau disease, and neurofibromatosis {568,1123, 1131,1134,1587}. Familial paragangliomas are associated with mutations of the mitochondrial complex II genes SDHD, SDHB, and SDHC {16,107,1599}. For details see Chapter 5.

Adrenal cortical carcinoma

L.M. Weiss
X. Bertagna
G.P. Chrousos
A. Kawashima
P. Kleihues
C.A. Koch

T.J. Giordano
L.J. Medeiros
M.J. Merino
N.G. Ordonez
H. Sasano

Definition
A malignant epithelial tumour of adrenal cortical cells.

ICD-O code   8370/3

Epidemiology
The incidence of adrenal cortical carcinoma has been stable, at about 0.1 cases per 100,000, accounting for about 3% of endocrine neoplasms. Most series report a predilection for females {2420}, although Surveillance, Epidemiology, and End Results (SEER) data from the United States suggest a higher incidence in males {417}. The SEER data also suggests a trend of increased rates among African Americans. There is a primary peak of incidence around age 70, with a secondary smaller peak in the first two years of life.

Clinical features
Signs and symptoms
The most common presentation is associated with glucocorticoid and androgen oversecretion by the tumour {1369,2342}; The first is responsible for Cushing syndrome: centripetal obesity, protein wasting with skin thinning and striae, muscle atrophy (myopathy), osteoporosis, impaired defense against infection, diabetes, high blood pressure, psychiatric disturbances, and gonadal dysfunction in men and women. Androgen oversecretion may induce virilisation in women. Mineralocorticoids, such as

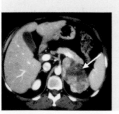
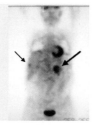

Fig. 3.01. Adrenal cortical carcinoma. CT scan (left) shows a large, irregular, non homogeneous adrenal tumour with high spontaneous density. PET imaging (right) demonstrates intense 18-FDG uptake in the adrenal tumour and in a hepatic metastasis (arrows).

DOC (deoxycorticosterone), may contribute a severe state of mineralocorticoid excess with high blood pressure and hypo-kalaemia. Exceptional tumours with estrogen secretion may provoke gynecomastia in men, metrorrhagia in post-menopausal women. A significant subset of ACCs secrete only (or predominantly) androgens; and some show no clinical features of hormone excess, although they may produce non-bioactive steroid precursors. The latter tumours may be discovered as "incidentalomas" {1109, 1370}, as mass lesions, or as metastatic disease.
ACCs tend to be large tumours (greater than 5-6 cm) that may provoke local or regional manifestations such as flank pain and/or fever, through local compression or in situ tumour necrosis.

Hormonal imbalance
Endocrinological investigations may establish the adrenal origin of the tumour. ACTH-independent cortisol oversecretion may be demonstrable by increased urinary cortisol excretion that is not suppressible with high doses of dexamethasone and is associated with undetectable ACTH plasma levels. The specific adrenal androgen dehydroepiandrosterone (DHEAS), is often elevated, which leads to increased plasma testosterone in females. Other steroids such as DOC, 17OH progesterone, Delta 4 androstenedione, and estrogens can be overproduced by the tumour. Twenty-four-hour urinary excretion of 17-ketogenic and 17-ketosteroids may be elevated. In "non-hypersecretory" ACCs, the entire hormonal work-up may be normal.

Imaging
Although imaging studies can provide vital information for detection and localization of adrenal cortical tumours and may suggest malignancy, the diagnosis of carcinoma must subsequently be determined by pathologic criteria.
Computed tomography (CT) scans and magnetic resonance (MR) images of

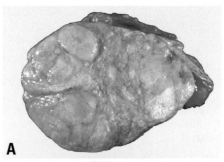

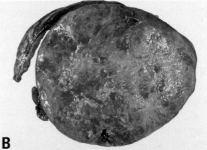

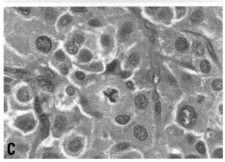

Fig. 3.02 **A** Adrenal cortical carcinoma. Gross appearance of adrenal cortical carcinoma. **B** Oncocytoma. **C** Adrenal carcinoma. A tripolar atypical mitotic figure is seen in this adrenal cortical carcinoma.

adrenal cortical carcinomas typically demonstrate a large (larger than 5 cm) inhomogeneously enhancing suprarenal mass, which may contain areas of decreased enhancement secondary to haemorrhage or necrosis {635}. Calcifications are present in 30% of the tumours on CT. Adjacent organs such as inferior vena cava, kidney, liver, and pancreas are frequently displaced or involved by the tumours. Hepatic and nodal metastases are common. Tumour extension to the inferior vena cava is best demonstrated on MR images.

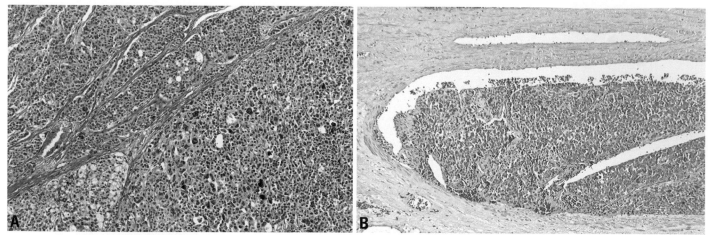

Fig. 3.03 Adrenal cortical carcinoma. **A** Note the nuclear pleomorphism. **B** Vascular invasion in the large vessel beyond the confines of an adrenal cortical carcinoma.

Ultrasonography with Doppler imaging is also valuable in evaluating the tumour thrombus. Iodo-cholesterol scintigraphy may help distinguish primary functional adrenal cortical lesions from medullary lesions and metastases to the adrenal gland, and may also be useful in the localization of metastatic adrenal cortical carcinoma. In the future, PET-scanning with 18FDG may help to characterize adrenal cortical tumours and identify distant metastases {145,2471}.

Tumour spread and staging
Invasion through the renal veins and the inferior vena cava can proceed up to the right atrium and result in metastatic tumour embolus to the lung {950}.
Adrenal cortical carcinomas most commonly spread to liver, lung, retroperitoneal lymph nodes, and bone, although practically any site may be involved at autopsy {1192}. The American Joint Committee on Cancer (AJCC) or International Union Against Cancer (UICC) do not recognize a specific staging system for adrenal cortical carcinoma. The staging system modified by Sullivan et al. is the system most commonly in use {2162}, although at least one group considers T3N1 disease to still represent Stage III since complete resection can theoretically be performed in such cases {950}. The majority of cases present with Stage IV disease, with about 40% of cases presenting with distant metastasis {417}.

Histopathology
Adrenal cortical carcinomas have architectural and cytologic features that gen-

erally recapitulate the normal adrenal cortex. The most common architectural pattern is that of patternless sheets of cells interrupted by a fine sinusoidal network. Other common patterns include broad trabeculae or large nests of cells. Although fine trabeculae or even serpiginous cords may be seen, true gland formation is not found. Broad fibrous bands may be present. Necrosis may be present and may be abundant, and myxoid change is occasionally seen {250}. Invasion of the capsule, sinusoids, or even large veins is commonly present. Cytologically, adrenal cortical carcinomas are composed of varying numbers of cells with eosinophilic or bubbly clear cytoplasm. Nuclear atypia varies from non-existent to highly pleomorphic. Similarly, the mitotic rate varies widely, from rare mitotic figures to several per high power field, with easily recognizable atypical forms. One group has proposed grading on the basis of mitotic rate, with tumours with >20 mitoses per high power field regarded as high grade {2372}. Rare variants of adrenal cortical carcinoma include adrenal cortical carcinomas with oncocytic features {554}, and carcinomas with sarcomatous areas, so-called adrenal carcinosarcomas {634}.

Immunohistochemistry
Immunostaining may be applied to tissue sections, core biopsies or fine needle aspiration cytology specimens. Immunohistochemical profiling may be helpful in separating adrenocortical carcinomas from renal cell and hepatocellular carcinoma, adrenal medullary and metastatic tumours. Immunoreactivity for α-inhibin

as well as for the A103 anti-melan-A antibody is sensitive but not specific for adrenal cortical carcinoma {270,1558}. Immunohistochemistry using antibodies to Ad4BP/SF-1 (Adrenal 4 Binding Protein / Steroidogenic factor 1) may be of use in the future in the specific identification of adrenal cortical cells {1945, 1946}. In contrast to other epithelial tumours, adrenal cortical carcinomas are variably reported to be negative to weakly positive for cytokeratin, and negative for epithelial membrane antigen, carcinoembyonic antigen, and glycoprotein HMFG-2 {676}. Adrenal cortical carcinomas are negative for chromogranin A, the most reliable marker for discriminating them from adrenal medullary tumours. Other neural markers have been reported to be variably positive in

Table 3.05
Histopathologic criteria proposed by Weiss {2372} for distinguishing benign from malignant adrenocortical neoplasms*, with modification proposed by Aubert {101}

1. High nuclear grade. Fuhrman criteria {769}
2. > 5 mitoses per 50 high-power fields
3. Atypical mitotic figures
4. < 25% of tumour cells are clear cells
5. Diffuse architecture (>33% of tumour)
6. Necrosis
7. Venous invasion (smooth muscle in wall)
8. Sinusoidal invasion (no smooth muscle in wall)
9. Capsular invasion

* The presence of three or more criteria highly correlates with subsequent malignant behaviour {2372}

Table 3.06
System of Van Slooten et al {2299} for distinguishing benign from malignant adrenocortical neoplasms

Histologic Criteria	Weighted Value
1. Extensive regressive changes (necrosis, haemorrhage, fibrosis, calcification)	5.7
2. Loss of normal structure	1.6
3. Nuclear atypia (moderate/marked)	2.1
4. Nuclear hyperchromasia (moderate/marked)	2.6
5. Abnormal nucleoli	4.1
6. Mitotic activity (≥2 per 10 HPF)	9.0
7. Vascular or capsular invasion	3.3

HPF = high-power fields
Histologic index >8 correlates with subsequent malignant behaviour.

cortical tumours. Ultrastructural studies usually reveal features typical of steroid-producing cells, with abundant rough and smooth endoplasmic reticulum, numerous mitochondria with well-developed tubular or lamellar cristae, and lipid.

Carcinoma vs. adenoma
The major differential diagnosis is with adrenal cortical adenoma. A variety of clinical, macroscopic, and microscopic features may be useful in this setting. Some of the proposed systems for distinguishing adrenal cortical carcinoma from adenoma are given in Tables 3.05-3.07 {923,2299,2372}. A recent publication has recommended a modification of the Weiss system, given in Table 3.05 {101}. Histologic criteria that are consistently useful across the classification systems include the mitotic rate, and the presence of vascular or capsular invasion. The MIB-1/Ki-67 labeling index may be of value and usually averages about 5-20%, with a wide range of variation {1472,1576,2214}. A labeling index for topoisomerase II alpha may also contribute to the differential diagnosis {952}. Insulin-like growth factor-2 may be of some help {101,574,1472,1576,2214}, while ploidy analysis is not helpful {385}. Some investigators believe that the criteria for malignancy differ for paediatric tumours, in which large tumour size or weight and age >3.5 years are associated with unfavourable outcomes {1818}, although a recent report has suggested that paediatric tumours may be evaluat-

ed using similar criteria as for adults {2383}. Findings favouring metastatic carcinoma rather than adrenal cortical carcinoma include bilaterality, evidence of any glandular, squamous, or small cell histology.

Somatic genetics
There are no known precursor lesions to adrenal cortical carcinoma and no specific genetic alterations have been identified to date in tumourigenesis or tumour progression {1122}.

Chromosomal imbalances
However, amplifications and losses of specific gene loci have been identified by comparative genomic hybridization or allelotyping {506,626,991,1100,1101, 2049,2491}. In these preliminary studies, the most frequent chromosomes with losses are 1, 2, 3, 4, 6, 9, 11, 13, 15, 17, 18, 22, and X. Gains occur most frequently on chromosomes 1, 2, 4, 5, 7, 8, 9, 12, 14, 16, 17, 19, 20, 22, and X. Some investigators found a correlation of chromosomal abnormalities with tumour size, i.e. adrenal cortical adenomas smaller than 5 cm had no detectable gains or losses, whereas adrenal carcinomas (the smallest being 7 cm) frequently had losses at chromosomes 2, 11q, and 17p as well as gains at chromosomes 4 and 5 {1100}. A recent study reported gain in chromosome 4 in benign adrenal cortical adenomas smaller than 5 cm, whereas adrenal carcinomas (>5 cm) had gains in chromosomes 5, 12, and 19 {2049}. Benign adrenal lesions had chromosomal losses only at 3q, whereas such losses occurred at 1p, 11, 17p, and 22 in adrenal carcinomas.

Molecular genetics
The most frequent molecular genetic alterations reported in preliminary studies of adrenal carcinomas are overexpression of IGF2 in sporadic tumours with duplication of the paternal allele {711-713,958}, loss of heterozygosity (LOH) at chromosomal subband 11p15 {711,1100,2491}, and low expression of *p57* {127,1312}. Overexpression of *EGFR* at 7p12 and of the tumour suppressor genes *p21* and *p16* are also frequent in adrenal carcinoma {127,1029,1742, 1948,2135}. A subset of sporadic adrenal carcinomas have LOH at the *TP53* locus 17p13 {711,1100,2337,2491} and somatic mutations in *TP53* {127,1636,

Table 3.07
System of Hough et al. {923} for distinguishing benign from malignant adrenocortical neoplasms.

Criteria	Value
Histologic Criteria	
1. Diffuse growth pattern	0.92
2. Vascular invasion	0.92
3. Tumour cell necrosis	0.69
4. Broad fibrous bands	1.00
5. Capsular invasion	0.37
6. Mitotic index (1 per 10 HPF)	0.60
7. Pleomorphism (moderate/marked)	0.39
Nonhistologic Criteria	
1. Tumour mass >100 g	0.60
2. Urinary 17-ketosteroids (10 mg/g creatinine/24 hours)	0.50
3. Response to ACTH (17-hydroxy-steroids increased two times after 50 mg ACTH IV)	0.42
4. Cushing syndrome with virilism, virilism alone, or no clinical manifestations	0.42
5. Weight loss (10 lb/3 months)	2.00

HPF = High-power fields; ACTH = adrenocorticotrophic hormone; IV = intravenous
The mean histologic index of malignant tumours was 2.91, indeterminate tumours 1.00, and benign tumours 0.17

1807}. Whereas LOH at the menin locus at 11q13 is frequent in sporadic adrenal carcinomas {870,1101, 2337}, somatic mutations in menin are uncommon {870,1101}. Rare alterations are somatic mutations in the *RAS* genes, *RET*, *EGF*, and *ATR1* {1887,1948,2450}.

Gene expression profiles
Preliminary DNA microarray analysis of a series of adrenal tumours revealed consistent gene expression differences between benign and malignant tumours, with increased IGF2 being the dominant transcriptional change among the approximately 10,500 genes surveyed in this study {721}. Interestingly, most growth factor receptors present on the microarray (e.g. EGFR and ERB-B2) were either not expressed or expressed at relatively low levels.

Genetic susceptibility
Almost all adrenal cortical carcinomas are sporadic. Among the extremely rare inherited cancer syndromes occasionally associated with adrenocortical carcinoma are two autosomal dominantly inherit-

ed syndromes, the Li-Fraumeni syndrome and the Beckwith-Wiedemann syndrome. Approximately one percent of patients with the classic Li-Fraumeni syndrome develop adrenal cortical carcinoma, usually before age 30 {1105,1919}. Most have germline mutations in the tumour suppressor gene *TP53* located at chromosomal subband 17p13 {2339}. Adrenal cancer as the sole manifestation of the Li-Fraumeni syndrome may be present in children with *TP53* germline mutations {1243}. Allele loss at 17p13 leading to biallelic inactivation of the tumour suppressor gene *TP53* is a frequent finding in tumours of patients with *TP53* germline mutations. The Beckwith-Wiedemann syndrome occurs sporadically or in an autosomal dominant pattern with variable expressivity. Family studies of such patients revealed a gene locus at chromosomal subband 11p15.5 {866}.

This locus includes the *IGF2* and the *p57/KIP2* genes. Uniparental paternal isodisomy for the *IGF2* locus is frequently found in individuals with Beckwith-Wiedemann syndrome. This often leads to overexpression of IGF2 in tumours including adrenal carcinoma from these patients {711,712}. The *p57* tumour suppressor protein inhibits G1 cyclin/cyclin-dependent kinase complexes and thereby negatively influences cell proliferation {235}.

Prognosis and predictive factors
The five-year survival rate is 50-70% and has been improving over time. This is possibly due to a detection of smaller lesions by advanced radiological techniques.
The most important prognostic factors for patients with a diagnosis of adrenal cortical carcinoma are age and stage.

Paediatric patients diagnosed with carcinoma have a relatively good prognosis as compared to adult patients, with 5-year survivals greater than 50% {2383}. Patients with tumours diagnosed in stages I and II have a far superior survival than those with tumours diagnosed in stages III and IV; in fact, the crucial factor may be whether neoplasms are completely resectable {950}. The most important pathologic prognostic factors include mitotic rate, tumour size and the Ki-67 index {838,2372}.

Adrenal cortical adenoma

H. Sasano
W.F. Young Jr.
G.P. Chrousos

C.A. Koch
T.J. Giordano
A. Kawashima

Definition
A benign epithelial tumour of the adrenal cortical cells.

ICD-O code　　　　　　8370/0

Epidemiology
The true incidence of adrenal cortical adenomas is unknown. Nodules are found commonly at autopsy and are more common with increasing age and with vascular diseases. Some of these may represent localized compensatory overgrowth of adrenocortical cells in response to localized ischaemic damage while others are true neoplasms. Size, weight and encapsulation are not reliable in differentiating adenomas from nodules. Adrenal cortical adenomas can occur in any age group including paediatric populations and in both sexes. The widespread use of computed abdominal imaging has resulted in increasingly frequent diagnosis of "adrenal incidentaloma", which may be associated with subclinical autonomous hormone secretion.

Localization
The great majority of adrenal cortical adenomas are unilateral. Precise localization to the zona glomerulosa, zona fasciculata, or zona reticularis cannot usually be established.

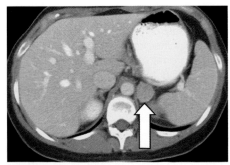

Fig. 3.04. Adrenal adenoma in a 24-year old woman with ACTH-independent Cushing syndrome. CT scan of the abdomen shows a 2.5 cm mass in the left adrenal gland. At laparoscopic left adrenalectomy a cortical adenoma (diameter, 2.4 cm) was found; the surrounding adrenal cortex was atrophic.

Clinical features
Clinical features associated with an adrenal cortical adenoma are dependent on the hormonal secretory status of the tumour.

Cortisol-producing adenoma
Cortisol hypersecretion may result in adrenocorticotropin hormone (ACTH) independent Cushing syndrome. Typical signs and symptoms include weight gain with central obesity, facial rounding and plethora, supraclavicular and dorsocervical fat pads, easy bruising, thin skin, poor wound healing, purple striae, proximal muscle weakness, emotional and cognitive changes, hypertension, osteoporosis, opportunistic and fungal infections (e.g., mucocutaneous candidiasis, tinea versicolor), altered reproductive function, and hirsutism. Hypercortisolism must be confirmed with baseline measurements of serum and 24-hour urine cortisol concentrations. Autonomous hypercortisolism should be confirmed with dexamethasone suppression testing {1597}. Undetectable plasma ACTH concentration classifies the subtype of hypercortisolism as ACTH-independent. In general, the cortisol production rate is correlated with adenoma size. Most adenomas that autonomously secrete enough cortisol to cause clinical Cushing syndrome are >2.5 cm in diameter. Patients that harbour cortisol-secreting adenomas that measure <2.5 cm in diameter may present with a milder symptom complex termed "subclinical Cushing syndrome" {1870,2202,2465}.

Aldosterone-producing adenoma
Aldosterone hypersecretion may result in hypertension and hypokalemia and is termed Conn syndrome or primary aldosteronism. Few symptoms are specific to the syndrome. Patients with marked hypokalemia may have muscle weakness, cramping, headaches, palpitations, polydipsia, polyuria, or nocturia. However, most patients with primary aldosteronism do not have hypokalemia {1869,2464}. There are no specific phys-

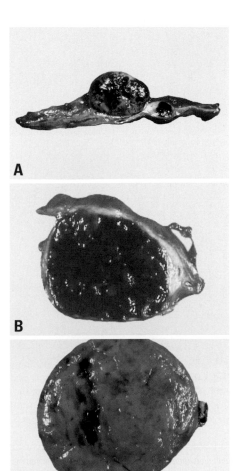

Fig. 3.05 A Cushing adenoma. The cut surface shows heterogenous tan and brown appearance. **B** Pigmented (black) adenoma. **C** Oncocytoma.

ical findings. The degree of hypertension is usually moderate to severe and may be resistant to the usual pharmacologic treatments. Screening for primary aldosteronism can be completed with a plasma aldosterone concentration to plasma renin activity ratio {684,1529}. The confirmation of primary aldosteronism is accomplished by demonstrating autonomous aldosterone secretion with sodium suppression testing {2464}. An apparent adrenal cortical adenoma on computerized imaging in a patient with primary aldosteronism is not necessarily an aldosterone-secreting adenoma. In addition, small nodules found on adrenal

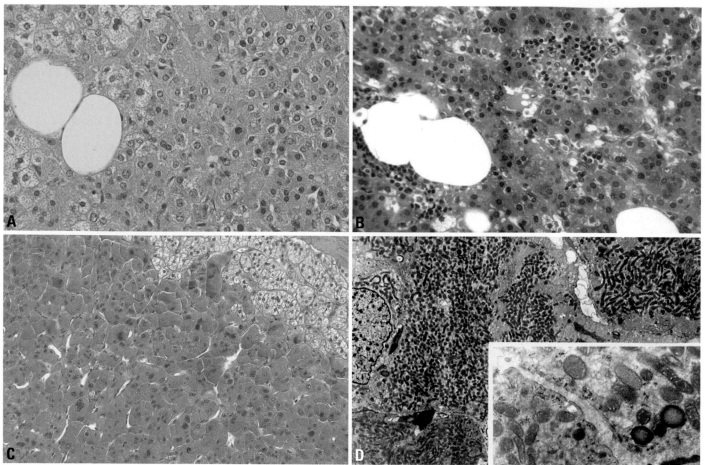

Fig. 3.06 A Cushing adenoma. This tumour is composed of tumour cells with eosinophilic cytoplasm. **B** Adrenal adenoma with varying proportions of clear cells with abundant intracytoplasmic lipid droplets and compact cells with lipid sparse eosinophilic cytoplasm. Note focal lymphocytic infiltrates. **C** Oncocytoma, composed of large cells with eosinophilic cytoplasm. **D** Electron microscopy of an adrenal oncocytoma. The tumour cells contain abundant mitochondria.

CT scan may be areas of hyperplasia or an aldosterone-secreting adenoma. Adrenal venous sampling helps solve these clinical dilemmas {2464}.

Androgen and estrogen secreting adenomas

Sex-hormone-secreting adrenal cortical tumours are rare {452,1175,1509} and when present are usually carcinomas {950} rather than adenomas. Patients with these tumours usually have symptoms referable to androgen excess in females (hirsutism, amenorrhea, virilization) or estrogen excess in males (gynecomastia, impotence). A testosterone-secreting adrenal tumour in adult males may be clinically silent.

Nonfunctioning adrenal cortical adenoma or "Adrenal incidentaloma"

An adrenal cortical incidentaloma is an adrenal mass that is discovered serendipitously by radiologic examination, in the absence of symptoms or clinical findings suggestive of adrenal disease {2465}. The introduction of abdominal ultrasound, computerized tomography, and magnetic resonance imaging has created the clinical dilemma of the adrenal incidentaloma. An adrenal incidentaloma should be characterized with respect to 1) functional status, with a medical history, physical examination, and hormonal assessment and 2) malignant potential, with an assessment of the imaging phenotype and mass size {2465}.

Imaging

Imaging procedures can greatly assist in localization of adrenal cortical adenoma. High resolution CT scanning of the abdomen can detect adrenal cortical adenomas less than 5 mm in diameter. MRI and ultrasonography are no better than CT in localization of adrenal cortical adenomas but T2-weighted MRI imaging may contribute to the differential diagnosis between adenomas and carcinomas. Arteriograms and venography usually provide little additional value. Scintigraphic imaging using ^{131}I-labeled cholesterol derivatives during dexamethasone suppression can provide a localization based on functional properties. Selective venous sampling of aldosterone can be of help in localization of small aldosterone-producing adenomas. Most adrenal masses incidentally found during CT or MR examinations in patients with indications other than suspected adrenal pathology are adrenal cortical adenomas. Adrenal cortical adenoma is typically a well-defined, rounded homogeneous mass. Intratumoural calcification, haemorrhage or necrosis is rare. CT and MR exams can be used to differentiate adenomas from non-adenomas (i.e., metastases). Most (80%) of adenomas contain sufficient intratumoural lipid ("lipid-rich" adenomas) to allow charac-

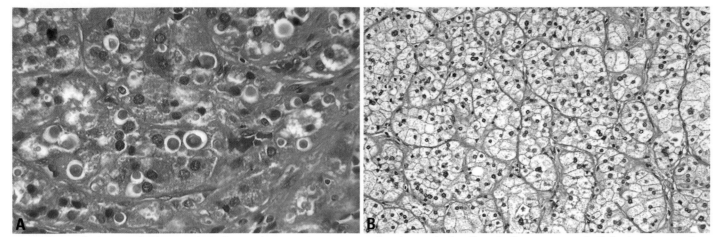

Fig. 3.07 Adrenal adenoma. **A** Adrenocortical adenoma demonstrating numerous spironolactone bodies. These bodies are concentrically laminated concretions frequently found in the zona glomerulosa of aldosterone producing tumours. **B** A benign adrenal cortical adenoma showing the characteristic microvesicular cytoplasm mimicking the adrenal zona fasciculata.

terization by means of unenhanced CT attenuation measurements and chemical-shift MR imaging.

Macroscopy
Most adrenal cortical adenomas are well-circumscribed intra-adrenal tumours, and some are encapsulated. Hormonally inactive adenomas cannot be differentiated from those that are hormonally active. The vast majority weigh less than 100 grams. Haemorrhage and necrosis are rarely observed. Adenomas associated with primary aldosteronism may appear bright yellow and well-circumscribed but not encapsulated, while those associated with Cushing syndrome may appear yellow to tan and encapsulated. A small number of adrenal cortical adenomas, usually clinically functional, have a homogeneous dark brown and black appearance. This variant is designated as black adenoma.

Histopathology
There are no definitive differences in histology, ultrastructure or expression of steroidogenic enzymes among the different clinically functional types of adenoma. Adrenal cortical adenomas usually consist of varying proportions of clear cells with abundant intracytoplasmic lipid droplets and compact cells with lipid sparse eosinophilic cytoplasm, occasionally with lipofuscin. Intermediate forms may also be observed. These cells form cords and/or nests with relatively abundant vasculature or sinusoidal structures. Eosinophilic whorled intracytoplasmic inclusions (spironolactone

bodies) may be seen in adenomas from patients with primary hyperaldosteronism treated with the drug. Adrenal cortical adenoma may show lipomatous or myelolipomatous metaplasia, which is not clinically relevant.

Oncocytoma
Among hormonally inactive adrenal cortical tumours are oncocytomas, which do not express steroidogenic enzymes and show histological features in common with oncocytic tumours at other sites {1947}. In principle, adrenal cortical oncocytoma is considered benign in its biological behaviour.

Immunohistochemistry
The compact cells usually express C17 or 17alpha-hydroxylase involved in cortisol production {1943} including aldosterone producing adrenocortical adenomas.

Electron microscopy
Ultrastructually adrenocortical adenomas demonstrate well-developed smooth endoplasmic reticulum and abundant mitochondria with well developed cristae.

Adjacent adrenal cortex
Non-neoplastic adrenals in Cushing adenoma usually demonstrate atrophy of the zonae fasciculata and reticularis, reflecting suppression of hypothalamo-pituitary-adrenal axis as a result of neoplastic cortisol secretion. In aldosterone-producing adenoma, there may occasionally be hyperplasia of the zona glomeru-

losa. This is termed "paradoxical hyperplasia" because the zona glomerulosa might be expected to be atrophic. In spite of the histological appearance, the cells appear to be nonfunctional as they do not express steroidogenic enzymes {1943}. These changes in the para-adenomatous gland may be the only indications of hormonal function of an adenoma.

Differential diagnosis
The main diagnostic problem in assessing adrenal cortical adenomas is the distinction from carcinoma. This is discussed in detail under adrenal cortical carcinoma.

Histogenesis
All adenomas derive from the normal adrenal cortex, including oncocytoma {1947}. This has been demonstrated by the expression of SF-1/Ad4BP (adrenal 4 binding protein), a marker of adrenocortical parenchymal cells, in all adrenocortical adenoma cells {1945}.

Somatic genetics
To date there are no consistent genetic changes that characterize adrenal cortical adenomas or distinguish between adenoma and carcinoma. The details are discussed under adrenal cortical carcinoma. Kjellman et al. {1100} reported adrenal cortical adenomas smaller than 5 cm had no detectable gains or losses, whereas adenomas larger than 5 cm had gain of 1q or 9q, or loss of 1p. These findings have clinical implications, since most experts recommend surgical

removal of an adrenal incidentaloma larger than 5 cm. However, incidental adrenal carcinomas as small as 1.7 cm have been reported {124}. Gene alterations such as LOH or somatic mutations in specific genes such as the *TP53*, *MEN1*, *GNAS1*, *GNAI2*, *ACTHR*, *ATR1*, and *RAS* genes are uncommon, whereas LOH at 11p15, the *P57* and *IGF2* locus, has been found in 32 of 94 adenomas {713}. Overexpression of IGF2 has been identified in 26 of 94 adenomas. Overexpression of *EGFR* at 7p12 is reported in 10 of 23 adenomas {1742}. DNA microarray analysis of normal adrenal cortex and adrenal cortical adenomas showed few transcriptional differences, a finding consistent with their similar histomorphology {721}.

Genetic susceptibility

Inherited syndromes that are associated with adrenal cortical adenomas or hyperplasias include Carney complex, multiple endocrine neoplasia type 1 (MEN 1), and the McCune-Albright syndrome. There are also congenital adrenal hyperplasia (CAH) and familial hyperaldosteronism (FH) type 1 and type 2. Carney complex is characterized by endocrine lesions including primary pigmented nodular adrenocortical disease (PPNAD) and pituitary tumours as well as spotty skin pigmentations, atrial and peripheral myxomas, and psammomatous melanotic schwannomas. Although most adrenal pathology in Carney complex is PPNAD, cortical adenomas that may be non-pigmented, may be seen in some patients. Two chromosomal loci of this autosomal dominant syndrome have been identified: 2p16 and 17q22-24 {327,2142}. *PRKAR1A*, a gene encoding protein kinase A regulatory subunit 1 alpha, is mutated in a subset of patients with Carney complex {1094}. MEN 1 is an autosomal dominantly inherited cancer syndrome in which up to 35% of patients with germline mutations in menin have adrenocortical nodules, most of them hormonally inactive {1122}. Familial hyperaldosteronism is a rare form of aldosterone excess caused by adrenocortical hyperplasia or nodules. The gene defect for FH type 1 is a hybrid gene at 8q24 {1300}. FH type 2 has been linked to 7p22 with a yet unidentified gene defect {1199}. Unilateral or bilateral adrenocortical hyperplasia or nodules develop in up to 80% of patients with CAH and germline mutations in the gene coding for 21-hydroxylase at 6p21.3 {995}. In these patients with CAH, adrenal cortical adenomas have been reported. Few patients with McCune-Albright syndrome, a sporadic postzygotic genetic disease, have adrenocortical adenomas {1122}.

Prognosis and predictive factors

Clinical prognosis for patients with adrenal cortical adenomas is determined by the severity of endocrine manifestations {1304,1740}. Histologically, the presence of severe cortical atrophy in adjacent non-neoplastic adrenal glands reflects significant suppression of the hypothalamic-pituitary-adrenal axis. These patients may need glucocorticoid supplementation {1944}. The presence of marked hypertensive changes in arterioles around the adrenals may be associated with persistent hypertension following surgery in primary aldosteronism. Therefore, it is important for the management of the patient that the pathologist reports the changes in the non-neoplastic adrenal cortex and in the vasculature around the gland.

Malignant adrenal phaeochromocytoma

L.D.R. Thompson
W.F. Young Jr.
A. Kawashima
P. Komminoth
A.S. Tischler

Definition

A malignant tumour of chromaffin cells of the adrenal medulla. Malignant phaeochromocytomas are currently defined by the presence of metastases. This definition does not account for the potentially lethal behaviour of tumours showing extensive local infiltration into adjacent organs or major blood vessels.

ICD-O Code
8700/3

Synonyms

Malignant paraganglioma; malignant chromaffinoma; phaeochromoblastoma; phaeochromocytoma with malignant features; phaeochromocytoma with atypical features; atypical phaeochromocytoma.

Epidemiology

Age and sex distribution for malignant phaeochromocytoma are not different from benign phaeochromocytoma. Malignant phaeochromocytomas comprise up to 10% of all phaeochromocytomas {1476,1478,1522,1650,1900, 1995,1997,1998,2229,2346}. There may be small differences in the frequency of malignancy between familial and sporadic phaeochromocytoma and between the different familial syndromes. NF1 tumours have a particularly low frequency of malignancy {2289}.

Localization

Localization is similar to benign phaeochromocytomas although extra-adrenal extension may be a clue to malignancy.

Clinical features

Signs and symptoms are similar to those found in patients with benign disease. Catecholamine excess and the degree of hypertension may be more marked in the patient with metastatic phaeochromocytoma. Patients with metastatic disease may have symptoms from mass effect and/or paraneoplastic syndromes due to peptide hormone secretion.

Imaging

Malignant phaeochromocytomas appear as large inhomogeneously enhancing masses. No imaging features can reliably distinguish common benign phaeochromocytomas from rare malignant phaeochromocytomas unless there is evidence of direct local invasion into the liver, kidney or pancreas, or distant metastases to the skeleton, lymph nodes, liver and lungs. Intratumoural necrosis, haemorrhage, and heterogeneity in imaging studies are common in both benign and malignant phaeochromocytomas. Bone scan and radiographs are useful for the evaluation of skeletal metastases. [123]I or ^{131}I-metaiodobenzylguanidine (MIBG) is useful for the detection of metastatic or locally recurrent disease.

Laboratory investigation

There are usually remarkably elevated levels of serum and/or urine catecholamines, norepinephrine, epinephrine, metanephrine, normetanephrine, dopamine, vanillylmandelic acid (VMA), or other metabolites. It has been suggested that dopamine values specifically may correlate with malignant phaeochromocytoma {1008,1774,2229}. Serum chromogranin A may be useful in monitoring the progression of disease.

Macroscopy

Several gross characteristics have been correlated with the propensity for malignant behaviour. The tumours tend to be larger than their benign counterparts. In addition, they may be nodular, lobulated, or bosselated, with a variegated cut surface showing mottled areas of haemorrhage and necrosis. The tumour can be fixed to the surrounding structures, occasionally infiltrating into the substance of the adrenal cortex and periadrenal adipose tissue {1476,1522,1914,1998,2035, 2229,2280}.

Tumour spread and staging

When metastatic deposits develop, the regional lymph nodes are most often affected, followed by the axial skeleton, liver, lung, and kidney {1476,1914,1974, 2023,2024,2229,2280,2281}. Malignant phaeochromocytomas may also show local invasion (capsular and periadrenal adipose connective tissue) and/or vascular invasion. However, these findings are not always present in tumours that

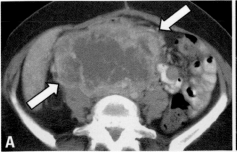
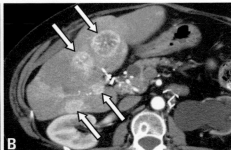
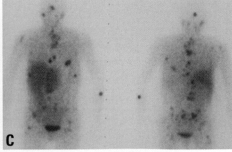

Fig. 3.08 Adrenal malignant phaeochromocytoma. **A** Abdominal CT scan from a 65-year-old woman shows massive locally recurrent malignant phaeochromocytomas. **B** Abdominal CT scan from this 72-year-old woman with malignant phaeochromocytoma with multiple liver metastases (arrows). **C** Scintigraphy with ^{123}I-meta-iodobenzylguanidine shows widespread metastatic disease.

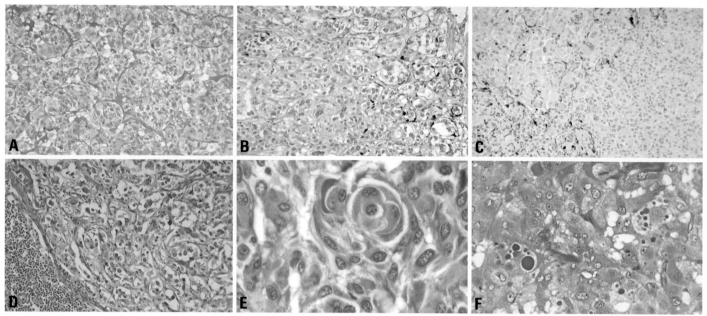

Fig. 3.09 Malignant phaeochromocytoma. **A** Mixed alveolar and trabecular architecture. **B** Lack of S-100 protein immunoreactivity in the large nests. **C** S-100 protein immunoreactivity is maintained in the nested (zellballen) area, while it is diminished or lost in the areas of large nests. **D** Metastatic phaeochromocytoma within a periadrenal lymph node. **E** A molded (morular) pattern is noted in a few cells within a malignant phaeochromocytoma. **F** Hyaline globules in a malignant phaeochromocytoma.

metastasize. There is currently no agreed upon staging system.

The most rigorous definition of malignancy requires that metastases must be present at a site where chromaffin tissue is not otherwise found thereby excluding the possibility of misclassifying multicentric primary lesions as metastases or the development of loco-regional recurrence {1476,1535,1760,1997,1998,2023,2035, 2280,2281}. An accumulation of specific histologic criteria has shown promise in the prospective diagnosis of a malignant phaeochromocytoma {1306, 1535,1974, 2229,2281}.

Histopathology

A number of histologic criteria have been identified in malignant phaeochromocytoma and include: 1) capsular invasion; 2) vascular invasion; 3) extension into the periadrenal adipose tissue; 4) expanded, large, and confluent nests; 5) diffuse growth; 6) necrosis; 7) increased cellularity; 8) tumour cell spindling; 9) profound cellular and nuclear pleomorphism; 10) cellular monotony (usually with smaller cells having high nuclear to cytoplasmic ratio); 11) nuclear hyperchromasia; 12) macronucleoli; 13) increased mitotic figures; 14) any atypical mitotic figures; 15) absence of hyaline globules.

Vascular invasion is defined by direct extension into the vessel lumen, intravascular attached tumour thrombi, and/or tumour nests covered by endothelium identified in a capsular or extracapsular vessel. Tumour plugs in vascular spaces within the tumour mass do not qualify as vascular invasion. No distinction is made between veins or lymphatic spaces. A "large nest" was defined as at least three times the size of the "zellballen" in a normal sympathetic paraganglion by the study in which the most precise definition

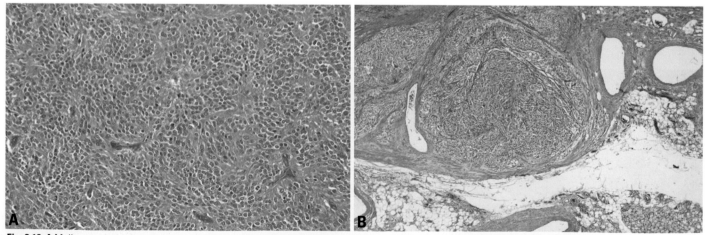

Fig. 3.10 A Malignant phaeochromocytoma. A diffuse pattern of growth seen in a malignant phaeochromocytoma. Focal tumour spindling is noted. **B** Vascular invasion identified in a malignant phaeochromocytoma of the adrenal gland. Note the brown fat in the surrounding soft tissue.

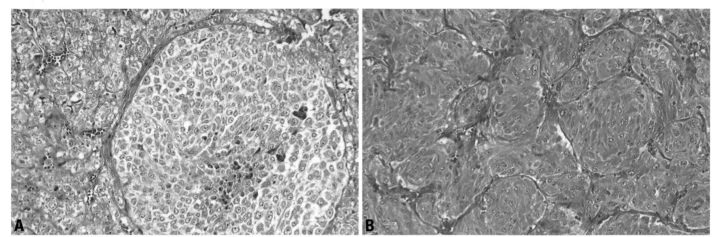

Fig. 3.11 Malignant phaeochromcytoma **A** The large nest is at least 3 times greater than the surrounding smaller zellballen. Note the central comedo-type necrosis. **B** Large nests with spindle tumour cells are characteristic of malignant phaeochromcytoma.

was employed {2229}. Necrosis may be focal within the centre of large nests, and / or confluent and diffuse. Degenerative changes are not considered as necrosis. Abnormal mitoses are defined by abnormal chromosome spread, tripolar, quadripolar or circular forms, or forms that are indescribably bizarre. Mitotic counts of >3 per 10 or 20 high power fields (magnification at x40 with a x10 objective lens) have been scored in different studies.

Several studies evaluating various combinations of the above criteria have been performed {1306,2229,2289} and have not reached entirely similar conclusions. For example, tumour size and necrosis but not local invasion or vascular invasion were found to be significant in a recent European study {2289}.

No one histologic feature is uniquely able to identify a tumour that will behave in an aggressive clinical fashion. As an alternative approach, a scaled score has been proposed to more heavily weight features that are statistically predictive of a poor biologic outcome {2229}. According to this approach, vascular invasion, capsular invasion, profound pleomorphism and nuclear hyperchromasia are weighted with one point, with the remaining features weighted with two points. A total score of ≥ 4 points suggested potentially malignant biologic behaviour. This system is at present not universally accepted.

In immunohistochemical studies, the sustentacular cells, demonstrable by S-100 protein reactivity, are diminished to absent in areas of large nests and diffuse growth {1329,1974,2229,2281}.

Some survey series have supported the utility of MIB-1 labeling in assessing malignancy, with thresholds for malignancy at mean labeling indices >2% {1571}, >10 % {2229}, or >20 cells / 200X field in fields of highest labeling {1081}. In two studies with cutoff points of 2.5 % {2289}, or 3% {392}, higher values had only a 50% sensitivity in identifying proven malignant tumours. Discrepancies between studies employing MIB-1 may result from different scoring protocols with counts derived from random fields, consecutive fields or fields of highest labeling density. Immunoreactivity for TP53 protein is present in some malignant phaeochromocytomas. However, it may not be related to patient outcome {1216,2229}.

Differential diagnosis

The principal differential diagnosis is between benign and malignant phaeochromocytoma, as discusssed above. The distinction from other neo-

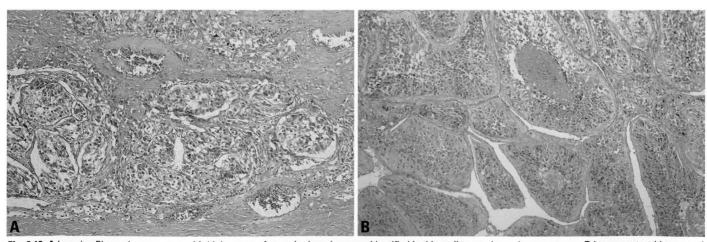

Fig. 3.12 A Invasive Phaeochromocytoma. Multiple areas of vascular invasion were identified in this malignant phaeochromocytoma. **B** Large nests with areas of central, comedo-type necrosis in a malignant phaeochromocytoma of the adrenal gland.

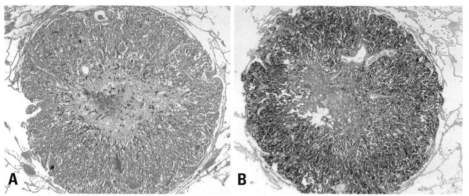

Fig. 3.13 Phaeochromocytoma. **A** A metastatic deposit in the parenchyma of the lung is identified in a patient who had a primary adrenal malignant phaeochromocytoma. **B** Diagnosis is confirmed by immunoreactivity for chromogranin.

plasms is addressed under benign phaeochromocytoma.

Somatic genetics

Somatic alterations reported in malignant phaeochromocytomas are similar to those reported in clinically benign tumours. However, in one CGH study, malignant tumours showed more frequently chromosome 11 alterations in malignant than in benign tumours {547}. In another study, losses on chromosomes 6q and 17p {456} were more common in malignancy. These results suggest that alterations of chromosomes 11, 6q or 17p may be involved in progression to malignancy. Furthermore, somatic *VHL* mutations are also reported to be more frequent in clinically malignant phaeochromocytomas when compared to their benign counterparts {453}.

Some authors have reported a high frequency of *TP53* mutations in malignant tumours {1303,2461}; however, others found no *TP53* mutations in sporadic phaeochromocytomas {446,871}. In immunohistochemical studies, loss of Rb protein (among other markers) was more frequently found in malignant tumours, however, larger molecular studies confirming these findings are still missing.

In contrast to sporadic medullary thyroid carcinomas, no significant frequency of somatic *RET* mutations was reported in malignant phaeochromocytomas {2290}. In immunohistochemical studies, loss of Rb protein and other markers were more frequently found in malignant tumours {790,1216}.

Molecular genetics

Tetraploid and aneuploid populations are present in both benign and clinically malignant phaeochromocytomas. Several studies employing flow cytometric DNA analysis have found non-diploid tumours to be more prone to aggressive behaviour and early recurrence than diploid tumours {688,860,1580,1679}. However, other studies have found no correlation between ploidy and malignancy {251}.

Genetic susceptibility

The genetic susceptibility of malignant and benign phaeochromocytomas is similar. Malignant tumours have been reported in patients with germline mutations of *RET*, *VHL*, *NF1* and the *SDH* genes {1123,1587}. Malignancy is less common in MEN 2-associated than in sporadic phaeochromocytomas {324,1476,1521, 1522,1650,1900,1995,2229,2346,2363, 2380}.

Prognosis and predictive factors

The usual prognosis of malignant phaeochromocytoma is poor, with a 45-55% 5-year survival {1522,1760,1997, 1998,2023,2024,2035,2229,2280,2296, 2297}. However, some patients may have indolent disease, with life expectancy of more than 20 years {2462}.

Until further studies identify precise biological markers that can accurately predict the clinical behaviour of catecholamine-secreting tumours, it may be advisable for all phaeochromocytoma patients to undergo lifelong hormonal monitoring and imaging studies to detect recurrence and metastasis {2195}.

Benign phaeochromocytoma

A.M. McNicol
W.F. Young Jr.
A. Kawashima
P. Komminoth
A.S. Tischler

Definition
A benign tumour of chromaffin cells (phaeochromocytes) of the adrenal medulla.

ICD-O code   8700/0

Synonyms and historical annotation
Paraganglioma; chromaffinoma.
A phaeochromocytoma is an intra-adrenal sympathetic paraganglioma. Historically, the term phaeochromocytoma ('dusky coloured tumour') is derived from the colour change that occurs when tumour tissue is immersed in chromate salts (chromaffin reaction) or in other weak oxidizing agents.

Epidemiology
Population studies report an annual incidence of between 0.4 {465} and 9.5 {143} per 1,000,000. Most are sporadic. Although 10% of tumours have classically been considered to be part of a syndromic association, recent evidence suggests the percentage of familial tumours is considerably higher {1585}. Phaeochromocytomas can occur at any age, but are most frequent in the fourth and fifth decades. Familial tumours tend to present at a younger age. The sex distribution is approximately equal. In the past, up to two thirds of cases were found only at autopsy {840,2123}, but more recently phaeochromocytomas account for 1.5–18% of adrenal 'incidentalomas', discovered when the abdomen is scanned for other intra-abdominal disease {74,259}.

Localization
Sporadic lesions are generally solitary. In contrast, in familial disease the majority are bilateral. They may occasionally coexist with extra-adrenal paragangliomas {1401}.

Clinical features
Signs and symptoms
Symptoms usually are present and are due to the pharmacologic effects of excess circulating catecholamines. Episodic symptoms include abrupt onset of throbbing headaches, generalized diaphoresis, palpitations, anxiety, chest pain, and abdominal pain. These "spells" can be extremely variable in their presentation and may be spontaneous or precipitated by postural changes, anxiety, exercise, or maneuvers that increase intra-abdominal pressure {2466}. The phaeochromocytoma "spell" may last 10 to 60 minutes and may occur daily to monthly. The clinical signs include hypertension (paroxysmal or sustained), orthostatic hypotension, pallor, retinopathy, tremor, and fever. Additionally, patients may present with secondary diabetes mellitus and/or paraneoplastic syndromes due to peptide hormone secretion.

Diagnosis of genetic susceptibility
Patients with genetic syndromes of multiple endocrine neoplasia type 2, von Hippel Lindau syndrome, or neurofibromatosis type 1 are at increased risk for phaeochromocytoma. Specific physical examination findings increase the pretest probability of sporadic phaeochromocytoma and familial phaeochromocytoma. For example, findings of a marfanoid body habitus and mucosal neuromas are highly suspicious, if not diagnostic, for multiple endocrine neoplasia type 2B; multiple large café au lait spots and or subcutaneous neuromas should increase the suspicion for neurofibromatosis type 1. However, it should be remembered that phaeochromocytoma may be the initial manifestation of some familial syndromes and may be the only manifestation of von Hippel Lindau syndrome Type 2c.

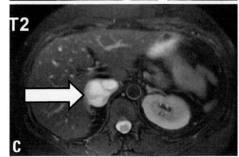
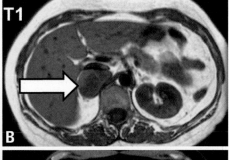
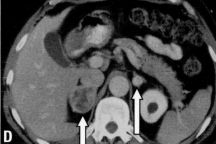

Fig. 3.14 Adrenal benign phaeochromocytoma. **A** CT scan of the abdomen shows a cystic 6.5 cm left adrenal phaeochromocytoma. Areas of cystic degeneration are typically seen on computed imaging in phaeochromocytoma. **B** T1-weighted MRI scan from a 54-yr-old-year old woman with a 4.5-cm right adrenal phaeochromocytoma (arrows). **C** MRI scan from a 54-yr-old-year old woman with a 4.5-cm right adrenal phaeochromocytoma (arrows). T2-weighted image shows increased signal intensity typical of phaeochromocytoma. **D** CT scan of the abdomen shows a vascular and cystic 4.5 cm right adrenal mass and a densely vascular 1.5 cm left adrenal mass in a patient with biochemically documented phaeochromocytoma. Bilateral phaeochromocytoma should raise the possibility of familial disease; this patient proved to have von Hippel Lindau disease.

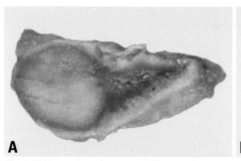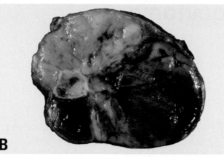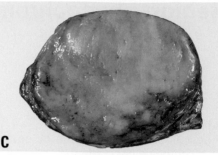

Fig. 3.15 Phaeochromocytoma. **A** The round tumour extends torwards the adrenal cortex but is macroscopically well defined. **B** Adrenal gland with phaeochromocytoma showing focal haemorrhages. **C** Phaeochromocytoma replacing most of the normal adrenal gland.

Frequently, patients are diagnosed with possible phaeochromocytoma before they are symptomatic because of genetic screening for hereditary endocrine syndromes or incidental discovery of adrenal masses on computerized abdominal imaging {1172}. These patients may harbor catecholamine-synthesizing neoplasms that are detected months or years before the onset of periodic hypersecretory states. Ten percent of benign sporadic adrenal phaeochromocytoma patients present with incidentally discovered adrenal masses {1172}.

Catecholamines and metanephrines
The diagnostic approach to catecholamine-producing tumours is divided into two series of studies. First, the diagnosis of a catecholamine-producing tumour must be suspected and then confirmed biochemically by the presence of increased urine or plasma concentrations of catecholamines or their metabolites {2203,2463}. Although convenient, plasma catecholamine measurements are not as sensitive (85%) {1276} or specific as the 24-hour urine measurements. Fractionated plasma metanephrines appear to be a product of intratumoural catecholamine catabolism and are currently proposed to be the most sensitive test to screen for phaeochromocytoma {1277,1953}.

Imaging
Computed tomography or magnetic resonance imaging should be the first localization test {1443}. Approximately 90% of catecholamine-secreting tumours occur in the adrenals and 98% occur in the abdomen. If the abdominal imaging is negative, the patient either has an extra-adrenal catecholamine-secreting paraganglioma or apparent catecholamine excess is not tumourous in nature.

Phaeochromocytomas are usually 3 cm or greater {1090} and vary from solid to complex to purely cystic, with areas of intratumoural necrosis, haemorrhage, or fluid-fluid levels {648}. Calcification may be present in a small percentage of cases on CT. Phaeochromocytomas appear hypo- to isointense on T1-weighted MR images and markedly hyperintense ("light-bulb") on T2-weighted images. Although the signal characteristics are not specific, they may be helpful in localising these tumours and eliminating some other types of mass lesions. {2302}.

Scintigraphy
The radiopharmaceutical guanethidine analogs [131]- and ^{123}I meta-iodobenzylguanidine (MIBG) have a remarkable affinity for adrenal medullary tissue. Scintigraphic localization with [^{123}I or ^{131}I]-meta-iodobenzylguanidine (^{123}I or [131]I -MIBG) is indicated to localize extra-adrenal catecholamine-secreting tumours (see chapters on extra-adrenal paraganglioma)

Macroscopy
Phaeochromocytomas are usually confined to the adrenal gland, and may appear encapsulated. Phaeochromocytomas are typically 3cm to 5cm in diameter but can be more than 10cm {1673}. The weight may range from < 5g to over 3,500g, the average in patients with hypertension being 100g {1810}. The cut surface is usually grey/white to tan and darkens on exposure to air. Focal haemorrhage, central degenerative change, cystic change and calcification may be present. The normal gland can be seen in most cases but is sometimes attenuated. An adrenal gland containing a phaeochromocytoma should be carefully dissected to look for evidence of diffuse and nodular adrenal medullary hyperplasia suggestive of familial disease.

Histopathology
Microscopic examination usually shows predominantly alveolar (zellballen) or trabecular architecture, or a mixture of the two. Diffuse or solid architecture can also be seen. A true capsule does not usually separate the tumour from the adjacent adrenal but a pseudocapsule may be present, or the tumour may extend to the adrenal capsule. The border with the adjacent cortex may be irregular, with intermingling of tumour cells with cortical cells.

The tumour cells typically either resemble normal chromaffin cells or are larger than normal chromaffin cells, with prominent nucleoli. The cytoplasm is granular and basophilic to amphophilic. Cellular and nuclear pleomorphism are sometimes prominent. Nuclear pseudoinclusions are present in some cases {482}. Spindle cells are present in about 2% of cases, usually as a minor component. A small cell variant is also described. Intracytoplasmic hyaline globules occur commonly. These are positive with periodic acid-Schiff stain and are diastase resistant. Small amounts of melanin-like pigment may be present {1223}, probably representing neuromelanin in most cases. Haemorrhage and haemosiderin deposits are common. Mitotic figures are rare, with an average of one per 30 high power fields reported in clinically benign lesions in one study {1306}.

Scattered ganglion cells may be present. Tumours containing such ganglion cells should not be interpreted as composite phaeochromocytomas {1306}. Sometimes the cells may undergo 'lipid degeneration', assuming a clear cell appear-

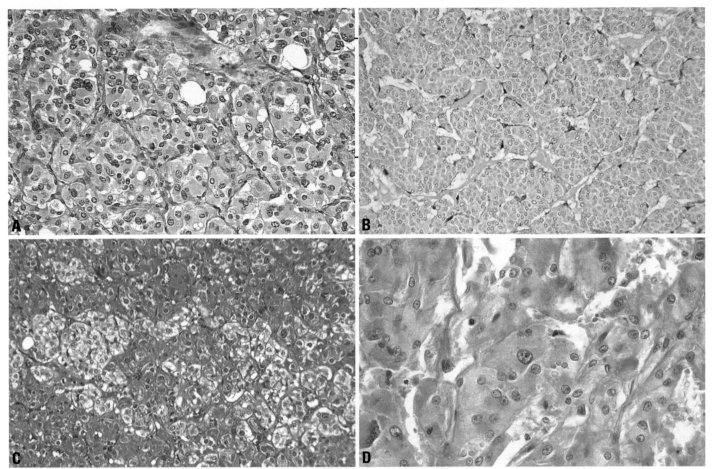

Fig. 3.16 Benign phaeochromocytoma **A** Characteristic "zellballen" architecture. A single, pleomorphic cell is noted in the right. **B** The S-100 protein highlights the supporting sustentacular framework surrounding the phaeochromocytes. **C** Adrenal mixed corticomedullary phaeochromocytoma with intermixed growth of medullary and cortical cells. **D** Benign PCC with intracytoplasmic hyaline globules.

ance, which may mimic an adrenal cortical tumour {1791,2282}. Oncocytic tumours have been described {1290}. Stromal sclerosis may be marked and amyloid has been reported. The vascular component is often prominent.

Specific diagnosis is usually based on morphology and confirmed by immunohistochemistry. Classic histochemical techniques such as the chromaffin reaction and silver stains are not specific and should be abandoned.

Immunohistochemistry

Phaeochromocytomas are positive for chromogranin A, the most reliable marker for discriminating them from adrenal cortical tumours and metastatic tumours that are not neuroendocrine. Phaeochromocytoma may be discriminated from other neuroendocrine tumours metastatic to the adrenal by staining for tyrosine hydroxylase {1339}. Other neural markers such as synapto-

physin have been reported to be variably positive in cortical tumours. The absence of positivity for epithelial membrane antigen (EMA) helps distinguish phaeochromocytoma from renal cell carcinoma. Electron microscopy can be of use in the differential diagnosis from renal cell and adrenal cortical carcinoma.

Immunostaining for S100 protein will demonstrate sustentacular cells {1329}, which are usually arranged around the periphery of the cell nests where there is an alveolar arrangement but are more randomly distributed in the other patterns. Interpretation can be difficult if the tumour cells are also positive. These tumours also produce a number of peptide hormones and cytokines. Although they are not normally documented as part of the diagnostic protocol, the exception would be in confirming the tumour as the site of hormone secretion in cases of ectopic hormone production (eg. ectopic ACTH syndrome).

Somatic genetics

Several studies have reported allelic losses at 1p, 3p, 17p, and 22q both in sporadic and familial phaeochromocytomas {1525,1555,2041} and a detailed analysis of 1p has revealed at least three putative tumour suppressor loci {166}.

Two studies have compared somatic alterations of VHL- or MEN 2- associated phaeochromocytomas with sporadic tumours and identified significant differences. Losses of chromosomes 3 and 11 appear to be very frequent and LOH at 1p and 22q infrequent in VHL phaeochromocytomas, when compared to MEN 2-associated or sporadic tumours. Furthermore, a low frequency of 3p LOH, a high frequency of 1p LOH and a moderate frequency of 22q LOH were also identified in sporadic phaeochromocytomas. These findings indicate that multiple genes other than VHL, especially on 1p, are significant for sporadic tumourigenesis and that distinct genetic pathways are involved in the development of sporadic *vs.* VHL phaeochromocytoma {164,1365}.

Two recent CGH studies on a total of 63 sporadic adrenal phaeochromocytomas and catecholamine-producing abdominal paragangliomas revealed similar patterns of copy number changes in both tumour groups. The most consistent findings included losses of 1p11-32 (82-86%), 3q (41-52%), 6q (34%), 3p and 17p (31% each), 11q (15-28%), 11p (26%), 3p13-14 (24%), 4q (21%) and 2q (15%). The most frequent gains included chromosomes 9q (38%), 17q (21-31%), 19p (26%), 19q (24%), 11cen-q13 (15%), and 16p (15%) {456,547}.

RET

Studies have suggested that the *RET* proto-oncogene is over-expressed in phaeochromocytomas, but does not have rearrangements {2179}. Approximately. 15% of sporadic phaeochromocytomas contain a somatic *RET* mutation {156,568, 1130,1131} and 2.1- 4.3% of tumours harbour a somatic *VHL* mutation {119,565, 907}. Furthermore, it was demonstrated that in addition, a *RET* variant with aberrant retention of intron 2 is enriched in phaeochromocytomas of both familial and sporadic origin, implicating *RET* as a target for RNA splicing deregulation {1254} in tumour cells.

VHL

In VHL- associated tumours the wild type allele is inactivated by LOH (51%), hypermethylation (33%) and intragenic somatic mutations {1773}.

GDNF / G protein / NF1

Other genes occasionally affected by somatic mutations include *GDNF* (1/28) {2418} and the G protein gene encoding for the G protein Gs alpha {2394}. One study employing RT-PCR and immunohistochemistry revealed loss of *NF1* in a small number of sporadic tumours {795}. However, a detailed mutation analysis has not yet been performed, probably due to the large size of the *NF1* gene.

Mitochondrial complex II genes

LOH of the *SDHD* locus on 11q23 was demonstrated in 30-72% of sporadic phaeochromocytomas but somatic mutations appear to be very rare (1/15) {16,97,717,1189,1721}. The same holds

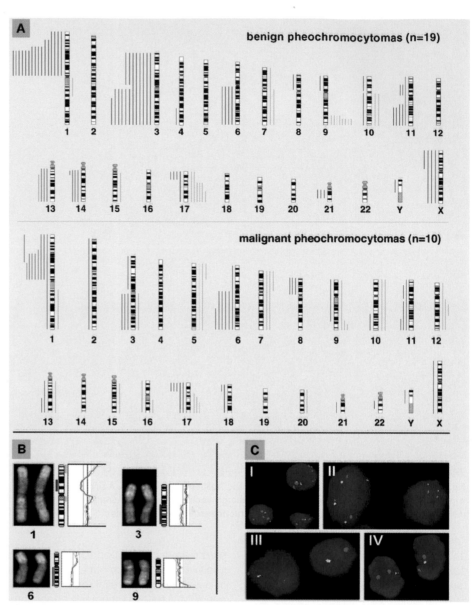

Fig. 3.17 Phaeochromocytoma. **A** Summary of comparative genomic hybridization (CGH). DNA copy number changes detected by CGH in 19 benign and 10 malignant sporadic PCCs. Red vertical lines on the left of the chromosomes ideograms indicate loss, green lines on the right gain of chromosomal material. **B** Details of CGH digital images (left) and fluorescent ratio profiles (right) illustrating genomic alterations of chromosomes 1 (loss of 1p with gain of the C-G rich telomeric region), 3 (loss of 3q), 6 (loss of 6q), and 9 (gain of 9q). **C** Fluorecence *in situ* hybridization (FISH) . I and II: interphase touch preparations of tumour number 8 analyzed using a centromeric probe for chromosome 1 (red signals) in combination with a 1p22ñ31-specific probe (green signals) (I) or a 1p36-specific probe (II), demonstrating aneuploidy of this tumour with loss of the 1p22ñ31 locus (I) but not of the 1p36 locus (II). III: Monosomy of chromosome 3 in case 4. IV: Diploid malignant tumour, showing the two copies of centromere 6 (red signals) and only one copy of the 6q22-specific locus (green signal), indicating loss of 6q. From H. Dannenberg et. al. {456}.

true for *SDHB*, which was found mutated in 1 of 24 sporadic tumours (4%) {97}. Thus far, no somatic mutations of *SDHC* have been described in sporadic phaeochromocytomas.

Genes that do not appear to be relevant in sporadic tumours include *RAS* {1546}, p16 {17} and the VHL-associated gene *CUL2* {532}.

Genetic susceptibility

Malignant and benign phaeochromocytomas are associated with a variety of inherited diseases including multiple endocrine neoplasia type 2 (MEN 2), von Hippel-Lindau (VHL) disease, neurofibromatosis type 1 (NF1), hereditary paraganglioma (PGL) syndromes, and Sturge-Weber disease, and are not uncommonly the first clinical manifestation of the syndromes {280}. In earlier reports it was estimated that 10% of phaeochromocytomas occur in the setting of an inherited disease. Recent data indicate that the frequency of familial tumours is considerably higher {1585}.

MEN 2

Approximately 50% of affected individuals develop phaeochromocytomas and a genotype-phenotype correlation has been established {564}. In the subtypes-both MEN 2A and 2B, phaeochromocytomas are an integral part of the syndrome and mutations of the *RET* codon 634 are more most frequently associated with adrenomedullary tumour development {564,1263}. The frequency of *de novo* germline mutations in MEN 2A and FMTC appears to be in the range of 6 % and in MEN 2B around 50 % {567,2404}.

VHL

The overall frequency of phaeochromocytoma in patients with von Hippel-Lindau (VHL) disease is 10-30% and is restricted to so called type 2 kindreds. It is the sole feature in so called type 2C families. Type 2 families more frequently exhibit germline missense mutations when compared to type 1 families (without phaeochromocytomas) which have deletions or premature termination mutations {658}. Occult germline mutations in patients with clinically sporadic

Table 3.08
Classification of von Hippel-Lindau disease

Type	Characteristics
1	Retinal angioma, haemangioblastoma, renal cell carcinoma
2 A	Retinal angioma, haemangioblastoma, phaeochromocytoma
2 B	Haemangioblastoma, renal cell carcinoma, phaeochromocytoma
2 C	Phaeochromocytoma

phaeochromocytomas were reported in 3-20% of patients {244,2291} and the frequency of *de novo* mutations was estimated to be 13% {1585}.

NF1

Phaeochromocytoma is clinically diagnosed in 1-4% of NF1 patients {1634, 1922}. However, the true prevalence is unclear due to lack of autopsy studies.

PGL

Phaeochromocytomas have recently been reported in patients with germline mutations in the mitochondrial complex II genes *SDHB* (PGL4) at chromosome 1p36 {97}, *SDHC* (PGL3) at 1q21 {1598} and *SDHD* (PGL1) at 11q23 {96} causing familial paragangliomas (PGL). As with NF1 the true prevalence of the association is unclear, in part because the genes have only recently been discovered. An additional confounding factor is that

most reports do not separate adrenal and extraadrenal sympathetic tumours but lump them into a single group 'phaeochromocytomas'. The estimated frequencies of occult germline mutations in *SDHB* and *SDHD* in sporadic phaeochromocytomas have been estimated to be 4.5% and 3.5%, respectively {142}. The combination of phaeochromocytoma with parasympathetic paragangliomas is particularly suggestive of these mutations.

Phaeochromocytomas have rarely also been reported in the setting of MEN 1 and other syndromes {445}.

Prognosis and predictive factors

The prognosis for patients with benign phaeochromocytoma is primarily dependent upon a successful surgical resection and extent of preoperative complications related to hypertension. There are no universally accepted histological criteria for the prediction of benign behaviour in phaeochromocytoma. For discussion of the features associated with malignancy see the section on malignant phaeochromocytoma.

Composite phaeochromocytoma or paraganglioma

A.S. Tischler
N. Kimura
R.V. Lloyd
P. Komminoth

Definition
A tumour that typically combines features of phaeochromocytoma or paraganglioma with those of ganglioneuroma, ganglioneuroblastoma, neuroblastoma or peripheral nerve sheath tumour. There have been reports of mixed medullary and cortical tumours {2382}, but in view of the distinct lineage of the cell types they are not considered as composite phaeochromocytomas in this section.

Synonyms
Compound or mixed adrenal medullary tumour or paraganglioma; mixed neuroendocrine-neural tumour.

Epidemiology
Composite phaeochromocytomas or paragangliomas are rare, with fewer than 40 cases in the literature {1082,1209, 1217,2244}. In a series of 120 sympathoadrenal paragangliomas from North America, areas of ganglioneuroma or ganglioneuroblastoma were encountered in 4 of 99 (4.0%) intra-adrenal and none of 21 extra-adrenal tumours {1306}. Four of 46 adrenal phaeochromocytomas (8.7%) showed composite features in a series from Hong Kong {1209}. Thoracic {2340} and retroperitoneal {1082,2191, 2459} extra-adrenal paragangliomas with

ganglioneuroma or ganglioneuroblastoma are reported occasionally. Phaeochromocytomas with malignant peripheral nerve sheath tumour comprise a distinct and even less common subset of composite tumour {1497,1505, 1900}. Composite tumours usually occur in adults, with a median age of approximately 50 years for all reported cases (range, 14-74 years for well-documented cases {1082,1209}) and with approximately equal frequency in males and females. Ganglioneuroblastoma was present in approximately 20% of all reported cases and ganglioneuroma in 80%.

Etiology
Apart from genetic susceptibility in some cases (see below), there are no factors known to contribute to the development of tumours with a composite phenotype.

Localization
All reported composite tumours for which the diagnosis is well documented by modern techniques appear to have arisen from paraganglia associated with the sympathetic nervous system. Approximately 90% were in the adrenal gland and the remainder in the urinary bladder {1217}, organ of Zuckerkandl

{2191} or elsewhere in the retroperitoneum {1082}.

Clinical features and investigations
Signs and symptoms associated with composite tumours are usually similar to those of ordinary phaeochromocytomas. The tumours may also cause the syndrome of watery diarrhea-hypokalemia-achlorhydria due to production of vasoactive intestinal peptide (VIP) {409,970,1248,1601,1911,2270}. Ultrasonography, computed tomography, magnetic resonance imaging (MRI) and MIBG scans aid in tumour localization. Tumour heterogeneity in imaging studies may suggest the presence of composite tumour {1217}. Plasma or urine levels of catecholamines or their metabolites are variably elevated {1082,1209}. Significant elevations of dopamine or homovanillic acid in blood or urine may suggest the presence of ganglioneuroblastoma {671,1082}.

Macroscopy
Gross examination of a composite tumour specimen may reveal patchy, pale, firm areas corresponding to ganglioneuroma {238}, or cystic, necrotic and haemorrhagic areas of ganglioneuroblastoma {1306}. In a high percentage

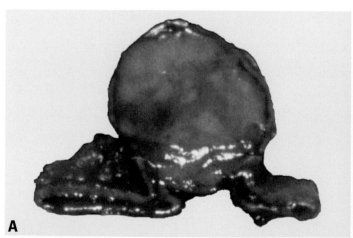 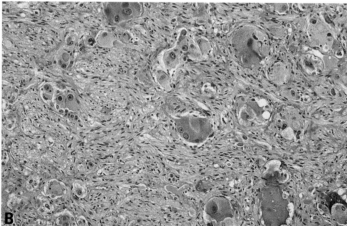

Fig. 3.18 Composite phaeochromocytoma. **A** Adrenal medullary tumour consisting of phaeochromocytoma (dark gray areas) and ganglioneuroma (pale gray areas). The heterogeneous gross appearance provides an important clue to the composite nature of the tumour. **B** Tumour area with feautures of ganglioneuroma. Note the numerous large, bizarre, multinucleated ganglion cells.

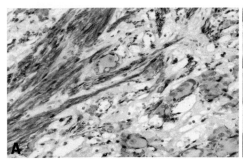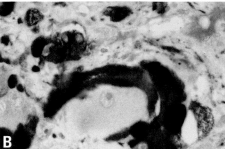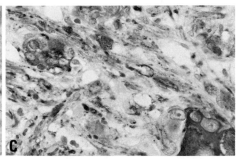

Fig. 3.19 Composite phaeochromocytoma. **A** Immunohistochemical staining for S-100 protein is positive for both, Schwann cells and sustentacular cells. **B** Chromogranin and **C** Synaptophysin are abundant in cell bodies of chromaffin-like cells but usually weakly expressed or absent in neurons, reflecting differing cellular content of secretory vesicles. Both neuronal marker proteins are irregularly distributed in neuronal processes, where vesicles tend to accumulate in varicosities. Greater abundance of synaptophysin may be due to small, agranular synaptic like vesicles, which do not contain chromogranin.

of cases, the composite phenotype is first noted during histological examination.

Tumour spread

Malignant composite phaeochromocytomas apparently metastasize both by haematogenous and lymphatic routes to liver, lung lymph nodes and bone {1209, 1573,1601,1949} and may cause seeding of the omentum and diaphragm {1601}.

Histopathology

Typical phaeochromocytomas or paragangliomas may contain scattered, neuron-like cells. The diagnosis of composite tumour requires both histoarchitecture and cell populations consistent with an additional type of tumour. Stromal features may provide a clue to the existence of a mixed phenotype. The tumours may be traversed by bundles of spindle cells that can be shown immunohistochemically to contain Schwann cells and axons, or there may be patchy areas with unusually prominent sustentacular cells. Stromal hyalinization occurs in some cases {2244}.

Immunohistochemistry

The individual components of composite tumours immunohistochemically resemble their normal counterparts or pure tumours of the same type. Useful functional markers include chromogranin A (CgA), synaptophysin (Syn) and the catecholamine biosynthetic enzymes tyrosine hydroxylase (TH) and phenylethanolamine N-methyltransferase (PNMT) {2242}. In addition, staining for S-100 protein will identify Schwann cells and sustentacular cells, while staining for neurofilament proteins will aid in identification of axon-like processes.

CgA is localized in the matrix of secretory granules, while Syn is a marker for the membranes of both secretory granules and small agranular synaptic-like vesicles {2400}. Because of their different distributions, CgA and Syn are complementary and may be differentially expressed. Both are strongly and diffusely positive in phaeochromocytoma and paraganglioma cells, which contain numerous secretory granules, while neuroblasts and mature neurons show weak or focal staining, often in a linear or punctate distribution corresponding to portions of axon-like processes where secretory organelles accumulate {238, 1975,2245}. This difference can be helpful for identifying foci of neuroblastoma in composite tumours {650} and for discriminating maturing neuroblasts from phaeochromocytoma cells of the same size.

Because TH and PNMT are cytosolic enzymes, staining is not dependent on storage of secretory granules. Almost all chromaffin cells in the human adrenal medulla are TH+/PNMT+, while extra-adrenal paraganglionic chief cells are usually TH+/PNMT-. Neurons both in the adrenal medulla and throughout the sympathetic nervous system are TH+/PNMT-. In three studies of phaeochromocytoma admixed with ganglioneuroma in which catecholamine-synthesizing enzymes were examined, most neurons were TH+/PNMT- as anticipated {238,364, 1082}. A few neurons in areas of ganglioneuroma may also be TH-, suggesting a switch to a non-catecholamine neurotransmitter such as acetylcholine. In contrast, ganglioneuroblastoma in composite tumours may be predominantly TH-, resembling some paediatric neuroblastomas {2243}.

The localization of VIP in composite tumours is of particular interest in cases of watery diarrhea-hypokalemia-achlorhydria syndrome. In the normal adrenal, VIP is a product principally of neurons and not of chromaffin cells, and immunoreactive VIP has been localized exclusively or predominantly to neuronal components of several composite tumours {1975,2245, 2270,2459}. However, occasional phaeochromocytoma cells do show VIP immunoreactivity {1082,2245}.

Precursor lesions and histogenesis

The available evidence favors an origin of the neurons in composite tumours from pre-existing phaeochromocytoma or paraganglioma cells. The alternative of a persistent pluripotent precursor has not been ruled out but there is no experimental evidence to support that possibility. In cell culture studies, both normal and neoplastic human chromaffin cells have been shown to be capable of undergoing neuronal differentiation, accompanied by decreased production of epinephrine and increased production of VIP {2246-2248}. Cells in composite tumours with intermediate features between neurons and chromaffin cells might therefore represent transitional phenotypes. As for paediatric neuroblastomas {48,49} it has been hypothesized that the Schwann cells in composite tumours may often not be neoplastic. In composite phaeochromocytoma/ganglioneuroma, benign-appearing Schwann cells may show more Ki67 labeling than any other cell type {238}.

Somatic genetics

No genetic abnormalities that distinguish composite tumours from typical phaeochromocytomas or paragangliomas have thus far been identified. Exon 31 of the neurofibromatosis gene *NF1*, which is involved in development of phaeochromocytomas showing focal composite features in a knockout mouse model {984,2249} has been shown to be normal in several human composite tumours {1085}.

Genetic susceptibility

Patients with composite tumours often have systemic disorders involving neuroectodermal and neuroendocrine tissues, most often neurofibromatosis type 1 (NF1) {364,377,1082,1573,1900}. Two patients had multiple endocrine neoplasia, type 2A {238,1431}, and one had a renal angiomyolipoma {1082}, suggesting a forme fruste of a neurocutaneous phakomatosis. Association of NF1 with the composite phenotype appears to be disproportionate to the overall association of NF1 with phaeochromocytoma, and bilateral composite phaeochromocytomas have been reported in one NF1 patient {364}.

Prognosis and predictive factors

Metastases from composite tumours almost always are derived from and have the histological characteristics of ganglioneuroblastoma. Very rarely, phaeochromocytoma or paraganglioma components metastasize together with ganglioneuroblastoma {1573}. Patients presenting with tumour confined to the adrenal and completely excised are reported to show no evidence of recurrence when followed for up to five years {671}, even when ganglioneuroblastoma is an extensive component of the tumour {289}. However, prolonged follow-up is required because neuroblastic tumours in adults may pursue an indolent course {649}. In one case, local recurrence developed after 15 years {1601}. Composite tumours containing ganglioneuroma without immature elements have the same prognosis as typical phaeochromocytoma or paraganglioma {1082,1306}. Metastasis of phaeochromocytoma from one such tumour has been reported {1209}.

Extra-adrenal paraganglioma: Carotid body, jugulotympanic, vagal, laryngeal, aortico-pulmonary

N. Kimura
R. Chetty
C. Capella
W.F. Young Jr.
C.A. Koch

K.Y. Lam
R.A. DeLellis
A. Kawashima
P. Komminoth
A.S. Tischler

Definition
Tumours arising from the paraganglia distributed along the parasympathetic nerves in the head, neck and mediastinum. These tumours are histologically identical and are named by anatomical site of origin.

ICD-O codes
Extra-adrenal paraganglioma
8693/1
Carotid body   8692/1
Jugulotympanic   8690/1
Vagal   8693/1
Laryngeal   8693/1
Aortico-pulmonary   8691/1

Synonyms
Nonchromaffin paraganglioma, Extra-adrenal phaeochromocytoma, Carotid body tumour, Carotid body paraganglioma, Chemodectoma, Glomus jugulare tumour, Glomus tympanicum tumour, Glomus vagale tumour, Glomus caroticum, Jugulotympanic paraganglioma, Aortic body tumour, Aortic body paraganglioma, Aorticopulmonary paraganglioma

Epidemiology
Parasympathetic paragangliomas are rare, with a prevalence of approximately 0.2-1.0/100,000 {569,1471}. Jugulotym-panic and carotid body tumours are the two most frequent, followed by vagal or aortic lesions {1154}. The average patient age is fourth and fifth decade of life. Overall gender distribution is almost equal {123,1195,1265}. Between 10-15% are bilateral or multiple, familial and malignant {1702,1754}. A significant increase in the incidence of carotid body paraganglioma has been reported in humans dwelling at high altitude, where a marked female predilection has been reported {1849}.

Localization
Carotid body paraganglioma: a paraganglioma arising from carotid body paraganglia located in or near the bifurcation of the common carotid artery.

Jugulotympanic paraganglioma: A paraganglioma arising from dispersed paraganglia in the base of the skull and middle ear. They can be quite small and located on the promontory of the middle ear or they can be larger, filling the cavity of the middle ear and protruding through the tympanic membrane.

Vagal paraganglioma: a paraganglioma arising from paraganglia located in the rostral vagus nerve, often close to the ganglion nodosum.

Laryngeal paraganglioma: a paraganglioma arising from paraganglia around the larynx.

Aorticopulmonary paraganglioma: a paraganglioma arising from dispersed paraganglia located at the base of the heart and associated with the great vessels.

Clinical features
Although they synthesize and store catecholamines, only about 1% of parasympathetic paragangliomas are clinically functional {2479}. This discrepancy may be attributed to the low production of catecholamines by most parasympathetic paragangliomas, which contrasts with the high production of catecholamines by sympathetic paragangliomas {1154}. Most patients are non-symptomatic and parasympathetic paragangliomas of the head and neck are increasingly incidental findings in imaging studies.

The most common presentation of a carotid body paraganglioma is a slow-growing, painless mass located deep to the anterior border of the sternocleidomastoid muscle in the upper or midneck. Only rarely the mass is painful with radiation into the head and shoulders.

Classical tympanic paragangliomas cause hearing disturbances, including tinnitus, aural pulsations or conduction-type of hearing loss, while classic jugular paragangliomas cause a jugular foramen

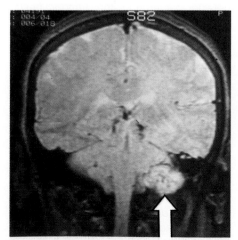

Fig. 3.20 MRI of a catecholamine-secreting jugulo-tympanic paraganglioma.

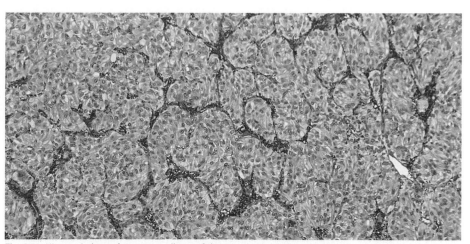

Fig. 3.21 Histopathology of a paraganglioma of the carotid body. Note the typical architecture with formation of zellballen.

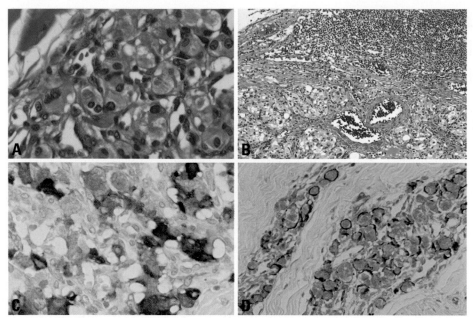

Fig. 3.22 Carotid body tumour. **A** Tumours are composed of two cell types: chief cells which have pale eosinophilic cytoplasm with slightly to moderately atypical nuclei and sustentacular cells which have spindle-shaped nuclei with scanty cytoplasm surrounding a nest of chief cells. **B** Lymph node metastasis of a carotid body tumour. **C** Chief cells of carotid body tumour are positive for chromogranin A. **D** Sustentacular cells of carotid body tumour are positive for GFAP.

syndrome with cranial nerves 9, 10, 11 and 12 palsies in various combinations. However, symptoms associated with tumours in the jugulotympanic region may overlap. More than one third of jugulotympanic paragangliomas present as a bluish mass behind the tympanic membrane or as a polyp in the external ear canal and a casual biopsy can lead to troublesome bleeding.

Patients with vagal paragangliomas present with a painless slowly growing mass, most often located in the parapharyngeal space above the carotid bifurcation. Cranial nerve involvement occurs in about 30% of patients, most frequently manifesting as vocal cord paralysis, hoarseness, or dysphagia due to vagus nerve damage {1195,1849}.

The most common symptom of laryngeal paragangliomas is hoarseness, but less common symptoms include spasmodic laryngeal pain and dysphagia. Clinical manifestations of mediastinal paraganglioma refer to space occupying mass and include: hoarseness, dysphagia, chest pain, cough and, occasionally, the superior vena cava syndrome.

Although approximately 10% of paragangliomas were traditionally thought to be familial, current evidence indicates that the percentage of inherited tumours is considerably higher {1585}. Multicentric

tumours occur in 10-20 % of apparent sporadic cases and in up to 80% of familial cases {7,1265,1754}.

Imaging and diagnosis

Initial imaging usually includes CT or MRI. The findings are similar to those of phaeochromocytomas. Dynamic enhanced CT and MRI may be used in detecting juxtacardiac or intracardiac paragangliomas. ^{123}I- or ^{131}I-metaiodobenzylguanidine (MIBG) is specific but not sensitive for the detection of parasympathetic paraglangliomas but correlation with CT or MR imaging is essential. False negative rates in one study were lowest for MRI, followed in ascending order by CT, angiography, ultrasonography, MIBG and Indium 111-pentreotide scintigraphy {569}. Fine needle aspiration and cytologic analysis can be helpful to confirm an imaging diagnosis of paraganglioma {637}. Open biopsy becomes necessary when the diagnosis is not achieved by these other means.

Macroscopy

Paragangliomas are solid tumours and are partially or completely encapsulated with a thin capsule. The cut surface is tan to red-brown, extremely vascular, homogeneous, or focally fibrotic.

Most paragangliomas are less than 6 cm

in size, although some are larger {2479}. Laryngeal paragangliomas average 2.5 cm {123}. Jugular paragangliomas may extend as finger-like projections into the lumen of the jugular vein. Paragangliomas appear as spherical, ovoid or fusiform encapsulated expansions in or around the carotid body, jugular, and laryngeal regions {1195}.

Tumour spread and staging

Aggressive growth with encirclement of blood vessels, incorporation of nerves, invasion of bone structures and intracranial extension is frequently observed in jugulotympanic, vagal and mediastinal paragangliomas and, less frequently, in carotid body tumours {1195}.

The incidence of metastazing paragangliomas varies according to the site and is reported to be up to 20% for mediastinal, up to 12.5% for carotid body, about 10% for vagal, and up to 3% for jugulotympanic and laryngeal paragangliomas. Metastases are mostly confined to regional lymph nodes. Distant metastases may involve bone, lung, liver and other sites {1195}.

Histopathology

Typically, the organoid pattern ("zellballen") of the normal paraganglion is seen in these tumours. However, a wide range of variant morphology may be observed, including trabecular, spindled, or angioma-like patterns {1195}. Tumours are composed of two cell types; chief cells which have pale eosinophilic cytoplasm with slightly to moderately atypical nuclei and sustentacular cells, accentuated by S-100 protein or GFAP immunostaining. There is a prominent vascular network separating the tumour nests. Extensive hyaline changes around vessels or broad band-like sclerosis intervening between tumour tissue may be helpful diagnostically. Mitotic figures are usually rare. There is no cellular polarity within the nests, helping to distinguish these tumours from other neuroendocrine tumours, such as carcinoid.

Immunohistochemically, neuroendocrine markers such as chromogranin A and synaptophysin are usually positive in chief cells.

Differential diagnosis

Tumours that should be differentiated from paragangliomas include carcinoid tumour, medullary thyroid carcinoma,

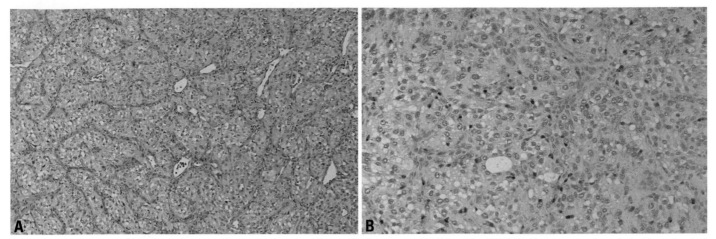

Fig. 3.23 Paraganglioma. **A** Mediastinal paraganglioma showing a prominent zellballen pattern. **B** S100 staining highlights the sustentacular cells in this mediastinal paraganglioma.

hyalinizing trabecular tumour of the thyroid gland, and rarely haemangiopericytoma and glomangioma. The combination of immunostaining with chromogranin A, synaptophysin, GFAP, S100 protein and tyrosine hydroxylase is helpful to distinguish paragangliomas from other tumours.

Somatic genetics

DNA copy number changes are infrequent in parasympathetic paragangliomas when compared to sympathetic paragangliomas. Loss of chromosome 11 may be an important event in their tumourigenesis, particularly in familial paraganglioma cases, along with 5p in sporadic tumours {141,191,454,492, 2298}. Flow cytometric DNA analyses are contradictory {744,1679} in determining the prognosis of paragangliomas.

In a study on 52 tumours from 44 patients it was demonstrated that *RET* is expressed but not mutated in parasympathetic paragangliomas {468}.

Genetic susceptibility

It has been estimated that 10-50% of parasympathetic paragangliomas are familial. Approximately 35% of individuals who present to an otolaryngologist with a head and neck paragangliomas have an inherited predisposition and individuals with carotid body tumours are 5.8 times more likely to have familial tumours than those diagnosed with paragangliomas at other anatomic locations {529}. The inheritance pattern of hereditary paraganglioma is autosomal dominant with age-dependent penetrance and maternal imprinting in patients with

SDHD mutations (the phenotype is expressed only if inherited paternally) in most kindreds {1600,1811}. Multicentricity is a strong predictive factor for the hereditary nature of the disorder in isolated patients.

Familial paragangliomas have been associated with germline mutations of *SDHD* (PGL1) on 11q23 (50%), *SDHB* (PGL4) on 1p36 (20%) {142} and rarely of *SDHC* (PGL3) on 1q21 {107,1599}. In a series of Dutch families, two founder mutations (Asp92Tyr and Leu139Pro) were described {2256}. In another study, the P81L germline mutation frequently encountered in North America was attributed both to a founder effect and recurrent mutations {142}. A novel mutation that causes skipping of exon 3 has recently been discovered in Belgium {1811}. A fourth possible gene that remains to be identified is located on 11q13 (PGL2) {1408}. The mechanism of tumour development in affected individuals with *SDHD*, *SDHB* and *SDHC* mutations appears to be caused by inactivating mutations which involve abolishion of the enzymatic activity of complex II in the mitochondrial respiratory chain by inactivating mutations and activation of the hypoxia pathway {715}.

Parasympathetic paragangliomas may also occasionally occur in other familial disorders. These include VHL disease {371,937} and von Recklinghausen disease (NF1) {104}. In addition, familial trait was suggested in a recent report on 79 affected individuals with Carney triad (paraganglioma, pulmonary chondroma and gastrointestinal stromal tumour) See Chapter 5 (Inherited tumour syndromes).

Prognosis and predictive factors

It is generally accepted that a paraganglioma is determined to be malignant only when metastases are demonstrated. The 5-year survival rate for patients with metastasis limited to regional lymph nodes is significantly higher than patients with distant metastases (approximately 80% versus 10%) {1265}. The median growth rate of paragangliomas has been estimated to be 1.0 mm/year with a median tumour doubling time of 4.2 years {993}, suggesting an indolent course.

Extra-adrenal paraganglioma: Gangliocytic, cauda equina, orbital, nasopharyngeal

A.S. Tischler
P. Komminoth
N. Kimura
W.F. Young Jr.

R. Chetty
J. Albores-
Saavedra
P. Kleihues

Definition
Extra-adrenal paragangliomas or paraganglioma-like tumours arising outside the usual distribution of sympathetic and parasympathetic paraganglia.

ICD-O codes
Gangliocytic   8683/0
Cauda equina   8693/1
Orbital nasopharynx   8693/1

Epidemiology
Orbital and nasopharyngeal paragangliomas are extremely rare tumours, reported from infancy to old age. Orbital paragangliomas show an equal sex distribution {72,150}, while those in the nasopharynx show a female predominance {887,1034,1174}. Paragangliomas of the cauda equina and gangliocytic paragangliomas are somewhat more common. The tumours occur throughout life with a median age of approximately 50 years and variably reported gender predilection {15,265,963,2101}. Orbital paragangliomas have occasionally been reported in association with parasympathetic paragangliomas in other locations {72}.

Localization
Orbital paragangliomas may arise anywhere in the orbit or in the retrobulbar space. In the nasal area, paragangliomas may arise both in the nasopharynx and the nasal cavity, including the vault and turbines {1034,1174}. In order to provide appropriate treatment, primary paragangliomas in those locations should be distinguished from secondary involvement by extension of jugulo-tympanic or vagal paragangliomas {569,1174}. Spinal paragangliomas usually arise from the cauda equina or filum terminale and are usually intradural and extramedullary. Occasionally the tumours show extradural extension, involve the conus medullaris or arise from caudal nerve roots {15,1532,2101}. Paragangliomas in the distal spinal area should not be confused with the glomus coccygium, which is a normal neuromyoarterial structure unrelated to pararaganglia. Gangliocytic paragangliomas almost always arise in the duodenum, particularly in the periampullary region {41,258,1904}, but have occasionally been reported in the jejunum {265}, pylorus {265} and pancreas {2252}. One case has been reported in the nasopharynx {2063}.

Clinical features
Orbital paragangliomas most commonly present with visual disturbance or with proptosis that may be pulsatile. Nasopharyngeal paragangliomas usually present with epistaxis or nasal obstruction. Cauda equina paragangliomas may be asymptomatic or present with low back pain, leg pain, difficulty walking, cauda equina syndrome, or increased intracranial pressure {843,1532,1677,1690}. Gangliocytic paragangliomas may present with gastrointestinal bleeding, abdominal discomfort, and/or obstructive jaundice {41,258,1904}. There have been no reports of signs or symptoms attributable to catecholamine secretion by any of the above tumours {569}. One patient with a gangliocytic paraganglioma presented with diarrhoea, steatorrhoea and weight loss that may have been caused by tumour-derived somatostatin {2252}.

Nasopharyngeal paragangliomas may be directly visualized as blue-gray to red, sometimes pulsatile, polypoid masses. Gangliocytic paragangliomas may be visualized directly by endoscopy or indirectly by barium swallow. Imaging with ultrasound, CT and MRI show a solid homogenous mass {258}. Magnetic resonance imaging is the optimal imaging technique for paragangliomas and has been applied to a number of cauda equina paragangliomas, typically showing a well-demarcated extradural mass with high signal on T-2 weighted images {15,2042,2170}.

Macroscopy
Orbital, nasopharyngeal and cauda equina paragangliomas are usually circumscribed, encapsulated or partially encapsulated tumours resembling paragangliomas in other locations. Gangliocytic paragangliomas are typically ulcerated, polypoid tumours that distend the submucosa of the bowel and may extend into the muscularis propria. They are usually 1-4 cm in diameter but may reach 7 cm or larger, and they are often non-encapsulated {265,1801}.

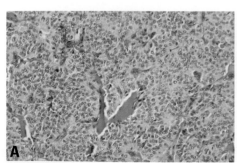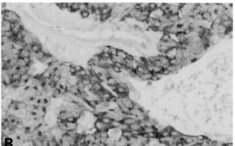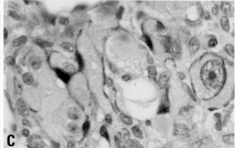

Fig. 3.24 Paraganglioma of the cauda equina. A Typical histopathologcal features with zellballen pattern. B Chromogranin staining of neural cells and C Immunoreactivity of sustentacular cells to S-100 protein.

Tumour spread and staging

There are no documented reports of metastases from paragangliomas originating in the orbit, nasopharynx or cauda equina. However, almost 40% of orbital paragangliomas {72} and occasional nasopharyngeal {1196} and cauda equina {15,1532,2101} paragangliomas recur locally. Approximately 8% of gangliocytic paragangliomas give rise to regional lymph node metastases {2252} and one tumour is reported to have infiltrated the mesentery {517}. There are no reports of distant metastases.

Histopathology

The histopathology of cauda equina and orbital paragangliomas is similar to that of carotid body and other parasympathetic paragangliomas.

Gangliocytic paraganglioma is a distinctive triphasic tumour consisting of epithelioid endocrine cells, spindled Schwann-like cells and ganglion cell-like elements. It thereby appears to be a hybrid tumour of a carcinoid, paraganglioma and ganglioneuroma. The proportion of the different elements varies within and between cases. The elements are haphazardly distributed and any one of them can predominate. The endocrine cells are polygonal or columnar and arranged in nests, trabeculae or gland-like structures. The endocrine cells are cytologically bland but they may exhibit focal mild atypia. The ganglion cells are reminiscent of their normal counterparts and may be uni- or multi-nucleated. They are distributed within the endocrine and spindle cell components. Spindle cells form the background and surround the nests of endocrine cells. Rarely, psammoma bodies and stromal amyloid can be encountered. The tumour is relatively well-circumscribed but an infiltrative growth margin is commonly seen.

In immuhistochemical studies, the endocrine cells are positive for the generic neuroendocrine markers synaptophysin and chromogranin A, although chromogranin A is not positive in all cases. In addition, they are positive for cytokeratins in contrast to typical paraganglion cells. Regulatory peptides such as pancreatic polypeptide, somatostatin, leu-enkephalin, serotonin, glucagon, vasoactive intestinal peptide (VIP), insulin and gastrin may also be present. The ganglion-like cells are also immunoreactive for neural and / or neuroendocrine markers, including neurofilament, and PGP 9.5. The spindle cells are positive for neurofilament, S-100 protein, neuron-specific enolase and PGP 9.5.

The growth fraction, as measured by Ki-67 or mitotic index is typically low.

Depending on which element dominates, the differential diagnosis varies. Considerations include carcinoid tumour, paraganglioma, ganglioneuroma, Schwannoma and carcinoma.

Genetic susceptibility

Gangliocytic paragangliomas may occasionally occur in the setting of patients with NF1 {329,1085,2124}.

Recently a patient with a spinal paraganglioma and a germline G12S *SDHD* mutation was described {1427}.

It is currently not clear whether this sequence variant is a polymorphism or a true tumour inducing mutation.

Prognosis and predictive factors

The prognosis for orbital paraganglioma is dependent on the extent of infiltration of local structures. Gangliocytic paragangliomas pursue an indolent course even in the presence of lymph node metastases. The prognosis of paraganglioma of the cauda equina after complete excision appears to be good, although there is local recurrence in approximately 4% of cases {2151}. This may be due to infiltration of caudal roots {1296}. Long-term follow-up of these tumours is required.

Extra-adrenal sympathetic paraganglioma: Superior and inferior paraaortic

N. Kimura
C. Capella
R.R. De Krijger
L.D.R. Thompson

K.Y. Lam
P. Komminoth
A.S. Tischler
W.F. Young Jr.

Definition
A paraganglioma arising from extra-adrenal paraganglia distributed along the sympathetic chains.

ICD-O codes
Extra-adrenal sympathetic paraganglioma
8693/1
Superior and inferior paraaortic paraganglioma
8693/1

Synonyms
Extra-adrenal phaeochromocytoma

Epidemiology
Most sporadic paragangliomas are solitary. The tumours arise in middle age and the distribution by sex is nearly equal {846,1994}.

Localization
Paragangliomas parallel the distribution of the paravertebral sympathetic chain. Paragangliomas of the retroperitoneum along the aorta including suprarenal, renal hilar and infrarenal sites are the highest in frequency.

Clinical features
These paragangliomas may be functionally active with excess secretion of catecholamines (usually norepinephrine) resulting in hypertension.

Macroscopy
Paragangliomas are solid tumours and are partially or completely encapsulated with a thin capsule. The cut surface of the tumour is tan to red-brown, extremely vascular, homogeneous, or focally fibrotic. Larger tumours may show haemorrhage and cystic degeneration. Tumours that produce substantial amounts of catecholamines change their colour from tan to brown in aldehyde-containing fixatives. Tumours that produce small amounts of catecholamines do not change colour.

Tumour spread and staging
Multiple extra-adrenal sympathetic paragangliomas may occur synchronously or metachronously anywhere along the sympathetic chains from the retroperitoneal to the cervical regions {605, 1038,2381}. Multiple paragangliomas should therefore be distinguished from metastatic paragangliomas. Reported frequency of distant metastasis is higher than that of adrenal phaeochromocytomas. The tumours metastasize to lymph nodes, lungs, bones, liver and occasionally to other unusual sites {1084,2023}.

Histopathology
The histology of functioning paragangliomas producing excessive catecholamines is very similar to that of the adrenal phaeochromocytomas. However, phenylethanol amine N-methyltransferase (PNMT), which synthesizes epinephrine from norepinephrine, is usually not detectable in extra-adrenal paragangliomas {1080}.
The differential diagnosis and the relevant histopathologic techniques for extra-adrenal paragangliomas are discussed in detail under adrenal phaeochromocytoma.
Electron microscopy is also useful to distinguish paragangliomas from tumours that are not neuroendocrine. Numerous membrane-bound secretory granules containing catecholamines, and other neuroendocrine components are observed. Neurotubules and neurofilaments are also observed and the endoplasmic reticulum is well developed.

Somatic genetics
Adrenal and extraadrenal sympathetic chromaffin tumours exhibit similar somatic defects and mutations (see phaeochromocytoma). Deletions of the short arm of chromosome 1 have also been identified in catecholamine-producing abdominal paragangliomas suggesting a common genetic etiology of both tumours {546}.

Genetic susceptibility
There are occasional multiple paragangliomas associated with SDH mutations, MEN type 2A and type 2B {1610}, von Recklinghausen disease (neurofibromatosis type 1) and von Hippel-Lindau syndrome {1803}. In Carney triad, functioning extra-adrenal paraganglioma is associated with epithelioid gastrointestinal stromal tumour (GIST) and pulmonary chondroma {307,309}.
Extraadrenal, parasympathetic paragangliomas are associated with germline

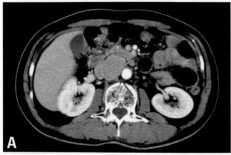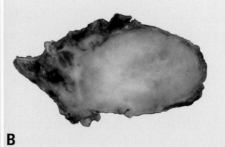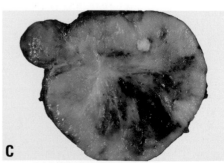

Fig. 3.25 Paraganglioma. **A** CT scan at the level of the renal hilum shows a well-defined, homogenous mass of soft tissue locating between the aorta and the inferior vena cava. **B** Well demarcated retroperitoneal paraganglioma **C** Paraganglioma of organ of Zuckerkandl showing focal areas of haemorrhage on cut section.

mutations in the three of the succinate dehydrogenase (SDH, mitochondrial complex II) subunits (*SDHD*, *SDHB* and probably *SDHC*) {1379,2462}. Furthermore, they are rarely associated with VHL and may be the sole or first manifestation of the disease {108,1543, 1803}.

Extra-adrenal sympathetic paraganglioma: Cervical, intrathoracic and urinary bladder

A.S. Tischler
P. Komminoth

Definition
Extra-adrenal paragangliomas arising from paraganglia that are distributed along the pre- and paravertebral sympathetic chains and the sympathetic nerve fibers innervating the pelvic and retroperitoneal organs. The definitions encompass "aortico-sympathetic" paragangliomas and a subset of "visceral-autonomic" paragangliomas {728}.

ICD-O codes
Urinary bladder   8693/1
Intrathoracic and cervical paravertebral
                                   8693/1

Synonyms
Extra-adrenal phaeochromocytoma

Epidemiology
Sympathetic paragangliomas usually present in the age range of 20-50 years. However, in some series up to 30% of patients are below 16 years. While almost 90% of tumours in adults are intra-adrenal (i.e., classic phaeochromocytomas), the distribution of intra- and extra-adrenal paragangliomas in paediatric patients is almost equal. As many as half of all paediatric patients develop multiple paragangliomas, sometimes both extra- and intra-adrenal. In contrast, adults more often present with solitary tumours. Sympathetic paragangliomas in different locations vary in age distribution, gender predilection and malignant potential.

Cervical sympathetic paragangliomas.
There are fewer than ten reported cases.

Prognosis and predictive factors
There are no established criteria to predict outcome. However, extra-adrenal location is associated with an increased risk of malignancy {1306,2289}. The definitive criterion of malignancy is the presence of lymph node or distant metastases. Other criteria for malignancy

Patients had an age range of 8-28 years, with a slight male predominance {660, 707,1490,1898,2079}; almost one half had additional paragangliomas at other sites. None of the cervical tumours was apparently malignant.
Thoracic sympathetic paragangliomas have been reported in patients 4 months to 64 years old (mean 29 years in one large series {685}) with a 2:1 male / female ratio. Approximately 7% {685} to 12% {1633} of the tumours gave rise to distant metastases. Approximately 20% of patients had multiple paragangliomas.

Paragangliomas of the urinary bladder.
These have been reported in patients 10-81 years old (mean approximately 39 years). The male/female ratio varies considerably between series. Although the ratio is roughly equal cumulatively {1269,1990}, some series show up to a 3/1 female predominance {359}. A review of all cases in Japan suggests distribution peaks for females 20-30 years old and for males older than 50 years {2046}. Approximately 5% of the tumours overall give rise to distant metastases {1217,1269,2046} but as many as 19% were malignant in some series {359}. Up to 18% were mutifocal within the bladder {359} and occasional patients had multiple or familial paragangliomas.

Localization
Approximately 85% of extra-adrenal sympathetic paragangliomas arise below the diaphragm (42 % in the vicinity of the

adrenal gland and renal hilum or pedicle, 28% in the vicinity of the organ of Zuckerkandl, 10 % in the urinary bladder and the remainder in varied locations). Approximately 12 % are intra thoracic and 2% cervical {660}.
Care must be taken not to confuse cervical or thoracic sympathetic paragangliomas with parasympathetic paragangliomas arising in nearby locations. Cervical sympathetic paragangliomas should be clearly documented as involving the cervical sympathetic chains and separate from the carotid body and other structures. Thoracic sympathetic paragangliomas typically arise in the posterior mediastinum, which should aid in distinguishing them from their typically anterior parasympathetic counterparts.
Urinary bladder paragangliomas may arise in any portion of the bladder and are occasionally multifocal {359,462, 1269,2046}.

Clinical features
Between 25 and 70% of extra-adrenal sympathetic paragangliomas are reported to present with signs and symptoms attributable to excess catecholamine secretion. The remaining cases usually present with pain or mass effects or as incidental findings. Clinically "non-functional" tumours are often biochemically functional and may release catecholamines during surgical manipulation or cystoscopy. Paragangliomas involving the cervical sympathetic chains frequently are associated with Horner's syndrome. Those involving the thoracic

chains have been reported to enter the spinal canal through the neural foramina and cause spinal cord compression {685}. In the bladder, paragangliomas are classically associated with a clinical triad defined by paroxysmal or persistent hypertension, haematuria and "micturitional attacks" with symptoms typical of phaeochromocytoma {462,1217,1269, 1550,2046}. However the complete triad is frequently not present, and hypertension or haematuria alone are the most prevalent complaints in recent reports. Ultrasonography, computed tomography, magnetic resonance imaging (MRI) and MIBG scans aid in tumour localization. In MRI scans the tumours appear bright in T2-weighted images. Plasma or urine levels of catecholamines or their metabolites are variably elevated, usually with a predominance of norepinephrine and normal or near-normal epinephrine {5,1038,1550}.

Macroscopy
Thoracic or cervical sympathetic paragangliomas are usually well circumscribed or encapsulated, with gray to tan cut surfaces that are focally or extensively haemorrhagic. They may firmly adhere to and occasionally invade adjacent tissues. Bladder paragangliomas are usually submucosal, appearing as fungiform, rounded or pedunculated masses that bulge into the lumen, with variable ulceration.

Tumour spread and staging
Sympathetic paragangliomas metastasize principally to bones, liver and lung. Seeding of the cerebrospinal fluid by thoracic paraganglioma has been reported {408}.

Histopathology
The histological appearances of extraadrenal sympathetic paragangliomas are indistinguishable from those of phaeo-

chromocytomas. Immunoprofiling serves to distinguish the tumours both from neoplasms that are not neuroendocrine and from other types of neuroendocrine tumours, particularly neuroendocrine carcinoma. The former objective is most specifically accomplished by positive staining for chromogranin A; the latter by positive staining for tyrosine hydroxylase (TH) and, in most cases, negative staining for cytokeratins. Other markers that may be helpful are synaptophysin as a generic neuroendocrine marker, S-100 protein to demonstrate sustentacular cells and, in some cases, specific peptide hormones. Although neuron-specific enolase has been employed as a marker in many studies, it is less specific than other markers now available and may arguably have outlived its utility.

TH, the rate-limiting enzyme in catecholamine synthesis, is expressed in all clinically functional paragangliomas and in a high percentage of those that are clinically silent {1083,1339,1661}. The precise prevalence of immunoreactive TH in silent tumours is uncertain because large series antedate current antigen retrieval methods. In contrast to TH, most series report little or no immunoreactivity for phenylethanolamine N-methyltransferase (PNMT) in extra-adrenal paragangliomas, consistent with the tumours' usually noradrenergic phenotype {1083, 1339,1661}. A notable exception is paragangliomas of the heart {1339}. Paragangliomas typically exhibit low mitotic counts and Ki67/MIB-1 labeling indices. MIB-1 labeling has been found to correlate with malignant potential in several recent studies (see below).

Somatic genetics
Adrenal and extraadrenal sympathetic paragangliomas exhibit similar somatic defects and mutations (see phaeochromocytoma). Little information is available on somatic genetic abnormalities specif-

ically in cervical or thoracic sites or in the urinary bladder.

Genetic susceptibility
Thoracic paragangliomas have been reported in some VHL patients {162}. Paraganglioma of the urinary bladder has been reported in neurofibromatosis {269}.

Prognosis and predictive factors
The general difficulties of diagnosing malignant paragangliomas are discussed in sections on phaeochromocytoma and parasympathetic paraganglioma. Although some survey series have generally supported the prognostic utility of MIB-1 {1081,1571}, a recent study focussed only on the urinary bladder found that no histologic criteria, including MIB-1 labeling, could distinguish benign from malignant paragangliomas. In that study, only patients with tumour of advanced stage (≥T3, tumour invading perivesical tissue) were found to be at risk of recurrence or metastasis, while patients with T1 or T2 disease had favourable outcomes after complete tumour resection {359}. Discrepancies between studies employing MIB-1 may result from different scoring protocols with counts derived from random fields, consecutive fields or fields of highest labeling density.

Adenomatoid tumour

L. Cheng
T.M. Ulbright

Definition
A rare benign tumour of mesothelial origin arising in the adrenal gland.

ICD-O code   9054/0

Epidemiology
Adenomatoid tumours of the adrenal gland usually occur in middle-aged men {59,693,727,1783,2060,2260}.

Localization
The tumour occurs as a solitary mass. Most tumours are intra-adrenal, but peri-adrenal localization may also occur {586}.

Clinical features
All tumours have been incidentally discovered at autopsy or during evaluation for other conditions. No syndromes or clinical symptoms have been linked to the tumour.

Imaging
Adenomatoid tumour of the adrenal gland has been reported as a solid enhancing mass with cystic components.

Macroscopy
Adenomatoid tumours range from 0.5 to 9 cm (mean, 3.9 cm) in largest dimension. The tumours are well circumscribed and usually discrete, white, solid or solid and cystic masses.

Histopathology
These tumours have the same microscopic, immunohistochemical and ultrastructural features as adenomatoid tumours of the urogenital tract.
Microscopic examination reveals a well-circumscribed lesion with variable combinations of adenomatoid, papillary, solid, and cystic patterns. Most typically, tubules having flattened to cuboidal cells with prominent cytoplasmic vacuoles are formed (adenomatoid pattern). The vacuoles cause the cells to have a "signet ring" appearance, but they lack intracellular mucin. In other cases similar cells are closely packed (solid pattern) or line papillae or cysts.

Differential diagnosis
The differential diagnostic considerations include metastatic adenocarcinoma, angiosarcoma, Kaposi's sarcoma, mesothelioma, lymphangioma, and cystic adenoma. The distinctive morphologic, immunohistochemical, and ultrastructural features of adenomatoid tumours allow ready distinction. A rare cytokeratin-positive epithelial lined cyst of the adrenal gland may represent a true mesothelial inclusion cyst that gives rise to adenomatoid tumour {1475,2060, 2260}. Some previously reported lymphangiomas of the adrenal gland {1750} may have been adenomatoid tumours that were misinterpreted {1783,2060}. The tumour cells have the usual immunohistochemical profile of mesothelial cells including strong immunoreactivity for cytokeratin and calretinin.

Histogenesis
The tumour is thought to originate from mesothelial inclusions localized within the adrenal gland; the immunohistochemical and ultrastructural findings support the mesothelial origin of these tumours. The growth of a mesothelial tumour in the adrenal gland may also be explained by the close embryologic relationship between the adrenal glands and the gonads.

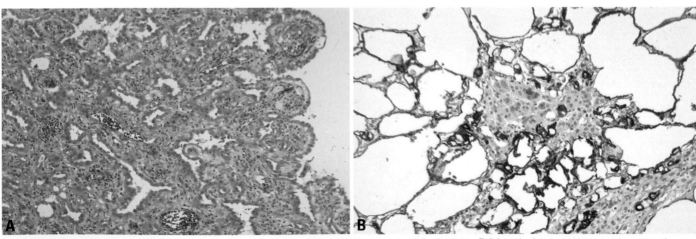

Fig. 3.26 Adenomatoid tumour of the adrenal gland. **A** Tubules and papillary structures in a hyalinized stroma. **B** Adrenal adenomatoid tumour demonstrating cystic dilation. Keratin immunohistochemistry highlights the neoplastic cells.

Sex cord-stromal tumour

L. Cheng
T.M. Ulbright

Definition
A tumour with sex cord-stromal differentiation, arising in the adrenal gland.

ICD-O code 8590/1

Epidemiology
All five documented cases of sex cord-stromal tumour of the adrenal gland occurred in post-menopausal women.

Etiology and cell origin
The histogenesis of sex cord-stromal tumour of the adrenal gland is uncertain {805,1660,1759,2262,2304}.

Clinical features
Patients with granulosa cell tumour of the adrenal gland present with irregular uterine bleeding and/or an abdominal mass {805,1660}. In contrast, patients with Leydig cell tumour of the adrenal gland present with virilization and have elevated serum testosterone and normal or slightly elevated urinary excretion of 17-ketosteroids.

Macroscopy
The tumours measure up to 9 cm in diameter. They are circumscribed, yellow to white or brown, and usually solid, but the granulosa cell tumours are occasionally cystic. Foci of haemorrhage may occur.

Histopathology
Only granulosa cell tumour and Leydig cell tumour have been reported {805,1660,1759,2262,2304}. Histologically, the tumours resemble their counterparts in the ovary. Germ cell tumours have not been documented at this site.

Prognosis and predictive factors
Two of the three patients with Leydig cell tumour were well on follow-up of two years each; no follow-up was available for the third. All three experienced decline in testosterone levels following tumour excision. No follow-up was available in the two patients with adrenal granulosa cell tumours. Exclusion of primary tumour in the ovary is essential for the diagnosis of these cases.

Adrenal soft tissue and germ cell tumours

R.V. Lloyd
A. Kawashima
A.S. Tischler

BENIGN LESIONS

Definition
A variety of benign tumours arising from components of the adrenal gland other than steroidogenic and catecholamine-producing cells.

Localization
Most of these tumours are unilateral and solitary, but they may be bilateral {1192,1211}.

Clinical features
Most tumours are small and asymptomatic. Larger tumours may be associated with symptoms related to the volume of the tumour.

Myelolipoma

ICD-O code   8870/0

The most common of these lesions is the myelolipoma which is variably classified as a tumour or tumour-like lesion. In a large recent series these account for approximately 2.5% of primary adrenal tumours {1211}. They are usually noted in mid to late adult life and there is no sex difference reported in most series. Although less common than myelolipomas, adrenal lipomas have a similar age and sex distribution {1205}.

Imaging
The characteristic CT and MR features of myelolipoma and lipoma are demonstration of areas of obvious fat within a well-defined adrenal mass {1057}. Calcification is present in a minority of cases on CT. Inhomogeneous attenuation within the tumours is common. The imaging diagnosis can be difficult when the amount of fat is poor or the lesion is complicated with haemorrhage, infarction, or calcification.

Macroscopy
Myelolipomas are soft and yellow to red, depending on the proportion of the components.

Histopathology
Myelolipomas comprise a mixture of mature adipose tissue and haematopoietic elements.

Haemangioma

Haemangiomas have been reported with a frequency of 0.01% in a series from the Armed Forces Institute of Pathology {1195,1673}. The age range for haemangiomas treated surgically has been from the third to eighth decade of life {1195}. In 11 surgically treated haemangiomas, nine patients were females {749,1659, 1675}.

Haemangiomas discovered at autopsy were usually 2 cm in size, while surgically removed lesions may be up to 22 cm in diameter {1195}.

Imaging
Adrenal haemangioma appears as a large inhomogeneously enhancing mass with variable areas of haemorrhage or necrosis. Progressive enhancement from the periphery to the center of the tumour may be present. Calcification is noted in approximately two-thirds of cases. The presence of phleboliths is a characteristic finding although uncommon. Non-enhanced T1-weighted MRI shows heterogenous low-signal intensity, while non-enhanced T2-weighted MRI shows marked high-signal intensity except in the central fibrotic areas {1664}.

Histopathology
Haemangiomas in the adrenal are usually of the cavernous type. Cystic haemangiomas and lymphangiomas should be differentiated from non-neoplastic cysts.

Leiomyoma

Adrenal leiomyoma has been reported as a soft tissue attenuation mass on CT and appeared isointense to hypointense to the liver on T1-weighted and on T2-weighted MR images but the imaging findings are not specific {1057,1611}.

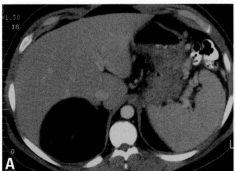 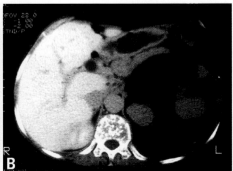 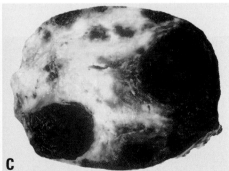

Fig. 3.27 Myelolipoma. **A** A myelolipoma of the right adrenal demonstrating an identical density to the subcutaneous fat. **B** Computed tomogram showing a well-demarcated mass in the adrenal region. The hypodense area is the adipose tissue and the dense areas are the bone marrow elements. **C** The adrenal gland shows a large well-demarcated mass composed of yellow adipose tissue and red bone marrow elements.

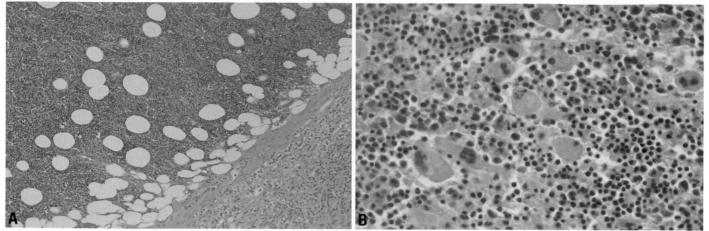

Fig. 3.28 Myelolipoma. **A** A mixture of mature adipose tissue and bone marrow cells including erythroid, myeloid and megakaryocytes are present in the tumour. There is compression of the adjacent adrenal cortex. **B** Higher magnification showing the same marrow cells.

Adrenal leiomyomas are usually associated with the adrenal vein or its tributaries {1673}.

Other benign lesions

Cystic lymphangioma appears as a thin-walled unilocular or multilocular cystic mass with or without fine calcification in the wall or septum. Cystic teratomas may have prominent rim calcification {151, 1210}. The most important differential diagnosis is non-neoplastic cysts {332}. Other rare lesions include schwannomas, ganglioneuroma, neurofibromas and teratomas. Any of these may present as incidental findings or with symptoms related to mass effect.

MALIGNANT TUMOURS

Definition

A variety of malignant tumours arising from components of the adrenal gland other than steroidogenic and cate-cholamine-producing cells. They usually carry a poor prognosis

Epidemiology

All of these tumours are rare. They include angiosarcoma, leiomyosarcoma, malignant peripheral nerve sheath tumour, primitive neuroectodermal tumour (PNET) and melanoma.

Localization

The tumours are usually large and unilateral and may extend beyond the adrenal.

Clinical features

Patients usually present with signs and symptoms from enlarging retroperitoneal masses with swelling, pain, weight loss, nausea, and vomiting, with or without metastatic disease.

Imaging

CT and MR imaging are helpful in assessing the extent of the tumour as well as hepatic, nodal, or venous spread but cannot prospectively define the tumour type {621}.

Macroscopy

The macroscopic appearance of these lesions is the same in the adrenal gland as at other sites.

Tumour spread and staging

Tumours may spread by direct invasion or haematogenous route. There is no universally accepted system for the staging of these lesions.

Histopathology

The histological and immunohistochemical features of these lesions are generally the same in the adrenal gland as at other sites. Angiosarcomas in the adrenal gland are usually of the epithelioid type {867,2375} and have a variable prognosis {2375}. Careful dissection may disclose an origin of leiomyosarcoma from the central vein. The diagnostic criteria for primary melanoma include presence of melanomas in only one adrenal; no prior or current pigmented lesions of the skin, mucosal surface, or eye, no history of removal of pigmented skin or eye lesions {321,458,867}.

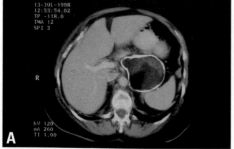
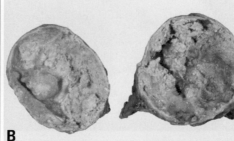
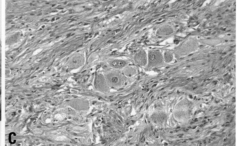

Fig. 3.29 Teratoma. **A** Cystic changes in the teratoma are prominent. **B** Benign cystic teratoma composed of a mixture of tissues. **C** Adrenal ganglioneuroma. An adrenal ganglioneuroma showing the characteristic ganglion cells separated by the background neural component. Pigment within the ganglion cells is seen.

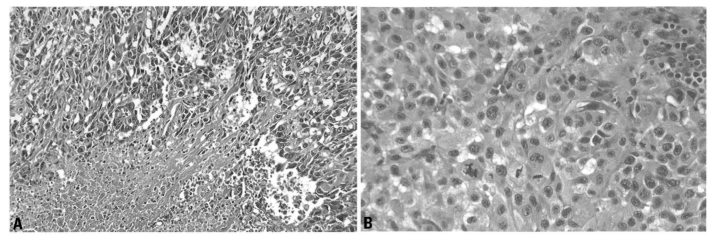

Fig. 3.30 A Angiosarcoma. An primary adrenal angiosarcoma demonstrates extensive necrosis in the lower part of the field. An anastamosing and arborizing vascular pattern is noted, lined by atypical endothelial cells with a hobnail appearance. **B** Melanoma. A primary adrenal gland melanoma identified at autopsy, demonstrates an epithelioid pattern of growth, reminiscent of an adrenal cortical carcinoma. Numerous atypical mitotic figures are seen.

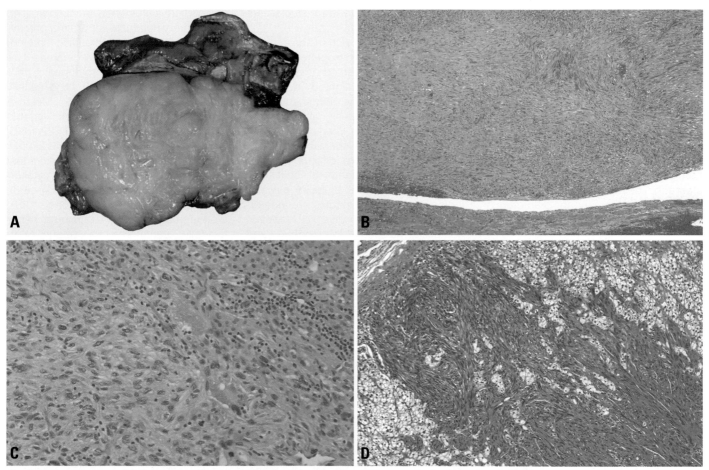

Fig. 3.31 Leiomyosarcoma **A** Leiomyosarcoma of adrenal forming a firm tan mass. **B** The central vein of the adrenal gland is seen to give rise to a leiomyosarcoma which demonstrates a spindle cell architecture. **C** High-grade leiomyosarcoma of adrenal. A few entrapped adrenal cortical cells are present. **D** Primary adrenal gland leiomyosarcoma invading into the surrounding adrenal cortical tissue. The spindle cells demonstrate atypical nuclei.

Secondary tumours

R.V. Lloyd
A. Kawashima
A.S. Tischler

Definition
Tumours that originate in extra-adrenal locations and spread to the adrenal either by metastasis or direct invasion.

Synonyms
Metastatic tumours.

Epidemiology
Secondary tumours of the adrenal increase in frequency with advancing age, and are most commonly diagnosed in the sixth to eighth decades {730, 1212}. Secondary tumours involving the adrenal are more common than primary tumours. The adrenal is the fourth most frequent site of spread of tumours after lungs, liver, and bone {2396}. In one autopsy series, metastases to the adrenals were present in 27% of patients dying with carcinomas {10}. The most common primary sites were the breasts, lung, kidney, stomach, pancreas, ovary, and colon. In a more recent series, the most common primary sites included the lung, stomach, oesophagus, and liver/bile duct {1212}. The mean diameter of metastases was 2 cm in one series {1212}.

Localization
Bilateral metastases are seen in almost half of the patients {1212,1894}. Spread of tumour within sinusoids of the involved adrenal gland may be present adjacent to the main metastatic focus, and these metastases may extend into several subcapsular extrusions of the cortex {1195}.

Clinical features
Signs and symptoms
Patients with metastatic tumour to the adrenals may present with adrenal cortical insufficiency {1212,1800,2002}. Because most of the adrenal cortex must be destroyed before secondary insufficiency develops {1195}, this finding is relatively uncommon. The most frequent tumours causing adrenal insufficiency are metastatic lung and breast carcinoma {2002}. Renal cell carcinoma, gastric, colonic, pancreatic, and transitional cell carcinoma do so less frequently {2002, 2029}.

Imaging
The first approach to imaging should be CT scan {1449}. On CT imaging the involved gland is usually round to oval and may be smooth or lobulated. Metastases usually look like soft tissue densities on CT scan {1449}, although this may be altered by extensive necrosis. CT is the study of choice to differentiate between a benign lesion (adenoma) and a metastasis in the patient with cancer {1449}. However, magnetic resonance imaging (MRI) and nuclear imaging may be advisable if CT studies are not diagnostic {1449}.
On MRI, the adrenal with metastatic disease usually has a heterogeneous signal intensity on T2-weighted images and sometimes on T1-weighted images. If there is haemorrhage into the tumour, there is usually a high signal on T1- and T2-weighted images. Imaging of certain primary lesions and specific metastatic lesions may be more difficult to diagnose, even with chemical shift MRI {1343,1449}. Adrenal biopsies may be indicated if imaging studies are indeterminate for metastatic disease. However, complications such as haemorrhage and infection may develop {1343}.

Macroscopy
The macroscopic appearance of metastatic malignancies in the adrenal is dependent on the primary sites; however, they are often grey-white with areas of necrosis, especially the larger metastases {1343}. If the lesion is dark brown to black, a malignant melanoma or extensive haemorrhage should be considered. The yellow colour of typical primary adrenal cortical tumours is usually absent except for a few tumours such as renal cell carcinomas {1627}. Secondary involvement by lymphomas, leukemias, and mesenchymal tumours such as leiomyosarcomas and angiosarcomas may have the characteristic appearance associated with the primary tumour.

Tumour spread and staging
The discovery of adrenal metastases in patients with primary tumours transfers them to an advanced stage. Because most of the tumours are asymptomatic, they are usually detected during the workup for disseminated disease {1212}.

Histopathology
Metastatic carcinomas, which constitute about 90% of the metastatic tumours, are usually easy to distinguish from adrenocortical tumours on H&E section. However, some tumours, such as renal cell carcinoma, large cell lung carcinomas, and hepatocellular carcinomas or even melanomas can simulate an adrenal cortical carcinoma. Immunoprofiling can be very helpful in separating primary adrenocortical from metastatic carcinomas. Adrenocortical carcinomas are always positive for steroidogenic transcription factor Ad4BP/SF1 and usually positive for inhibin-alpha, Melan-A (A103), D-11, vimentin, with variable staining for keratin {270,622,1496, 1713,1814,1946,1983,1984,2043,2200}.
Other immunohistochemical markers that may be helpful include: TTF-1, cytokeratin-7, surfactant proteins for lung carcinomas; HEPPAR-1, polyclonal CEA, alpha-fetoprotein and albumin for hepatocellular carcinoma; CD10 and NCL-RCC (Clone 66.4C2) for renal cell carcinoma {103,2445,2456,2457}. Melanomas can be readily diagnosed with S100 protein, tyrosinase, HMB-45, vimentin, and Melan-A.
Secondary involvement of the adrenals by malignant lymphomas has been reported in 18-25% of patients at autopsy {1823,1866}. This usually occurs in patients with widespread disease. Bilateral involvement may be present with both Hodgkin and non-Hodgkin lymphomas in 10-12% of patients {1823}. Immunohistochemical and flow cytometric studies for T and B cell markers can readily assist in making the diagnosis {1866,1978}.
Other metastatic malignancies to the adrenal include sarcomas such as angiosarcoma and Kaposi sarcoma, which usually occurs in the setting of acquired immunodeficiency syndrome {1195}. Rare cases of metastatic leiomyosarcoma and malignant nerve sheath tumours to the adrenals have

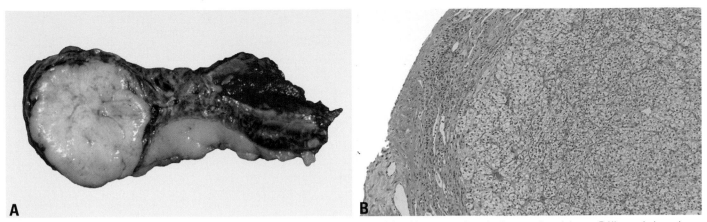

Fig. 3.32 Metastatic renal cell carcinoma. **A** The metastasis forms a discrete pale tan nodule with compression of adjacent adrenal tissue. **B** Histopathology showing that the tumour compresses the adjacent adrenal cortex.

been reported {1195}. Immunohistochemical markers for CD-31, CD-34, HHV-8, C-Kit, S100 protein, smooth muscle actin, and CD-57 can assist in the differential diagnosis when only small biopsy specimens are available for diagnosis {1481}.

Prognosis and predictive factors

Although many patients with secondary adrenal involvement are upgraded to a higher stage when the metastases are uncovered, patients may benefit from surgical resection of adrenal metastases with improved long-term survival {106,243,471,1342,1367,1751,1893,2275}. Survival for five years or longer has been reported more frequently after resection of adrenal metastases of lung carcinomas, renal cell carcinomas, and melanomas. However, in the most recent series {1212}, the median survival after resection was eight months, and survival over five years was present in only 5% of patients with symptomatic adrenal metastases {1212}.

CHAPTER 4

Tumours of the Endocrine Pancreas

Tumours of the endocrine pancreas are much less frequent than those of the exocrine pancreas and usually have a much better prognosis. Hormones secreted by endocrine neoplasms include insulin, glucagon, somatostatin, gastrin, vasoactive intestinal polypeptide (VIP), pancreatic polypeptide (PP), serotonin, ACTH, and calcitonin. Depending on the peptide hormones produced, they may cause distinct clinical syndromes, including life-threatening hypoglycaemia, gastric and/or duodenal ulcers, or dehydration due to diarrhoea.

Most pancreatic neuroendocrine tumours can be surgically resected and this leads to a rapid regression of clinical symptoms. Poorly differentiated neoplasms may be metastatic at the time of clinical presentation, and this is associated with a poor prognosis.

Genetic susceptibility may play an important role. Up to 20% of gastrinomas are associated with the inherited MEN-1 syndrome.

WHO histological classification of tumours of the endocrine pancreas

Well-differentiated endocrine tumour	8150/1[1]
Functioning	
Insulin-producing (insulinoma)	8151/1
Glucagon-producing (glucagonoma)	8152/1
Somatostatin-producing (somatostatinoma)	8156/1
Gastrin-producing (gastrinoma)	8153/1
VIP-producing (VIPoma)	8155/1
Others	
Non-functioning	
Microadenoma (<0.5 cm)	8150/0
Others	

Well-differentiated endocrine carcinoma	8150/3
Functioning	
Insulin-producing (insulinoma)	8151/3
Glucagon-producing (glucagonoma)	8152/3
Somatostatin-producing (somatostatinoma)	8156/3
Gastrin-producing (gastrinoma)	8153/3
VIP-producing (VIPoma)	8155/3
Serotonin producing with carcinoid syndrome	8241/3
ACTH producing with Cushing syndrome	8150/3
Non-functioning	8150/3
Poorly-differentiated endocrine carcinoma - small cell carcinoma	8041/3
Mixed exocrine – endocrine carcinoma	8154/3

---

[1] Morphology code of the International Classification of Diseases for Oncology (ICD-O) {664} and the Systematized Nomenclature of Medicine (http://snomed.org). Behaviour is coded /0 for benign tumours, /3 for malignant tumours, and /1 for borderline or uncertain behaviour.

Pancreatic endocrine tumours: Introduction

Ph.U. Heitz
P. Komminoth
A. Perren
D.S. Klimstra
Y. Dayal

C. Bordi
J. Lechago
B.A. Centeno
G. Klöppel

Terminology

In this chapter the term "pancreatic endocrine tumour" replaces earlier terms, e.g. pancreatic neuroendocrine tumour, islet cell tumour, and APUDoma.

Epidemiology

Pancreatic endocrine tumours are uncommon and represent 1-2% of all pancreatic neoplasms. The tumours show no significant gender predilection and occur at all ages, with a peak incidence between 30-60 years. Clinically unrecognised or asymptomatic, and usually small tumours (diameter less than 1 cm) have been found in 0.4-1.5% of unselected autopsies {779,1086,1154,1356, 1874, 2097}.

The reported overall incidence of tumours of the endocrine pancreas has increased during recent years. This is probably due to the application of more sensitive diagnostic approaches such as imaging techniques, reliable laboratory tests and careful "morphofunctional" analysis by immunohistochemical and molecular biological techniques {2097}.

Endocrine function

Pancreatic endocrine tumours are separated based on their clinical manifestation, into functioning and non-functioning.

Functioning tumours are associated with clinical syndromes caused by inappropriate secretion of hormones. Within this group are insulinomas, glucagonomas, somatostatinomas, gastrinomas, VIPomas, and other less common tumours. The clinical syndromes are described under the headings of the various functioning tumours.

Non-functioning tumours (or inactive, clinically silent, nonsyndromic) are not associated with a distinct hormonal syndrome but may still show elevated hormone levels in the blood or immunoreactivity in tissue sections. For this reason, the term "nonsyndromic" pancreatic endocrine tumour may more accurately describe this group, but is not widely used {2094}. Therefore, tumours with the majority of cells expressing (and often secreting) pancreatic polypeptide (PP), or neurotensin are included in the group of non-functioning tumours (as are many "D-cell tumours" or "somatostatin producing tumours"), because they do not cause a distinct hormonal syndrome. Non-functioning tumours only become clinically apparent due to their large size, to invasion of adjacent organs, or the occurrence of metastases. Rarely they may present as acute pancreatitis.

Increasingly, they are incidentally detected on imaging tests.

Tumours with a diameter of less than 0.5 cm, the minimum size required for gross detection, are defined as microadenomas and are, as a rule, non-functioning.

Macroscopy

The majority of the tumours are well demarcated and solitary, showing a white-yellow or pink-brown colour. The consistency is variable. Rarely, they are cystic {1301}.

Their diameter ranges usually around 1-5 cm. Among the functioning tumours, insulinomas are usually smaller (less than 2 cm in diameter) than glucagonomas, somatostatinomas, gastrinomas or VIPomas, but the size of the tumours is not related to the severity of the hormonally induced symptoms.

Non-functioning tumours are generally larger than 2 cm in diameter (often 5 cm or more). They are probably detected relatively late because they do not induce a clinical syndrome due to inappropriate hormone secretion.

Tumours with a diameter of more than 2 cm have an increased risk of malignant behaviour and those over 3 cm are usually malignant.

Cytopathology

Fine needle aspiration biopsy (FNAB) is a useful method for investigating pancreatic endocrine tumours and their metastases. Guidance techniques include computed tomography (CT), transabdominal ultrasonography (TUS) and, more recently, endoscopic ultrasonography (EUS). The cytomorphological features of pancreatic endocrine tumours are the same for functioning and non-functioning tumours {25, 161,401,2072}. Smears are usually uniformly cellular and composed of a relatively monotonous population of cells predominantly arranged singly, but also in loose clusters or pseudorosettes. The round to ovoid, smoothly contoured nuclei demonstrate a salt-and-pepper chromatin pattern. The cytoplasm is

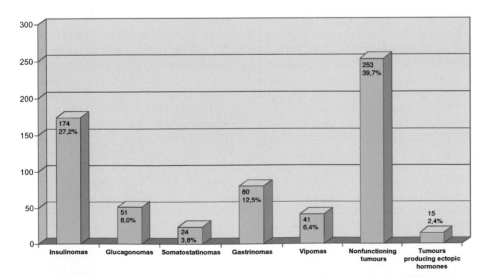

Fig. 4.01 Frequency of various types of pancreatic endocrine tumours, based on a series of 638 cases.

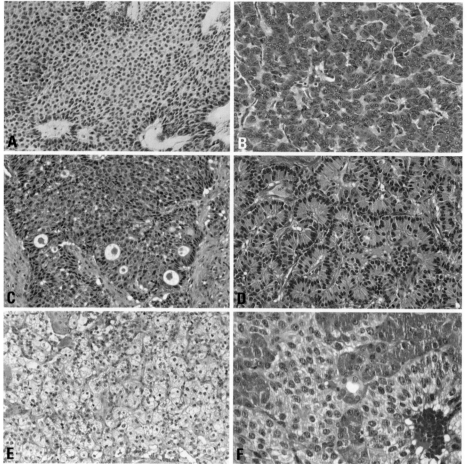

Fig. 4.02 Growth patterns of pancreatic endocrine tumours. **A** Solid growth pattern. **B** Trabecular growth pattern. **C** Gland formation. The cells lining the lumina are cytologically identical to those of the remainder of the tumour. **D** Gyriform growth pattern: Nested architecture and peripheral palisading of nuclei. **E** Clear lipid-rich cells.H&E. **F** Solid growth pattern and focal oncocytic metaplasia.

amphophilic and varies in quantity and density. Some cells may be stripped of their cytoplasm whereas others may have abundant cytoplasm and a plasmacytoid appearance.

Histopathology

Most pancreatic endocrine tumours are well differentiated showing various histological patterns, characterised by a solid, trabecular, glandular, gyriform, tubuloacinar or pseudorosette arrangement of their cells. The cells are relatively uniform, show finely granular eosinophilic cytoplasm and a centrally located round to oval nucleus that may display a distinct nucleolus. Occasionally, clear cells, vacuolated lipid-rich cells, oncocytes or"rhabdoid" features {1717} may be observed. The amount of stroma and degree of fibrosis vary. These patterns differ considerably from one tumour to another and may vary within the same

tumour. However, in most instances these features are sufficiently distinctive to permit recognition of the endocrine nature of a given tumour.

In general, the histological pattern of a tumour does not allow a conclusion as to its functional state or type of the hormone produced. There are two exceptions to this rule: amyloid deposits are indicative of insulinomas, and glandular structures containing psammoma bodies are commonly observed in somatostatin producing tumours of the periampullary duodenum.

Poorly differentiated endocrine carcinomas are uncommon. These highly aggressive neoplasms are hardly recognizable as endocrine tumours at first sight and require immunohistochemical examination to reveal their neuroendocrine phenotype. They show rather pleomorphic cells, usually in a solid arrangement, with hyperchromatic nuclei

and an elevated mitotic index (>10 per 10 HPF).

Markers of neuroendocrine differentiation

Pancreatic endocrine tumours can clearly be identified by using antibodies to markers common to all or most neuroendocrine cells, i.e. synaptophysin, an integral membrane glycoprotein of synaptic vesicles, or protein gene product (PGP) 9.5, a cytoplasmic protein. Neuron specific enolase (NSE) is widely reported to stain these tumours, but the results should be interpreted with caution in light of the low specificity of this marker. The presence of immunoreactive chromogranins, which are glycoprotein components of the matrix of neuroendocrine secretory granules, indicates the presence of secretory granules, i.e. some degree of differentiation of the tumour cells {1874,2097}. In less well granulated examples, chromogranin staining is generally less intense and extensive, despite diffuse strong staining for synaptophysin. Pancreatic endocrine tumours also contain cytokeratins 8, 18 and 19 and may often contain neurofilaments as well.

Hormonal markers

The use of these markers is helpful in characterizing tumour cell types and their specific hormonal products. However, functioning tumours are defined on the basis of clinical symptoms due to inappropriate hormone secretion rather than immunohistochemical findings.

In the majority of functioning tumours, the hormone causing the syndrome can be detected by immunohistochemistry. However, staining intensity or the number of positive cells is not related to the severity of symptoms. This is in part due to the impairment of the genetic and posttranslational regulation of hormone synthesis and secretion. There is a high degree of heterogeneity among the individual tumour cells in the content of immunoreactive peptide hormones and corresponding mRNA. In addition, immunoreactive hormones with reduced biological activity or with a greatly shortened or prolonged half-life in the serum may be produced. Highly functioning tumours may paradoxically lack immunohistochemically detectable hormones, presumably due to their rapid secretion. In such cases, mRNA detection techniques may be useful. On the other hand, an immunoreactive hormone may not be secreted due to an impaired secretory pathway. Thus, immunoreactive hormones very often can be localized to cells of non-functioning tumours.

Upon careful investigation it has become obvious that many tumours are composed of more than one phaenotype (multihormonal tumours). As a rule however, only one cell type correlates with an associated syndrome of endocrine hyperfunction. The classification of the tumours must therefore be "morphofunctional", i.e. not only based on cell typing. It must primarily take into consideration the clinical signs and symptoms, and determination of circulating hormone concentrations. Metastases may produce hormones other than those found in the primary {2097}.

Staging and prognosis

No staging system, such as the UICC TNM system, has been applied to pancreatic endocrine tumours.

The most reliable evidence of malignant behaviour in pancreatic endocrine tumours is metastasis to the regional lymph nodes or the liver or gross infiltration of adjacent organs. Many of the smaller examples, including most insulinomas, probably have malignant potential, but interruption of their natural history by surgical resection prevents the expression of such potential. A proposal has been made to separate pancreatic endocrine tumours into prognostic groups based on mitotic rate and necrosis {899}.

Among the functioning tumours, most insulinomas show benign behaviour. In contrast, the other types of functioning tumours fall either into the categories of well-differentiated tumours with uncertain behaviour (approx. 10-15%) or, more fre-

Table 4.01
Immunophaenotyping of pancreatic endocrine tumours.

General neuroendocrine markers
Synaptophysin
Protein Gene Product (PGP) 9.5
CD56
MAP18

Markers of the matrix of secretory granules
Chromogranins

Hormone (cell type) – specific markers
Insulin
Glucagon
Somatostatin
Gastrin
Vasoactive Intestinal Polypeptide (VIP)
Pancreatic Polypeptide (PP)
Serotonin
ACTH
Neurotensin
Calcitonin

Table 4.02
Criteria for the clinicopathological classification of pancreatic endocrine tumours.

1 Well-differentiated endocrine tumour

1.1 'Benign' behaviour
Confined to the pancreas, non-angioinvasive, no perineural invasion, <2 cm in diameter, <2 mitoses/10 HPF and <2% Ki-67 positive cells

1.2 Uncertain behaviour
Confined to the pancreas and one or more of the following features: ≥2 cm in diameter, 2-10 mitoses/10 HPF, >2% Ki-67 positive cells, angioinvasion, perineural invasion

2 Well-differentiated endocrine carcinoma
Low grade malignant
Gross local invasion and/or metastases

3 Poorly-differentiated endocrine carcinoma
High grade malignant
>10 mitoses / 10 HPF

quently, of well-differentiated carcinomas (approx. 85-90%).

A small number of non-functioning tumours are well-differentiated tumours showing benign or uncertain behaviour; however, the vast majority (approx. 90-95%) are well-differentiated carcinomas. Poorly differentiated endocrine carcinomas are uncommon {2097}.

Clinicopathological correlations

There is an obvious need to establish a close correlation between morphological classification and tumour-associated syndromes. This is emphasized by the difficulty in predicting the biological behaviour of well-differentiated endocrine tumours based on histological criteria alone. In addition, available follow-up studies most often refer to tumours

diagnosed according to the associated clinical syndrome due to inappropriate hormone secretion.

To definitely establish the benign nature of a tumour, a long clinical follow-up period is needed, because metastases may develop years after removal of the primary lesion.

With the exception of the poorly differentiated endocrine carcinomas, the progression of the disease is often remarkably slow. Survival for five to ten years after appearance of liver metastases is not uncommon. However, inappropriate secretion of hormones may cause life-threatening hypoglycaemia, gastric and/or duodenal ulcers, or important loss of fluid by watery diarrhoea.

The final 'morpho-functional' classification of an endocrine tumour of the pan-

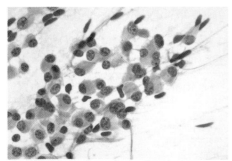

Fig. 4.03 Fine needle aspiration (FNA) of a pancreatic endocrine tumour. Amphophilic cytoplasm, uniform nuclei and finely granular chromatin, imparting a salt-and-pepper appearance.

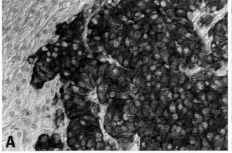
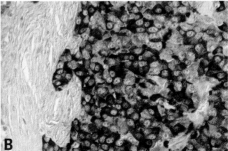

Fig. 4.04 Gastrinoma. Endocrine differentiation is more universal than cell-specific hormone production. **A** Virtually all tumour cells contain synaptophysin. **B** The majority, but clearly fewer cells contain chromogranin A.

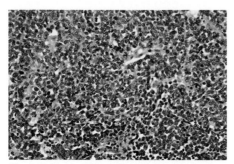

Fig. 4.05 Poorly differentiated endocrine carcinoma. Diffuse sheets of cells with nuclear pleomorphism, necrosis and a high mitotic rate.

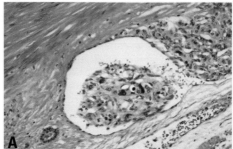

Fig. 4.06 **A** Pancreatic endocrine tumour. Vascular invasion. **B** Well differentiated endocrine carcinoma with massive vascular invasion.

creas should take into consideration (1) the clinical syndrome induced by or associated with, a tumour, (2) determination of the blood concentration of hormone(s) to identify the hormone(s) secreted by the tumour, (3) the size (mass) of the tumour, (4) the histological differentiation and probable biological behaviour of the tumour, (5) the phaenotype(s) of the various tumour cells and, if necessary and feasible, (6) molecular genetic analysis of the tumour.

Differential diagnosis
Histopathology
Most pancreatic endocrine tumours are recognizable without much difficulty. The use of immunohistochemical markers of the neuroendocrine phenotype and of hormonal content most often can establish the diagnosis unequivocally.

An important differential diagnostic problem is to distinguish solid-pseudopapillary neoplasms from endocrine tumours of the pancreas. Solid-pseudopapillary neoplasms morphologically resemble endocrine tumours, and furthermore, produce CD56, NSE and sometimes synaptophysin, as has been demonstrated by immunohistochemistry. Arguments in favour of the diagnosis of a solid-pseudopapillary neoplasm of the pancreas are the following: 1) it does not produce a hormonal syndrome but only local symptoms, 2) it is usually large, with a diameter often over 5 cm, 3) it contains clusters of cells with a clear foamy cytoplasm, 4) it often shows aggregates of PAS-positive hyaline globules in and between the tumour cells, 5) it contains broad, hyalinized septa including small blood vessels, 6) it displays haemorrhages, necrotic foci and occasionally cholesterol crystals, 7) it lacks expression of chromogranin and usually also

cytokeratin, but expresses vimentin, alpha-1-antitrypsin and CD10, 8) it lacks immunohistochemical expression of peptide hormones, 9) it occurs predominantly in young women, and 10) most tumours show a benign biological behaviour {1874}.

Further tumours which may be confused with pancreatic endocrine tumours are acinar cell carcinoma, pancreatoblastomas {1537}, poorly differentiated ductal adenocarcinoma, clear cell carcinoma, epithelioid gastrointestinal stromal tumours, primitive neuroectodermal tumours (PNET) and pancreatic metastases (e.g., renal cell carcinoma, small cell lung carcinoma, melanoma)

Acinar cell carcinomas, which histologically may be very difficult to distinguish from endocrine tumours of the pancreas, usually produce trypsin (-ogen) and other pancreatic (pro-) enzymes. The same is true for pancreatoblastomas. Both neoplasms may contain scattered endocrine cells. Truly mixed acinar-endocrine or ductal-endocrine carcinomas are very rare. In these tumours the endocrine cell component should account for at least one third of the entire cell population. Poorly differentiated ductal adenocarcinomas as well as clear cell carcinomas reveal focal expression of

mucin (MUC1) and carcinoembryonic antigen (CEA). Most epithelioid gastrointestinal stromal tumours (GIST) are characterized by the expression of C-KIT (CD117) and absence of staining for neuroendocrine markers. PNETs express a set of markers, including CD99. Metastases of clear cell carcinomas of the kidney lack neuroendocrine markers, but in addition to cytokeratins frequently express vimentin and CD10.

Cytopathology
The key entity in the differential diagnosis is acinar cell carcinoma. It can be distinguished from pancreatic endocrine tumours by its arrangement in loose, grapelike clusters, granular cytoplasm and prominent cherry red nucleoli {1191}. The neoplastic cells from a solid-pseudopapillary tumour, when detached from the fibrovascular cores may be mistaken for those of a pancreatic endocrine tumour. A search in the remainder of the smear for structures with the characteristic three-layered papillary architecture (a central capillary, a middle layer of myxoid stroma and an outer layer of neoplastic cells) will yield the correct interpretation {760}.

Pancreatic endocrine tumours may be mistaken for lymphomas because they

Table 4.03
Adverse prognostic factors of well-differentiated pancreatic endocrine tumours.

Metastasis	Regional lymph nodes, liver
Gross invasion	Adjacent organs
Tumour diameter	2 cm or more
Angioinvasion	Veins, lymphatic vessels
Perineural invasion	Intrapancreatic nerves
Mitoses	>2 per 10 HPF
Proliferative index Ki-67 / MIB-1	>2%
Necrosis	
Functioning tumours except insulinoma	

Table 4.04
Genetic alterations detected by loss of heterozygosity analysis (LOH), comparative genomic hybridization (CGH) and mutation analysis.

Locus	LOH	Gene	Mutation	CGH {2105,2107,2154,2490}	Reference
1p36-	10/29 (34%)			21/102 (21%)	{541}
1q32-	8/29 (28%)			16/102 (16%)	{1830}
3p23-	23/31 (74%)			19/102 (19%)	{120}
3p25-26-	31/73 (42%)	VHL	1/75 (1%)	19/102 (19%)	{382,879,1530,1830}
6q22-	43/69 (62%)			29/102 (28%)	{121,1830}
9p-	12/37 (32%)	CDKN2A/p16	1/44 (2%)	0/102 (0%)	{1531,2008}
9q+				29/102 (28%)	
10q23-	8/16 (50%)	PTEN	1/31 (3%)	14/102 (14%)	{1723}
11p14-				28/102 (27%)	
11q13	75/111 (67%)	MEN1	33/155 (21%)	31/102 (30%)	{441,750,879,880,1530,2018,2350,2495}
11q22-23	20/37 (54%)	SDHD	0/20 (0%)	31/102 (30%)	{1721,1830}
12p12+		K-Ras	1/39 (3%)	23/102 (23%)	{1531}
15q-		SMAD3	0/18 (0%)	6/102 (6%)	{2025}
17p13-	15/40 (38%)	TP53	1/40 (3%)	2/102 (2%)	{1531,1830}
17p+				32/102 (31%)	
18q21-	23/68 (34%)	DPC4	0/41 (0%)	6/102 (6%)	{879,1531,1722}
22q12.1	9/12 (75%)			4/102 (4%)	{2385}
Xq-	11/23 (48%)			14/46 (30%)	{1512}
Y-	5/14 (36%)			14/56 (25%)	{1512}

are dyscohesive and may lack much cytoplasm {161}. However, an absence of lymphoglandular bodies in the background and the formation of loosely cohesive epithelial structures will exclude the diagnosis of lymphoma. Possibly more likely to occur is the misdiagnosis of a pancreatic endocrine tumour as a plasmacytoma, since pancreatic endocrine tumours may have a very plasmacytoid appearance {505}. Features that will help to avoid this error are the presence of a salt-and-pepper chromatin pattern in the nuclei rather than the clock-face chromatin pattern seen in a plasmacytoma, greater variability in nuclear size and shape, and an absence of a paranuclear halo in the pancreatic endocrine tumour.

Molecular genetic analysis

Whereas the molecular basis of familial pancreatic endocrine tumours associated with multiple endocrine neoplasia type 1 (MEN 1) and von Hippel-Lindau (VHL) syndrome has recently been established {351,1241}, little is known about the oncogenesis and the molecular basis of progression of sporadic tumours.

A small number of published studies indicate that, in contrast to other human tumours, the activation of oncogenes is not a common event in pancreatic endocrine tumours {903,980,1346}. In particular, the common genetic muta-

tions identified in pancreatic ductal adenocarcinomas (e.g., TP53, K-RAS, CDKN2A/p16, DPC4) are not found in pancreatic endocrine tumours {931}.

Molecular and cytogenetic analyses have identified a number of chromosomal alterations in pancreatic endocrine tumours.

Chromosomal imbalances

Comparative genomic hybridization (CGH) studies of 102 pancreatic endocrine tumours revealed that chromosomal losses occur slightly more frequently than gains, while amplifications are uncommon {2105,2107,2154,2490}. Furthermore, the total number of genomic changes per tumour appears to be associated with both tumour volume and disease stage, indicating that genetic alterations accumulate during tumour progression {2105}. Thus, large tumours or those with increased malignant potential, and especially metastases, harbour more genetic alterations than small and clinically benign neoplasms {2105,2490}. These findings point toward a tumour suppressor pathway and genomic instability as important mechanisms associated with tumour progression.

In the majority of tumour types chromosomal alterations are not randomly distributed but are particularly common in certain chromosomal regions, including 4pq (17%), 5q (25%), 7pq (41%), 9q (28%), 12q (23%), 14q (32%), 17pq

(31%) and 20q (27%) (gains) and 1p (21%), 3p (19%), 6q (28%), 10pq (14%), 11q (30%), Y (31%) and X (31%) (losses). Additional losses of 3p, 6pq, 10pq and gains of 5q, 12q, 18q and 20q are associated with malignant behaviour {2490}.

Losses of chromosome 1 and 11q as well as gains of 9q appear to be early events in the development of pancreatic endocrine tumours, since they are already present in a substantial number of small (<2 cm) tumours {2490}. The other aforementioned alterations appear to occur later, accumulating during progression and are frequently associated with malignant biological behaviour. Prevalent chromosomal aberrations common in metastases include gains of both chromosomes 4 and 7, and losses of 21q {2490}, implying that these chromosomal

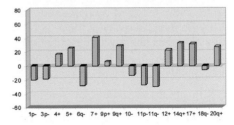

Fig. 4.07 Pancreatic endocrine tumours. Summary of the results obtained by CGH. Gains of chromosomal material are prominent on chromosomes 4, 5, 7, 9, 14, 17 and 20, while losses are concentrated on chromosomes 1, 3, 6 and 11.

imbalances may contribute to tumour dissemination.

Loss of heterozygosity (LOH)

When comparing the results of LOH studies using PCR microsatellite markers with those of CGH, similar chromosomal regions exhibit genetic losses. However, in general the rate of LOH is roughly twice that of allelic losses detected by CGH. At regions 3p23, 6q22, 9p, 11q13, 18q21 and 22q12.1 the differences are even more pronounced, indicating that small deletions, not detectable by CGH, are involved {2385}. Only a small number of candidate genes located at some of the above mentioned chromosomal loci have been thoroughly investigated and many genes remain to be identified.

Pooled data indicate that somatic *MEN1* mutations are present in 21% (33/155) of spontaneous neoplasms and that 68% (75/111) harbour losses of 11q13 and/or of more distal parts of the long arm of chromosome 11. These findings indicate that another yet unknown tumour suppressor gene might be involved {441, 443,750,879,880,1530,1721,1830,2018, 2350,2495}. However, the *SDHD* gene has recently been excluded as a candidate gene {1721}.

Point mutations

Point mutations in tumour-associated genes, including *VHL*, *CDKN2A/p16*, *PTEN*, *K-RAS*, *TP53* appear to be extremely rare (1-3%) {382,750,1531, 1723, 2008}. Mutations have not been identified in *DPC4/SMAD4*, *RET*, *ZAC*, *BRAF* and *SMAD3* {1131,1531,1722,1725,2025}.

Synopsis

When comparing molecular data of the different types of sporadic tumours it appears that (1) the highest average number of chromosomal aberrations and allelic losses are present in non-functioning tumours, followed by glucagonomas and VIPomas, (2) many of these aberrations are associated with malignant clinical behaviour, (3) insulinomas and especially gastrinomas exhibit fewer genetic

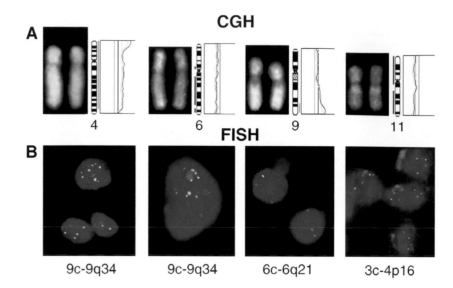

Fig. 4.08 Pancreatic endocrine tumour. Analysis by comparative genomic hybridization(CGH) and fluorescence in-situ hybridization (FISH). Small functioning and non-functioning tumours of the pancreas: Gain of 9q34 is an early event in insulinomas (green fluorescence in FISH; red: centromere of chromosome 9). There is a deletion of one copy of 6q21 (green fluorescence) in the presence of both centromeres of chromosome 6 (red). A duplication of 4p16 as shown by FISH (green) is present as compared with the centromere 3 (red). From: E.J. Speel et al. {2107}.

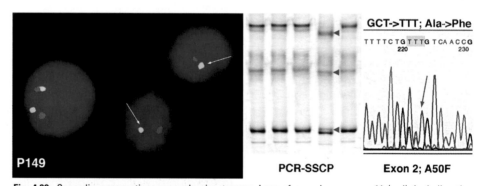

Fig. 4.09 Sporadic pancreatic neuroendocrine tumour. Loss of one chromosome 11 (red), including the MEN-1 locus (green) in the majority of tumour cells. PCR-SSCP shows a band shift in exon 2 (red arrow heads) which is caused by a A50F missense mutation as shown by sequence analysis. From: B. Gortz et al. {750}.

alterations than the other tumour types, (4) the frequency of *MEN1* mutations in insulinomas is remarkably low, (5) functioning tumours other than insulinomas exhibit a higher frequency of *MEN1* mutations and associated LOH at 11q13 than non-functioning tumours.

These observations indicate that different types of pancreatic endocrine tumours evolve along different genetic pathways and that somatic inactivation of *MEN1* is involved in a significant proportion of functioning tumours, but only exceptionally in insulinomas.

Insulinoma

P. Komminoth
A. Perren
K. Öberg

G. Rindi
Ph.U. Heitz
G. Klöppel

Definition

An insulinoma is a functionally active and commonly benign endocrine tumour of the pancreas with evidence of B-cell differentiation and clinical symptoms of hypoglycaemia due to inappropriate secretion of insulin.

ICD-O code

Insulin producing tumour
8151/1
Insulin producing carcinoma
8151/3

Synonyms

Related, but not universally applicable terms for these tumours include "functioning beta-cell tumour", "insulin producing pancreatic endocrine tumour" or "insulin producing islet cell tumour".
Symptoms of hypoglycaemia due to inappropriate secretion of insulin were first described by Harris in 1924 {836} and three years later the association between insulin secreting pancreatic endocrine tumours and hypoglycaemia was reported by Wilder et al {2386}.

Epidemiology

Insulinomas are the most frequent of all functioning pancreatic endocrine tumours (see Pancreatic endocrine tumours) {1154,1874}. The incidence of insulinoma was reported to be 2-4 patients per million population per year {1207,2012}. Insulinomas have been diagnosed in all age groups but rarely occur below the age of 15. The highest

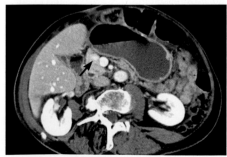

Fig. 4.10 Abdominal CT of a patient with a small insulinoma (arrow).

incidence is found between 40-60 years. Approximately 10% of the patients are younger than 20 years and 10% older than 60 {603,714,2011,2120}. Females seem to be slightly more frequently affected (1.5:1 ratio) in most reported series {682,714,729,1255,2011,2012, 2295}.

Etiology

The etiology and pathogenesis of insulinomas are unknown. No risk factors have been associated with these tumours. Embryologically, pancreatic tumours arise from similar precursor cells as pancreatic islet cells which are derived from the endoderm {1253}. The results of a recent clonality study on pancreatic endocrine tumours are consistent with the hypothesis that these tumours primarily might be polyclonal or oligoclonal neoplasms which are eventually outgrown by a more aggressive cell clone that may give rise to invasive growth and/or metastasis {1724}.

Localization

The majority of insulinomas are located in the pancreas or are directly attached to it. Ectopic (extrapancreatic) insulinomas with symptoms of hypoglycaemia are extremely rare (1.8%) and are most commonly found in the duodenal wall {627,2120}. Other reported locations include the ileum, jejunum, gastric wall, hilus of the spleen, gastrosplenic ligament, lung, cervix and ovary {11,1075, 1124,1714,2017,2036,2458}.
Compiled data indicate that insulinomas are equally distributed between the head, body and tail of the pancreas with a slight predominance in the head and tail region {516,627,925,1542,2120}. Approximately 85% of insulinomas occur singly, 6-13% are multiple and 4-6% are associated with MEN1 {516,682,714, 729,1255,2011,2120,2295}.

Clinical features

Signs and symptoms

Patients with insulinoma manifest symptoms that can be grouped into two major categories: neurological symptoms and the autonomic nervous system response. The most common and convincing symptoms result from neuroglucopenia, followed by the catecholamine response. Most prominent are symptoms of central nervous system dysfunction including diplopia, blurred vision, confusion, abnormal behaviour and amnesia. Some patients may develop loss of consciousness and coma or even permanent brain damage. Sometimes the patients also present with focal seizures. When triggered by hypoglycaemia the release of catecholamines produce symptoms such as sweating, weakness, hunger, tremor, nausea, anxiety and palpitation. These symptoms, although highly suggestive, are not pathognomonic for hypoglycaemia and a low blood glucose level must be demonstrated during their occurrence. The Whipple triad includes: (1) symptoms of hypoglycaemia, (2)

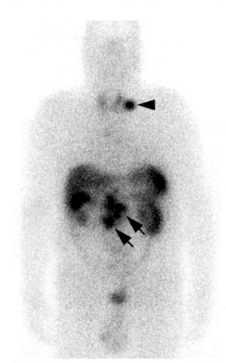

Fig. 4.11 Octreoscan of a patient with an endocrine tumour of the ileum. Note paraaortal metastases (arrows) and infraclavicular lymph node metastases (arrowhead). The latter were confirmed by cytology.

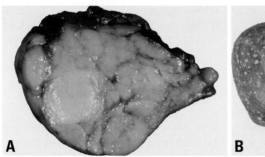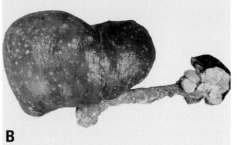

Fig. 4.12 A Insulinoma. The tumour is small, sharply demarcated. B Malignant insulinoma invading the spleen. Numerous small liver metastases are present.

plasma glucose levels <3.0 mmol per litre; and (3) relief of symptoms with administration of glucose {1620,2010, 2120, 2497}.

Imaging
Transabdominal ultrasonography yields a sensitivity of 20-65% in various series, CT scan 25-60%, angiography 35-75%, and intraoperative ultrasonography 90-100%. More specific methods include octreoscan and PET-scan.

Diagnostic procedures
Determination of plasma insulin and proinsulin concentrations by radioimmunoassay has greatly facilitated and simplified the diagnosis of insulinoma. Usually insulin, proinsulin, C-peptide and blood glucose are measured together to demonstrate an inappropriately high secretion of insulin in relation to blood glucose and to distinguish endogenous

from factitious hyperinsulinaemia. In general, 80-85% of all insulinomas are diagnosed by these measurements. Inappropriately high plasma insulin levels, during 48-72 hour fasting, is also regarded as a sensitive diagnostic test. Alternatively, C-peptide suppression is also a valuable screening or confirmatory test for insulinoma.

Macroscopy
Grossly, insulinomas are well-circumscribed tumours, softer than the surrounding pancreatic parenchyma and have a red-brown cut surface. Tumours with abundant stroma or amyloid are firmer. Insulinomas are frequently discovered while still small with 75% of the tumours measuring 0.5-2 cm in diameter and less than 2 g in weight. The reported diameter ranges from 0.5-11 cm {1154}. Tumour size is unrelated to severity of symptoms. Degenerative, necrotic and

cystic changes are uncommon and most often restricted to large tumours. Insulinomas producing a hypoglycaemic syndrome in MEN1 patients are usually larger than 1 cm. Microadenomas, i.e. tumours below 0.5 cm in diameter, with insulin expression, no matter how numerous they are, seem to remain functionally silent {1114}. This implies that the insulinomas in MEN1 patients are among the grossly apparent and palpable pancreatic tumours. If there are several large tumours usually only one of them is an insulinoma.

Tumour spread and staging
Malignant insulinomas may show gross local invasion of peripancreatic fatty tissue and/or adjacent organs such as the duodenum or the spleen. The first metastases are usually found in regional lymph nodes (peripancreatic, coeliac, periaortic) and the liver. Spread to other distant sites is unusual. So far there is no staging system that specifically applies to insulinomas (see Pancreatic endocrine tumours).

Histopathology
Insulinomas exhibit four main histological patterns including a solid, trabecular, gland-like (tubular or acinar) tumour growth and mixed forms {858,1154}. Larger tumours are encapsulated but the capsule is usually incomplete. Smaller tumours and microadenomas (see Nonfunctioning tumours, microadenomas, others) are rarely encapsulated. Tumour cells frequently exhibit a bland cytology and cells with large, pleomorphic nuclei are rare. If present, these features are not predictive of malignant behaviour. A relatively uncommon, but characteristic finding in insulinomas is the deposition of amyloid. Its major component is islet amyloid polypeptide (IAPP) or amylin, that can be visualized by immunohistochemistry {2388}. Calcifications and intracytoplasmatic pigment may rarely be seen in insulinomas {957,2405}.

Immunohistochemistry
Almost all insulinomas exhibit immunoreactivity for insulin and proinsulin. The intensity and extent of this immunoreactivity, however, does not correlate with circulating insulin levels. Strong positivity for insulin at the secretory pole of the cells and proinsulin in the perinuclear

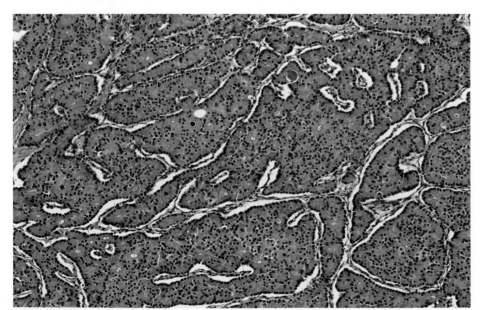

Fig. 4.13 Insulinoma with trabecular architecture.

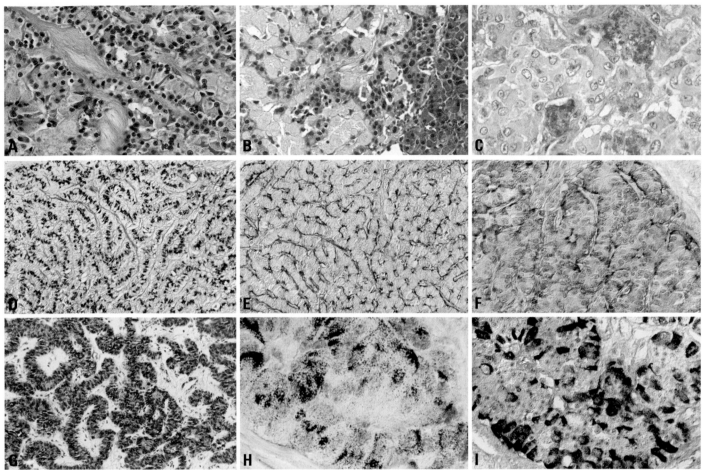

Fig. 4.14 A Insulinoma with trabecular architecture. **B** Insulinoma. Stroma-containing amyloid. **C** Amyloid visualized by Congo red staining. **D** Insulinoma, highly differentiated, trabecular architecture. Proinsulin localized to the paranuclear Golgi area. Antibody specific for proinsulin. **E** Insulin predominantly localized at a secretory pole of the tumour cells. **F** Insulinoma with a trabecular growth pattern. Localization of insulin at the secretory pole of the tumour cells and partly within the cytoplasm. Antibody to insulin. **G** mRNA for insulin visualized by in-situ hybridization. **H** Proinsulin is partly located in the paranuclear Golgi area but also in the cytoplasm and at the secretory pole of the tumour cells. Proinsulin is secreted together with insulin in these tumours. Antibody specific for proinsulin. **I** Insulin is localized within the entire cytoplasm and at the secretory pole of the cells.

region, i.e. the Golgi region can be seen in some highly differentiated insulinomas. More often, however, an abnormal staining pattern for insulin and proinsulin is found {1871,1872}. About 50% of insulinomas are multihormonal. In such tumours insulin positive cells are admixed with cells expressing glucagon, somatostatin, pancreatic polypeptide or other hormones {1154}.

Useful additional immunohistochemical markers for the classification of insulinomas are MIB-1 (to assess proliferation index), CD31 (to visualize angioinvasion) and somatostatin receptor subtypes {1681}. In cases with non-detectable insulin by immunohistochemistry in-situ hybridization may be helpful to identify insulin mRNA in tissue sections {2106}.

Electron microscopy
There are several classifications of insulinomas based on the ultrastructrural shape of their secretory granules {174, 429,430,2164}. However, as it has become more and more obvious that insulinomas are extremely heterogeneous, containing poorly and well-granulated cells in the same tumour, the use of these classifications is limited. In a more recent study it was demonstrated that the pathophysiology of insulinomas is less likely caused by decreased storage capacity for insulin, as proposed earlier, than by impaired conversion of proinsulin to insulin {1873}.

Precursor lesions
No definite precursor lesion has been identified for insulinoma. Proliferation of β

cells (β cell hyperplasia, nesidioblastosis), in patients with persistent hyperinsulinaemic hypoglycaemia cannot be considered a precursor lesion of insulinoma because it is genetically different {2006}.

Histogenesis
The histogenesis of insulinoma is uncertain {1835}. Ductal proliferation may sometimes be associated with insulinoma, suggesting a potential duct cell origin. Alternatively, an islet origin of β cell tumours is suggested by histology in MEN1 patients {2094} and is supported by observations that transgenic mice consistently developed islet B-cell hyperplasia, dysplasia and insulinomas, in the absence of ductuloinsular proliferation {815,1834,1835,1837}.

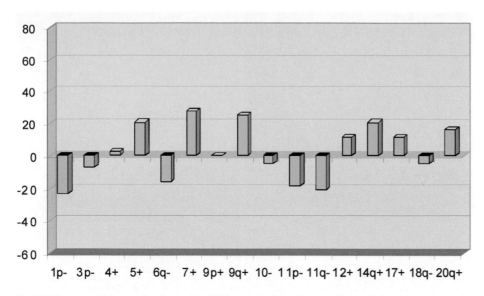

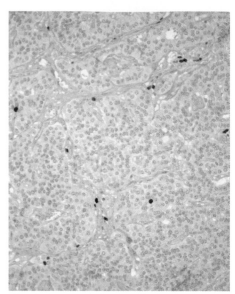

Fig. 4.15 Summary of the results obtained by CGH analysis of insulinomas. Gains of chromosomal material mainly occur on chromosomes 5, 7, 9q, 14q and 20q while losses are shown on 1p, 6q, 11p and 11q.

Fig. 4.16 Insulinoma. The proliferative index is less than 2 %. Antibody Ki-67.

Somatic genetics

Compiled data from 43 analysed tumours indicate that as compared to other pancreatic endocrine tumours, insulinomas exhibit fewer genomic alterations by CGH (see Pancreatic endocrine tumours) {2105,2107,2154, 2490}. In particular, losses of 3p and other malignancy-associated alterations are rare. Losses of 3q and gains of 15q appear to be more frequently encountered in insulinomas than in the other pancreatic endocrine tumour types. Gains of 9q34 and losses of 1p36 and 11q appear to be early alterations already detectable in tumours smaller than 2 cm.

Despite allelic losses of up to 40% at 11q13 (the locus of *MEN1*), somatic mutations of the *MEN1* gene appear to be rare when compared to the other endocrine tumour types. They were identified in only 7.7% (5/65) of sporadic insulinomas {750,879,1530,2018,2105, 2350,2495}. Somatic mutations in other genes such as *VHL* and *CDKN2A/p16* are only occasionally encountered (1/22 and 1/9) {1530,1531}.

Genetic susceptibility

Insulinoma is the second most frequent functioning enteropancreatic tumour in MEN1 patients after gastrinoma, the latter often arising in the duodenum {1250}. Rare examples of insulinomas have also been described in patients suffering from NF1 {672}. Approximately 4-7% of unselected patients with insulinomas suffer

from MEN 1 {2012} .Between 10 and 30% of the pancreatic endocrine tumours in MEN1 patients are associated with symptoms of hypoglycaemia due to inappropriate insulin secretion {757, 1154,1939}. Between 12 and 17% of VHL patients develop pancreatic endocrine tumours which may show focal insulin immunoreactivity {1357}. However, most of these tumours are clinically non-functioning.

Prognosis and predictive factors

In contrast to the other types of pancreatic endocrine tumours, the vast majority of insulinomas are benign at the time of diagnosis {2094}. This may be due in part to their early detection as they already become symptomatic when still small {1113,2092}. The percentage of malignant insulinoma ranges from 2.4-17.9 % with an average of 8.4 % {682, 714,729,1255,2011,2092,2120,2295}. Malignant insulinomas occur in an older age group and are rare in children {426,2152}. It appears that males are more frequently affected than females {449}.

Insulinomas of less than 2 cm in diameter without signs of angioinvasion, gross invasion or metastases and showing a mitotic rate of <2 mitoses per 10 HPF or <2% Ki-67 (or MIB-1) staining index are considered benign (macroadenomas) {2097}. There are no immunohistochemical markers available which reliably predict the biological behaviour of insulino-

mas {1133,1190,1291}. Risk factors in insulinomas that are not overtly malignant include: diameter larger than 2 cm, high mitotic/MIB1 index and necrosis {899}. Malignant insulinomas contain a higher number of genetic alterations than benign tumours {2106,2107}. Furthermore, it has been shown that losses of chromosomes 3pq and 6q as well as gains of 17pq and 20q are associated with malignant behaviour {2107}. The involved genes, however, remain to be identified.

Glucagonoma

G. Klöppel   K. Öberg
P. Komminoth   X. Matias-Guiu
A. Perren   Ph.U. Heitz

Definition

A glucagonoma is a functionally active and usually malignant endocrine tumour of the pancreas with evidence of A-cell differentiation and clinical symptoms of the glucagonoma syndrome, due to inappropriate secretion of glucagon, and including a skin rash (necrolytic migratory erythema), stomatitis, mild diabetes mellitus and weight loss.

Pancreatic endocrine tumours with A-cell differentiation but without a glucagonoma syndrome should not be considered glucagonomas, but non-functioning pancreatic endocrine tumours.

ICD-O code

Glucagon producing tumour
                    8152/1
Glucagon producing carcinoma
                    8152/3

Epidemiology

Glucagonomas represent about 5% of all clinically relevant pancreatic endocrine tumours and 8-13% of functioning tumours (see Pancreatic endocrine tumours) {2094}. The estimated incidence of the glucagonoma syndrome is 1 per 20 million per year {1771}. Patients most often present between the ages of 40-70 years (range 19-72 years) and women are slightly more often affected {1885}.

Etiology

Glucagonomas are occasionally part of MEN1 {2112,2355}.

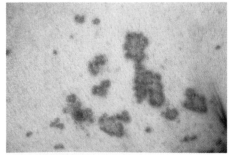

Fig. 4.17 Glucagonoma syndrome: necrolytic migratory erythema. From E. Ruttman et al. {1885} .

Localization

Glucagonomas commonly occur in the tail of the pancreas or attached to the pancreas {1885}. Extrapancreatic glucagonomas are extremely rare {1852}.

Clinical features

Signs and symptoms

The *glucagonoma syndrome* was described in detail in 1974 {1397} but had already been observed in 1960 {752}. The glucagonoma syndrome is thought to reflect the catabolic action of excessively elevated glucagon levels {883,1397,1771}.

The most common presenting feature of the glucagonoma syndrome is *necrolytic migratory erythema* found in about 70% of all patients. The rash usually starts in the groins and the perineum and migrates to the distal extremities. The syndrome also includes mild glucose intolerance, normochromic normocytic anaemia, weight loss, depression, diarrhoea and a tendency to develop deep vein thrombosis. The skin rash may be associated with angular stomatitis, cheilitis, atrophic glossitis, alopecia, onycholysis, vulvovaginitis and urethritis. The cause of the rash is still unknown. A direct effect of glucagon on the skin, prostaglandin release, deficiency of amino acids, free fatty acids or zinc have been proposed as the underlying mechanisms. Marked weight loss occurs in around 65% of all patients and diabetes mellitus is seen in about 50% of all cases. Normochromic and normocytic anaemia occurs in about 1/3 of patients and is probably due to direct bone marrow suppression by glucagon or to the deficiency of amino acids. Diarrhoea occurs in 1/5 of the cases as do psychiatric disturbances. A tendency to venous thrombosis is increased, occurring in around 10-15% of all patients and may be life-threatening {53, 201,1185,2111}.

Imaging

Imaging procedures include helical CT, ultrasonography, MRI and somatostatin receptor scintigraphy and PET-scan.

These tumours are usually large at diagnosis unless they occur in patients with MEN 1. Somatostatin receptor scintigraphy (octreoscan) is the most sensitive localization procedure and also an important method for staging of the disease. Small tumours may be detected by endoscopic ultrasonography.

Diagnostic procedures

The diagnosis of glucagonoma is made on the basis of raised fasting plasma glucagon concentration together with demonstrable tumour and characteristic clinical features. Fasting plasma glucagon concentration is usually elevated 10 to 20 fold; however, in some patients it may be only marginally so. Tolbutamide or arginine stimulation tests may be used to confirm the diagnosis. Approximately 1/5 of glucagonoma patients also have raised fasting plasma gastrin concentration.

Macroscopy

Most glucagonomas are rather large, solitary pancreatic tumours reaching up to 35 cm in greatest diameter. The mean diameter is approximately 7 cm {1885,2094}. The colour of the cut surface is brown-red to pink, and the consistency is usually soft. Because of their large size, degenerative changes, such as haemorrhage, necrosis and cystic change are frequently seen in these tumours.

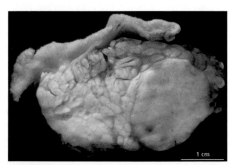

Fig. 4.18 Glucagonoma within the head of the pancreas. The tumour is sharply demarcated.

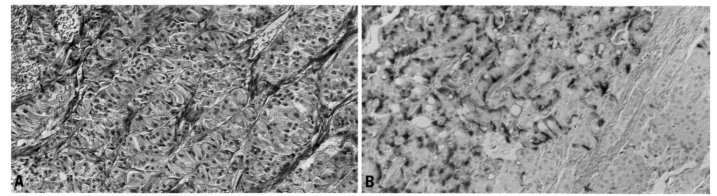

Fig. 4.19 A Glucagonoma with a trabecular architecture. **B** Glucagonoma. Intense glucagon production by tumour cells.

Tumour spread and staging

As in other endocrine tumours of the pancreas, glucagonomas spread by local invasion into surrounding tissues and metastasize to the regional lymph nodes and the liver. So far there is no staging system that specifically applies to glucagonomas (see Pancreatic endocrine tumours).

Histopathology

The histological features of glucagonomas do not differ fundamentally from those of other pancreatic endocrine tumours {230,1885,2094}. They do, however, show a predominance of a mixed trabecular-solid patterns. The tumour cells show faintly granular, often abundant cytoplasm.

Immunohistochemistry

Glucagonomas often stain weakly for glucagon, but also show reactivity for peptides derived from proglucagon (glycentin, glucagon-like peptides 1 and 2) {230,806,1885}. In addition, numerous PP immunoreactive cells can often be identified. Mitoses are noted infrequently.

Electron microscopy

Electron microscopically, glucagonomas show atypical secretory granules {230, 2355}.

Somatic genetics

CGH reveals frequent chromosomal gains and losses involving different chromosomes. Only a small number of tumours (12) have been investigated, however, and the results may not be representative. The chromosomal loci involved are similar to those involved in non-functioning tumours, and gains of chromosome 7 are present in up to 80%

of cases {2105,2107,2154,2490}. Using LOH analysis corresponding allelic imbalances have been described, though with higher frequencies of losses at 1p36, 3p25-26, 6q22, 10q23 and 11q13 {120,750,879}.

Somatic *MEN1* mutations were reported in 2 of 3 investigated tumours. No mutations could be identified in the genes *VHL, PTEN, SDHD* and *DPC4* {382,1721, 1722}.

Genetic susceptibility

Glucagon-immunoreactive tumours may occur in the setting of MEN1 {1114,1250, 1941}. In a series of 100 pancreatic tumours in 28 patients with MEN1, 37 displayed glucagon immunoreactivity, and one patient presented with the glucagonoma syndrome {1250}. In MEN1, these tumours tend to be multiple (59%) and benign (75%) {2089}. A glucagon-immunoreactive tumour was associated with familial adenomatous polyposis {2131}. In contrast, glucagon

production seems to be uncommon in pancreatic tumours occurring in patients with von Hippel-Lindau disease {1357}.

Prognosis and predictive factors

Approximately 60-70% of glucagonomas are already metastatic at the time of diagnosis {883,1771,1885}. Even small glucagonomas are considered tumours of uncertain behaviour or well-differentiated endocrine carcinomas (see Pancreatic endocrine tumours). These tumours tend to grow slowly and patients may survive for many years.

Occasionally, in multihormonal tumours, the glucagonoma syndrome may be associated with, or followed by, another syndrome, such as a hypoglycaemia syndrome or VIPoma syndrome {333, 1640,2447}.

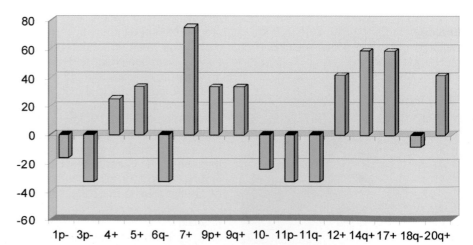

Fig. 4.20 Analysis of genetic alterations of glucagonomas by CGH. Chromosomal gains are frequent on chromosomes 4, 5, 7, 9, 12, 14, 17 and 20 while losses occur at 1p, 3p, 6q, 10, 11p & q.

Somatostatinoma

Y. Dayal
K. Öberg
A. Perren
P. Komminoth

Definition

A somatostatinoma is a functionally active and usually malignant endocrine tumour with evidence of D-cell differentiation and clinical symptoms reflecting the diverse pathophysiologic effects of chronic inappropriate secretion of somatostatin (hypersomatostatinemia; somatostatinoma syndrome). Extrapancreatic endocrine tumours such as those of the duodenum, lung, thyroid and paraganglia composed either exclusively or predominantly of somatostatin immunoreacticve cells, but unassociated with the somatostatinoma syndrome should therefore be more appropriately designated as somatostatin producing endocrine tumours (or D-cell tumours).

ICD-O code

Somatostatinoma producing tumour
        8156/1
Somatostatinoma producing carcinoma
        8156/3

Historical annotation

Somatostatinomas were independently described by Ganda et al. {687} and Larsson et al. {1236}.

Epidemiology

Somatostatinomas account for between 1 to 2% of endocrine tumours of the gastroenteropancreaticohepatic (GEPH) axis. Duodenal somatostatin producing tumours appear to be as common as their pancreatic counterparts. Unlike other gastrointestinal and pancreatic endocrine tumours that may occur at any age, somatostatinomas generally arise in adults 25-85 years of age. The vast majority occur between the fourth and sixth decades and are twice as common in females as in males {464,2323}.

Etiology

While some somatostatinomas are associated with NF1, MEN1 and Von Hippel-Lindau syndromes, the etiology of their sporadic counterparts is unclear, similar to that of endocrine tumours of the GEPH axis.

Localization

Although somatostatinomas may arise anywhere within the pancreas, they are most commonly located in the head.

Clinical features

Signs and symptoms

The subtle and nonspecific somatostatinoma syndrome consists of markedly elevated somatostatin concentrations in plasma and/or tumour, diabetes mellitus of recent onset, hypochlorhydria, gallbladder disease (cholelithiasis, suppression of gallbladder motility), diarrhoea, steatorrhoea, anaemia and weight loss {1164}. Although each of these syndromic components can be due to the inhibitory effects of somatostatin on the secretory activity of various endocrine and exocrine cell types and the suppression of gallbladder motility, the very existence of the somatostatinoma syndrome has been questioned on the ground that these features are non-specific and very common in the older age group in which these tumours most often arise.

Imaging

Ultrasonography is the most sensitive method to demonstrate somatostatinomas of the pancreas and duodenum. Extrapancreatic and metastatic lesions can be detected by ultrasonography, CT scan, and MRI. Somatostatin receptor scintigraphy and PET-scan have proven to be the most sensitive methods to demonstrate extrapancreatic and extraduodenal somatostatinomas.

Diagnostic procedure

The diagnosis is confirmed by documentation of elevated plasma concentrations of somatostatin and the presence of the somatostatinoma syndrome.

Macroscopy

Irrespective of whether they are pure or mixed, somatostatinomas usually occur as solitary, well-circumscribed, but not encapsulated, soft, grey-white to yellow-tan tumours {2091}, that are generally large (average diameter 5-6 cm) by the time they are discovered {1064,2091}.

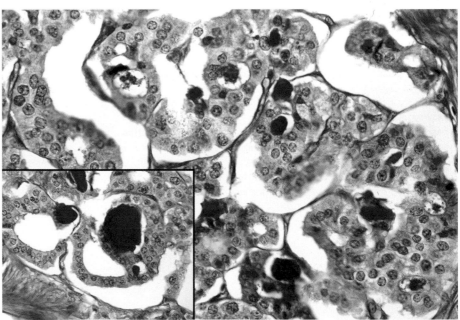

Fig. 4.21 Somatostatinoma. Tumour with a predominant trabecular growth pattern and glands containing several psammoma bodies. High power micrograph of tumour stroma including psammoma bodies.

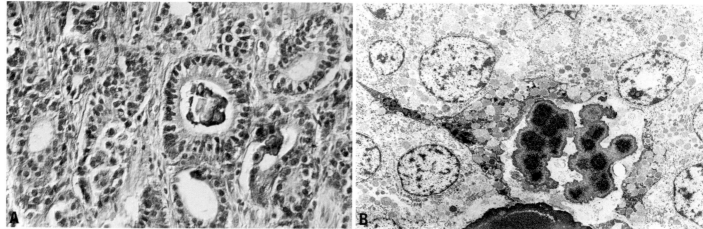

Fig. 4.22 Somatostatinoma. **A** Tumour with glandular architecture and psammoma bodies producing somatostatin as shown by immunophenotyping. **B** Psammoma body at transmission electron microscopy level. The psammoma body shows a coral-like configuration. There is an electron-dense central portion surrounded by a paler peripheral area with needle-like crystal structures arranged radially.

Tumour spread and staging

Because somatostatinomas are generally large by the time they are detected, nearly two-thirds have already metastasized to the regional lymph nodes or the liver {105,2045}.

Histopathology

Somatostatinomas share histologic features with other pancreatic endocrine tumours. In contrast to duodenal somatostatin producing tumours, they often lack the prominent gland formation and psammoma bodies.

Somatostatinomas usually show fairly uniform histochemical reactions. The tumour cells are uniformly non-argentaffin and show argyrophilia only with the Hellerstrom-Hellman technique that is selective for somatostatin-producing cells. Some tumours may show focal Grimelius-positive argyrophilia in a small number of cells.

Immunohistochemistry

Synaptophysin is strongly and diffusely positive in almost all tumour cells, while chromogranins are less consistently expressed. Stains for somatostatin show an intense immunoreactivity in a dominant population of the tumour cells. Cytoplasmic staining for such products as ACTH, calcitonin, insulin, glucagon, *etc.* may be found in a variable, but small proportion of the tumour cells and may correlate with the focal Grimelius-positive argyrophilia seen in those tumours {292, 464,776}.

Electron microscopy

The tumour cells contain large numbers of intracytoplasmic membrane-bound neurosecretory granules in which two distinct populations can be identified. The majority of the secretory granules are large (range of diameter 250-450 nm), round and moderately electron-dense. The second subset consists of smaller granules (range of diameter 150-300 nm), with somewhat denser cores.

Precursor lesions

Somatostatinomas have not been associated with any precursor lesion.

Somatic genetics

Very little information is available on somatic genetic alterations in these rare tumours. One tumour listed as somatostatinoma, analyzed by CGH showed a loss of chromosome X and gains of chromosomes 7, 11, 14 and 18pter-q11.2 {2154} and a second exhibited allelic loss together with a somatic mutation of *MEN1* {750}.

Genetic susceptibility

Pancreatic somatostatinomas have occasionally been reported in patients with MEN1 {1878}, Von Hippel-Lindau syndrome {1389} and in a small subset of NF1 patients {2217}.

Prognosis and predictive factors

As somatostatinomas are usually large tumours, most are considered endocrine tumours of uncertain behaviour or well-differentiated endocrine carcinomas. The largest experience with these uncommon endocrine tumours estimates a 75.2% 5-year survival overall, with a 59.9% in patients with and 100% of the patients without metastases {2091}. However, in retrospect not all of these cases may have been functioning tumours.

Gastrinoma

P. Komminoth   C. Bordi
A. Perren   G. Klöppel
K. Öberg   P.U. Heitz
G. Rindi

Definition

A gastrinoma is a functionally active and usually malignant endocrine tumour with clinical symptoms due to inappropriate secretion of gastrin (Zollinger Ellison syndrome; ZES) {2094}. Tumours with immunohistochemical expression of gastrin but without evidence of ZES should not be designated gastrinomas. Two types of gastrinomas can be distinguished, sporadic, non-familial gastrinoma with ZES (≈80% of cases), and familial gastrinoma with ZES in the setting of MEN 1 (≈20%).

ICD-O code

Gastrin cell tumour   8153/1
Gastrin cell tumour, malignant
                             8153/3

Synonyms and historical annotation

Ulcerogenic tumours. The syndrome was named after R.M. Zollinger and E.H. Ellison who first described the association between "islet cell tumours" and ulcerogenic disease in 1955 {2498}. The peptide hormone gastrin was isolated by R. A. Gregory et al. in 1960 {771} and the pathogenesis of ZES was elucidated in 1964 {556}.

Epidemiology

The majority of patients with ZES suffer from a gastrinoma of the pancreas or duodenum. Gastrinomas are relatively common functionally active endocrine tumour of the pancreas accounting for about 20% of cases, second in frequen-cy only to insulinomas {858}. In some series they are approximately half as common as insulinomas {255,858,1111}, whereas in other series gastrinomas and insulinomas have a similar incidence {577}. In the United States, approximately 0.1% of patients with duodenal ulcers have evidence of ZES {577}.

The reported incidence of gastrinomas is between 0.5-4 per million population per year {255,463,987,2094}. ZES is more common in males than in females with a ratio of 3:2. The mean age at the onset of symptoms is 38 years (range 7-83 years) in some series {556,2398} and 50 years (range 45-51 years) in others {220,281, 1001,1802,2114}.

Etiology

The etiology and pathogenesis of sporadic gastrinomas are unknown. Approximately 20% of gastrinomas are part of MEN 1. No other risk factors are known.

Localization

Substantial variation has occurred in the distribution of pancreatic versus non-pancreatic gastrinomas with the passing of time, possibly related to the refinement of clinical and pathological (immunohistochemical) diagnostic procedures. Indeed, the collection of 800 cases in the Zollinger-Ellison Tumour Registry up to 1973 demonstrated localization of gastrinomas to the pancreas in 53% of patients and to the duodenum and jejunum in 13% {644}. In contrast, the recent experience of a large reference center in the United States revealed an overall incidence of pancreatic localization of 24% with a drop to 14% in sporadic cases whereas a duodenal localization was found in 49% of cases (47% in sporadic ones) {1619}.

Pancreatic gastrinomas more frequently occur in the head of the gland {515,2109}. More than 90% of duodenal gastrinomas are located in the first and second parts of the duodenum and limited to the submucosa in 54% of patients {2227}. The anatomical area comprising the head of the pancreas, the superior and descending portion of the duodenum and the relevant lymph nodes has been called the "gastrinoma triangle" since it harbors the vast majority of these tumours {926,1002,1617,1618,2109}.

Other primary sites of gastrinomas are being identified increasingly {1619}, including stomach, jejunum, biliary tract, liver, kidney, mesentery and heart {62, 374,709,1237,1416,1616,2109,2236}. Some peripancreatic and periduodenal lymph node gastrinomas are thought to represent primary tumours rather than metastases from an occult primary in the duodenum {184,477,2409} and some patients have been cured after resection of the tumourous lymph nodes {51,1617, 1618}. This hypothesis of primary lymph node gastrinomas has been challenged {515,2235}. In two recent studies, however, neuroendocrine and gastrin expressing cells were identified in peripancreatic and duodenal lymph nodes of patients without neuroendocrine tumours, provid-

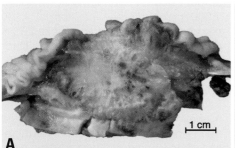 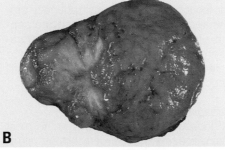

Fig. 4.23 Malignant gastrinoma. **A** Ill-defined gastrinoma in the head of the pancreas invading the papilla Vater and the duodenal wall. **B** Large, malignant gastrinoma with areas of necrosis and fibrosis.

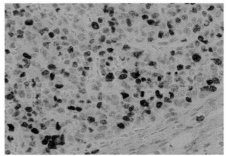

Fig. 4.24 Liver metastasis of a gastrinoma. High proliferative index (Ki-67 labeling).

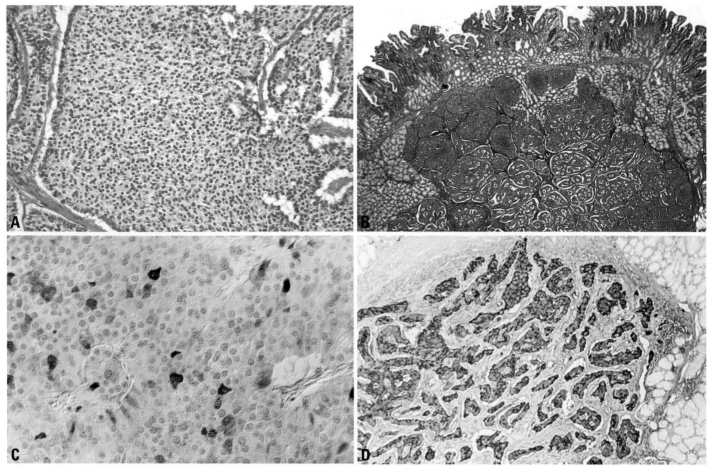

Fig. 4.25 A Gastrinoma. Solid growth pattern. **B** Duodenal gastrinoma. Tumour with a partly solid partly trabecular growth pattern invading duodenal glands and the muscularis mucosae. **C** Gastrinoma. Production of gastrin by numerous tumour cells shown by immunophaenotyping. **D** Massive gastrin production by the majority of tumour cells is shown by immunophenotyping.

ing evidence that these embryonic rests might be precursors of nodal gastrinomas {875,1726}. Still, gastrinomas arising from lymph nodes are extremely uncommon. The diagnosis can be made only after exclusion of a primary gastrinoma at another localization. Rarely, ovarian or pancreatic mucinous cystadenomas or -carcinomas may secrete enough gastrin to cause ZES {211,1406}.

Clinical features

Signs and symptoms

Most patients with gastrinomas suffer from typical duodenal ulcer at presentation, but about 20% have no ulcer. In almost every patient the initial symptoms are caused by gastric acid hypersecretion. Abdominal pain from either peptic ulcer disease or gastroesophageal reflux disease remains the most common symptom occurring in more than 75% of patients. Diarrhoea initially may be the only symptom in 10-15% and occurs with abdominal pain in about 50% of patients.

Diarrhoea is caused by high gastric acid output in the duodenum, thereby neutralizing the pancreatic enzymes necessary for digestion. This will cause malabsorption. In late stages of the disease symptoms may be caused by the tumour itself, e.g. right upper quadrant abdominal pain and weight loss.

In early studies more than 90% of patients with gastrinoma and the Zollinger-Ellison syndrome at presentation had a peptic ulcer and in more than 25% the ulcers were multiple or in unusual locations. Past patients frequently presented with complications or severe peptic ulcer disease (e.g. bleeding, perforation, oesophageal strictures) and although this is less common today it still occurs.

Imaging

Endoscopic ultrasonography is the most sensitive method to demonstrate small gastrinomas of the pancreas and duodenum. Extrapancreatic and metastatic

lesions can be detected by ultrasonography, CT scan, MRI. Most recently, somatostatin receptor scintigraphy and PET-scan have proven to be the most sensitive methods to demonstrate gastrinomas. The sensitivity is about 70% and specificity 85%. It is even higher for metastatic liver disease, with a sensitivity of 92% and a specificity of 90-100%.

Diagnostic procedures

If the gastric pH is below 2.5 and the serum gastrin concentration above 1,000 picogram per ml (normal <100 picogram per ml) the diagnosis of ZES is confirmed and no other diagnostic studies are actually needed. Unfortunately, the majority (40–50%) of patients present serum gastrin concentrations between 100 and 500 picogram per ml. In these patients a secretin test should be performed in addition to a determination of basal acid and pentagastrin stimulated acid output. Most patients with ZES have a basal acid output above 15 mEq per hour if they have not undergone previous acid-reductive surgery. The secretin test is considered positive when an increase in serum gastrin over the pretreatment value is more than 200 picogram per ml.

Macroscopy

Most sporadic gastrinomas are solitary tumours. In the pancreas tumours are usually well-circumscribed, non-encapsulated and their diameter generally exceeds 2 cm. Their texture varies from soft to firm depending on the amount of fibrous stroma. Multiple pancreatic tumours are more common in patients with MEN 1 associated ZES {1748}. However, most of these MEN associated tumours exhibit immunoreactivity for peptides other than gastrin and, thus, are not causative of ZES {229,1748}.

In the duodenum most gastrinomas are less than 1 cm in diameter. Microgastrinomas (<0.5 cm) are easily overlooked. The size of the tumours is not related to the severity of hormonally induced symptoms. Duodenal gastrinomas appear as well circumscribed, soft, grey to yellow, often polypoid tumours with or without ulcerated overlying mucosa. In older series 13% of tumours were multiple {266}. Multiplicity of tumours, however, is indicative for an associated MEN 1 syndrome {1128, 1129}.

Tumour spread and staging

Duodenal gastrinomas can metastasize while still very small, and give rise to paraduodenal lymph node metastases, which may be larger than the primary. It has, therefore, been suggested that the so-called lymph node gastrinomas are metastases of occult duodenal microgastrinomas {515,2235}. The exact percentage of malignant gastrinomas is unclear. In early studies 60-90% of gastrinoma patients had metastatic disease at the time of diagnosis but in recent studies the percentage has dropped to 34% (range 13-52%) probably due to earlier diagnosis {1002}. Metastases to the liver generally occur late and are only seen in a small percentage of patients at the time of surgery, mostly in patients with with pancreatic tumours {477,515, 2110}.

So far there is no staging system that specifically applies to gastrinomas (see Pancreatic endocrine tumours).

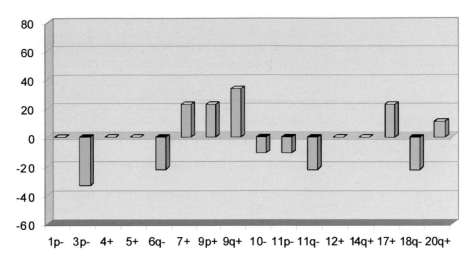

Fig. 4.26 Analysis of chromosomal alterations of gastrinomas, using CGH. Chromosomal gains are prominent on chromosomes 7, 9p, 9q and 17, while chromosomal losses are shown in 3p, 6q and 11q.

Histopathology

The histopathological findings of gastrinomas, either pancreatic or extrapancreatic, almost invariably correspond to those of well differentiated endocrine tumours according to the WHO classification {2097}. As with other pancreatic endocrine tumours malignancy cannot be predicted histologically in most instances, except in the rare tumours in which angioinvasion or infiltration of peripancreatic tissues can be documented {2094}. The growth fraction of gastrinomas was found to be similar to that of other functioning but lower than that of non-functioning pancreatic endocrine tumours whereas a MIB-1 index >10% was invariably associated with development of metastases {391}.

Due to their substantial differences pancreatic and extrapancreatic gastrinomas are described separately as are the histopathological features of extratumoural pancreatic tissue.

Pancreatic gastrinomas

The histological arrangement of pancreatic gastrinomas has no distinctive features with respect to other functioning or non-functioning differentiated endocrine tumours of the pancreas. The early observation of an abundance of glandular like structures {773} was not confirmed by further studies. Actually, pancreatic gastrinomas are predominantly arranged in a mixed trabecular and solid pattern with varying amount of intervening stroma. Tumours with pure, gyriform/ribbon pattern, especially if multi-

ple, are likely to be accompanying neoplasms that are shown by immunohistochemistry to produce nongastrin hormones, mostly glucagon and/or pancreatic polypeptide {229,1748}. Necrosis is uncommon in gastrinomas. Tumour cells tend to show regular round or ovoid nuclei with minimal atypia and well-represented cytoplasm with faint eosiniphilic granularity. Mitoses are infrequent.

Immunohistochemistry. Although gastrinoma may react with Grimelius silver stain or with a number of general neuroendocrine markers, the conclusive evidence for the diagnosis is provided by gastrin immunohistochemistry, which may react diffusely in most tumour cells or in discrete cells or cell clusters. In cases in which the tumours are mostly or entirely unreactive to gastrin antiserum, the use of a panel of antibodies directed against specific sequences of the gastrin molecule may be necessary. Detection of gastrin mRNA by in situ hybridization is recommended in tumours in which constitutive secretion of the hormone results in undetectable or absent gastrin storage in tumour cells.

Electron microscopy. Showing varying proportions of cells either devoid of granules or with nondiagnostic granules {431}, EM has virtually no diagnostic relevance.

Duodenal gastrinomas

These tumours are mostly confined to the mucosa and submucosa and their predominant patterns include broad trabeculae and glandular-like structures.

Immunohistochemistry. Gastrin immuno-staining is usually intense and diffuse whereas electron microscopy shows more abundant and typical G cell granules {2094}.

Non-tumour pancreatic tissue.
Islet cell hyperplasia and nesidioblastosis (i.e., budding off of islet cell clusters from ductal pancreatic epithelium) is frequently encountered in the pancreas of gastrinoma patients {431,2094}. Gastrin has never been convincingly demonstrated in these lesions that may possibly depend on the trophic effect of tumour dependent hypergastrinaemia. A morphometric study of the PP-rich pancreatic region of ventral embryological origin in patients with sporadic gastrinomas showed pronounced PP cell hyperplasia, possibly as a manifestation of a more diffuse disorder of PP cells in this condition {1414}.

Histogenesis
Gastrin gene expression in endocrine pancreas of mammals is restricted to fetal life {240}, and gastrin-containing G-cells are normally not encountered in the postnatal human pancreas. Therefore pancreatic gastrinomas are considered "ectopic" tumours, whereas gastrinomas arising from the duodenum, jejunum or stomach, where G-cells are normally found, are considered "eutopic" tumours. Similar to all pancreatic endocrine tumours the histogenesis of gastrinoma is uncertain.

Somatic genetics
The number of gastrinomas investigated by molecular methods is relatively small and the majority of these studies have focused on the mutational state and allelic loss of the *MEN1* gene on 11q13. Furthermore, many studies did not clearly separate between pancreatic and duodenal tumours and, thus, the results might not be fully representative. Compiled results of CGH studies on 9 pancreatic gastrinomas revealed that chromosomal alterations are less often present than in other types of pancreatic endocrine tumours (including insulinomas), with the exception of losses of 3p and 18q21 which occur more frequently {2105,2107,2154,2490}. The rates of allelic losses at 11q13 and mutations of the *MEN1* gene are the highest of all pancreatic endocrine tumours and have

been found in 90% (28/31) and 37% (19/51) of tumours, respectively {750, 879,2350,2469,2495}. Somatic *MEN1* mutations in primary pancreatic gastrinomas are mostly located in exon 2 and in duodenal tumours they are mainly found in other exons of the gene {734}. Mutations of other genes have not been described.

Genetic susceptibility
Approx. 20-25% of patients suffering from ZES have MEN 1 {1002,2094}. The prevalence of MEN 1 in patients with gastrin producing tumours of the duodenum and upper jejunum has been reported to be 5.3% {2093}. Pancreatic endocrine tumours in the setting of VHL disease consistently lack gastrin immunoreactivity {1357}.

Prognosis and predictive factors
Gastrinomas show a high risk of malignant behaviour independent of size and should therefore be classified as tumours with uncertain behaviour or as well-differentiated endocrine carcinomas when gross invasion and/or metastases are present. Gastrinomas in patients with liver metastases seem to behave more aggressively than those with lymph node metastases only {477,2110} and regional lymph node metastases appear to have little influence on the overall survival of patients suffering from ZES {477,2365}. The risk for liver metastases increases with tumour size and pancreatic location of the primary. It is low in MEN 1 patients. Thus, the frequency of liver metastases is 30% in patients with pancreatic gastrinomas and 3% in patients with duodenal tumours {2094}. The growth rate of hepatic metastases as revealed by modern, sensitive imaging studies, also has important predictive relevance. It has been used to separate aggressive from non-aggressive variants of gastrinomas, the former showing a tumour size increase of at least 50% in volume per month {2163} (25% in MEN 1 cases {710}) and the latter no or lower growth. In spite of the occurrence of liver metastases also in the group of indolent gastrinomas, tumour related deaths were almost entirely confined to the aggressive growth group {710,2163}. Metastases to other organs such as lung, pleura, skin, bone and spleen occur very rarely {463}. It has been reported that duodenal gastrinomas are less malignant

(38%) than pancreatic ones (60-70%) {960,2098}. However, recent studies reported a more than 50% malignancy rate of duodenal gastrinomas {1748, 2227}. It may be that the reported less malignant behaviour of duodenal gastrinomas is only due to the earlier detection. The same holds true for the proposed lower malignancy rate of duodenal gastrinomas in MEN 1 patients.

In general, the progression of gastrinomas is relatively slow with a combined 5-year survival rate of 65% (62-75%) and 10-year survival rate of 51% (47-53%) {1002}. Even with metastatic disease a 10-year survival of 46% (lymph node metastases) and 40% (liver metastases) has been reported. Patients with complete tumour resection have excellent 5 and 10-year survival rates (90-100%). Again, patients with pancreatic tumours have a worse prognosis than those with primary tumours in the duodenum (10-year survival 9% versus 59%) {2365}. The rate of tumour related death in aggressive forms of gastrinomas ranges from 38% in MEN 1 cases {710} to 62% in sporadic cases {2163}.

There are no established markers to predict the biological behaviour of gastrinomas. However, some have found that Her2/neu amplification and overexpression of EGF and hepatocyte growth factor (HGF) are associated with aggressive growth {735,1707}.

VIPoma

J. Lechago
E.J.M. Speel
A. Perren
M. Papotti

Definition

A VIPoma is a functionally active and usually malignant endocrine tumour, arising mostly in the pancreas, which secretes mainly vasoactive intestinal peptide (VIP). VIP-secreting tumours have been associated with the watery diarrhoea syndrome. Additional substances produced by VIPomas, possibly contributing to the clinical syndrome, include peptide histidine methionine (PHM), pancreatic polypeptide (PP), neurotensin, and others.

ICD-O code

VIP-producing tumour
                                    8155/1
VIP-producing carcinoma,
VIPoma, malignant   8155/3

Synonyms

VIPomas have also been referred to as diarrhoeogenic tumours of the pancreas and islet cell tumours of the pancreas with watery diarrhoea {2094}. The syndrome associated with VIPomas, originally known as Verner-Morrison syndrome recognizing its discoverers {2312}, has also been called pancreatic cholera {1437} and WDHA (watery diarrhoea, hypokalemia, achlorhydria) syndrome {1410}.

Epidemiology

Pancreatic VIPomas constitute about 80% of diarrheogenic neoplasms and 3-8% of all endocrine tumours in the pancreas {1111}. Approximately 50% of pancreatic VIPomas are malignant (metastatic) at the time of diagnosis {2090}. Females are affected more often than males and the age of the patients ranges from 19-79 years (mean: 48 years) {294,1539}. By contrast, two thirds of the neurogenic VIPomas are found in paediatric patients {1036,1349}. VIPomas are not familial, except for some tumours associated with MEN 1 {949,1649}.

Etiology

With the exception of those associated with the MEN 1, no etiologic factors are known for VIPomas.

Localization

VIPomas are located in the pancreas in about 80% and outside the pancreas in the remaining 20% {2094}. Pancreatic VIPomas are located more often in the tail (47%) than in the head (23%) or the body (19%) {294,1111,1649}. Extrapancreatic VIP-secreting epithelial tumours are exceedingly rare and include lesions in the small intestine {294}, oesophagus {2360}, and kidney {808}. Neurogenic tumours such as ganglioneuromas, ganglioneuroblastomas, neuroblastomas, and phaeochromocytomas constitute the bulk of the extrapancreatic VIP secreting tumours and are located more commonly in the retroperitoneum (65%) than in the mediastinum (35%) {1126,2094}.

Clinical features

Signs and symptoms

The Verner-Morrison syndrome is characterized by Watery Diarrhoea, Hypokalaemia and Achlorhydria or more often hypochlorhydria (WDHA syndrome) {1538,2313}. The secretory diarrhoea ranges between 0.5-6.0 litres per 24 hours and is usually the most prominent symptom at presentation. It results in severe loss of potassium and bicarbonate, which, in turn, lead to metabolic acidosis and dehydration. Additional features include hypercalcaemia with normal parathormone levels, hyperglycaemia, and occasionally flushing of the face and the chest. Rare instances of tetany have been reported, explained by hypomagnesaemia with normal or elevated calcium levels {949,1163}.

Imaging

As in other endocrine tumours of the pancreas, ultrasound, CT-scan, MRI, octreoscan and PET-scan are the methods currently utilized to localize pancreatic VIPomas and their metastases.

VIP in plasma

Plasma VIP assay should be carried out to confirm the VIPoma diagnosis, a level above 60 pmol/L being virtually diagnostic. Additional corroboration may be afforded by evaluation of plasma PHM levels, as this peptide is more resistant to proteolysis than VIP {202}.

Macroscopy

Pancreatic VIPomas do not present gross features that distinguish them from other endocrine tumours. These neoplasms are generally solitary, except in rare cases associated with MEN 1. They appear as sharply demarcated, but unencapsulated, masses ranging between 2-20 cm in maximum diameter (median diameter: 4.5 cm). The cut surface is variable, generally pink-tan or grey, and may display focal haemorrhage, fibrous septa, cystic change, or even gross calcifications {1552,1649}. Most VIP-producing neurogenic tumours are encapsulated {2094}.

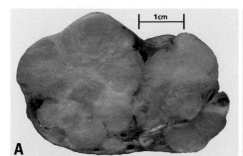
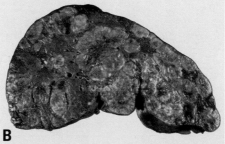

Fig. 4.27 VIPoma. **A** Large multinodular tumour with partly visible capsule and some necrotic and fibrotic areas. **B** Multiple liver metastases.

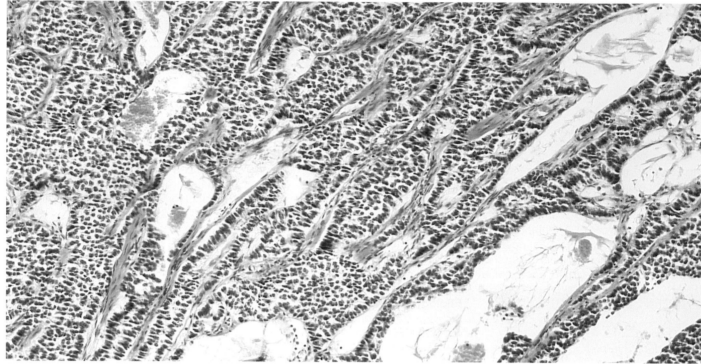

Fig. 4.28 VIPoma. Trabecular and gyriform architecture and partly peripheral palisading of nuclei.

Tumour spread and staging

Metastatic spread of VIPomas is found in about one-half of the pancreatic tumours at the time of diagnosis {1538,2094}. Metastases are more commonly found in the liver (haematogenous spread) than in the regional lymph nodes (lymphatic spread) {294,2090}. Indeed, vascular and perineural permeation is found at the periphery of one-half of the pancreatic VIPomas, generally in association with metastatic spread {2094}. So far there is no staging system that specifically applies to VIPomas (see Pancreatic endocrine tumours).

Histopathology

The microscopic appearance of pancreatic VIPomas does not present distinguishing traits. The tumour cells are rounded or polygonal, with a moderate amount of well-demarcated, faintly granular, eosinophilic cytoplasm. The nuclei may be regular, but often exhibit mild to occasionally moderate pleomorphism: they may be hyperchromatic or display a stippled chromatin pattern, and nucleoli are inconspicuous {294,2094}. Even significant nuclear atypia does not have prognostic significance applicable to a grading system. The mitotic count is usu-

ally low (<2 per 10 HPF), even in malignant tumours, although in about 12% of the tumours it may be relatively high and include the presence of atypical mitoses {2094}. The tumour cells grow in an organoid fashion and may be arranged in solid, trabecular and tubuloacinar patterns. The intervening stroma varies widely, ranging from delicate fibrovascular septa to broad, richly vascularized collagenous bands {294,2094}. Occasional examples of calcium {1552} or amyloid deposits {435} have been reported, the latter being of the islet amyloid polypeptide (IAPP; amylin) variety.

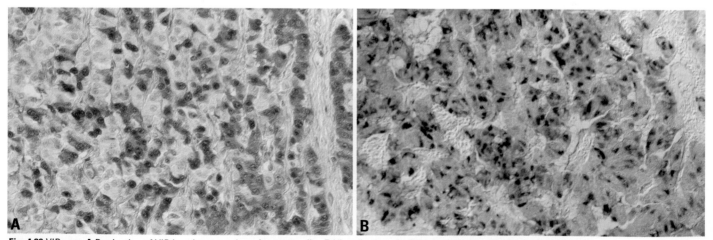

Fig. 4.29 VIPoma. **A** Production of VIP by a large number of tumour cells. **B** Visualization of mRNA for VIP shown by in-situ hybridization.

Immunohistochemistry

Generic endocrine markers, such as synaptophysin, chromogranins and others are positive in more than 90% of the tumours. In multiple studies, VIP has been immunolocalized in 87% of diarrhoeogenic tumours, peptide histidine methionine (PMH), a flanking sequence within the VIP precursor polypeptide, in 57%, PP in 53%, GH-releasing hormone in 50%, and the alpha chain of hCG in 48% {294,1649,2094,2095}. Other pancreatic hormones are expressed in less than 20% of the tumours, and the gastrin-related peptide ghrelin has been found recently in one VIPoma {2328}. All but type 4 somatostatin receptor subtypes have been demonstrated in individual VIPomas {1681,1815}.

Electron microscopy

Whereas the ultrastructure of pancreatic and neurogenic VIPomas has been characterized in numerous publications {1, 294,631,1649}, including the use of immunoelectron microscopy, such techniques are not essential for diagnosis.

Precursor lesions

No precursor lesions are known for VIPomas. Whereas early reports attributed some cases of WDHA syndrome to islet cell hyperplasia {2313}, such association has not been reported in the recent literature {2094

Histogenesis

The histogenesis of the pancreatic VIPomas is obscure since, as pointed out above, no normal or neoplastic islet cells appear to produce VIP. A somewhat perplexing finding is that, in spite of the existence of VIP-containing neurons in the normal pancreas, all neurogenic tumours associated with VIP-hypersecretion so far have been extrapancreatic {1238}.

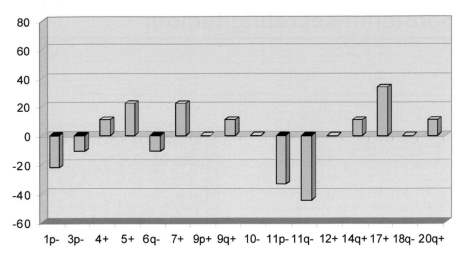

Fig. 4.30 Analysis of chromosomal alterations of VIPomas, using CGH. Chromosomal gains are shown on chromosomes 5, 7 and 17 while losses occur predominantly on 1p, 11p and 11q.

Somatic genetics

The CGH data on nine examined VIPomas exhibited frequent chromosomal gains and losses involving various chromosomes in all but one. The chromosomal loci involved were similar to those of other malignant pancreatic endocrine tumours. However, LOH analysis revealed a higher frequency of corresponding allelic imbalances {2105,2107, 2490}.

MEN1 mutations have been found in 4 of 9 examined sporadic VIPomas {95, 2018}. No mutations could be identified in the genes *VHL*, *PTEN*, *SDHD* and *DPC4* {382,1721,1722}.

Genetic susceptibility

VIPomas are very rarely associated with MEN 1 {949,1649}. No association has been described with VHL or NF1.

Prognosis and predictive factors

As outlined in the Introduction, most VIPomas confined to the pancreas are classified as well-differentiated endocrine tumours with uncertain behaviour. Those exhibiting metastatic activity fall into the well differentiated endocrine carcinoma variety. Poorly differentiated, small cell (high grade) endocrine carcinomas have not been reported in association with the VIPoma syndrome.

After treatment, a meta-analysis study reported a 59.6% 5-year survival for patients with metastases and 94.4% for patients without metastases {2090}.

Little is known with respect to the prognosis of VIPomas in particular. It is understood that, like most endocrine tumours of the pancreas, VIPomas tend to have an indolent biological behaviour, even when metastatic {1858}. The massive diarrhoea with ensuing electrolyte imbalance associated with these tumours may initially pose a higher threat to the patient's life than the growth and spread of the tumour itself. No histopathologic criteria for prognosis have been developed so far.

Serotonin-secreting tumour

R.Y. Osamura
K. Öberg
E.J.M. Speel
M. Volante
A. Perren

Definition
A serotonin-secreting tumour is a usually malignant neoplasm of the pancreas that may become functionally active (syndromic) only after metastasizing to the liver. It produces the clinical symptoms of the carcinoid syndrome.

ICD-O code   8241/3

Synonyms
Carcinoid (obsolete); Carcinoid-islet cell tumour (obsolete)

Epidemiology
The actual incidence of serotonin secreting tumours of the pancreas is not known because evidence of serotonin production iis not routinely sought. Pancreatic tumours causing the carcinoid syndrome are extremely rare {508,1498,1656,1730, 2096,2294,2384}.

Clinical features
When a patient develops liver or retroperitoneal metastases, the carcinoid syndrome may occur with typical flushing, diarrhoea and bronchoconstriction, accompanied by elevated plasma 5-HT levels and urinary 5-HIAA excretion. In the absence of metastases, the tumour remains clinically silent, and the production of serotonin is only demonstrable by immunohistochemistry {614}. The carcinoid syndrome is due to a variety of factors released, including serotonin, kallikreins, substance P, and other tachykinins and prostaglandins.

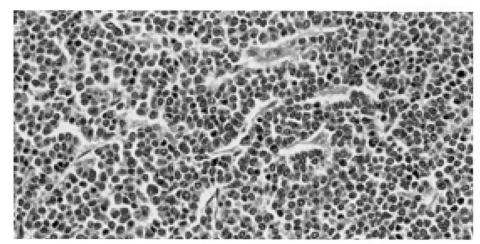

Fig. 4.31 Serotonin-secreting tumour. High-grade small cell carcinoma with solid architecture.

Imaging
Ultrasonography, CT scan, MRI, somatostatin receptor scintigraphy and PET-scan are currently the most sensitive methods for the detection of these tumours and their metastases.

Plasma / urine
The diagnosis is confirmed by documentation of elevated plasma levels of 5-HT and/or high urinary 5-HIAA excretion {615}.

Macroscopy
The tumours are usually large at diagnosis and do not present gross features that distinguish them from other pancreatic endocrine tumours.

Tumour spreading and staging
The tumours are frequently malignant and metastasize to lymph nodes and liver.

Histopathology
Most serotonin secreting tumours share histological features with other well differentiated pancreatic endocrine tumours and do not resemble midgut endocrine tumours (carcinoids). In one report, a poorly differentiated (small cell) endocrine carcinoma secreted serotonin {1701}.

Immunohistochemistry
The tumour cells are immunopositive for serotonin and may express other hormones as well.

Somatic genetics
Somatic genetic alterations in serotonin-producing endocrine tumours of the pancreas have not been reported.

Genetic susceptibility
No association with MEN 1, Von Hippel Lindau or NF1 has been documented {1250,1357,1989}.

Prognosis and predictive factors
All syndromic examples have liver metastases and therefore the ultimate prognosis is poor; however, the disease may progress very slowly.

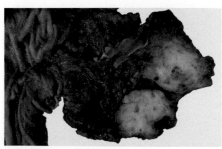

Fig. 4.32 Serotonin secreting tumour in the head of the pancreas.

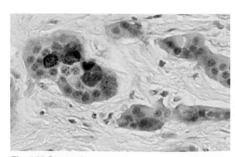

Fig. 4.33 Serotonin secreting tumour. Serotonin production shown by immunohistochemistry.

ACTH and other ectopic hormone producing tumours

R.Y. Osamura
K. Öberg
A. Perren

Definition
Tumours that secrete ectopic hormones (e.g. ACTH, GHRH, PTHrP, calcitonin) are usually malignant neoplasms of the pancreas that produce clinical symptoms related to the specific peptide.

ICD-O code   8150/3

Epidemiology
ACTH-secreting pancreatic endocrine tumours comprise about 10% of ectopic Cushing syndrome cases and occur predominantly in women (64% of cases).

Etiology
The etiology of these tumours is unclear.

Localization
No preferential localization has been reported.

Clinical features
Ectopic secretion of ACTH may lead to Cushing syndrome with some or all of its features. However, the clinical symptoms generally appear within a shorter period of time than those caused by an ACTH-secreting tumour of the pituitary or a cortisol-secreting tumour of the adrenal cortex. In 5% of patients with ZES and 14% of those with Cushing syndrome, the same tumour produces both syndromes {1436,2094}.

The other ectopic hormones which may be secreted by pancreatic endocrine tumours and may produce a syndrome include growth hormone releasing hormone (GHRH) and growth hormone (GH)

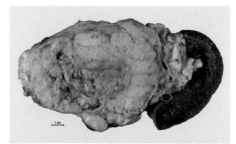

Fig. 4.34 Large, multi-nodular, focally necrotic, ACTH secreting tumour invading the spleen.

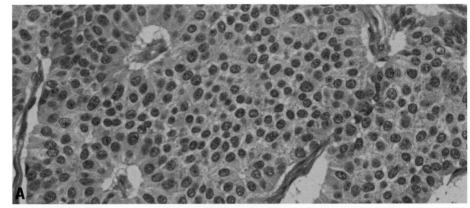

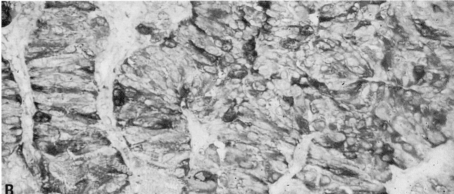

Fig. 4.35 ACTH-secreting tumour. **A** Partly solid, partly glandular architecture. **B** Immunophenotyping shows ACTH production by the tumour.

(acromegaly) {592,1928,1929}, corticotropin releasing hormone (CRH) (Cushing syndrome) {1436}, parathyroid hormone (PTH) and PTH-related peptide (PTHrP) (hypercalcemia) and calcitonin (diarrhoea) {78}.

Imaging
Ultrasonography, CT scan, MRI, somatostatin receptor scintigraphy (octreoscan) and PET-scan are currently the most sensitive methods for the detection of these tumours and their metastases.

Diagnostic procedures
The diagnosis is confirmed by documentation of elevated plasma levels of the appropriate hormone.

Macroscopy
Ectopic hormone producing tumours do not present gross features that distin-

guish them from other pancreatic endocrine tumours. They are generally solitary and large. In rare cases they are associated with MEN 1 {507,1219,1905, 2155}.

Tumour spread and staging
Because ectopic hormone producing tumours are large by the time they are detected, the majority have already metastasized to the regional lymph nodes or the liver {507,1905}.

Histopathology
The microscopic appearance of ectopic hormone producing tumours is not distinctive.

Immunohistochemistry
The hormone causing the syndrome can be detected by immunostaining, but the number of immunoreactive cells may

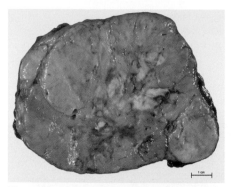

Fig. 4.36 Calcitonin-secreting tumour. Large, sharply defined tumour surrounded by a capsule showing necrotic and small haemorrhagic areas.

vary greatly. In addition to this hormone there may be other peptides identified {87,390,969}.

Somatic genetics
LOH of 3p was found in 3 of 3 PTHrP producing tumours, but in none of the two investigated ACTH-producing tumours {382}.

Genetic susceptibility
No association with MEN 1, VHL or NF1 has been documented.

Prognosis and predictive factors
Ectopic hormone producing tumours tend to be large, malignant and already metastatic to the liver at the time of diagnosis. Their ultimate prognosis is, therefore, poor {390,519}.

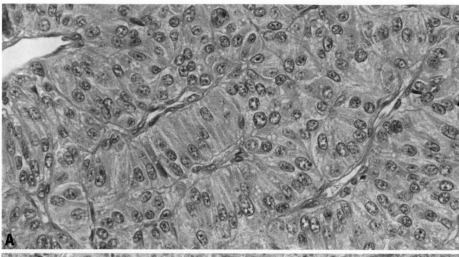
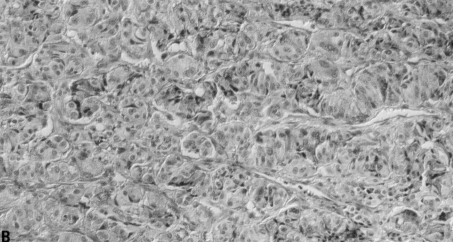

Fig. 4.37 Calcitonin-secreting tumour. **A** Well differentiated tumour displaying a trabecular architecture. **B** Calcitonin immunoreactivity in a large number of tumour cells.

Non-functioning tumours and microadenomas

D.S. Klimstra
A. Perren
K. Öberg
P. Komminoth
C. Bordi

Definition

A non-functioning pancreatic endocrine tumour (NF-PET) is a usually malignant low grade endocrine neoplasm from which the patient suffers no paraneoplastic symptoms referable to the inappropriate secretion of any of the hormones or bioamines produced by functioning pancreatic endocrine tumours. For this reason, the term "nonsyndromic" pancreatic endocrine tumour may more accurately describe this group, but this term is not widely used. Since no specific clinical syndrome has been reported with inappropriate secretion of PP, these tumours are designated "PPoma" based only on their immunohistochemical profile and high levels of circulating PP, and are included with the NF-PETs.

Within the group of NF-PETs, examples measuring less than 0.5 cm are regarded as microadenomas and are clinically benign.

ICD-O code

Non-functioning pancreatic endocrine tumour   8150/1
Non-functioning pancreatic endocrine carcinoma   8150/3
Microadenoma   8150/0

Synonyms

Islet cell tumour, insuloma (obsolete), non-functioning pancreatic endocrine neoplasm.

Epidemiology

The prevalence of NF-PETs differs between incidental microadenomas and clinically relevant NF-PETs. Microadenomas rarely come to clinical attention; their prevalence has been estimated based on autopsy studies to be 0.4–1.5% {779,1086,2094} depending upon the amount of pancreatic tissue examined. Clinically relevant NF-PETs are much less common, with a prevalence of approximately 0.2-2 per million population {2094}. Based on surgical series, NF-PETs constitute 30-40% of all PETs (see Introduction, page 177) {248, 1069,1111,2094}, although their com-

mon incidental detection during diagnostic imaging procedures is expected to increase their frequency in future studies. Clinically significant NF-PETs may occur at any age but are rare in childhood {2048}. The age range is 12-79, with a mean age of 49.7 years {494,543,1 069,1314,2307}. Both sexes are equally affected (male to female ratio is 1:1.15). NF-PETs in patients with MEN 1 occur at a younger age.

Etiology

No etiologic factors are known with the exception of those tumours associated with MEN 1 {580,1114,1741} and VHL {896,938}. There is a suggestion of an association with tuberous sclerosis as well {2311}.

Localization

NF-PETs are more common in the head of the pancreas, with approximately two-thirds of surgically resected tumours

occurring there {494,543,1069,1314, 2307}. Because these tumours are hormonally silent, the lesions most likely to cause local symptoms (i.e., those in the head of the gland) are most commonly detected.

Clinical features

Signs and symptoms

These tumours are hormonally silent and are initially asymptomatic. When they grow large, they present with symptoms due to local disease or distant metastases. Lesions in the pancreatic head may induce back pain or jaundice, but much less commonly than pancreatic adenocarcinoma. Often NF-PETs in the body and tail of the pancreas do not present with symptoms but the mass may be palpated on examination. In addition, patients may complain of nausea, vomiting, diarrhoea and lethargy. Approximately 15-20% of the patients are asymptomatic {1069}.

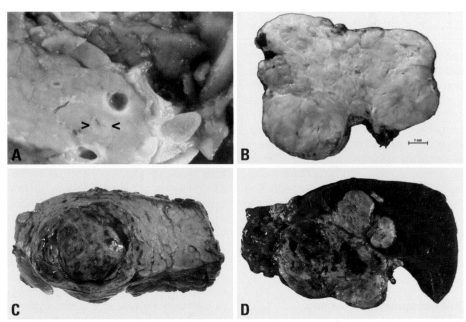

Fig. 4.38 A Circumscribed microadenoma (between arrows) with tan-cut surface (diameter, 0.2 cm). **B** Large, malignant non-functioning tumour with areas of necrosis and fibrosis. **C** Gross appearance of cystic pancreatic endocrine neoplasm (PEN). Note the large central cyst with minimal yellow tumour parenchyma surrounding the cavity. **D** Gross appearance of malignant NF-PET. The tumour is multinodular and invades the spleen.

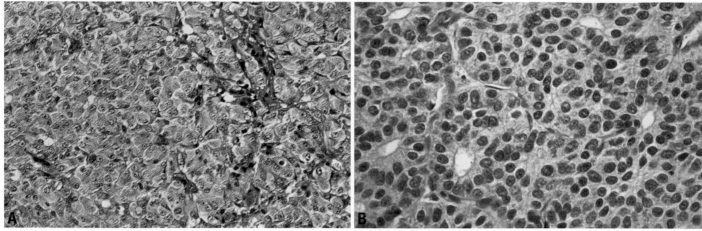

Fig. 4.39 Non-functioning tumour. **A** Liver metastasis displaying solid and trabecular architecture. Pan. **B** Solid and glandular architecture.

Imaging

Ultrasonography, CT scan, MRI, somatostatin receptor scintigraphy (octreoscan) and PET-scan are currently the most sensitive methods for the detection of these tumours and their metastases {1165, 2068}.

Diagnostic procedures

These tumours can be diagnosed by measurement of levels of circulating chromogranins, HCG-alpha-subunit, PP and others. Pancreatic hormone levels may be elevated despite the absence of a functional syndrome.

Macroscopy

Since microadenomas measure by definition less than 0.5 cm, most examples are not grossly detectable. Those that are identified on macroscopic examination of the pancreas appear as circumscribed, but unencapsulated red to tan soft nodules.

Larger NF-PETs may exhibit a wide range of gross appearances. Some tumours are sharply circumscribed and partially or entirely surrounded by a fibrous capsule. The consistency is often soft and fleshy and the tumours vary from red-tan to yellow. Other examples have a more pronounced fibrous consistency, and gross lobulation may occur. Areas of necrosis are uncommon, but degenerative cystic change may be found {1301}.

Tumour spread and staging

NF-PETs grow initially by direct extension into local structures, including peripancreatic soft tissues and spleen for tumours in the tail of the gland and duodenum or common bile duct for tumours in the head. Tumour thrombi within large veins may be found. Metastases occur both to regional lymph nodes as well as to the liver; distant metastases are usually limited to the later stages of the disease {494,543,1069,1314,2307}.

So far there is no staging system that specifically applies to NF-PETs (see Pancreatic endocrine tumours).

Histopathology

NF-PETs have organoid growth patterns typical of differentiated endocrine tumours and are not significantly different from most types of functioning PETs {439}. A nesting growth pattern is most common, but trabecular and gyriform patterns may also occur. Intratumoural heterogeneity is common, particularly in larger examples {1111,1112}. The stromal component varies considerably, from simple fine capillary-sized vessels between tumour cell nests to broad areas of dense, hyalinized collagen. Some tumours exhibit amyloid-like stroma, and stromal calcifications (exceptionally including psammoma bodies) may be found. Most cells contain moderate amounts of amphophilic to slightly basophilic, finely granular cytoplasm. The nuclei are generally centrally located without apparent polarization with respect to the fibrovascular stroma, although eccentric nuclei may be found, imparting a rhabdoid configuration to the cells {1717}. Nuclei are generally round to oval with minimal atypia and coarsely clumped ("salt-and-pepper") chromatin. Some examples demonstrate more nuclear abnormalities, including enlarged nuclei and irregular nuclear membranes {2485}; prominent nucleoli

may also be found. Most NF-PETs have very few mitotic figures. In many examples, they are essentially undetectable, but as many as 10 mitoses per 10 HPF are allowable in a NF-PET (more than 10 mitoses per 10 HPF qualifies the tumour as a well-differentiated endocrine carcinoma). Necrosis is highly variable; many NF-PETs have none, but punctate foci or larger, infarct-like areas may be found.

In some NF-PETs, small ductules may be found between nests of endocrine cells. These ductular cells have more abundant cytoplasm and round nuclei without endocrine cytologic features. Although there may be close juxtaposition of these ductules to the neoplastic endocrine cells, the two cell types remain immunohistochemically distinct, and the ductules are likely entrapped and non-neoplastic. True glandular differentiation may also occur in NF-PETs, with luminal spaces being formed within nests of endocrine cells. In contrast to entrapped ductules, these lumina are lined by cells cytologically indistinguishable from the surrounding tumour cells.

Immunohistochemistry

NF-PETs express general markers of endocrine differentiation including synaptophysin, chromogranins, CD56, and CD57 {858,1336,1551}. Although NF-PETs are not associated with clinical syndromes due to inappropriate hormone secretion, it is common for immunohistochemical staining to demonstrate peptide hormones or serotonin in highly variable proportions of the tumour cells. For example, PPomas have expression of PP in the majority of the tumour cells {1239,2253,2255}. Many tumours with predominant expression of somatostatin (D-cell tumours) fall into the non-functioning category as well. In all NF-PETs, there is often expression of more than one peptide, including insulin, glucagon, somatostatin, pancreatic polypeptide, vasoactive intestinal polypeptide, gastrin, adrenal corticotrophic hormone, or others. {899,1235, 2094}. In only rare cases will the entire tumour fail to stain for any of these peptides, although occasionally only scattered cells are positive. Microadenomas are more likely to show diffuse expression of a single peptide, most often glucagon or PP {2094}.

Microadenomas may be difficult to distinguish from enlarged but non-neoplastic islets. Microadenomas normally exceed 500 μm in maximum diameter; in addition, immunohistochemical staining for islet peptides is helpful, since they lose the normal proportion and distribution of peptide cell types that are retained in enlarged non-neoplastic islets.

Many NF-PETs also express glycoproteins including CEA and CA19.9 {899, 1030}. Tumours demonstrating gland formation are particularly likely to stain for glycoproteins. Focal acinar differentiation may also be detected, generally in single widely scattered cells (less than one third) that stain for trypsin (-ogen) or chymotrypsin (-ogen) {1030,2448}.

Immunohistochemical staining for MIB-1 may be used to demonstrate the proliferative rate of NF-PETs. Most tumours show a low proliferative rate, with a labeling index of 1-5%, but staining of up to 10% of the tumour cell nuclei is acceptable {2094}. A greater percentage of immunoreactivity for MIB-1 suggests a diagnosis of high grade endocrine carcinoma.

Electron microscopy
Electron microscopy is generally not necessary for diagnostic purposes. If ultrastructural examination is performed, the tumour cells contain relatively abundant dense core neurosecretory granules that vary in size and shape from one tumour to another. Most have a nonspecific morphology, with a dense granule core separated by a halo from the limiting membrane. The granules are randomly distributed in the cytoplasm, and usually measure only 100-350 nm, easily separating them from larger, apically polarized zymogen granules of acinar cell carcinomas {578,772}. Characteristic secre-

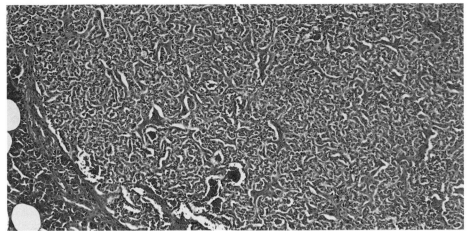

Fig. 4.40 Microadenoma. The tumour lacks a capsule and shows an uniform trabecular architecture.

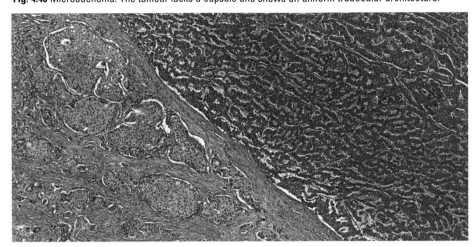

Fig. 4.41 Pancreatic endocrine tumour. Heterogeneity of architecture: nested vs. trabecular pattern.

tory granules of α cells or β cells are usually absent in NF-PETs.

Morphologic variants
A number of morphologic variants of NF-PETs have been described. Oncocytic PETs have cells with abundant granular eosinophilic cytoplasm in the majority of the tumour {320,753,1786}. These cells are filled with mitochondria. In many oncocytic PETs, the nuclei are enlarged

and moderately atypical, frequently with a prominent nucleolus. Some PETs demonstrate marked nuclear pleomorphism, with very large irregular and anaplastic forms {2485}. These tumours have been designated pleomorphic PETs and are frequently confused with higher grade lesions such as anaplastic carcinomas or ductal adenocarcinomas. Although the nuclei are markedly atypical, the cells generally also have abun-

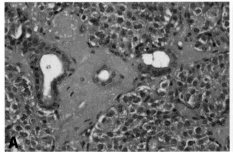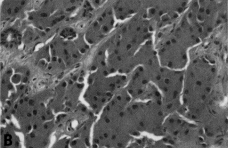

Fig. 4.42 A Non-functioning tumour showing entrapped non-neoplastic ductules. **B** Non-functioning tumour showing oncocytes with abundant granular eosinophilic cytoplasm.

dant cytoplasm, and the mitotic rate is not increased relative to other NF-PETs (distinguishing them from high grade endocrine carcinomas). This type of endocrine pleomorphism has not been shown to have adverse prognostic significance {2485}. Clear cell change may also occur in NF-PETs. In many of the reported examples, the cytoplasm contains innumerable clear vacuoles, sometimes scalloping the nucleus. Clear cell PETs have been reported more frequently in patients with VHL and may be confused with metastatic renal cell carcinoma {896}. None of these variants appear to have any prognostic significance.

Precursor lesions

There is no generally accepted precursor lesion for sporadic NF-PETs. Patients with MEN 1 have been reported to demonstrate islets with altered morphology, possibly representing precursors of NF-PETs.

Somatic genetics

CGH data from 28 tumours indicate that NF-PETs harbour the highest number of different chromosomal gains and losses compared to the other tumour types. These genetic aberrations involve chromosomal loci that are generally enriched in clinically malignant tumours {2490}. Gains of chromosome 4 and losses of 6q appear to be early events as they are already detectable in 40% and 50% of tumours with a diameter of less than 2 cm, respectively {2107}. Results of LOH and CGH studies correspond well and a variety of allelic imbalances have been described {120,121} indicating a high degree of genomic imbalance in these tumours.

Rarely identified somatic mutations in non-functioning PETs include genes such as *MEN1* (2/26) {750,880,1530, 2350}, *PTEN* (1/6) {1723}, *K-RAS* (1/30) {1531} and *TP53* (1/30) {1531}. No mutations could be found in *VHL* {382,1530}, *CDKN2A/p16* {1531}, *SMAD3* {2025} and *DPC4* {1722}.

Genetic susceptibility

NF-PETs occur in MEN 1 patients and multiple microadenomas ("microadenomatosis") are the hallmark of pancreatic involvement in this syndrome {1129}. Approximately 12-17% of VHL patients develop multiple NF-PETs that typically have a clear-cell cytology {811,896}.

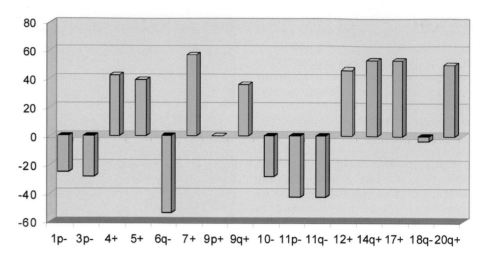

Fig. 4.43 Summary of chromosomal alterations of non-functioning tumours, using CGH. Chromosomal alterations are more numerous than in functioning pancreatic endocrine tumours. Chromosomal gains occur predominantly on chromosomes 4, 5, 7, 9q, 12, 14q, 17 and 20q, while losses are frequent at 1p, 3p, 6q, 10, 11p and 11q.

Prognosis and predictive factors

Pancreatic endocrine microadenomas are benign tumours {2094} and there is no evidence that they progress to clinically relevant malignant PETs.

NF-PETs are relatively aggressive neoplasms. Approximately 65-80% of cases are associated with clear-cut evidence of malignant behaviour (gross invasive growth or metastasis), and tumour recurrence following resection is common {494,543,1069,2094,2307}. With current earlier detection on imaging techniques this figure may decrease. Once distant metastases occur, cure is highly unlikely, although the rate of tumour progression may be slow. Most patients with metastatic NF-PETs survive for several years, and in some instances survival for a decade or more in the presence of hepatic metastases may occur. Following surgical resection, the five year survival for NF-PETs is reportedly 65%, but the ten year survival is only 45% {899}. In addition, a sizeable proportion of patients with NF-PETs present initially with distant metastases, perhaps because there is no paraneoplastic syndrome to draw clinical attention to the tumour early in its course.

In NF-PETs, specific peptide production has no impact on survival {899}. Some studies have demonstrated a correlation between overall nuclear grade and prognosis {899}. Other factors reportedly predictive of more aggressive behaviour include loss of progesterone receptor

expression {1715,2314}, aneuploidy {1068}, increased Ki-67 or PCNA labeling index {391,1715,2330}, increased fractional allelic loss {1830}, upregulated CD44 isoform expression {959}, and immunohistochemical expression of CK19 {491}. Loss of heterozygosity (LOH) at several chromosomal loci has also been reported to correlate adversely with prognosis, including chromosomes 1p {541}, 3p {120,382}, 6q {121}, 17p {788}, 22q {2385}, and X {1749}.

Mixed exocrine-endocrine carcinomas

C. Capella
K. Öberg
M. Papotti
M. Volante
C. Bordi

Definition

Mixed exocrine-endocrine carcinomas of the pancreas are malignant epithelial neoplasms in which the exocrine and endocrine cells are intimately admixed in the primary tumour as well as in its metastases and each component comprises at least one third of the tumour tissue. They include mixed ductal-endocrine carcinoma and mixed acinar-endocrine carcinoma. Exocrine tumours in which the endocrine component is represented by scattered individual cells should not be included in this category. Endocrine tumours with entrapped non-neoplastic ducts or other parenchymal elements of the pancreas are also not considered mixed tumours.

ICD-O code   8154/3

Synonyms

Mixed exocrine-endocrine tumour, duct-islet cell tumour, mixed carcinoid-adenocarcinoma

Epidemiology

Mixed ductal-endocrine and mixed acinar-endocrine carcinomas are exceedingly rare in the pancreas {1110}. Mixed ductal-endocrine carcinomas account for approximately 0.5% of all ductal adenocarcinomas {1638} and mixed acinar-endocrine carcinomas for 15% of all acinar cell carcinomas {1106}. These tumours mostly occur in the in the 7th or 8th decades of life {1638}. Mixed acinar-endocrine carcinomas also rarely occur in childhood. Acinar-endocrine carcinomas have a slight female predominance {1106}, while ductal-endocrine carcinomas occur more frequently in males {1638}.

Localization

The majority of mixed ductal-endocrine carcinomas occur in the head of the pancreas {1110,1638}, while acinar-endocrine carcinomas are evenly distributed in the pancreas {1106}.

Clinical features
Symptoms and signs

Presenting symptoms are, in the majority of patients, non-specific and include obstructive jaundice, abdominal pain and weight loss. Only one patient with a mixed ductal-endocrine carcinoma presented with a hormonal syndrome: ZES due to inappropriate gastrin secretion {2212}.

Imaging

Ultrasonography, CT scan, MRI, somatostatin receptor scintigraphy (octreoscan) and PET-scan are currently the most sensitive methods for the detection of these tumours and their metastases.

Diagnostic procedures

There are no specific laboratory tests to diagnose these tumours.

Macroscopy

Mixed ductal-endocrine carcinomas present as solid masses, showing grey-white or yellow colour, with areas of necrosis and measure 3-10 cm in diameter {1110,2212}. Mixed acinar-endocrine carcinomas are tan to yellow, circumscribed with a soft, fleshy cut surface. Their diameter ranges around 3-11 cm, with a mean of 8 cm {1106}.

Tumour spread and staging

Metastases affect the liver and regional lymph nodes, although distant spread to other organs is reported in some patients {1106,2212}. Mixed ductal endocrine carcinomas are staged using the same criteria as ductal adenocarcinoma.

Histopathology
Mixed ductal-endocrine carcinoma

The exocrine component of these tumours is represented by moderately to poorly differentiated ductal or glandular structures or mucinous (colloid) carcinomatous structures. The ductal carcino-

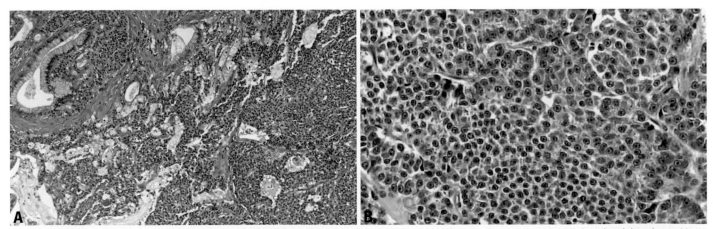

Fig. 4.44 Mixed ductal endocrine carcinoma. **A** Solid architecture with rare glandular formations in the endocrine part of the tumour (right) and ductular architecture (center and upper left corner). Large entrapped pancreatic duct. **B** Mixed acinar-endocrine carcinoma with solid areas composed of small endocrine cells and acinar formation by larger cells of the acinar phaenotype.

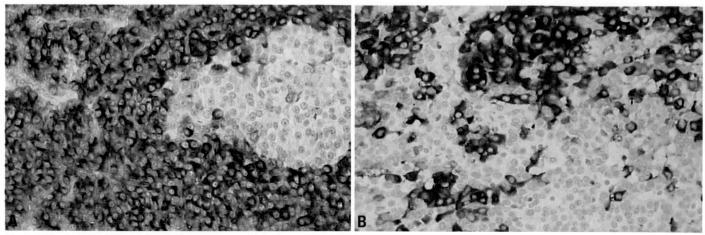

Fig. 4.45 Mixed acinar-endocrine carcinoma. **A** Immunostaining for trypsin labels the acinar component of the tumour. **B** Immunostaining for chromogranin A labels the endocrine component.

matous cells are columnar, with pale cytoplasm, ovoid or round nuclei and distinct nucleoli. In some cases, scattered goblet cells are also present. Histochemically, the ductal cells stain for neutral and acid mucins (positive for periodic acid-Schiff and alcian blue). The endocrine component can be well or poorly differentiated. The well differentiated endocrine component is represented by solid, trabecular or acinar structures formed by small to medium sized cells, with granular eosinophilic or amphophilic cytoplasm and nuclei smaller than those of ductal cells. The endocrine cells are positive for Grimelius' stain, while they are negative for mucin stains. The cell population and growth pattern of the poorly differentiated endocrine component are similar to those of small cell carcinoma of the lung {1638}. Simple lumen formation in a pancreatic endocrine tumour is not sufficient evidence of a neoplastic ductal component.

Immunohistochemistry. Neoplastic duct cells are strongly positive for cytokeratins 7 and 19, carcinoembryonic antigen and CA 19.9 {1110,1280,1638}. The endocrine cells consistently express synaptophysin and often chromogranins. Among hormones somatostatin is the one most often detected {1110,1280, 1638}, whereas gastrin was detected in the single tumour that presented with a functional syndrome {2212}.

Mixed acinar-endocrine carcinoma
In many mixed acinar-endocrine carcinomas both tumour components can be convincingly identified only with immuno-

histochemical staining. In some cases the acinar component can be recognized in H&E stained sections due to the organization of neoplastic cells in small glandular units with basal nuclei and apical cytoplasmic granularity. The endocrine component in contrast, consists most frequently of solid nests or trabecula of cells with randomly oriented nuclei and amphophilic cytoplasm.

Immunohistochemistry. The acinar differentiation is defined by immunoreactivity for pancreatic enzymes including trypsin, chymotrypsin and lipase {1106}. Chromogranins are expressed in most tumours. A minority of cases also show focal staining for hormones such as glucagon, somatostatin, gastrin and pancreatic polypeptide {1106}. A few cells may coexpress both acinar and endocrine markers ("amphicrine cells").
The only study reporting Ki67 labelling index of mixed ductal-endocrine carcinomas indicated different values varying from very low, in a case of moderately differentiated carcinoma, to 67.1%, in a case of mixed carcinoma with a poorly differentiated (small cell) endocrine component {1638}.
Electron microscopy. Ultrastructurally, ductal cells with mucingranules, acinar cells with characteristic zymogen granules ranging from 250-525 nm, or endocrine cells with small dense core granules measuring from 100-300 nm can be identified. Some cases may show amphicrine cells with an admixture of intracytoplasmic mucin or zymogen granules with small endocrine granules {582,1106}.

Precursor lesions
No precursor lesions are known for these tumours.

Somatic genetics
Detailed genetic studies on mixed exocrine-endocrine carcinomas of the pancreas have not been reported. No somatic or germline mutations in the *MEN1* gene were detected in four tumours analysed (Papotti M and Bussolati G, unpublished observations).

Genetic susceptibility
A genetic susceptibility for mixed exocrine-endocrine pancreatic carcinomas has not been reported.

Prognosis and predictive factors
The behaviour of mixed exocrine-endocrine carcinomas is dictated by the exocrine component. Mixed ductal-endocrine carcinomas and mixed acinar-endocrine carcinomas, both have the same poor prognosis as ductal adenocarcinoma and acinar cell carcinoma, respectively {1106,1110}.

Poorly differentiated endocrine carcinoma

C. Bordi
K. Öberg
M. Papotti
M. Volante
C. Capella

Definition

A poorly differentiated endocrine carcinoma (PDEC) of the pancreas is a highly malignant neoplasm composed of small to intermediate-size cells showing endocrine differentiation and a high proliferative rate (>10 mitoses per 10 HPF).

ICD-O code   8041/3

Synonyms

Small cell carcinoma, high grade neuroendocrine carcinoma, neuroendocrine carcinoma, oat cell carcinoma (obsolete).

Epidemiology

PDECs are rare tumours accounting for about 1% of all malignant pancreatic tumours {1536,1629} and no more than 2-3% of pancreatic endocrine neoplasms {2094}. They invariably arise in elderly patients, with a male predominance {1817}. The rate of identification of these neoplasms may, however, be influenced by several factors: (1) the endocrine nature of these tumours may have been unrecognized, with most of them having been misclassified as exocrine tumours in the past; (2) alternatively, some PDECs have been incorrectly diagnosed as pancreatic "carcinoid" tumours; and (3) a metastatic PDEC from an occult primary has been mistaken for a primary pancreatic PDEC {2094}, (4) conversely a primary pancreatic PDEC has been interpreted as a metastasis from an occult pulmonary small cell carcinoma.

Etiology

An association with cigarette smoking has been reported {363} but requires confirmation.

Localization

A predominant location in the pancreatic head has been reported {1817}.

Clinical features

Signs and symptoms

PDECs may present with symptoms similar to those of the exocrine pancreatic tumours {473,1000,1069}. Presentation with widespread metastases may occur. Lesions in the pancreatic head may induce back pain and jaundice due to obstruction of the common bile duct. Rarely these tumours may present with massive haemorrhage as a result of either penetration into the gastrointestinal tract or erosion of vessels in the retroperitoneum. Individual tumours were associated with Cushing syndrome {418}, carcinoid syndrome {747} and another with hypercalcaemia {897}.

Imaging

A majority of these tumours are large and thereby detected by standard procedures such as ultrasonography, CT scan of the abdomen as well as MRI {2005}. Smaller tumours in the head of the pancreas can be detected by endoscopic ultrasonography {53}. Somatostatin receptor scintigraphy (octreoscan) is often negative due to lack of expression of somatostatin receptor types 2 and 5.

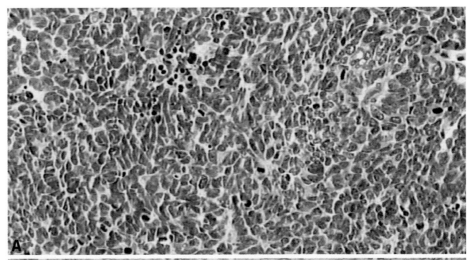

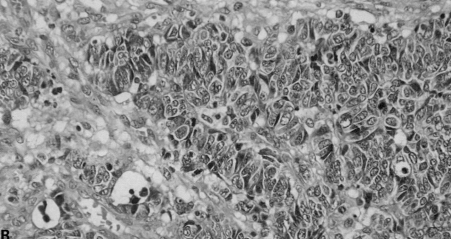

Fig. 4.46 Poorly differentiated endocrine carcinoma. **A** Solid sheets of poorly differentiated endocrine cells with brisk mitotic activity and apoptotic cells. **B** Higher magnification detailing the solid pattern of the poorly differentiated endocrine carcinoma.

Diagnostic procedures

In general serum concentrations of chromogranins A and B are normal but neuron specific enolase (NSE) may be elevated. Other markers such as CA 19-9, CA 50 and 5-HT may also show increased serum levels.

Macroscopy

The tumours have an average diameter of approximately 4 cm {1817}. They appear as firm, white-grey masses with ill-defined borders, often showing areas of necrosis and haemorrhage.

Tumour spread and staging

Invasion of the adjacent duodenum or of other peripancreatic tissues is frequent. Extensive, widespread metastases are the rule, involving regional and distant lymph nodes, as well as intra- and extra-abdominal organs such as liver and lung {1817.2094}.

Histopathology

The tumours commonly consist of tightly packed nests and diffuse irregularly shaped sheets of cells, often, with extensive central necrosis. Tumour cells are of small to intermediate size with hyperchromatic, round to oval nuclei and scanty, poorly defined cytoplasm and closely resemble those of the small cell carcinoma of the lung. {1817.2094}. Mitoses are abundant (>10 per 10 HPF). Some examples also have a more organoid architecture and moderately abundant cytoplasm.

Immunohistochemistry

PDECs stain diffusely for cytosolic/ microvesicular markers such as synaptophysin or PGP9.5 but are negative or only focally and weakly positive for granular markers such as chromogranins {812}. As a rule no reactivity for peptide hormones is found. Abnormal nuclear accumulation of TP53, a feature virtually absent in low-grade endocrine carcinomas, is commonly though not invariably found. The Ki67-MIB1 labelling index is consistently above 10% and often exceeds 50%. Tumours with more abundant cytoplasm have more intense immunoreactivity for neuroendocrine granule markers and for peptide hormones {2094}.

Electron microscopy

The diagnostic finding is the presence of sparse small (100-200 nm in diameter), round, membrane-bound, dense-cored secretory granules in the tumour cells. In addition there are free ribosomes, poorly developed rough endoplasmic reticulum and intermediate filaments {812.2094}.

Differential diagnosis

As is usually the case for small cell carcinomas of whatever origin, cytokeratin immunostaining and lack of reactivity for common leucocyte antigen may be crucial in the differential diagnosis with non-Hodgkin lymphoma. PNET can be distinguished by diffuse immunoreactivity for CD99 (O13), although both tumours may strongly express cytokeratins {1371, 1549}.

Prominent cytologic atypia, extensive necrosis, a Ki67 index above 10% and diffuse nuclear expression of TP53 are useful in differentiating PDECs with intermediate sized cells from well differentiated endocrine carcinomas.

Finally, the distinction of a metastasis from an extra-pancreatic PDEC may be difficult by histological and/or immunohistochemical criteria. This situation demands accurate clinical evaluation of the patients.

Somatic genetics

Specific molecular alterations are so far unrecognised in PDECs. The most important differential molecular feature, as compared to well-differentiated endocrine tumours and carcinomas, is the presence of alterations of TP53 gene {1838}, leading to nuclear protein accumulation, as in most small cell carcinomas of other sites.

Genetic susceptibility

As opposed to well-differentiated endocrine tumours and carcinomas, PDECs have been very infrequently associated with MEN 1 {1628}. No data are available on their occurrence in the setting of VHL.

Prognosis and predictive factors

The highly aggressive behaviour of PDECs and the usually advanced and unresectable stage at the time of diagnosis make the mortality of these tumours virtually 100%. The survival time ranges from 1 month to one year, despite initial favourable response to chemotherapy {1533,1629}.

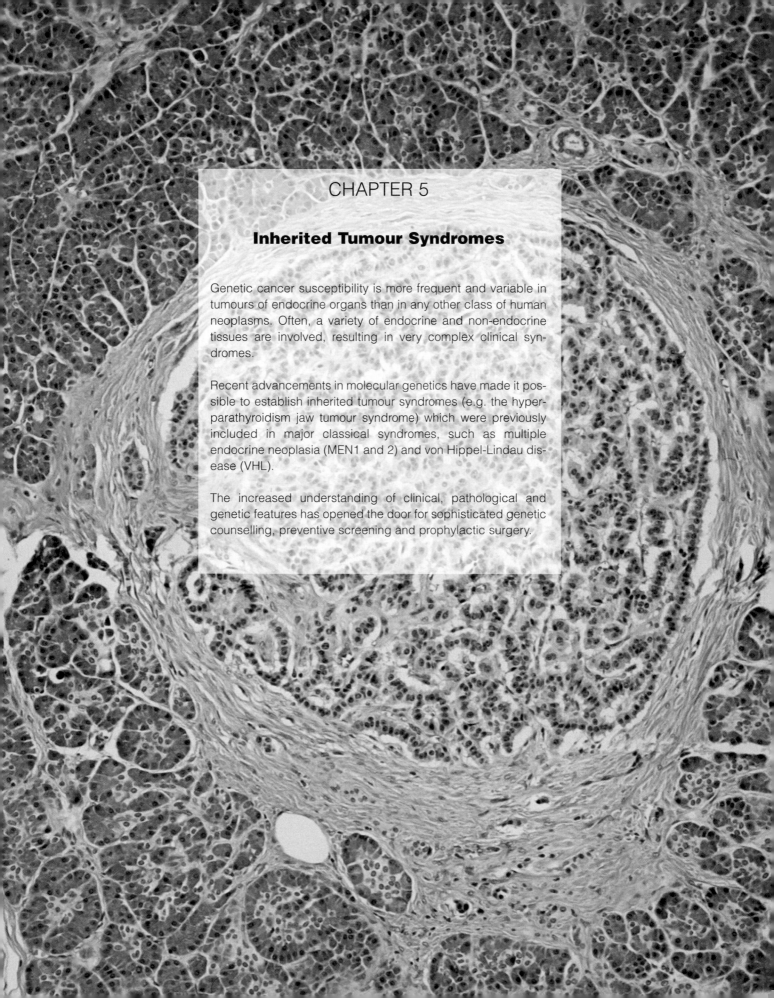

CHAPTER 5

Inherited Tumour Syndromes

Genetic cancer susceptibility is more frequent and variable in tumours of endocrine organs than in any other class of human neoplasms. Often, a variety of endocrine and non-endocrine tissues are involved, resulting in very complex clinical syndromes.

Recent advancements in molecular genetics have made it possible to establish inherited tumour syndromes (e.g. the hyperparathyroidism jaw tumour syndrome) which were previously included in major classical syndromes, such as multiple endocrine neoplasia (MEN1 and 2) and von Hippel-Lindau disease (VHL).

The increased understanding of clinical, pathological and genetic features has opened the door for sophisticated genetic counselling, preventive screening and prophylactic surgery.

Introduction

C. Eng

This chapter discusses the clinical, genetic and pathologic details of endocrine tumours which are components of inherited neoplasia syndromes. In addition to the classical syndromes, such as the two multiple endocrine neoplasia syndromes (MEN) and von Hippel-Lindau disease (VHL), this chapter also contains such entities, which in the past, had been part of sections dedicated to the more "traditional" syndromes. For example, there is a separate section on hyperparathyroidism jaw tumour syndrome which would previously have been discussed with MEN 1. However, with the recent isolation and partial characterisation of the susceptiblity gene, *HRPT2*, this syndrome has come into its own. Similarly, non-MEN 2, non-VHL heritable phaeochromocytoma and paraganglioma would have been briefly discussed in the sections on MEN 2 and VHL. Given the discovery and characterisation of the autosomal genes encoding three of the four subunits of mitochondrial succinate dehydrogenase as susceptibility genes for phaeochromocytomas and paragangliomas, this syndrome was felt to deserve a distinct section as well. Because this is a chapter in a book dedicated to endocrine tumours, a conscious decision was made not to assign Cowden syndrome its own section, but instead to discuss it with all familial non-medullary thyroid carcinoma predisposition. Finally, there are two particularly notable features in this chapter. Each section discussing a particular type or group of inherited syndrome(s) ends with a subsection on genetic counselling and preventative measures written by a cancer genetic counselor or a practising physician-clinical cancer geneticist. There is also a reference table (below), which gives genetic differential diagnoses based on organ-specific endocrine neoplasias.

Table 5.01
Genetic differential diagnoses by endocrine organ system.

Organ	Histologic Type	Syndromes	Gene
Adrenal	Adrenocortical neoplasia	Li-Fraumeni syndrome	*TP53*
		Carney Complex	*PRKAR1A*
		Beckwith-Wiedemann syndrome	*CDKN1C / NSD1*
		MEN1	*MEN1*
	Phaeochromocytoma	Von Hippel-Lindau disease	*VHL*
		Pheochromocytoma-paraganglioma syndrome	*SDHD, SDHC, SDHB*
		MEN2	*RET*
		Neurofibromatosis type 1	*NF1*
Pancreas	Islet cell neoplasias	MEN1	*MEN1*
		Von Hippel-Lindau disease	*VHL*
Paraganglia	Paraganglioma	Phaeochromocytoma-paraganglioma syndrome	*SDHD, SDHC, SDHB*
		Von Hippel-Lindau syndrome	*VHL*
		MEN2	*RET*
		Neurofibromatosis type 1	*NF1*
Parathyroid	Adenoma / Hyperplasia	MEN1	*MEN1*
		MEN2	*RET*
	Carcinoma	Hyperparathyroidism-jaw tumour syndrome	*HRPT2*
Pituitary	Adenoma	MEN1	*MEN1*
		Carney complex	*PRKAR1A*
Thyroid	Papillary carcinoma ^	Familial adenomatous polyposis syndrome	*APC*
		Cowden syndrome*	*PTEN*
		Carney complex ?	*PRKAR1A*
		Familial site specific non-medullary thyroid cancer syndromes	None yet
	Follicular carcinoma	Cowden syndrome*	*PTEN*
		Werner syndrome	*WRN*
	Medullary carcinoma	MEN2	*RET*

MEN1/2, multiple endocrine neoplasia syndromes.
* The great majority of epithelial thyroid carcinomas seen in Cowden syndrome are folllicular thyroid carcinomas. Occasionally, papillary thyroid carcinomas (PTC) are seen in this syndrome. There is anecdotal evidence that what is commonly referred to as 'PTC' in familial adenomatous polyposis syndrome (FAP) is not identical to classic PTC. However, reclassification awaits systematic studies. For patient care, and hence purposes of differential diagnosis, FAP is still listed under the differential diagnosis of PTC.

Multiple endocrine neoplasia type 2

O. Gimm
C.D. Morrison
S. Suster

P. Komminoth
L. Mulligan
K.M. Sweet

Definition

The multiple endocrine neoplasia type 2 (MEN 2) syndrome is an inherited tumour syndrome with an autosomal dominant pattern of inheritance, caused by germline mutations of the *RET* gene. It is characterised by the coexistence of various endocrine tumours involving the thyroid, the adrenal, and the parathyroids {2121}. In addition, abnormalities affecting various non-endocrine organs/tissues (e.g. intestine, mucosa, cornea, skeleton) may be present. MEN 2 has been clinically subdivided into 3 groups: familial medullary thyroid carcinoma (FMTC), MEN 2A and MEN 2B.

MIM Number

The Mendelian Inheritance in Man (MIM) number for FMTC is 155240, the MIM number for MEN 2A is 171400, and the MIM number for MEN 2B is 162300.

Synonyms

MEN 2 has also been named multiple endocrine adenomatosis (MEA) type 2 or previously abbreviated MEN II, which should no longer be used. MEN 2A is also known as Sipple syndrome {2064}. MEN 2B was also termed MEN 3 {1092}; even less common is the term Wagenmann-Froboese syndrome {665, 2338}.

Incidence / Prevalence

The incidence of MEN 2 is unknown. The hereditary form of medullary thyroid carcinoma (MTC) has been assumed to account for about 25% of all MTCs. MTC is believed to account for 5-10% of all thyroid malignancies. The incidence of thyroid cancer has been assumed to be 1-3/100,000 per year. Hence, MEN 2 may have an incidence of approximately 1.25–7.5/10,000,000 per year. Its prevalence is believed to be about 1/35,000. The female to male ratio in MEN 2 is roughly 1:1, in some studies a slight predominance of the female gender has been reported.

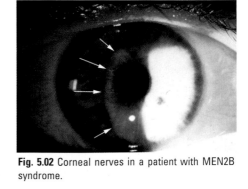

Fig. 5.02 Corneal nerves in a patient with MEN2B syndrome.

Diagnostic criteria

Besides MTC, patients with MEN 2A may develop phaeochromocytoma and/or primary hyperparathyroidism. Patients with MEN 2B may develop phaeochromocytoma, neuromas of the tongue and/or ganglioneuromatosis of the intestine, a marfanoid habitus and/or medullated corneal nerve fibres. None of these latter phenotypes need be present in MEN 2B nor are they pathognomonic {742,746, 1778}, i.e. they have been also been reported in patients without MTC or MEN 2B-specific *RET* mutations although it is difficult to determine if such clinical features are "over-called" once a clinical suspicion of MEN 2 is raised. Clinically evident primary hyperparathyroidism is not part of MEN 2B. By definition, patients with FMTC develop MTC only.

Since the identification of RET as the MEN 2 susceptibility gene in 1993, the definitive diagnosis of MEN 2 relies almost exclusively on germline RET mutation analysis. Of note, RET mutation analysis has to be performed in any patient with MTC and is also recommended in patients with phaeochromocytoma {1585}, irrespective of age of the patient, the absence of accompanying disease features or family history in order to identify index patients (probands) and to enable at-risk relatives timely diagnosis and therapy.

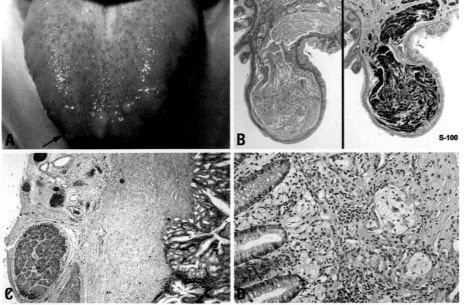

Fig. 5.01 Multiple endocrine neoplasia type 2b. **A** Ganglioneuromatosis of the tongue in a MEN2B patient (arrows). **B** Histology of ganglioneuroma of the tongue. **C** S100 Immunostaining of ganglioneuromatosis of the gallbladder. **D** Microscopic aspect of a ganglioneuromatosis in the appendix of a MEN2B patient.

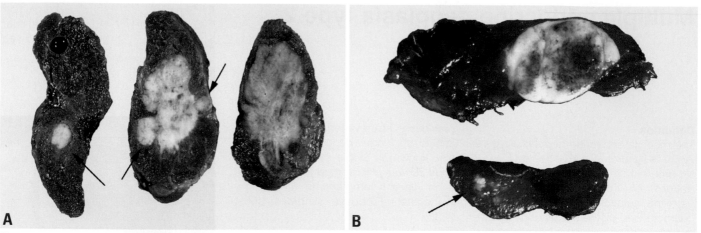

Fig. 5.03 Multiple endocrine neoplasia type 2 (MEN 2). **A** Macroscopic aspect of a multifocal (arrows) familial medullary thyroid carcinoma. **B** Bilateral medullary thyroid carcinoma.

Medullary thyroid carcinoma

Age distribution / penetrance

About 70% of patients with MEN 2A develop clinically apparent MTC by the age of 70 years {1762}. By the age of 35 years, the biochemical penetrance reaches 100%. Of note, MTC has been found in young children age 10 years and below {526,1309,2373}, in MEN 2B even at the age of 6 months {2210}. Patients with FMTC diagnosed with thyroid tumours are on average older than patients with MEN 2A.

Clinical features

Thyroid nodules may be the first clinical sign of MTC. Routine preoperative calcitonin measurement in any patients having a thyroid nodule may identify MTC preoperatively {1670,1828,2318}. Medullary carcinoma of the thyroid metastasizes early to lymph nodes and distant organs (mainly liver, lung and bone). At primary operation, generally more than 50% of index patients already have lymph node metastases. Hence, metastases may be the initial symptom of patients with MTC. In the case of high serum calcitonin levels, symptoms may arise from diarrhoea not responding well to common anti-diarrhoeic drugs. It is relatively rare to present with phaeochromocytoma or hyperparathyroidism.

Pathology

The histopathologic features of MTC in MEN 2 are virtually indistinguishable from those observed in the sporadic cases. Certain features, however, differ in the two ways. As noted earlier, MTC in

MEN 2 tends to occur at a younger age and is typically bilateral and multicentric {190,200}. The tumours are typically well circumscribed but unencapsulated, with a tan-pink, soft to rubbery cut surface. The smaller lesions tend to arise at the junction of the upper and middle third of the thyroid lobes, corresponding to the areas containing the highest concentration of C cells. Larger lesions can occupy the entire lobe and infiltrate the perithyroidal tissue.

Another feature that distinguishes the sporadic form of MTC from that in MEN 2 is the frequent presence of *C-cell hyperplasia* in the latter {200,1728,2407}. In MEN 2 patients, foci of C-cell hyperplasia are typically present in the vicinity of the tumours as well as in areas away from the main tumour mass. The finding of C-cell hyperplasia may thus serve as a morphologic marker for MEN 2-associated MTC. The definition of C-cell hyperplasia remains controversial. Morphologically, the process can be nodular or diffuse {480,2406}. In diffuse hyperplasia, C-cells are increased and diffusely scattered throughout the thyroid parenchyma. In nodular hyperplasia, C-cells occur in clusters that may obliterate the follicular spaces. Most authors require the presence of clusters of more than 6 cells in several foci from both lobes to make the diagnosis of nodular C-cell hyperplasia {1470,2408}. In the diffuse form, an increase of over 50 C-cells per low-power field in both thyroid lobes is the most commonly accepted criterion {1862}. Use of special stains, including calcitonin and chromogranin immunostains, may be of aid for high-

lighting these cells in cases of C-cell hyperplasia. However, at present, genetic testing is the most accurate method for identifying familial and MEN 2-associated C-cell lesions, and is more reliable than morphologic identification of C-cell hyperplasia {1309,1734,2373}. C-cell hyperplasia has also been described in association with non-medullary thyroid carcinoma, follicular adenoma, lymphocytic thyroiditis and solid cell nests {30,345,797}. Such cases have been regarded as a reactive physiologic process unassociated with malignant potential {1728}.

The histologic appearance of MTC in MEN 2 mirrors that of the sporadic cases. A wide range of cytologic features and histologic growth patterns characterize the tumours. As with the sporadic cases, a solid or compartmentalized ("organoid") growth pattern predominates. The tumour cells may be round, oval, polygonal or spindled, and generally contain abundant granular eosinophilic cytoplasm. The nuclei are uniform, round to oval, with occasional pleomorphism and multinucleation. Mitotic figures are usually scarce, particularly in the smaller tumours. Stromal deposits of amyloid and calcium deposits resembling psammoma bodies are also frequent findings. Unusual morphologic variants that can mimic other tumours have also been described.

The histologic diagnosis of MTC can be confirmed with the use of immunohistochemical stains. Calcitonin and calcitonin gene-related peptide (CGRP) represent the most sensitive markers for these tumours, although they are not

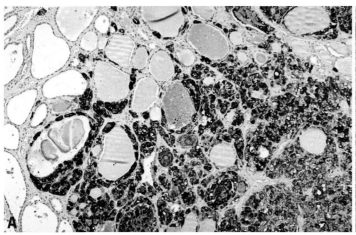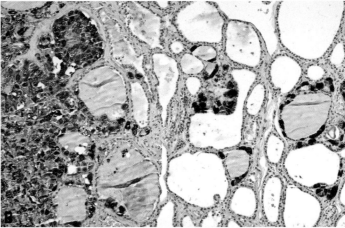

Fig. 5.04 Multiple endocrine neoplasia type 2 (MEN 2). **A** Medullary thyroid carcinoma in a MEN2 patient. Calcitonin immunohistochemistry. **B** C-cell hyperplasia adjacent to a medullary thyroid carcinoma of a patient with MEN2 (calcitonin immunostaining).

entirely specific and can be expressed in other conditions {481,2051,2477}. Calcitonin positivity can be focal and restricted to only a few tumour cells. Also, a small subset of MTC (approximately 1.5%) may be negative for calcitonin {909}.

Two additional markers of value for the diagnosis of MTC are chromogranin and CEA; strong expression of the latter has been identified in some studies as associated with a worse prognosis {1981}. A variety of other markers, including low-molecular weight cytokeratin, vimentin, neuron-specific enolase, synaptophysin, somatostatin, and numerous other peptides have been identified in these tumours but are not specific for MTC and are therefore of limited diagnostic value {1862}.

Prognosis and prognostic factors

Patients with hereditary MTC overall appear to have a better prognosis than patients with sporadic MTC. However, this may be due to the younger age at diagnosis because of surveillance, i.e. lead time bias. Patients with MEN 2B are believed to develop the most aggressive form of MTC; however, a recent study did not confirm this assumption {1259}. The 5-year survival rate in MTC is about 80-90%, the 10-year survival rate is about 60-70% {177,877}. Prognostic factors may be tumour stage {177,525}, and postoperative calcitonin level {525,724}. The studies that tie the presence of somatic M918T mutation and prognosis {817,1347} are deeply flawed as somatic mutation analyses were performed on either primary MTC or metastases.

Phaeochromocytoma

Clinical features

The most common symptoms are hypertension, headache, tachycardia, and sweating. Patients with phaeochromocytoma may present with orthostatic dysregulation. In patients with MEN 2, phaeochromocytoma rarely (10%) precedes the development of MTC {324} and, hence, is either diagnosed synchronously or metachronously during follow-up. Due to the genetic origin of the disease, both adrenal glands may be affected.

Biochemically, phaeochromocytoma can be diagnosed by measuring elevated levels of free catecholamines (epinephrine, norepinephrine) in 24-hour urine. Alternatively, their metabolites (e.g. vanillylmandelic acid) may be measured. Even more sensitive (>95%) seems to be the determination of plasma metanephrines or chromogranin A {550}. Once diagnosed biochemically, the localization and the extent of the phaeochromocytoma needs to be determined. Enlarged adrenal glands are almost always present if the patient is symptomatic. In these cases, computed tomography and/or magnetic resonance imaging may be helpful in determining both localization and extent of the phaeochromocytoma. While both imaging techniques have a high sensitivity (reaching up to 100%), their specificity is rather low (70%). Also, they may fail to identify extra-adrenal phaeochromocytoma. However, extraadrenal phaeochromocytomas are a relatively unusual event in MEN 2. In these instances, ^{131}I-meta-iodobenzylguanidine (MIBG) may be very helpful. While its sensitivity is only about 80%, its specificity reaches nearly 100%.

Pathology

The majority of patients with MEN 2A and MEN 2B exhibit bilateral diffuse or nodular adrenal medullary hyperplasia as a precursor of phaeochromocytoma. Adrenomedullary involvement is not a feature of true FMTC. Diffuse medullary hyperplasia is defined as the expansion of the medulla into the alae or tail of the gland with or without nodule formation, enlargement of the adrenal medulla beyond the normal ratio of cortical area to medullary area of 4:1 and a two- to three-fold increase in medullary volume and weight as compared to age- and sex-matched controls {483,1881}. Nodules larger than 1 cm in diameter are considered phaeochromocytomas, while smaller nodules are defined as nodular medullary hyperplasia {316}. However, these criteria are arbitrary and remain to be confirmed by molecular analyses. Macroscopically, nodules of adrenomedullary hyperplasia are typically grey to tan and soft in texture. On microscopic examination there is often a mixed pattern of diffuse and nodular hyperplasia expanding into the tail of the gland and there may be intermingling of medullary and adrenocortical cells. Nodules vary in size, usually lack true encapsulation, may show a "nodule in nodule" appearance and outlines of neighbouring nodules may be partially molded {1192}. Cellular, architectural and immunohistochemical features of hyperplastic lesions are similar to those

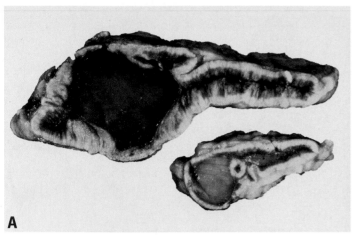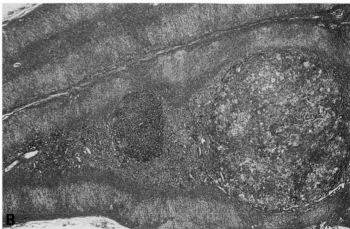

Fig. 5.05 Multiple endocrine neoplasia type 2 (MEN 2). **A** Macroscopic view of multifocal phaeochromocytoma and adjacent nodular adrenomedullary hyperplasia in a patient with MEN2. **B** Close up of nodular adrenomedullary hyperplasia (nodules < 1 cm) adjacent to phaeochromocytoma in a patient with MEN2.

seen in phaeochromocytomas. Phaeochromocytomas in MEN 2 patients are mostly multicentric and bilateral, vary in size and are confined to the adrenal medulla {2363}. However, some extraadrenal tumours and a phaeochromocytoma arising from an accessory adrenal gland have also been described {1048,1610}. Smaller tumours are often accompanied by diffuse and nodular adrenomedullary hyperplasia but larger tumours, as sporadic phaeochromocytomas, show expansive growth with compression of the adrenal cortex and overgrowth of the hyperplastic medulla. Histologically, MEN 2-associated phaeochromocytomas are similar to sporadically occurring counterpart tumours. However, some studies reported a higher frequency of insular pattern, large or pleomorphic cells with vacuolated or granular cytoplasm, prominent nucleoli and hyaline globules in MEN 2A tumours than in sporadic phaeochromocytomas {751,1121}. Occasionally, lipid degeneration may histologically mimic an adrenal cortical tumour {2282}. Melanin pigmentation, the presence of phaeochromoblasts as well as calcospherites have also been described {1221}.

Immunohistochemically, MEN 2-associated phaeochromocytomas exhibit a similar expression pattern of neuroendocrine and other markers as sporadic tumours {1132}. However, some have reported differences including higher levels of corticotrophin hormone, lower levels of VIP and more S100 protein-positive cells in familial tumours when compared to sporadic phaeochromocytomas {1329,1534}. RET immunostaining is not

helpful to distinguish MEN 2-associated from sporadic phaeochromocytomas since the latter may also harbour gain-of-function *RET* mutations with consequent RET overexpression {1430}. In contrast to MEN 2-associated tumours, which harbour germline RET alterations, the *RET* mutations in sporadic tumours are somatic in nature {1131}.

Most series report a very low malignancy rate for phaeochromocytomas in MEN 2 patients when compared to sporadic tumours, but metastasizing tumours do occur {370,697,888}. In two series of 100 and 300 MEN 2 patients with phaeochromocytomas, a frequency of 3% and 4%, respectively, of malignant tumours was reported {324,1521}.

As in sporadic tumours, histological criteria to predict malignancy in tumours without metastases are not reliable in all cases and unequivocal immunohistochemical or molecular markers of malignancy are not yet available {1974,2229}. Malignant tumours are usually heavier, show coarse nodularity, confluent necrosis, absence of hyaline globules, higher mitotic rates, small cell morphology, reduced numbers or absence of sustentacular cells and may exhibit a different immunohistochemical expression pattern than benign tumours {392,469,790,1909, 1910,1979,2281,2289}.

In addition to phaeochromocytomas, so called composite phaeochromocytomas (with additional components of neuroblastoma, or ganglioneuroma, or ganglioneuroblastoma) arising in the adrenal medulla of MEN 2 patients have been described {238,1431}.

Prognosis and prognostic factors

Phaeochromocytoma as part of MEN 2 is almost always benign, with less than 5% reported to be malignant {324,1521}. Hence, the prognosis of patients with MEN 2 is mainly determined by the clinical course of their MTC. However, patients with phaeochromocytoma harbour a high risk of developing a hypertensive crisis, which may be lethal, during operations or childbirth. Hence, the presence of phaeochromocytoma needs to be excluded prior to a surgical procedure for MTC. If present, phaeochromocytoma has to be treated first.

Hyperparathyroidism

Clinical features

The symptoms of primary hyperparathyroidism (pHPT) are very well known as 'moans, groans, stones and bones'. In the 21st century, in countries where clinical surveillance and genetic testing are routine, patients with MEN 2 rarely present with these signs and symptoms. In comparison to sporadic pHPT and pHPT related to MEN 1, the disease appears to be rather mild and is generally diagnosed during follow-up.

The diagnosis is made based on the co-presence of elevated parathyroid hormone and elevated serum calcium levels. The risk of untreated pHPT is diverse. Severe osteoporosis and osteopenia followed by bone fractures may develop. Besides kidney stones, patients may present with abdominal pain due to peptic ulcers and/or pancreatitis. Further, fatigue and lethargy may be present in the case of severe pHPT.

Prior to primary surgery, no preoperative imaging techniques are necessary. In the case of persistent or recurrent pHPT, however, sestamibi scanning, having a high sensitivity (90%) and specificity (almost 100%), is the preferred imaging technique to identify the responsible parathyroid tissue {2364}.

Pathology

The gross findings of parathyroid hyperplasia in MEN 2 do not differ from those of hyperplasia in a non-familial association. All four glands are generally enlarged and hypercellular with a relative paucity of intraparenchymal fat (classic or usual type hyperplasia). There can be considerable variation in the size of individual glands from a given case, as well as variation in the degree of intraparenchymal adipose tissue. Occasionally, one may find two glands that are markedly enlarged and two glands of near normal size (pseudoadenomatous hyperplasia), which does not preclude the diagnosis of parathyroid hyperplasia particularly in the setting of MEN 2. In a subset of cases, there is little variation from normal parathyroid glands grossly or histologically, with an abundance of intraparenchymal fat in all glands examined (occult hyperplasia) {196,1892}. Regardless of the disparity of size or degree of cellularity between one or more parathyroid glands from a patient with known MEN 2 the diagnosis of parathyroid adenoma should not be used.

Generally, the histological findings are the same as those described for hyperplasia occurring in a non-familial setting {478}. The predominant cell type is the chief cell, which has faintly eosinophilic cytoplasm and a centrally placed round relatively monotonous nucleus without conspicuous nucleoli. There is generally some variation in the amount of cytoplasm present, which often occurs in discrete foci creating a slightly nodular appearance at low power magnification. Some chief cells have more abundant cytoplasm with a lesser degree of eosinophilia that results in varying degrees of cytoplasmic clearing and are referred to as clear cells. This is not to be confused with diffuse water-clear („wasserhelle") cell hyperplasia, which is generally not associated with MEN 2 {478}. Oxyphil cells are the result of an increased number of mitochondria in the cytoplasm that results in a granular eosinophilic appearance. Regardless of the variation in cytoplasmic features the nuclear characteristics are remarkably similar among all cell types, although as in other endocrine organs, it is not uncommon to see focal nuclear atypia in benign parathyroid neoplasia. While nuclear atypia is more frequent in adenomas than hyperplasia {1245}, it is not uncommon to see nuclear enlargement with some degree of hyperchromasia or occasional multinucleated cells in parathyroid hyperplasia. Rarely does one see diffuse atypical nuclear changes from an MEN 2 family with particularly aggressive parathyroid disease.

The architectural pattern in all cases of parathyroid hyperplasia consists of cords or nests or cells in a glandular pattern as well as foci of solid sheets of cells (nodular hyperplasia), although these findings are not specific for MEN 2 and can be seen in parathyroid adenoma as well as non-familial hyperplasia. Occasionally the overall architectural pattern is predominantly follicle-like with a single or few rows of chief cells surrounding a centrally located pseudolumen that generally contains a slight amount of eosinophilic debris. The intraparenchymal fat content is generally reduced in parathyroid hyperplasia, but there is a great deal of variation in this finding.

The presence of mitotic figures in the absence of malignancy is a frequent finding in benign parathyroid neoplasia {1924} and this applies equally well in MEN 2 associated parathyroid hyperplasia {2073}.

Prognosis and prognostic factors

MEN 2A-related primary hyperparathyroidism is generally mild, however, single cases with severe forms have been observed.

Other component features of MEN 2

Hirschsprung disease

Hirschsprung disease (HSCR) (MIM #142623) is a congenital abnormality characterised by absence or hypoplasia of neurons and ganglia of the submucosal and myenteric plexuses along variable lengths of the hindgut {1698}. Loss-of-function mutations of the RET proto-oncogene may be the single most common cause of HSCR {544}. Co-segregation of MEN 2 and HSCR has been recognised in a small subset of MEN 2 cases (<1%) {1533,2173}. In these cases, both disease phenotypes arise from a single mutation of RET, generally affecting the extracellular cysteine codons 609, 611, 618 or 620. Although the mutant protein is constitutively active, reduced levels are expressed on the cell surface, leading to both loss-of-function (HSCR) and gain-of-function (MEN 2) phenotypes associated with a single RET mutation {1553,2173}.

Cutaneous lichen amyloidosis

In a few families with MEN 2, cutaneous lichen amyloidosis has been described {514,1623}. In these instances, cutaneous lichen amyloidosis has been assumed to be a paracrinopathy {1151}.

Genetics

MEN 2 is inherited as an autosomal dominant disease, caused by germline mutations of the RET (REarranged during Transfection) proto-oncogene.

Chromosomal location

All three disease phenotypes have been mapped to a single locus on chromosome 10q11.2 by linkage analyses, and RET mutations have been identified in each disease subtype {512,564,1556}.

Gene structure

The RET gene spans 21 exons, and encodes a transmembrane receptor tyrosine kinase with three protein isoforms of 1072, 1106 and 1114 amino acids that differ in their C-terminal residues {1566, 1697,2172}. All RET receptors have a large extracellular domain, involved in recognition and binding of RET-ligands and co-receptors, a transmembrane domain, and an intracellular tyrosine kinase domain which is required for autophosphorylation of the receptor and initiation of downstream signalling.

Gene expression

The RET tyrosine kinase is essential for the development of the kidney, central and peripheral nervous systems, and some neuroendocrine tissues, as well as for maturation of spermatogonia {102, 533,1485,1669}. Its expression is highest in neural crest cells and neural crest

Table 5.02
Genotype-phenotype correlation in MEN 2.

Exon	Codon	FMTC	MEN 2A	MEN 2B
10	609	609	609	
	611	611	611	
	618	618	618	
	620	620	620	
11	630	630		
	634	634	634	
13	768	768		
	790	790	790	
	791	791	791	
14	804	804	804#	804†
	844	844		
15	883			883
	891	891	891¶	
16	918			918
Mean age at diagnosis§ (yrs)		45-55	25-35	10-20
Medullary thyroid carcinoma (MTC)		90-100%*	90-100%*	100%
Phaechromocytoma		-	40-60%	40-60%
Primary hyperparathyroidism		-	10-30%	-
Ganglioneuromatosis		-	-	+
Multiple mucosal neuromas		-	-	+
Marfanoid habitus		-	-	+
Thickened corneal fibers		-	-	+

§ The age at diagnosis has become younger since the identification of RET
# based on one report with MTC and adrenal and extra-adrenal phaeochromocytoma {1610}
† based on several reports with additional germline *RET* mutation {1046,1486,1516}; however, it appears that the phenotype is rather MEN 2B-like than typical MEN 2B
¶ based on one personal communication
* since the identification of *RET*, many patients undergo surgery before MTC occurs
− = disease/finding absent or frequency observed not higher that in the general population
+ = disease/finding present in most cases but neither required nor pathognomonic {742,746,1778}.

derived structures during embryogenesis and in the earliest stages of kidney induction and morphogenesis, but decreases to low levels in adult tissues {102,533,1669}.

Gene function

RET plays a role in development and maturation of peripheral nerves and in kidney induction but is also an important mechanism of neuronal survival in the peripheral nervous system, and particularly in the enteric nerve plexuses {226}. In normal cells, RET is activated by interaction with a multicomponent complex including members of both a soluble ligand family, the glial cell line-derived neurotrophic factors (GDNF), and also a family of cell surface bound co-receptors, the GDNF family receptors α (GFRα) {1886}.

Mutation spectrum

Activating germline mutations of *RET* are identified in >95% of all MEN 2 cases {564}. These are generally missense mutations clustered in only a few codons of *RET*, and there are strong correlations of specific disease phenotypes with subsets of these changes. As *RET* acts as an oncogene, a second somatic mutation of that locus is generally not part of MEN 2 tumourigenesis.

Genotype vs phenotype

Mutations of cysteine residues in the extracellular domain of *RET* (codons 609, 611, 618, 620 and 634) are found in most patients with MEN 2A and are strongly linked to the presence of phaeochromocytoma and hyperparathyroidism (HPT) {564,1554}. These mutations result in replacement of a cysteine normally involved in intramolecular bonds, leaving an unpaired cysteine residue available to form intermolecular bonds with other RET receptors, leading to constitutive dimerization and activation of RET signalling in the absence of its ligands and co-receptors {93,231,1934}. Patients with FMTC may have germline mutations of the same cysteine codons or may alternatively have mutations of intracellular residues (768, 790-91, 804, 844, 891) {564,982,1696}. The latter variants appear to alter RET binding of ATP and are reportedly associated with later onset, less aggressive disease phenotypes. The MEN 2B phenotype is associated almost exclusively with mutations of codons 918 (>95% cases) or 883 in the intracellular domain of RET {564,568, 718,906}. These mutations appear to alter *RET* substrate specificity and may result in stimulation of aberrant downstream signals which leads to the broader and more severe phenotype associated with this disease subtype {2100}.

Genetic counselling

All of the MEN 2 subtypes are inherited in an autosomal dominant manner with age-related penetrance.
MEN 2A. Almost all (>98%) affected individuals have an affected parent. Penetrance is at least 70% by 70 years of age with MTC as the usual first manifestation {562,1554,1761,1985}. In MEN 2A (and FMTC), *RET* mutation analysis can be restricted to exon 10, 11, 13, 14, and 15 (Table 5.02) {179,208,512,905,1556}.
MEN 2B. About 40% of affected individuals have *de novo* mutations {1621}. Thyroid carcinoma and multiple mucosal neuromata occur in virtually all affected individuals {1540}. If MEN 2B is suspected, mutation analysis should include exon 16 (M918T, >95%) {306,568,906} and 15 (A883F, 2-3%) {718,2069}.
FMTC. The presence of two or more MTC individuals on the same side of the family with objective evidence against phaeochromocytoma and hyperparathyroidism suggests FMTC. Age related penetrance is likely lower than MEN 2A {562}. However, FMTC is a clinical diagnosis and mutation carriers must not forego surveillance for other features although it is tempting to postulate that *RET* 768 and 804 mutations only result in FMTC.
Since *RET* gene mutations can be identified in >98% of all MEN 2 families, DNA-based diagnostic testing is considered standard of medical care in many countries worldwide {241,2223}. Gene testing should be offered to at-risk children in MEN 2A/FMTC families by age 6

{241,562}. For children at risk of MEN 2B, gene testing should be immediate, and certainly prior to age 2 {1259}. Prenatal testing is technically possible when a *RET* mutation has been identified in an affected family member.

Preventive measures
Prophylactic thyroidectomy
For those individuals who test positive for a *RET* mutation, a total prophylactic thyroidectomy is recommended for all subtypes and is safe for all ages. This should be done prior to age 6 for MEN 2A and by the age of 6 months, certainly before 2 years of age, for MEN 2B {192,241, 526,1259,1308,1595,2374}. Surgical intervention at an early age may be less imperative in the codon 768 and 804 mutation families due to the lower penetrance and later onset of the thyroid disease {562,2022}, however, clinical variability has been reported {613,666, 1259}.

Screening recommendations following surgery depends on the pathology. If an individual has overt MTC at the time of surgery, screening should include calcium- or pentagastrin-stimulated calcitonin testing every 3-6 months for the first 2 years, every 6 months from 3-5 years after surgery, and then annually. If only a small focus of MTC is found at the time of surgery, follow-up screening should involve annual basal (unstimulated) calcitonin for 5-10 years. If no cancer is present in the thyroid, no follow-up screening is indicated, even if C-cell hyperplasia is present. All individuals who have undergone thyroidectomy need thyroid hormone replacement therapy and monitoring {241,562,716}.

Screening for phaeochromocytoma
In MEN 2, phaeochromocytomas rarely occur before the presence of MTC {324}. However, at-risk individuals should undergo yearly screening for phaeochromocytoma, beginning at age 6. This consists of abdominal ultrasound or CT scans and 24-hour urine studies (vanillyl mandelic acid, metanephrines and catecholamines) {550}. Annual blood tests for chromogranin A and free catecholamine levels may be considered. Phaeochromocytoma should always be excluded in at-risk individuals prior to any surgery to avoid a life-threatening hypertensive crisis {241,562,716}.

Screening for parathyroid adenoma or hyperplasia
Screening for parathyroid hyperplasia in MEN 2A includes annual blood tests measuring ionized calcium and intact parathyroid hormone (iPTH) levels beginning at the time of MEN 2 diagnosis. Once hyperplasia is diagnosed, surgery to remove the parathyroid glands is necessary. At that time or when thyroidectomy is performed, whichever occurs first, all 4 parathyroid glands and the thymus should be removed. Half of a parathyroid gland should be pulverized and autografted into a muscle in the arm or neck to control the body's calcium levels and can be easily removed if indicated {241,562,716,2373}. Since parathyroid involvement in MEN 2B is rare or absent, parathyroid screening is generally not recommended unless otherwise indicated {562}.

RET mutation negative families
For *RET* mutation negative families, at-risk individuals should undergo annual screening for MTC, phaeochromocytoma and parathyroid hyperplasia from the age of 6 to the age of 35 years as above. Prophylactic thyroidectomy would not be routinely offered to this subgroup {562}.

Multiple endocrine neoplasia type 1

A. Calender
C.D. Morrison
P. Komminoth

J.Y. Scoazec
K.M. Sweet
B.T. Teh

Definition

Multiple endocrine neoplasia type 1 (MEN 1) is an autosomal dominant disease characterised by multifocal endocrine tumours affecting parathyroids, endocrine pancreas, anterior pituitary, cortical areas of the adrenal glands, diffuse endocrine tissues in thymus, bronchial tubes and various uncommon tumoural lesions in the skin, central nervous system and soft tissues.

MIM No. 131100 {1468}

Synonyms

The following terms should no longer be used: MEN I, Wermer syndrome, multiple endocrine adenomatosis type 1, familial Zollinger-Ellison syndrome.

Incidence

The prevalence in most populations is estimated to be between 1:40000 and 1:20000. About 10% of the patients have germline *MEN1* mutations arising de novo without any previous familial history {130}. Germline *MEN1* mutations have been found in about 5% of patients with sporadic primary hyperparathyroidism, a common disease occurring with a prevalence of 1:2000 to 1:1000 {2277}. Nevertheless, MEN 1 prevalence might be underestimated based on the observation that most patients predisposed to MEN 1 share at initial diagnosis a single endocrine lesion {2034}.

Diagnostic criteria

The diagnosis of MEN 1 should be suggested in individuals with newly diagnosed endocrine neoplasia component of MEN 1 (e.g., primary hyperparathyroidism, gastroenteropancreatic tumour, pituitary adenoma, adrenocortical and thymic endocrine tumours). This diagnosis is further strengthened if additional criteria commonly related to inherited cancers are met (e.g., age <50 years; positive family history; multifocal or recurrent neoplasia; two or more endocrine organs or systems affected). The diagnostic criteria for MEN 1 are given in Table 5.03.

Hyperparathyroidism

Age, distribution and penetrance

MEN 1 has a very high penetrance and an equal sex distribution. Although rare in early teens or younger, the cumulative percentages of patients who develop biochemical evidence of hyperparathyroidism increase with age. They reach 43%, 85%, and 94% at the ages of 20, 35, 50 years, respectively {2269}.

Clinical features

MEN 1-related parathyroid disease manifests as a multiglandular disorder rather than solitary adenoma, the latter of which is a common feature in sporadic primary hyperparathyroidism. As a result, recurrence is common in patients who only have partial parathyroidectomy. Parathyroid carcinoma, a feature of familial hyperparathyroidism-jaw tumour syndrome, however, is not known to be associated with MEN 1 and shown related to the HRPT2 locus on chromosome 1 {319}. Although "moans, groans and stones" are the hallmarks of severe or longstanding hypercalcemia, the majority of MEN 1 cases are asymptomatic and commonly detected through routine biochemical investigations.

Pathology

The gross findings of parathyroid hyperplasia in MEN 1 do not differ from those of hyperplasia in a non-familial association. All four glands are generally enlarged and hypercellular with a relative paucity of intraparenchymal fat (classic or usual type hyperplasia). There can be considerable variation in the size of individual glands from a given case, as well as variation in the degree of intraparenchymal adipose tissue. Occasionally, one may find two glands that are markedly enlarged and two glands of near normal size (pseudoadenomatous hyperplasia), which does not preclude the diagnosis of parathyroid hyperplasia particularly in the setting of MEN 1. In a subset of cases there is little variation from normal parathyroid glands grossly or histologically, with an abundance of intraparenchymal fat in all glands examined (occult hyperplasia) {196,1892}. Regardless of the disparity in size or degree of cellularity between one or more parathyroid glands from a patient with known MEN 1, the diagnosis of parathyroid ade-

Table 5.03
Diagnostic criteria for MEN 1.

The presence of two or more of the following signs identifies the MEN 1 patient:

1. Primary hyperparathyroidism with multiglandular hyperplasia and/or adenoma or recurrent primary hyperparathyroidism
2. Duodenal and/or pancreatic endocrine tumours, both functioning (gastrinoma, insulinoma, glucagonoma) and non-functioning or multisecreting tumours as proven by immunohistochemistry, gastric enterochromaffin-like tumours
3. Anterior pituitary adenoma, both functioning (GH-secreting tumours or acromegaly, prolactinoma) and non-functioning or multisecreting (GH, PRL-prolactin, LH-FSH, TSH) lesions as proven by immunohistochemistry
4. Adrenocortical tumours, both functional and non-functioning
5. Thymic and/or bronchial tubes endocrine tumours (foregut carcinoids)
6. A first-degree relative (parent, sibling, or offspring) with MEN 1 according the above criteria.

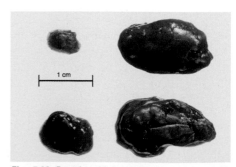

Fig. 5.06 Parathyroid hyperplasia. Macroscopic aspect of the parathyroid glands of a normal individual (left) and a MEN1 patient (right).

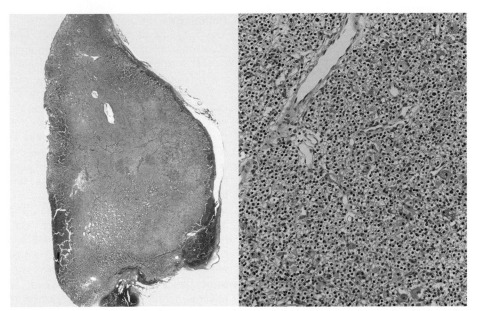

Fig. 5.07 Parathyroid hyperplasia. Gross section and histopathological features of a parathyroid gland of a MEN1 patient.

noma should not be used.

Generally, the histological findings are the same as those described for hyperplasia occurring in a non-familial setting {478}. The predominant cell type is the chief cell, which has faintly eosinophilic cytoplasm and a centrally placed round relatively monotonous nucleus without conspicuous nucleoli. There is generally some variation in the amount of cytoplasm present, which often occurs in discrete foci creating a slightly nodular appearance at low power magnification. Some chief cells have more abundant cytoplasm with a lesser degree of eosinophilia that results in varying degrees of cytoplasmic clearing. This is not to be confused with diffuse water-clear (wasserhelle) cell hyperplasia, which is generally not associated with MEN 1 {1245}. Oxyphil cells are the result of an increased number of mitochondria in the cytoplasm that results in a granular eosinophilic appearance. Regardless of the variation in cytoplasmic features, the nuclear characteristics are remarkably similar among all cell types, although, as in other endocrine organs, it is not uncommon to see focal nuclear atypia in benign parathyroid neoplasia. While nuclear atypia is more frequent in adenomas than hyperplasia {1245}, it is not uncommon to see nuclear enlargement with some degree of hyperchromasia or occasional multinucleated cells in parathyroid hyperplasia.

The architectural pattern in all cases of parathyroid hyperplasia consists of cords or nests or cells in a glandular pattern as well as foci of solid sheets of cells (nodular hyperplasia). These findings are not specific for MEN 1 and can be seen in parathyroid adenoma as well as non-familial hyperplasia. Occasionally, the overall architectural pattern is predominantly follicle-like with a single or few rows of chief cells surrounding a centrally located pseudolumen that generally contains a slight amount of eosinophilic debris. The intraparenchymal fat content is generally reduced in parathyroid hyperplasia, but there is a great deal of variation in this finding.

The presence of mitotic figures in the absence of malignancy is a frequent finding in benign parathyroid neoplasia {1923} and this applies equally well in MEN 1 associated parathyroid hyperplasia {2073}.

Prognosis and prognostic factors

The patients are treated by surgery, either a total parathyroidectomy with autotransplantation or subtotal resection of three and a half parathyroid glands. The prognosis for these patients after such treatment should be no different from sporadic counterparts. However, because of the genetic basis of their parathyroid disease, half glands left behind in the neck or autotransplated glands are still at risk for rehyperplasia.

These patients are believed not to develop malignancy.

Pituitary tumours

Clinical features

Anterior pituitary adenoma is the first clinical manifestation of MEN 1 in around 10% and 20% of familial and sporadic cases, respectively {322,2310}. Its prevalence in MEN 1 varies from 20-60% with a mean estimate value of 42% in largest studies. Mean age of onset of pituitary tumours is 38 ±15 yr with rare occurrences in children younger than 5 yrs {2149}. Of the various subtypes of MEN 1-related pituitary adenomas, prolactinomas (PRL) are the most commonly seen (≈60%), followed by growth hormome (GH) secreting (≈10%), adrenocorticotropin (ACTH) secreting (≈5%) and nonsecreting (≈15%) adenomas. Around 10% of MEN 1 pituitary adenomas show cosecreting immunohistochemical reactivities including PRL, GH, ACTH and less commonly LH, FSH and TSH. More than 80% of MEN 1-related pituitary lesions are macroadenomas including 30-35% of invasive cases. MEN 1 pituitary adenomas are significantly more frequent in women than in men (50% versus 30%) the easier recognition of clinical signs related to an excess of prolactin secretion in women may account for this sex-ratio. When present, major clinical signs are those observed in sporadic counterparts of these tumours: amenorrhea, infertility, galactorrhea in women, hypogonadism in

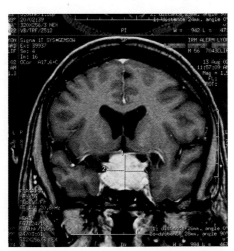

Fig. 5.08 MEN 1. Frontal magnetic resonance imaging showing a MEN1-related pituitary macroadenoma.

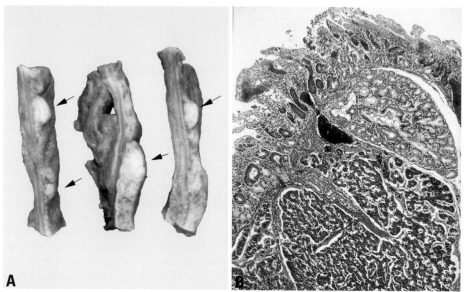

Fig. 5.09 Multiple endocrine neoplasia type 1 (MEN 1). **A** Multiple endocrine tumours in the mucosa/submucosa (see arrows) of a MEN1 patient suffering from Zollinger Ellison syndrome. **B** Well differentiated endocrine carinoma in a submucosa of the duodenum in a patient with MEN1 with Zollinger-Ellison syndrome.

men, related to prolactinomas, acromegaly secondary to excess GH and Cushing disease related to overproduction of ACTH and secondary adrenal hyperplasia. About one-third of tumours are invasive macroadenomas {2310} which can cause morbidity due to mass effects, leading to hypopituitarism and compression of adjacent structures, especially of the optic chiasm. The diagnosis of MEN 1 pituitary tumours requires a careful clinical history, including family history, basal hormone (PRL, GH, IGF-1) levels and radiological screening of the pituitary gland by magnetic resonance imaging.

Pathology

The majority of MEN 1 patients with involvement of the anterior pituitary exhibit a single adenoma and multicentricity appears to be extremely rare {1033,2044}. Convincing evidence for isolated diffuse hyperplasia of one of the cell types, similar to findings in the parathyroid and endocrine pancreas of MEN 1 patients, has not yet been reported; however, PRL or GH cell hyperplasia of the peritumoural parenchyma has been described {295,1626}.

In general, all types of adenomas and immunohistochemical expression patterns may be encountered in MEN 1 patients and the morphological features are not different from those seen in sporadic pituitary adenomas. However, in several series, a higher frequency of functionally active tumours with a high proportion of prolactinomas was reported when compared to sporadic pituitary adenomas {295}. A substantial proportion of tumours are microadenomas (<10 mm), but in one series from 1987, thrice the frequency of macroadenomas (≥10 mm) was reported {1967}. Immunohistochemically, approximately one third of adenomas produce more than one hormone and the majority exhibit a positive prolactin immunostaining (73-76%), followed by growth hormone (14–37%) or both {295,1960,1960}. Tumours expressing ACTH or other hormones {2426} are less frequent and non-functioning adenomas are rare.

Prognosis and prognostic factors

Treatment of pituitary tumours in MEN 1 varies according to the type and staging of the adenoma and is identical to that applied in sporadic counterparts. There is no good data to suggest that prognostic outcome is any different from the sporadic counterpart. However, because clinical surveillance may be routine, the MEN 1-related pituitary tumours may be detected at an earlier stage {412A,2310}.

Duodenal and pancreatic endocrine tumours

Clinical features

Endocrine tumours of the duodenum and pancreas are common manifestations in MEN 1 disease. Clinical expression of these tumours is highly variable and related to the extent, localisation, nature

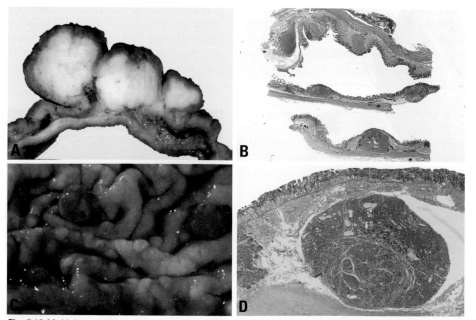

Fig. 5.10 Multiple endocrine neoplasia type 1 (MEN 1). **A** Cut surface of the wall of the stomach from a patient with MEN1 and Zollinger Ellison syndrome, showing multiple endocrine tumours in the mucosa and submucosa (ECLomas). **B** Microscopic sections of the duodenum from a MEN1 patient. In the mucosa and submucosa there are multiple endocrine tumours (gastrinomas). **C** Microcarcinoidosis of the stomach. **D** Two adjacent gastrinomas in the mucosa/submucosa of a MEN1 patient.

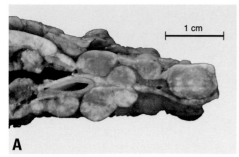

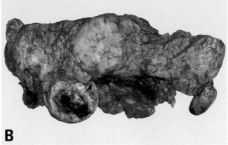

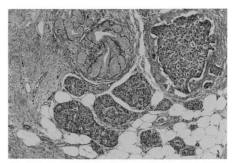

Fig. 5.11 Multiple endocrine neoplasia type 1 (MEN 1). **A** Adrenal nodular hyperplasia. **B** Resection specimen from the tail of the pancreas from a patient with MEN1. The cut surface shows three well demarcated tumours.

Fig. 5.12 Multiple endocrine neoplasia type 1 (MEN 1). Microadenoma (upper right) adjacent to a group of islets.

and level of hormone(s) secreted by tumoural cells. Predominant hormone secretion may occur and leads to a specific clinical syndrome.

Zollinger-Ellison syndrome (ZES)

This is the most frequent clinical state related to duodenal and/or pancreatic gastrinoma observed in MEN 1 patients and due to excessive production of gastrin by tumour cells. Initial symptoms are caused by gastric acid hypersecretion {556}. Abdominal pain or gastro-oesophageal reflux disease or both can occur in up to 80% of patients, while diarrhoea occurs in 10-20%. Atypical peptic ulcer disease with multiple lesions or ulcers in unusual locations should suggest the diagnosis of MEN 1-related ZES {1003}. Gastrinomas occur in 20-60% of MEN 1 patients and management of gastric acid secretion by H⁺-K⁺ ATPase inhibitors (proton pump inhibitors) has significantly reduced or abrogated the risk of severe complications of ZES such as bleeding, perforation and esophageal strictures. In about 90% of MEN 1 patients with ZES, the source of gastrin excess is usually multiple small duodenal tumours. Diagnosis of gastrinomas

includes measurement of specific biological and hormonal levels, such as fasting gastrin levels, measurement of gastric pH and gastrin provocative secretin test {668,1003}.

The early diagnosis of pancreatic endocrine tumours is enhanced by a standardised meal stimulation test and further measurement of serum gastrin and pancreatic polypeptide (PP) {2066}. Radiological imagine of the upper abdomen are performed every third year in *MEN1* gene carriers and include percutaneous and endoscopic echography, spiral computed tomography (CT), and somatostatin receptor (octreotide) scintigraphy.

Insulinomas

These are the second most frequent pancreatic tumours observed in the setting of MEN 1. Among large series of patients tested, one would expect that about 5-10% of patients with insulinomas belong to a MEN 1 genetic background {2012}. Common and convincing symptoms result from hypoglycaemia, followed by a catecholamine response. The mean duration of symptoms in patients without previous clinical history before diagnosis

has ranged from 1 year to 3-5 years and early recognition of *MEN1* gene carriers may now avoid long delays in insulinoma recognition. Various short and long term fasting tests and concomitant determinations of serum glucose and insulin levels are the most reliable biological procedures for insulinoma diagnosis. Apart from standard abdominal radiological examinations such as CT and ultrasonography, specific techniques for tumour localization including arteriography, trans-hepatic portal venous sampling, selective arterial calcium stimulation with hepatic venous sampling and intraoperative ultrasonography have been shown to represent reliable procedures {1620}.

Glucagonoma, *VIPoma* and other uncommon pancreatic endocrine tumours occur in less than 5% of MEN 1 patients but are characterised by a high malignant potential {1000}. More than 70% of glucagonomas and 40% VIPomas are malignant. Glucagonomas induce a necrolytic migratory erythema associated with diabetes mellitus secondary to abnormal glucagon secretion, VIPomas clinical expression is related to excessive production of vasoactive intestinal pep-

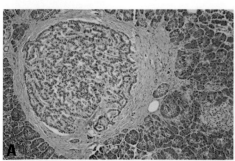

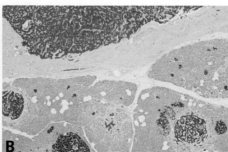

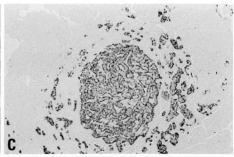

Fig. 5.13 Multiple endocrine neoplasia type 1 (MEN 1). **A** Microadenoma (< 5 mm) in a MEN1 patient. In comparison note the normal islet on the right. **B** Synaptophysin immunostaining exhibits parts of an encapsulated macrotumour (top) as well as several microadenomas. Same case as figure A. **C** Pancreatic microadenoma immunostained for glucagon.

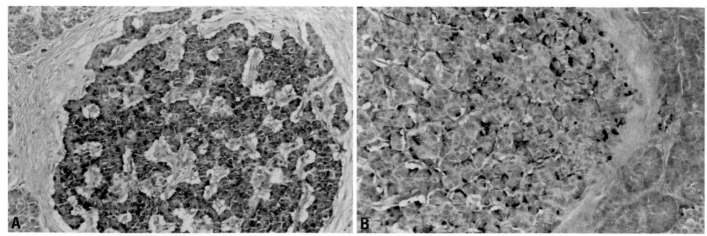

Fig. 5.14 Multiple endocrine neoplasia type 1 (MEN 1). **A** Pancreatic microadenoma exhibiting PP immunoreactive cells. **B** MEN1 microadenoma exhibiting cells immunoreactive for glucagon. [Immunostains using DAB as chromogen, followed by nickle-cobalt intensification and nuclear red as counterstain.]

tide (VIP) with the classical Verner-Morrison syndrome associating watery diarrhoea, hypokaliemia and achlorhydria (WDHA) {354,1691}. Very rare tumours observed in MEN 1 or a sporadic context are somatostatinoma and those secreting ACTH, calcitonin or GRF (Growth Releasing factors). Radiological diagnosis is performed with previously described methods.

Non-functional pancreatic endocrine tumours are characterised by the absence of any symptoms related to hormone hypersecretion. Nevertheless, they may have in situ production of hormones and peptides without biological effects (NSE) {1250}. Fortuitous diagnosis of non-functioning tumours is common mainly in the context of MEN 1 clinical surveillance protocols. Measurement of serum insulin, proinsulin, PP, glucagon and gastrin both in basal and provocative conditions may be useful, but repeated assessment of of serum chromogranin A (CgA) levels is considered more accurate (about 70% senstivity) for an earlier diagnosis of these insidious tumours {135}. Non-functioning pancreatic endocrine tumours may occur in 20-40% of MEN 1 patients {1753}. When misdiagnosed, they are often discovered after local compression and/or hepatic metastases occur.

Pathology

Pancreatic involvement in MEN 1 patients occurs in 30-75% of patients when assessed by clinical screening methods and approaches 100% in autopsy series {1388}. The majority of affected patients exhibit numerous non-functioning microadenomas (<0.5 cm) spread throughout the pancreas {1114} with a predominance of the pancreatic tail {881}. The small tumours usually display a distinct trabecular pattern and may show conspicuous connective tissue stroma {1114}. Immunohistochemically, they express one or several hormones and usually stain for pancreatic polypeptide, glucagon and/or insulin, but are functionally silent {229,1114,1741}. At the time of diagnosis, larger endocrine pancreatic tumours are usually multiple, vary in size {1950} and may be cystic {1301}. Clinically they can secret different hormones. Hyperinsulinism is seen in about one fourth of patients. Histologically they show a solid, adenomatous or trabecular pattern. Tumours with amyloid deposition usually exhibit insulin production. Similar to pituitary lesions, endocrine pancreatic tumours in MEN 1

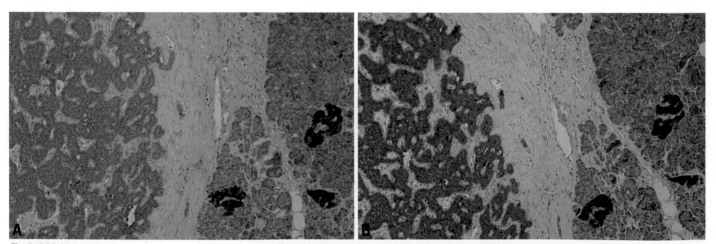

Fig. 5.15 Multiple endocrine neoplasia type 1 (MEN 1). **A** Menin (C-terminal epitope) immunohistochemistry in a MEN1-associated pancreatic endocrine tumour (left). Note the weak immunohistochemical signal in the tumour compared to the strong signal in the adjacent islets. **B** Menin (N-terminal epitope) immunohistochemistry in a MEN 1 associated pancreatic endocrine tumour. Note the retained immunohistochemical signal in the tumour and the strong signal in the adjacent islets.

patients consistently express multiple hormones {2171} but one hormone usually predominates {1111}. However, similar to sporadic endocrine pancreatic tumours, immunohistochemical expression patterns do not necessarily correlate with blood hormone levels or clinical syndromes due to possible impaired hormone secretion of tumour cells or the production of functionally inactive but immunoreactive molecules. Pancreatic polypeptide and glucagon containing tumours are most often found {1741} while tumours expressing predominantly or exclusively insulin are less common {1250}. Tumours with main immunoreactivity for somatostatin, vasointestinal polypeptide or other hormones are rare {173,552,1264,1741} and those with pure gastrin expression are an exception. The pancreatic tumours only rarely give rise to metastases and criteria to define malignancy are the same as for sporadic tumours. As for other endocrine tumours no reliable markers of malignancy are available {1214,1836}. In addition to microadenomas and endocrine macrotumours, the pancreas' of MEN 1 patients frequently exhibit small nests of endocrine cell budding from ducts as well as ill shaped islet-like cell clusters with cellular irregularities and abnormal distribution of the four islet cell types. These nesidioblastosis-like features are mainly seen in cases with additional severe obstructive pancreatitis due to duct stenoses by large endocrine tumours and should therefore not be regarded as the precursor lesion of the pancreatic endocrine tumours in MEN 1 {1180}. The Zollinger-Ellison syndrome occurring in approximately 50% of MEN 1 patients is mainly due to functioning gastrinomas located in the duodenum and is only exceptionally associated with pancreatic tumours. The gastrinomas are mostly located in the mucosa and submucosa of the proximal duodenum, are multiple and very small (<1 cm) and thus difficult to localise clinically, at surgery or autopsy {515}. Immunocytochemically, they stain almost exclusively for gastrin. They may give rise to periduodenal-parapancreatic lymph node metastases, which can be found in 60-80% of the cases and may be much larger than the primary tumour {1748}. The development of liver metastases occurs late in the course of the disease. Multiple somatostatinomas of the duodenum have also

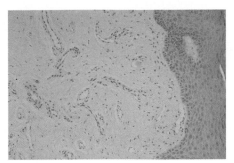

Fig. 5.16 Microscopic aspect of an angiofibroma in the skin of a MEN1 patient.

been described in MEN 1 pancreas' but appear to be very rare {1037,2451}.

Prognosis and prognostic factors
Malignancy of duodenal and pancreatic endocrine tumours has been recognized for all subtypes and mainly for gastrinomas (≥40%), glucagonoma (≥80%), VIPoma (≥40%) and non-functional tumours (≥70%). Malignant insulinomas are less common and may represent 5-10% of patients. Cure is highly dependent of tumour size and early diagnosis in asymptomatic gene carriers is a prerequisite for medical and/or surgical treatment success. Long-term studies suggest that about 23% of MEN 1-related gastrinomas develop liver metastases and 14% demonstrate aggressive growth. After a mean follow-up of 8 years, 4% of patients had died {710}. In a large study of patients who underwent surgery, 34% of patients with sporadic gastrinomas were free of disease at 10 years, as compared with none of the patients with MEN 1 {1619}. The overall 10-year survival rate was 94%.

Other component features of MEN 1

Adrenal cortical lesions
Adrenal cortical lesions are observed in 20-40% of MEN 1 patients and commonly hyperplastic, bilateral and nonfunctional {2067}. Most of MEN 1 adrenal enlargements and tumours remain asymptomatic and are commonly diagnosed 5 years later than MEN 1 {1231}. Median tumour diameter at diagnosis is 3.0 cm, with most tumours being 3 cm or smaller. In rare cases, hyperaldosteronism and Cushing syndrome have been reported {148,1231}. Most tumours are non-functioning and about 15-20% of

them become malignant. The lesions are often small and non-functioning and can therefore be managed by close surveillance but others have significant malignant potential and should be considered for surgery (subtotal adrenalectomy) when they are 3 cm or larger.

Cutaneous proliferations
Cutaneous lesions are present in 40-80% of MEN 1 patients, with variable histological forms {459}. Nodular lipomas are usually multicentric and show no recurrence after surgery. Large visceral lipomas have been also reported. The most common lesions are collagenomas and multiple and facial angiofibromas {459,1907}. Careful attention to cutaneous lesions in patients with endocrine tumours may be relevant for an earlier clinical diagnosis of MEN 1. Angiofibromas are clinically and histologically identical to those in individuals with tuberous sclerosis. Less common cutaneous lesions observed in MEN 1 are cafe au lait macules, confetti-like hypopigmented macules and multiple gingival papules in 2 patients {459}. Primary malignant melanomas have been observed in patients with MEN 1 belonging to large families {1615}. This highlights a possible role of the MEN1 gene in the tumourigenesis of a small subgroup of melanomas and conversely suggests that MEN 1 patients have a slightly increased predisposition to cutaneous and uncommonly choroidal melanoma.

Thymic and bronchial neuroendocrine tumours
These tumours are observed in about 5-10% of MEN 1 patients. As for duodenal and pancreatic endocrine tumours, they originate in the foregut. Thymic neuroendocrine tumours (carcinoids) are observed predominantly in males and carry a poor prognosis {2209}. MEN 1-related thymic carcinoids constitute approximately 25% of all cases of thymic carcinoids. In patients with MEN 1, this is an insidious tumour not associated with Cushing or carcinoid syndromes {708, 2209}. Local invasion, recurrence, and distant metastasis are common, with no known effective treatment. Computed tomography or magnetic resonance imaging of the chest, as well as octreoscanning, should be considered as part of clinical screening in patients with MEN 1. Prophylactic thymectomy during sub-

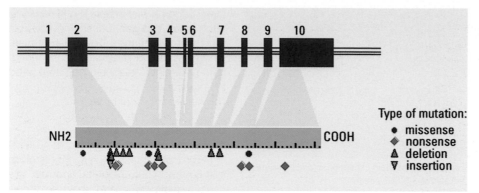

Fig. 5.17 MEN 1. Structure of the *MEN1* gene and examples of germline mutations spread over the coding sequence. From I. Lemmens et al. {1272}.

total or total parathyroidectomy should reduce the risks of thymic carcinoid. Bronchial carcinoids are less common in MEN 1 and occur predominantly in women {1560}. Most bronchial tumours in MEN 1 are typical carcinoids and treatment requires curative resection with a risk of locoregional failure.

Gastric ECLomas

ECLomas are presumed to originate from proliferation of enterochromaffin-like (ECL) cells in gastric mucosa and such tumours are mainly recognized during gastric endoscopy for Zollinger-Ellison syndrome (ZES) in MEN 1 {228}. These tumours are often small and multiple and they may be observed in about 10% of MEN 1 patients. ECLoma may be found in antro-pyloric and fundus mucosa and may be induced both by hypergastrinaemic conditions and genetic predisposition to MEN 1 {227}. Prognosis of ECLomas in patients with ZES-MEN 1 is good. Metastases are rare and tumour-related deaths are exceptional. ECLomas measuring less than 1 cm should be treated by endoscopic polypectomy and survey {274}. Considering the good prognosis of these tumours, aggressive surgery could be limited to selected patients.

Central nervous system tumours

Spinal ependymomas have been observed in rare MEN 1 patients and localize mostly in intratentorial cervical or lumbar regions {723,1049}. They are rapidly symptomatic and need surgery. One epidemiological study of a large series of MEN 1 patients has assessed that uncommon forms of meningioma and astrocytoma may occur in the context of genetic predisposition to MEN 1 {277}.

Soft tissue tumours

Oesophageal leiomyoma and renal angiomyolipoma have been described in rare MEN 1 cases {1466,2333}. Malignant gastrointestinal stromal tumour (GIST) represents an atypical presentation of MEN 1 syndrome but has been considered as non-fortuitous {1680}.

Genetics of MEN1

Chromosomal location

The *MEN1* gene (GenBank acc.no. U93237) is localized on chromosome 11q13 {1234}. This has mainly been shown by deletion mapping in tumours from MEN 1 patients {272}. Most tumours in MEN 1 affected patients, including less common lesions such as thoracic and gastric carcinoids, ECLomas and cutaneous tumours, show somatic loss of the wild-type allele (loss of heterozygosity (LOH) at 11q13 {558}. This observation is consistent with the fact that *MEN1* is a tumour suppressor gene with most pathogenic mutations corresponding to a loss of function.

Gene structure

The *MEN1* gene consists of 10 exons, spanning ~9 kb of genomic sequence, and encoding a protein of 610 aminoacids, menin {351,1272}. The first exon is noncoding and constitutes most of the 111 nt 5'-UTR. The sequence around the start codon (gccATGg) of the 610-amino acid open reading frame (ORF) is identical to the "Kozak consensus". The 797 nt 3' UTR has an unusual polyA signal (AATACA) located at –13. The exon sizes range from 41 bp to 1296 bp, and the introns range in size from 79nt to 1,563nt. Menin does not reveal

homologies to any other known proteins. The only motifs which have been recognised in the menin sequence are two leucine zippers, and two nuclear localization sequences (NLS) in the carboxyterminal part of the protein {791}. Menin has orthologs not only in mouse and rat, but also in zebrafish and drosophila (98%, 97%, 75%, and 47% homology, respectively), but there is no homologue known in the yeast Saccharomyces cerevisae {792,1072, 2130}.

Gene expression

The *MEN1* transcript is 2.9 kb (GenBank acc.no. U93236) in all tissues, with an additional 4.2 kb transcript also being present in the pancreas and thymus {1272}. Western blot analysis showed strong expression of menin as a 68 kDa protein in all types of human cell lines and tissues tested, and mostly in brain cortex, kidney, pituitary, testis, thymus adrenal glands with lower or undetectable levels in pancreas, liver, lung and skin {2361}. Menin is a nuclear protein whose expression is cell cycle regulated {1020}. In all cell lines tested, menin is found both in the nucleus and the cytoplasm, but its localization depends on the phase of the cell-cycle: during interphase, menin localizes in the nucleus; during and immediately after cell division, it migrates in the cytoplasm {933}. Various transcripts of *MEN1* vary in the content of their 5'-untranslated region. All transcript variants display upstream exons correctly spliced to *MEN1* exon 2. Further identification of 5' promoting regions will be relevant to identify tissue-specific promotion and the promoter(s) of the menin minor 4,2 Kb transcript in pancreas and thymus {1071}. Mouse models of MEN 1 have produced via inactivation of the mouse *Men1* gene through homologous recombination (knock-out mice) {425}. Homozygous inactivation of the *Men1* gene is lethal early during embryogenesis. *Men1*+/- heterozygotes develop mostly hyperplastic pancreatic islets and small tumours from 9 months of age. Other tumours were also observed in these mice, e.g. parathyroid hyperplasia and adenoma, pituitary adenoma, and adrenocortical adenoma/carcinoma.

Gene function

Menin is supposed to play a role in control pathways of cell growth and differen-

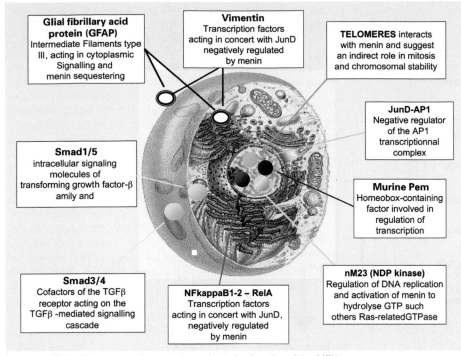

Fig. 5.18 MEN 1. Menin interacting proteins and putative function of the *MEN1* gene.

tiation during embryogenesis and post-natal life. To date, menin has been shown to interact with a subset of proteins involved in regulation of transcription, DNA replication, mitosis, apoptosis, genome integrity, growth factors signalling pathways and extracellular matrix organization. The first discovered was JunD, a transcription factor belonging to the AP1 transcription complex family {12}. Wild-type menin represses transcriptional activation mediated by JunD, may be via a histone deacetylase-dependent mechanism {733}. There may be an antagonistic action of Menin towards JunD with its tumour suppressive function. JunD has a reported effect in the inhibition of cell growth inside the AP1 complex. Menin represses the inducible activity of the c-fos promoter and inhibits Jun N-terminal kinase (JNK)-mediated phosphorylation of both JunD and c-Jun {686}. This occurs through two independent mechanisms uncoupling ERK and JNK activation from phosphorylation of their nuclear targets Elk-1, JunD and c-Jun, hence inhibiting accumulation of active Fos/Jun heterodimers. This provides molecular insights into the tumour suppressor function of menin and suggests a mechanism by which menin may interfere with Ras-dependent cell transformation and oncogenesis. Menin

interacts directly with three members of the NF-KappaB family of transcription regulators, NF-KappaB1 (p50), NF-KappaB2 (p52), and RelA (p65) {868}. These proteins are known to play a central role in oncogenesis of various organs, as they modulate the expression of numerous genes. NF-KappaB and JunD cooperate – and interact directly - to activate transcription in rat hepatocytes {1789}. Menin interferes with the TGFß signaling pathway at the level of Smad3 {1021} and probably with Smad1 and Smad5 {2103}. The latter interactions have been implicated in menin-specific inactivation of the commitment of pluripotent mesenchymal stem cells to the osteoblast lineage. Through TGFβ pathways, menin is important for both early differentiation of osteoblasts and inhibition of their later differentiation, and it might be crucial for intramembranous ossification. Smad-mediated TGFß signaling and Ras phosphorylation pathway may be related and lead for instance to activation of AP-1 complexes in which JunD is a primary component. This may be a relevant core action of menin action which has been shown to share an intrinsic GTPase activity {2436}. Last in this series, the rodent protein Pem has been shown to bind Menin directly {1273}. Pem is a homeobox-containing protein,

expressed mostly in testis, which plays a role in the regulation of transcription. However, Pem has no known homolog in the human genome. Menin may also be present in the cytoplasm and interact with two intermediate filaments proteins, glial fibrillary acidic protein (GFAP) and vimentin {1353}. These interactions suggest that intermediate filament network may serve as a cytoplasmic sequestering network for menin. The binding of menin to GFAP raises the issue of a putative role of this tumour suppressor in glial cell oncogenesis such as ependymoma. Interestingly, menin interacts with Nm23, a nucleoside diphosphate kinase ß isoform 1 which was first isolated as a metastasis suppressor {1639}. Nm23 associated to GFAP-containing intermediate filaments and enables menin to hydrolyze GTP, hence linking menin to Ras-related GTPases. This suggest again atypical GTPase activity of Menin may play a central role through multiple factors in the cell with specific actions depending the cellular type and physiological context. Menin may play a role in synapse formation and plasticity during embryonical organization. Lastly, menin might control genome stability through interaction with Nm23 which isoform 1 is associated to the centrosomes in dividing cells. Centrosomes regulate chromosome integrity and orchestrate the formation of GFAP and vimentin containing filaments through protein phosphorylations regulated by GTPases. The direct or indirect role of menin in maintaining genome stability and DNA integrity has been assessed by numerous reports which show evidence that normal cells from MEN 1 patients present with an elevated level of chromosome alterations {975, 2251}. These aberrations might be related to the increase of premature centromere division observed in cell lines from patients with a heterozygous MEN 1 gene mutation when compared to normal controls {1906}. Recently, another molecular link between the MEN 1 pathogenic context and cellular DNA replication has been found through the demonstration that menin was found to interact with the 32-kDa subunit (RPA2) of replication protein A (RPA), a heterotrimeric protein required for DNA replication, recombination and repair {2161}. *In vitro* and *in vivo* biological assays have shown that stable overexpression of Menin partially suppresses the *RAS*-mediated tumour phe-

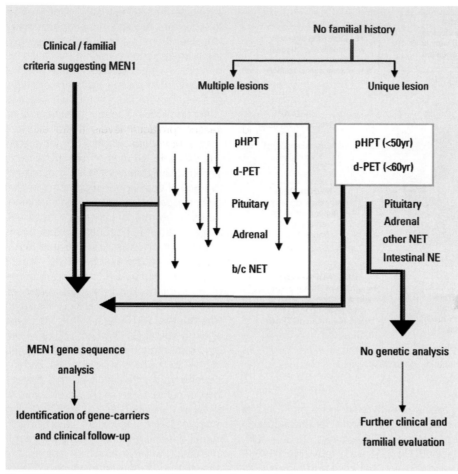

Fig. 5.19 MEN 1. A schematic view of *MEN1* gene testing in clinical practice.

notype directly supporting *MEN1* gene function as a tumour suppressor gene {1078}. In pancreatic islet cells, menin inhibits insulin promoter activity, hormonal secretion and cell proliferation through a mechanism which might involve suppression of AP-1 activation by menin either by direct inhibition on AP-1-mediated transcription and suppression of c-Fos induction {1954,2470}.

Mutation spectrum
Germline and somatic mutations in the *MEN1* gene do not appear to cluster in hot spots and are spread over the entire coding and intronic sequences {2362}. More than 400 different mutations have now been described. Approximatively 60% are truncating mutations, either frameshift (~40%) or nonsense (~20%) mutations, 20% are missense mutations, 10% are in frame deletions or insertions and about 10% are intronic and splice-site mutations. Large germline deletions encompassing the whole *MEN1* locus

have also been shown {278,1096}. The frequencies of mutations detected in different studies vary, and range from 75-95% of the MEN 1 kindreds analyzed. Non-familial presentations of at least one or two MEN 1-related endocrine lesions have germline *MEN1* mutations in 5-10% of cases. Taken together, it has been shown that genetic analysis of the *MEN1* gene may be helpful in 8% of all-comers with primary hyperparathyroidism, in those younger than 50 years and in about 6% of subjects affected by duodenal and/or pancreatic endocrine tumours.

Genotype vs phenotype
Penetrance of MEN 1 at age 50 years is about 85% in gene-carriers. To date, there is no clear-cut genotype-phenotype correlation in MEN 1 patients {2362}. The clinical presentation, age of onset and natural history of the disease have been known to vary extensively even among members of the same family. The mutations spread throughout the 9 transcribed

exons making any correlation study even more difficult. However, the findings of predominantly missense mutations in familial isolated hyperparathyroidism, especially in large families, may be the exception. For example, in two large autosomal dominant familial isolated hyperparathyroidism (FIHP) families, which are characterized by multiglandular disease (one with 7 affected and the other 14 affected), two distinct missense mutations in close proximity in exon 4, E255K and Q260P were identified {1047, 2206}. Nevertheless, even if specific point mutations might be related to mild phenotype, this has no accurate incidence in clinical follow-up of MEN 1 patients. In the same family, expressivity of MEN 1-related lesions is highly variable {322,723}. Specific mutations have been conversely related to uncommon expression of the disease, such as the Burin-variant of MEN 1, characterized by the absence of pancreatic tumours {1647}. Nevertheless, this correlation may be related to founder effects in related families living in the same region. More than 10% of the mutations arise de novo {130} and despite typical expression of the disease, about 5-10% of MEN 1 patients do not share germline mutations in the coding region or intronic borders of the *MEN1* gene, suggesting that some of the mutations occur in unknown parts or regulatory regions of the *MEN1* gene.

Genetic counselling and preventive measures

Genetic counselling
MEN 1 is inherited in an autosomal dominant manner with an age related penetrance and variable expression. Clinical primary hyperparathyroidism is present in at least 50% of the patients by age 20 years {130,1989}. Penetrance is more than 80% by age 50 years, although blood and urine tests could detect 90% by this age {130,322,1421}. Most individuals with MEN 1 will have an affected parent (90%) although onset of symptoms can be quite variable, even within the same family {350,1421}. DNA-based testing is recommended for index patients and their relatives to establish the diagnosis by molecular means and for medical management rather than to determine major prophylactic interventions {262,350}. DNA-based diagnostic

testing is useful for individuals and families who have some of the components of MEN 1 but are not classic {319,1423}. The appropriate age for offering *MEN1* genetic testing remains controversial, however, given the significant early morbidity that can occur, testing of at-risk children should be strongly considered {241,1308}. Prenatal testing is possible when a *MEN1* mutation has been identified in an affected family member.

Preventive measures

Although early pre-symptomatic biochemical screening for MEN 1 does significantly improve diagnosis, decrease morbidity, and is considered standard of care by most practising clinical cancer geneticists, there is no general consensus as to what management protocol is most beneficial and cost-effective. There is agreement that regular biochemical screening for high-risk individuals should be every 6-12 months, selected imaging studies less often (every 3-5 years), and this should continue for life {241,758, 1421,2358}.

Screening for primary hyperparathyroidism

Blood tests measuring ionized calcium and intact parathyroid hormone (iPTH) levels should be done at 6-12 month intervals, beginning by 8-10 years of age. Elevated ionized calcium and/or elevated parathyroid hormone levels confirm the presence of hyperparathyroidism, at which point surgical resection should be discussed. As parathyroid tumours are multiple in MEN 1 some groups practice complete parathyroidectomy with fresh parathyroid auto-transplantation to the forearm, or cryopreservation of a portion of a parathyroid gland. Others try to leave a parathyroid remnant although the possibility of recurrence remains high. All agree that transcervical thymectomy should be done as part of the initial parathyroidectomy.

Screening for islet cell tumour

Although primary hyperparathyroidism is the usual first presenting sign, this is not always so. Moreover, MEN 1-related islet cell tumours typically present with symptoms of hormone release rather than bulk disease. Thus annual pre-symptomatic screening should include, at a minimum, fasting and secretin-stimulated gastrin levels beginning at age 20. Many practitioners also do fasting glucose, insulin and glucagon, as well as albumin, prolactin and chromogranin-A. Given that one fourth of tumours are non-functional, abdominal imaging studies (CT, MRI or Octreotide scan) should be done every 3-5 years. In general, surgery in MEN 1 is indicated for most symptomatic MEN 1-related islet cell tumours, as these are usually benign. The exception is gastrinoma, which in MEN 1 is usually multiple and/or metastatic, and the role of surgical versus non-surgical management remains controversial.

Screening for pituitary tumour

The management of pituitary tumour in MEN 1 involves annual screening for fasting prolactin levels (PRL) although some advocate monitoring insulin-like growth factor (IGF-1) as well. Most begin regular biochemical screening by age 8-10; some wait until early adulthood. CT scan or gadolinium-enhanced MRI of the pituitary gland is usually not routinely done in the United States, but some physicians will do them every 3 years.

Other screening

Gastroduodenal, thymic and bronchial carcinoid tumours can occur in patients with MEN 1, and are usually more aggressive than sporadic cases. Thus some groups have advocated baseline CT or MRI scan with follow-up imaging studies every 3 years.

Hyperparathyroidism-Jaw tumour syndrome

B.T. Teh
K.M. Sweet
C.D. Morrison

Definition
Hyperparathyroidism-jaw tumour syndrome (HPT-JT) is an autosomal dominant disorder characterised by parathyroid adenoma or carcinoma, fibro-osseous lesions (ossifying fibroma) of the mandible and maxilla, and renal cysts and tumours.

MIM No. 145001

Synonyms
Familial isolated hyperparathyoridism; familial cystic parathyroid adenomatosis

Incidence or prevalence
It is a relatively recently described entity and its incidence or prevalence is unknown.

Diagnostic criteria
Unlike the MEN 1 patients who invariably develop multiglandular disease, the HPT-JT patients present with hereditary solitary (occasionally double) adenoma or carcinoma. The latter is a rare entity and is not associated with other forms of hereditary endocrine neoplasia syndromes and should lead to strong suspicion of this syndrome. About 30% of patients also develop fibro-osseous lesions, primarily in the mandible and maxilla. Kidney lesions have been reported including bilateral cysts, renal adenoma, hamartomas and papillary renal cell carcinoma. It is important to be aware that in some families, only parathyroid lesions are present. As more families are currently being tested genetically, it is expected that the incidence and spectrum of its associated clinical features will be better known in due course.

Hyperparathyroidism

Age distribution/penetrance
About 80% of patients present with hyperparathyroidism, that may develop in late adolescence, similar to the presentation in MEN 1. There is a reduced penetrance in females {2207}, and parathyroid carcinoma occurs in approximately 10-15% of affected individuals {319}.

Clinical features
Compared with MEN 1-related hyperparathyroidism, HTP-JT syndrome appears to run a more aggressive course: the patients tend to have more severe hypercalcemia and some actually present with hypercalcemic crisis. In addition, there appears to be a much higher incidence of parathyroid carcinoma than in other endocrine related disorders.

Pathology
Primary hyperparathyroidism in HPT-JT syndrome is more often one or two gland involvement (adenoma or double adenoma) that may or may not present synchronously {985}. One unique feature of the parathyroid neoplasia is the high incidence of cystic change {1396}, but such changes also occur in sporadic parathyroid adenoma or hyperplasia. The diagnosis of parathyroid carcinoma remains a challenge, and the only indisputable proof for parathyroid malignancy is extensive local invasion and/or metastasis. The finding of parathyroid carcinoma in the small number of reported families with HPT-JT syndrome is significant considering the rarity of parathyroid carcinoma in sporadic parathyroid tumours.

Prognosis and prognostic factors
The majority patients with adenoma can be cured by surgery and recurrence is not as common as in MEN 1 patients. Prognosis is guarded once parathyroid carcinoma is confirmed, but it is unclear whether the prognosis is any different from sporadic parathyroid carcinoma.

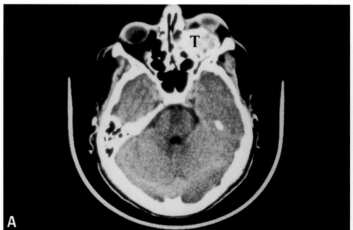 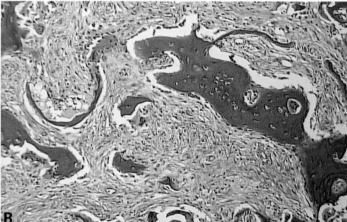

Fig. 5.20 Hyperparathyroidism - jaw tumour syndrome (HPT-JT). **A** CT showing a well demarcated fibroosseus lesion in the maxillary antrum. **B** Typical jaw lesion from a patient with HPT-JT syndrome with a dense, relatively avascular fibroblast-rich stroma and irregular spicules of woven bone, some of which show at least a focal rim of osteoblasts.

Jaw tumours

Clinical features
Some cases are fast growing while some are insidious and slow growing. Radiographic features generally show a well-demarcated osseous lesion of the mandible or maxilla.

Pathology
The usual case is described as having a relatively avascular cellular fibroblast-rich stroma, sometimes with a storiform pattern, admixed with bone trabeculae and/or cementum-like spherules. Some of the bone trabeculae generally show at least focal osteoblastic rimming. It is distinct histologically from the classical bone lesion of hyperparathyroidism, *osteitis fibrosa cystica*, which tends to resolve slowly after correction of the hyperparathyroidism, albeit over a course of months to years {1993}. In contrast, the fibroosseous lesions of HPT-JT do not resolve with correction of the hyperparathyroidism. While most of these lesions involve either the mandible or maxilla of one side, bilateral or multifocal lesions have been described {331, 2354}.

Prognosis and prognostic factors
While none of the described jaw tumours have behaved in a malignant fashion, some have recurred {1864,2207} although it is difficult to discern if this is due to incomplete initial resection or development of a new lesion.

Other features

In addition to cystic adenomatosis and jaw lesions, a wide spectrum of tumours has been associated with HPT-JT syndrome but most notable is the association of various renal lesions, which occurs in approximately 20% of patients {319,1022,2166,2207}. In the two families reported, 5 individuals in one kindred and 2 in the other had renal lesions. In the latter kindred, polycystic kidney disease was the predominant finding, while in the other kindred in addition to renal cysts there were several individuals with renal hamartomas described as cystic tumours with mesenchymal, blastemal, and epithelial elements. Another renal tumour that has been reported with HPT-JT syndrome is Wilms tumour {1022,

2166}, which has been reported in three separate individuals from three separate families.

Genetics

Chromosomal location
The *HRPT2* gene is mapped to 1q25-q31 {2166}.

Gene structure
The *HRPT2* gene contains 17 exons spanning 18.5 kb of genomic distance and predicted to express a 2.7kb transcript. It encodes a protein of 531 amino acids {319}.

Gene expression
The gene is ubiquitously expressed including kidney, heart, liver, pancreas, skeletal muscles, brain and lung {319}.

Gene function
The function remains unknown although the gene has moderate (32%) identity to a yeast protein Cdc73p, which is an accessory factor associated with an alternative RNA polymerase II {319}.

Mutation spectrum
The vast majority of mutations are frameshift and nonsense loss-of-function mutations found in several exons. The most common exon involved is exon 1 {319}.

Genotype vs phenotype
To date, it remains unknown if there is a genotype-phenotype correlation.

Genetic counseling

When HPT-JT is suspected in a family, DNA-based testing is recommended for index patients and their relatives to establish the diagnosis and for medical management. As the *HRPT2* gene was recently identified, testing for each of the complex syndromes associated with hereditary primary hyperparathyroidism has become possible {319}.

Screening for primary hyperparathyroidism
Annual blood tests measuring ionized calcium and intact parathyroid hormone (iPTH) levels should begin by 15 years of age. Surgical intervention should occur once serum levels confirm the presence of HPT. Parathyroid disease in HPT-JT is typically represented by asynchronous adenomas although the potential for malignancy needs to be considered {2055,2356}. While some groups advocate removal only of the enlarged parathyroid gland with continued regular monitoring {1423,2055}, the alternative approach would be complete parathyroidectomy with fresh parathyroid auto-transplantation to the forearm (or sternocleidomastoid), or cryopreservation of a portion of a parathyroid gland.

Screening for jaw manifestations
Orthopentography of the jaw every three years.

Screening for renal manifestations
At-risk individuals should receive annual abdominal ultrasound or CT scan with and without contrast at least every other year to screen for polycystic disease, Wilms tumour or carcinoma, and renal hamartomas {1993}.

Table 5.04
Tumours and cysts reported in association with HPT-JT syndrome.

Lesions	Reference
Renal cysts, polycystic kidney disease, renal hamartoma	{2207}
Wilms tumour	{1022,2166}
Renal cysts	{331}
Renal cysts, papillary renal cell carcinoma, multiple renal cortical adenomas, Hurthle cell adenoma, clear cell pancreatic adenocarcinoma	{845}
Adenomyomatous polyps of endometrium	{669}
Papillary thyroid carcinoma, uterine leiomyoma	{965}
Cellular neurofibroma	{1396}

Von Hippel-Lindau syndrome (VHL)

E.R. Maher
K. Nathanson
P. Komminoth
H.P.H. Neumann

K.H. Plate
T. Bohling
K. Schneider

Definition
Von Hippel-Lindau (VHL) disease is a dominantly inherited familial cancer syndrome caused by germline mutations in the *VHL* tumour suppressor gene. VHL disease demonstrates marked phenotypic variability and age-dependent penetrance. The most frequent tumours are retinal and central nervous system haemangioblastomas, renal cell carcinoma, phaeochromocytoma and pancreatic endocrine tumours. Families with VHL disease may be subdivided according to clinical phenotype, and this subdivision forms the basis for genotype-phenotype correlations (see later).

MIM No. 193300 {1862}

Synonyms
Von Hippel-Lindau syndrome

Incidence/prevalence
VHL disease was estimated to have an incidence of 1/36000 live births in Eastern England {1383} and a prevalence of 1/39000 in South-West Germany {1590}.

Diagnostic criteria
If there is a confirmed family history of VHL disease, a clinical diagnosis can be made in a relative with a single typical VHL tumour (e.g. retinal or central nervous system haemangioblastoma, clear cell renal cell carcinoma, phaeochromocytoma, pancreatic endocrine tumour or endolymphatic sac tumour). In isolated cases without a family history, two tumours (e.g. two haemangioblastomas or a haemangioblastoma and a visceral tumour) are required for the diagnosis. Genetic studies allow a molecular-based diagnosis of VHL in atypical cases and early diagnosis in patients who do not satisfy clinical diagnostic criteria.

Phaeochromocytoma

Age distribution and penetrance
The association of phaeochromocytoma with VHL is strongly dependant upon genotype (Table 5.06). More than 95% of patients with truncating or null mutations have VHL type 1 (low risk of phaeochromocytoma) {358,433} Patients with VHL type 2 (high risk of phaeochromocytoma) have primarily missense mutations. The penetrance of phaeochromocytoma in those with missense mutations of VHL is high: one large series estimated a 59% risk by age 50 years {1381}. Risks for specific missense mutations vary, with risks of 82% for type 2B codon 167 mutations and 50% for the "Black Forest" c.505 type 2A mutation at 50 years being reported {163,1381}. In series of VHL patients with phaeochromocytomas, the age range of diagnosis is from 5-64 years, starting notably younger and with a younger average at diagnosis than in

other hereditary syndromes with phaeochromocytoma (MEN 2, SDHD, SDHB) {119,244,565,962,1585,1587, 2291,2348}.

Clinical features
Patients with VHL and phaeochromocytoma commonly have multi-focal disease, both adrenal and extra-adrenal. Extra-adrenal disease has been particularly associated with a mutation at nucleotide 505 {2348}. As noted above, early age at diagnosis of phaeochromocytoma is a predominant feature, however, there is some genotype-phenotype correlation with individuals with mutations at nucleotides 595 and 695 presenting with phaeochromocytomas at a younger age than those with other mutations (p<0.025) {2348}. As mutations in *VHL* can lead to phaeochromocytoma alone, it is difficult to define the frequency of phaeochromocytoma as the first sign of VHL. However, depending on the mode of ascertainment, *VHL* mutations have been identified from 2-50% of the patients with sporadic or isolated phaeochromocytoma in hospital based series {119,244,565,1587,2291}. In the recent study of 271 sporadic phaeochromocytomas in a population-based series, mutations in VHL were found in 11% of cases and accounted for almost half of the germline mutations identified (30/66) {1585}. The biochemical findings found in phaeochromocytomas due to VHL

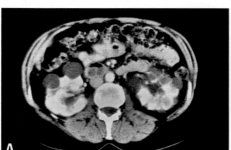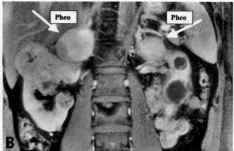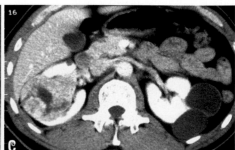

Fig. 5.21 von Hippel-Lindau syndrome. **A** Multiple bilateral renal cysts without tumours in a patient with Von Hippel-Lindau disease. **B** Bilateral multiple renal cysts and multiple renal carcinomas and bilateral adrenal phaechromocytomas (arrow and "Pheo") in a 36 year old patient with Von Hippel-Lindau disease; initially the diagnosis was missed and the adrenal tumours summarized among the tumours originating from the kidneys. **C** A 40 year old patient with Von Hippel-Lindau disease. Note a huge tumour of the right kidney and cysts of the left kidney. The extent of the tumour made nephrectomy necessary.

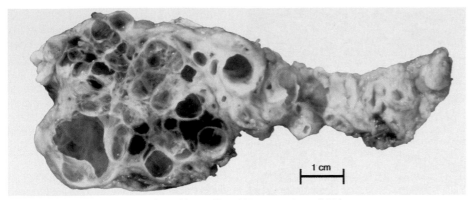

Fig. 5.22 Pancreatic cysts in a patient with von Hippel-Lindau syndrome (VHL).

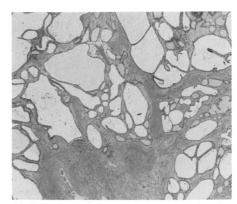

Fig. 5.23 Microscopic aspect of a microcystic adenoma of the pancreas in a VHL patient.

have been elucidated recently. Phaeochromocytomas associated with VHL are noradrenergic due to decreased expression of phenylethanolamine-N-methyltransferase (PNMT) in the tumours, which converts norepinephrine to epinephrine {551}. As a result, patients with phaeochromocytoma due to VHL usually demonstrate an increase only in normetanephrines, reflected in both plasma and urinary measurements.

Pathology

Patients of type 2 families {258} often present with multiple, bilateral phaeochromocytomas, which can be accompanied by extra adrenal chromaffin tumours and parasympathetic paragangliomas {902,937,1564,2480}. A study of 14 phaeochromocytomas in eight patients with VHL disease demonstrated that VHL-associated phaeochromocytomas have a distinct histologic phenotype as compared with phaeochromocytomas in patients with MEN 2. VHL tumours are characterised by a thick vascular tumour capsule; myxoid and hyalinized stroma; round, small to medium tumour cells intermixed with small vessels; cells with predominantly amphophilic and clear cytoplasm; absence of cytoplasmic hyaline globules; and lack of nuclear atypia or mitoses. In contrast to MEN 2 {483}, there is frequently no extratumoural adrenomedullary hyperplasia in the VHL adrenal gland {1121}. Another study on 30 VHL-associated phaeochromocytomas revealed lower total tissue contents of catecholamines and expression of TH as well as negligible stores of epinephrine and expression of PNMT when compared to phaeochromocytomas

MEN 2 patients {551}. Occasional tumours with melanin-like pigment or lipid degeneration have also been described in VHL patients {1223,1791}. A study has shown that immunohistochemistry is not helpful for the discrimination of VHL-related from sporadic tumours since both tumour types demonstrated positive staining for the VHL protein, suggesting that the antibody also recognizes the mutated VHL protein {1354}.

As in sporadic and other familial forms of phaeochromocytomas, malignant transformation may also occur in VHL-associated tumours {1026,1543,1777}.

Prognosis and prognostic factors

Phaeochromocytomas associated with VHL are frequently asymptomatic; studies have reported symptoms in 16-30% of patients {551,2348}. While the low frequency of symptoms may in part be because many tumours are detected on routine screening, the frequency is still lower than that in other comparable syndromes, such as MEN 2. The prognosis associated with phaeochromocytoma is quite good, with the rate of malignancy

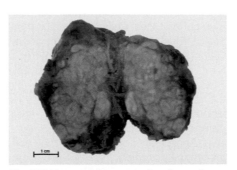

Fig. 5.24 Macroscopic aspect of a clear-cell pancreatic endocrine tumour in a VHL patient.

less frequent (<5%) than in sporadic disease {2348}. In one study, 12 VHL patients with 17 adrenal masses were followed for a median of 35 months with no morbidity {2346}. Laparoscopic partial adrenalectomy has been advocated as a means to preserve adrenal function. Partial adrenalectomy has been reported to have similar clinical results to complete adrenalectomy with less morbidity {2346}. Due to the high rate of phaeochromocytoma in patients with VHL type 2, many patients develop contralateral phaeochromocytomas or phaeochromocytoma in remaining adrenal tissue several years after their initial surgery {2348}. However, metastatic disease has not been reported after partial adrenalectomy for phaeochromocytoma {2346}.

Renal cell carcinoma

Clinical features

In cross-sectional studies, the frequency of renal cell carcinoma (RCC) in VHL disease is ~35%, although the risk of RCC in type 1 kindreds and type 2B kindreds

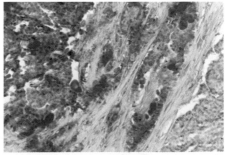

Fig. 5.25 Fat staining of a clear-cell pancreatic endocrine tumour in a VHL patient.

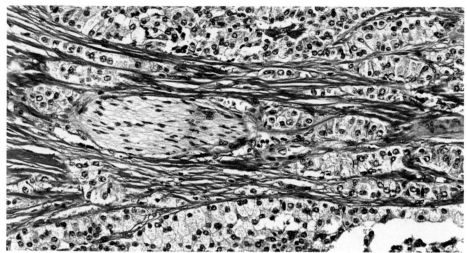
Fig. 5.26 Pancreatic endocrine tumour with clear cell features in a VHL patient.

approaches 70% at age 60 years {1380}. Men and women are equally affected. Mean age of clinical manifestation is 35-45 years. Asymptomatic small RCC have been detected as early as 16 years of age {1061}. Thus VHL-associated RCC is different from sporadic RCC, which is more frequent in males, and detected, on average, about 15 years later than in VHL disease {357,1586}. Similar to patients with sporadic RCC, VHL-associated RCC may become symptomatic with gross hematuria or metastases, but the majority of these tumours are now detected in an asymptomatic stage by renal imaging in VHL patients and at-risk individuals. Renal function is normal in patients with VHL-associated RCC. If one kidney has been already removed, there may be mild impairment of renal function. Acute renal failure can occur in a remnant kidney after hematuria and pelvic clotting. RCC can be the first manifestation of VHL, although this occurs in <20% of cases.

Pathology
VHL-associated RCC is always a clear cell carcinoma {1589}. Sporadic and VHL-associated clear cell tumours are often indistinguishable but certain criteria are frequently observed in VHL.

Macroscopy
VHL-associated RCC can occur as a single carcinoma of a kidney, but multifocal tumours are more frequently observed. Typically, both tiny and large tumours are found. Most tumours are surrounded by a marked pseudocapsule. The tumours are often heterogenous; they comprise cystic areas of serous liquid or blood. In addition to solid tumours, renal cysts are a typical component of VHL-involvement of the kidney {1586}. Both kidneys are usually affected, but the number and size of tumours and cysts differ. Most of these characteristics can be demonstrated in a surgical specimen. However, preoperatively, this can be demonstrated also by CT scanning or MR imaging {379}.

Histology
The dominant finding by conventional haematoxylin and eosin staining is a tumour composed of cells with clear cytoplasm and small nuclei. Most tumours can be classified as grade 1, sometimes, in part, as grade 2, but rarely, as grade 3. Typical is a microcystic growth pattern. The cystic structures contain liquid or blood. Endothelial or epithelial cells are mostly absent. Fibrotic stroma can show incorporation of iron. Necrotic tumour areas are rare. Most tumours have a marked pseudocapsule {1586}. Renal cysts occurring in patients with VHL may contain small foci with atypical epithelial cells or even incipient carcinomas {1765}. By long-term observation, however, most cysts do not transform into cancer. Similar to sporadic RCC, in VHL, RCC tumour invasion into the veins can be observed. This may be evident in small veins of the renal parenchyma or branches of the renal vein. Apparently normal kidney may contain many microfoci of RCC on microscopic examination {2347}.
Histologically, VHL-associated RCC and haemangioblastoma of the CNS can appear with a remarkably similar pattern. In fact, such CNS tumours have been interpreted as metastases of RCCs. Spinal tumours may produce similar diagnostic difficulties. Immunohistochemical staining may be helpful but inconclusive results may be obtained in some instances. It is important to be aware of such problems {1588}.

Prognosis and prognostic factors
Differential diagnosis
Tumourous and cystic involvement of the kidneys can lead to misinterpretations. Tuberous sclerosis complex and autosomal dominant polycystic kidney disease should be excluded. Clinical presentation, radiology and pathology can contribute to the differential diagnosis.

Prognosis and prognostic factors
RCC is the only frequent lesion in VHL that truly constitutes a carcinoma. However, as the diagnosis and treatment of CNS tumours have improved with MR imaging and microsurgical techniques, RCC has emerged as an important cause of morbidity and mortality {1380}. Nevertheless, growth of VHL-associated RCC seems to be slower compared to sporadic RCC. Metastases are associated with large tumours {1586}. One surgical series reported that 25% of VHL patients with a RCC >3 cm at surgery developed metastatic disease, but none with smaller tumours {2344}. Hence, it appears that tumours can be observed up to a diameter of 3 cm, and in many centres nephron sparing surgery is performed in when lesions reach 3 cm. When bilateral nephrectomy has been performed, kidney transplantation is a good option for patients with VHL {737}. So far, there are no clear data demonstrating that specific germline mutations correlate with the prognosis of VHL-associated RCC. However, mutations leading to truncation of the putative VHL protein may be associated with a more aggressive clinical course.

CNS haemangioblastomas

Clinical features
CNS haemangioblastomas are a cardinal feature in VHL disease. The lifetime risk of cerebellar haemangioblastoma is ~70% by age 60 years and symptomatic

spinal cord lesions occur in ~25% of patients {1383}. Supratentorial lesions are rare. Approximately 30% of all patients with cerebellar haemangioblastoma have VHL disease and the mean age at diagnosis of those with VHL disease is considerably younger than in sporadic cases {1382}. Patients with cerebellar haemangioblastomas typically present with symptoms of increased intracranial pressure and limb or truncal ataxia (depending on the location of the tumour).

Pathology
Macroscopically, capillary haemangioblastomas appear as well circumscribed, highly vascularised red tumour nodules, often within the wall of large cysts. Multiple haemangioblastomas occur in patients with VHL disease. This reflects numerous independent tumour sites and is not a sign of metastasis.

Histologically, capillary haemangioblastomas consist of large vacuolated stromal cells embedded in a rich capillary network. The distinction of cellular and reticular variants, based on the abundance of the stromal cells appears not to be of clinical significance.

Current evidence suggests that the stromal cells represent the neoplastic component of the tumour, whereas the capillary network forms as a consequence of aberrant gene expression in stromal cells {2150}. The stromal cell nuclei may vary in size, with occasional hyperchromatic nuclei. The typical "clear cell" morphology of capillary haemangioblastoma is based on numerous lipid-containing cytoplasmic vacuoles. This feature can sometimes lead to differential diagnostic problems between capillary haemangioblastoma and metastatic renal cell carcinoma. Immunohistochemistry for cytokeratins and EMA may facilitate the differential diagnosis, because stromal cells do not express epithelial marker proteins.

Ultrastructurally, the most prominent feature of the stromal cells is an abundant electron-lucent cytoplasm containing lipid droplets. Some studies have demonstrated electron-dense bodies, reminiscent of Weibel-Palade bodies, and small granules, reminiscent of neuroendocrine granules. The histogenetic origin of stromal cells is currently unclear. Sources of origin that have been proposed include microglia, histiocytes, neuroendocrine cells, endothelium, astrocytes, choroid plexus epithelium and haematopoietic cells {1167}.

Stromal and capillary endothelial cells differ significantly in their antigen expression patterns. Stromal cells lack endothelial cell proteins, and no consistent antigen expression profile has been established for these cells. The expression of pVHL in stromal and not in endothelial cells, however, supports the notion that only the stromal cells are neoplastic {1354}. Stromal cells may express neuron-specific enolase, neural cell adhesion molecule, transthyretin, epidermal growth factor receptor and ezrin {198}. Vimentin is the major intermediate filament expressed by stromal cells {207}.

The stromal cells express high levels of the hypoxia-inducible transcription factors (HIF) –1 and –2 {636}. Constitutive HIF expression in stromal cells is a consequence of increased stability of this protein. HIF-1 and –2 are rapidly degraded by an oxygen-dependent process involving several enzymes, transcription factors and the proteasomal complex {1166,1448}. Proteosomal degradation of HIF-1 and –2 is also dependent on functional pVHL, in stromal cells, the inactivated pVHL leads to HIF-1 and –2 accumulation. As a consequence, HIF target genes such as vascular endothelial growth and erythropoietin are upregulated on the transcriptional level, partly explaining the vascular and cystic phenotype of the tumours and the high incidence of erythocytosis in patients with VHL disease {1167}.

The high expression of VEGF in stromal cells and of VEGF-receptors in both vascular endothelial cells and in stromal cells argues for paracrine and autocrine growth mechanisms of haemangioblastomas {207,844,2403}.

In accordance with the highly vascular nature of capillary haemangioblastoma, intratumoural haemorrhage may occur. Cysts are common, but necrosis or calcification are usually absent. In adjacent reactive tissues, particularly the cyst walls, gliosis with Rosenthal fibres may occur. The tumour edge is generally well demarcated, and infiltration into surrounding neural tissues rarely occurs. Mitoses are rarely seen and the MIB-1 labelling index is below 1%.

Prognosis and prognostic factors
Haemangioblastomas are benign tumours and the results of surgery for single peripherally located cerebellar lesions are often excellent. However, the treatment of multicentric tumours, and particularly, brain stem and spinal tumours may be difficult, and significant morbidity may result. It is hoped that antiangiogenic therapy may offer a medical approach to the treatment of inoperable CNS and retinal haemangioblastomas and early clinical trials are in progress.

Retinal angiomas

Clinical features
Retinal angiomas are the most common presenting feature of VHL disease and are multiple and bilateral in many cases. Retinal angiomas (mean 1.85 lesions, range 0-15) are found in almost 70% of cases {2366}. Patient management is directed towards identifying asymptomatic angiomas as early treatment reduces the risk of visual loss. Approximately 15% of patients have an optic disc angioma. Intraretinal exudation is a common complication of retinal angioma, but may be transient.

Pathology
The benign vascular lesions characteristic of VHL disease are often referred to as "retinal angiomas", but their histopathological appearance is identical to CNS haemangioblastomas (see above).

Prognosis and prognostic factors
The cumulative risk of visual loss has been estimated as 35% in gene carriers and 55% in patients with retinal angiomas at age 50 years {2366}. Potentially sight-threatening complications such as exudation, retinal traction or hemorrhage tend, on average, to be associated with larger angiomas.

Pancreatic endocrine tumours and pancreatic cysts

Clinical features
Pancreatic cysts and tumours are both features of VHL disease. Multiple cysts are the most frequent pancreatic manifestation but are rarely of clinical significance and impairment of pancreatic function is uncommon. Pancreatic tumours occur in 5-10% of cases and are

usually non-secretory islet cell tumours. A high frequency of malignancies has been reported in VHL associated islet cell tumours. Surgery is indicated in tumours >3 cm while tumours <1 cm may be monitored {1295}.

Pathology

Endocrine pancreatic tumours

Approximately 5-10% of VHL patients develop endocrine pancreatic tumours, which may be multiple. The tumours are typically well circumscribed and vary in size from 0.4 to 8 cm (median 2 cm). They are usually confined to the pancreas and exhibit a tan, red/brown, gray or yellow colour.

Morphologically, the endocrine pancreatic tumours are characterised by solid, trabecular, and/or glandular architecture and prominent stromal collagen bands with no detectable amyloid on congo red stains. Sixty percent of the tumours reveal focal or general clear-cell cytology {896}; however, glycogen is detectable in a minority of cases. There may be marked focal nuclear atypia but mitoses seldom exceed 2 per 10 high-power fields. Immunohistochemically most tumours are positive for panneuroendocrine markers (chromogranin A and/or synaptophysin), cytokeratin and S-100; 35% demonstrate focal positivity for pancreatic polypeptide, somatostatin {1389, 1951}, insulin, and/or glucagon; and no immunostaining for pancreatic and gastrointestinal hormones is observed in the remaining 65% of tumours {1357}. Clinically, the majority of tumours are functionally inactive {811}. Dense core neurosecretory granules are evident by electron microscopic examination, and the clear cells additionally exhibit abundant intracytoplasmic lipid. By molecular analysis, tumours show allelic loss of the second copy of the VHL gene {1357}.

No nesidioblastosis-like proliferations or islet cell hyperplasia are seen in the nonneoplastic pancreatic tissue. Occasionally, VHL patients present with pancreatic masses, which are due to metastases of renal cell carcinoma {340,1125}.

Pancreatic cystic disease

Microcystic adenoma and benign serous cysts of the pancreas may occur in 35-75% of VHL patients {811}, usually with coexisting renal lesions. Virtually all affected individuals develop multiple lesions, which may grossly be seen as cysts and microcystic adenomas as conglomerate of cysts ranging from 0.5 to 18 cm or subtotally replacing the pancreatic parenchyma. A histopathological analysis of 21 cysts and 98 microcystic adenomas in nine VHL patients with a known germline mutation revealed 21 benign serous cysts, 63 microscopic microcystic adenomas (size <0.4 cm), and 35 macroscopic microcystic adenomas (size >0.5 cm) {1523}. The average number of lesions per patient was 2.1 benign cysts (range, 0-8), 7.7 (1-37) microscopic microcystic adenomas, and 3 (0-21) macroscopic microcystic adenomas. All cystic lesions show similar histology. They exhibit prominent fibrous stroma containing small vessels and smooth muscle cells. The epithelial lining of cysts consists of cells with clear and/or amphophilic cytoplasm, abundant intracytoplasmatic glycogen on PAS/PAS-D stain, absence of acidic mucin on mucicarmine stain and positive immunoreactivity for cytokeratin and MAK6.

VHL deletions were detected in all types of pancreatic cystic lesions providing direct molecular evidence of their neoplastic nature and integral association with VHL disease {1523}. Interestingly, VHL gene alterations may also be detected in some sporadic microcystic adenomas of the pancreas {2332}.

Other rarely encountered lesions in the pancreas of VHL patients include haemangioblastoma and ductal adenocarcinoma {810}.

Prognosis and prognostic factors

Endocrine pancreatic tumours are usually confined to the pancreas and exhibit a slow growth rate but metastatic tumours have been described {340,416,810, 1125,1357,1523,2332}. Metastasising tumours show a mean diameter of 5 cm. All types of cystic lesions are clinically benign and follow an indolent course. They have an excellent prognosis because malignant transformation is very rare.

Other component features

Papillary cystadenoma of the epididymis

Papillary cystadenoma of the epididymis account for <10% of benign epididymal tumours and an association with VHL disease is well recognised. Although often asymptomatic, they may present as an intrascrotal mass or be detected during investigations for infertility. A survey of 56 male patients with VHL disease revealed evidence of epididymal cystadenomas in 54% and two-thirds of these had bilateral lesions.

Histopathology

Epididymal papillary cystadenomas (ECs) are found in 54% of male VHL patients and 2/3 of all tumours are associated with VHL. They are unilateral in 33% and bilateral in 67% of cases and are mostly located in the head of the epididymis. They usually grow as 1.5 to 2.0 cm solid tan-brown masses with small cystic components {378}. Histologically, the tumours consist of solid cords of cells and dilated ducts outlined with papillae. The cells are cuboidal to low columnar with a ciliated surface and exhibit a glycogen-rich cytoplasm with secretory droplets.

Prognosis

Epididymal cystadenomas are benign and usually do not require treatment. Although no association between epididymal cysts and clinical subtype of VHL disease has been detected, one study {378} found a suggestive (p=0.06) correlation with truncating VHL gene mutations.

Endolymphatic sac tumours (ELST)

Endolymphatic sac tumours (ELST) have only been recognized as a specific component of VHL disease in the last decade. In a large survey of VHL patients using MRI and CT scans, Manski et al. {1402} found that 11% patients with VHL disease had an ELST. Hearing loss is the most common symptom of an ELST, but tinnitus and vertigo also occur in many cases. Mean age at onset of hearing loss was 22 years and in 62% of patients with ELSTs, hearing loss was the first manifestation of VHL. Therefore, endolymphatic sac tumours should be considered as a cause of hearing loss in VHL disease. Hearing loss is associated with larger tumours.

Histopathology

Endolymphatic sac tumours (ELST) are rare intracranial tumours originating from the pars rugosa of the endolymphatic sac, which can grow bilaterally in VHL patients and lead to hearing loss {2240}.

However, they also may occur sporadically. Histologically, the tumours exhibit papillary structures containing non-ciliated cuboidal or columnar cells occasionally with PAS positive globules. Glandular structures containing colloid like fluid may also be encountered. Mitoses and necrosis are rare. A thick fibrous stroma with numerous microvessels, haemorrhage and haemosiderin deposits is frequently seen.

The cells show a distinct expression of CKs (CAM 5.2, 34betaE-12, CK7, CK8 and CK19), but not for CK10/13 or CK20. Vascular endothelial growth factor (VEGF) and neuron specific enolase are usually strongly positive and there is also a weak CD34 immunoreactivity. CEA, GFAP, S-100, synaptophysin and thyroglobulin are negative {913}.

Papillary cystadenomas of the broad ligament and mesosalpinx

In female VHL patients, benign papillary cystadenomas of the broad ligament and mesosalpinx have been described {700}. The tumours are probably of mesonephric origin and manifest as cystic lesions up to 3 cm in diameter. They are bilateral in 50% of cases and exhibit complex papillae lined by a mostly single layer of bland cuboidal to columnar, non-ciliated cells. More recently a broad ligament tumour of probable Müllerian origin and papillary tumours in the retroperitoneum have also been reported {2031, 2379}.

A study on allelic deletion of the VHL gene in papillary tumours of the broad ligament, epididymis and retroperitoneum provided evidence that these rare benign neoplasms are a phenotypic manifestation of the VHL disease {2031}.

Haemangioblastomas

Capillary haemangioblastoma are benign, highly vascular tumours limited almost exclusively to the central nervous system, however, they are occasionally also found at other sites such as peripheral nerves {704}, the pancreas {810}, liver {1853} and spinal nerve roots {973}. Morphologically, they are indistinguishable from their CNS counterparts. The tumours are well circumscribed and contain many small calibre vessels lined by endothelial cells and surrounded by pericytes. They are rich in large, often vacuolated stromal cells which stain strongly for vimentin and neuron-specific enolase

and only occasionally for S100 protein.

Cysts of the pancreas, kidney, adrenal, testis and ovary

Rarely, benign epithelial cysts are found in locations such as testis {252}, ovary {1564}, adrenal, kidney and pancreas in VHL patients. However, in the latter two locations, lesions have to be separated from microcystic adenomas and cystic clear cell carcinomas, respectively.

Genetics

Chromosomal location
The VHL tumour suppressor gene maps to chromosome sub-band 3p25.

Gene structure
The VHL coding sequence is represented in three exons and encodes two VHL transcripts. The major transcript (isoform I) represents all 3 exons, whereas exon 2 is absent from isoform II {1820}. To date, no isoform 2-encoded protein product has been detected and the identification of VHL patients with germline deletions of exon 2 (resulting in the expression of isoform II only from the mutant allele) suggests that isoform II does not encode a functional gene product. The VHL gene specifies two translation products: a full length 213 amino acid protein (pVHL30) which migrates with an apparent molecular weight of ~28-30 KDa, and a shorter protein (~18-19 KDa; pVHL19), which is translated from an internal translation initiation site at codon 54 and produces a 160 amino acid protein. Evolutionary conservation of VHL amino acid sequence is very strong over most of the sequence included in pVHL19, but the first 53 amino acids included in pVHL30 are much less conserved {2417}. The primary sequence of pVHL19 shows little

homology to any known protein.

Gene expression
The 4.7 kb mRNA is widely expressed in both fetal and adult tissues. In particular, the tissue expression of the VHL mRNA and protein does not reflect the limited number of organs affected in VHL disease {415,1241,1354,1822}.

Gene function
The VHL gene product appears to have multiple functions, the best characterised of which is the role of pVHL in regulating proteolytic degradation of the a subunits of the HIF transcription factors, HIF-1 and HIF-2. The VHL gene product has two well-defined protein binding domains. The pVHL a domain interacts with the elongin C protein and this interacts with two further proteins, elongin B and cullin-2 to form a tetrameric VCBC complex {1348,1704}. Structural and sequence motif homologies between the VCBC complex and the yeast SCF (Skp1-Cdc53/Cul1-F-box) complex suggested that VCBC might have a SCF-like function and target specific proteins for ubiquitination and protosomal degradation {1348}. In particular, pVHL was predicted to have a "F-box function" and to determine which proteins were targeted. This model was supported by the observation that the Rbx-1 protein, an essential general component of SCF complexes, associated with the VCBC complex {1031}. Furthermore, the elucidation of the crystal structure of the pVHL/elonginB/elonginC complex demonstrated structural analogy between the F-box protein in SCF complexes and the elongin C binding site in pVHL {2118}. Thus, there was strong circumstantial evidence that pVHL might target specific proteins for polyubiquitination. VHL-related tumours such as RCC, hae-

Table 5.05
Comparison of clinical features of VHL disease, tuberous sclerosis (TSC) and autosomal dominant polycystic kidney disease (PKD). SEGA, subependymal giant cell astrocytoma.

	VHL	TSC	PKD
Renal cancer	+++	(+)	(+)
Angiomyolipoma	-	+++	-
Renal cysts	+	+	+++
Renal insufficiency	-	(+)	++
Cranial lesions	Haemangioblastoma	Calcifications Tubera, SEGA	Aneurysms
Liver lesions	Rarely cysts/angioma	Rarely hamartoma	50% cysts
Pancreas lesions	Cysts Infrequently islet	Rare	Rarely cysts

mangioblastoma and phaeochromocytoma are highly vascular and overexpress a wide range of hypoxia-inducible mRNAs, including VEGF and VEGF receptor, in normoxic conditions {1448, 2050,2403}. Normal oxygen-dependent regulation could be restored by re-introducing wild-type pVHL into VHL null RCC cell lines {731,955,1286,2050}. Many hypoxia-inducible genes are regulated by the HIF-1 and HIF-2 heterodimeric transcription factors. Whilst the β-subunits of HIF-1 and HIF-2 are constitutively expressed, their α-subunits are degraded rapidly by the proteasome under normoxic conditions, but are stabilised by hypoxia. pVHL plays a critical role in regulating proteosomal degradation of HIF-1 and HIF-2α subunits {1448}. Thus, under normoxic conditions, pVHL binds to HIF-1α (or HIF-2α) (via a β-domain surface binding site on pVHL) and promotes polyubiquitylation and proteosomal degradation of HIF-1α {396, 1031,1448,2196}. In the absence of a functioning pVHL, HIF-1α is not destroyed resulting in HIF-1 (and HIF-2)-mediated upregulation of hypoxia-inducible mRNA expression. Thus, the VHL-HIF-α interaction links the SCF-like function of the VCBC complex to the angiogenic phenotype of VHL-associated tumours. While HIF dysregulation associated with VHL-inactivation provides a plausible explanation for the vascular nature of VHL tumours, the relevance to growth suppression is less clear. However, recent reports suggest that HIF-2 may be oncogenic per se {1134,1404}.

The ability of pVHL to bind HIF-1α is dependent on the hydroxylation status of specific proline residues in the HIF-1α protein. Hydroxylation of these prolines is oxygen-dependent and so under hypoxic conditions, the prolines are not hydroxylated and pVHL is unable to bind HIF-1α {977,983}.

In addition to its role in regulation of HIF-1 and HIF-2, pVHL has been implicated in a variety of cellular processes including cell cycle control, regulation of mRNA stability, fibronectin metabolism and microtubule stability {872,1637,1703, 1747}. In view of the role of pVHL in targeting HIF-1 α-subunits for ubiquitylation and proteolysis, it might be expected that further such targets would be identified. However, although some additional targets for pVHL targeted ubiquitylation

Table 5.06
Clinical subtypes of VHL disease and their association with *VHL* gene mutations and pVHL function.

Subtype	Tumour frequency			Mutations	Effect on HIF
	HAB	RCC	PCC		
Type 1	High	High	Rare	Mainly deletions, truncations or missense mutations that affect protein folding	Upregulation of *HIF-α* and *HIF-1* target genes
Type 2A	High	Rare	High	Missense mutations	Upregulation of *HIF-α* and *HIF-1* target genes
Type 2B	High	High	High	Mainly missense mutations	Upregulation of *HIF-α* and *HIF-1* target genes
Type 2C	Nil	Nil	High	Missense mutations	No evidence of HIF dysregulation
Key: HAB = haemangioblastoma, RCC = renal cell carcinoma, PCC = phaeochromocytoma					

have been suggested (e.g. a novel deubiquitinating enzyme and an atypical protein kinase C (PKClambda) {1294, 1645}, the relevance of these to VHL tumour suppressor activity has not been established. In particular, it may be difficult to elucidate whether pVHL functions are independent of HIF dysregulation. Thus, while cyclin D1 transcription appears to be regulated by pVHL, the evidence that this is HIF-independent is equivocal {194,2481,2482}. Although a 1999 report suggested that folding and assembly of pVHL into a complex with elongin B and C is directly mediated by the chaperonin TRiC/CCT {612}, it has since been suggested that retention of TriC/CCT binding is not of primary importance in VHL tumour suppressor activity {816}.

Mutation spectrum

Germline *VHL* gene mutations have been identified in >500 kindreds {358,433, 1381,1821,2483} (http://www.umd.necker.fr). Although a wide variety of mutations have been described, no mutations have been reported in the first 53 amino acids of pVHL30. Germline *VHL* mutations may be divided into three broad groups. Large genomic deletions account for up to 40% of all mutations and the rest are divided approximately equally between intragenic missense mutations and protein truncating mutations (nonsense, frameshift insertions and deletions, splice site mutations). Molecular genetic analysis of the com-

plete *VHL* coding region by direct sequencing and large deletion detection (e.g. quantitative Southern blot and FISH analyses) has been reported to detect mutations in up to 100% of cases {1672,2137}. VHL patients without detectable mutations may be mosaic {2013}. Recurrent *VHL* gene mutations (e.g. C694T, C712T, G713A) mostly represent multiple *de novo* mutations at hypermutable sequences (e.g. CpG dinucleotides, small repeats) {1821}. However, the T505C (Y98H) "Black Forest" mutation common in Southwest Germany and in North American kindreds of German origin is a founder mutation in these communities {245}.

Genotype vs phenotype

VHL disease kindreds have been divided into type 1 (no [or rare] phaeochromocytoma) and type 2 (phaeochromocytoma) subsets. Large deletions and truncating mutations typically predispose to haemangioblastomas and RCC but not phaeochromocytomas (PCC) (type 1 phenotype) {433,1381,2483}. Certain missense mutations that are predicted to disrupt pVHL protein folding may produce a type 1 phenotype, but the majority of type 2 kindreds have a missense mutation. Type 2 families are further subdivided according to the presence or absence of RCC and haemangioblastomas {245,1589,2418}. These genotype-phenotype correlations may be helpful in clinical management with regard to the risk of phaeochromocytoma, but missense mutations are heterogeneous, the tumour risks associated with specific mutations may differ markedly and so risk estimates should be used with caution. Patients presenting with a familial phaeochromocytoma only history (type 2C) may have a mutation that has been detected in other type 2 subsets (e.g. R167Q which is seen in type 2B) suggesting that these kindreds are also at risk for haemangioblastomas and RCC. However, some missense mutations are restricted to type 2C kindreds suggesting that they do not predispose to other VHL tumours. These complex correlations are consistent with the hypothesis that the VHL gene product has multiple and tissue specific functions.

Structural analysis of the VCBC complex {2118} demonstrated that missense mutations associated with a type 1 phenotype often occur at codons within the hydrophobic core mutations and are predicted to cause complete disruption to the pVHL structure. In contrast, type 2A/2B mutations show a trend against hydrophobic core mutations, causing mostly local effects, suggesting that type 2 mutations have a strong bias against total loss of function {2118}. These observations are consistent with the high frequency of loss of function deletion (and truncating mutations) in type 1 families and the rarity of such mutations in type 2 kindreds. Furthermore, in vitro analysis of pVHL function demonstrates partial retention of pVHL binding to elongin C or HIF-1 with phaeochromocytoma-associated missense mutations {393,394}. These findings would suggest that complete loss of pVHL function (generally) does not predispose to, or is incompatible with phaeochromocytoma development. Analysis of HIF-1 regulation by overexpression of mutant VHL proteins demonstrated complete or partial dysregulation with Type 1, 2A and 2B associated mutations, but Type 2C mutants retained the ability to regulate HIF-1 (although fibronectin binding was impaired) {393,394,901}. These findings suggest that HIF-1 dysregulation is not necessary for phaeochromocytoma development in VHL disease.

Further evidence of the complexity of genotype-phenotype correlations has emerged with the demonstration that homozygous missense VHL mutations may cause congenital polycythaemia

syndromes without evidence of VHL disease {58,1700}.

In addition to the phenotypic variability associated with allelic heterogeneity, genetic modifiers may influence the phenotypic expression of VHL disease. Thus, one series suggested that patients with retinal angiomas had a higher risk of cerebellar haemangioblastoma and RCC than those without retinal involvement {2367}. Evidence for genetic modifiers was provided by the observation that there was a significant correlation between numbers of retinal angiomas in close relatives but not between distant relatives. Recently, allelic variants in the cyclin D1 gene have been reported to influence haemangioblastoma development {2481}.

Genetic counselling

VHL disease is a pleotropic autosomal dominant disorder with age-dependent penetrance (penetrance is >95% at age 60 years). Individuals known or suspected of having VHL should be provided genetic counselling. Genetic counselling consists of collecting a detailed family medical history, providing a risk assessment, and arranging genetic testing {1732,1977}. The genetic testing process involves discussing the implications of test results to the patient and other family members, and facilitating appropriate follow-up care {696}. Providers should be sensitive to the possible emotional sequelae of positive test results and the burden of sharing this information with other at-risk relatives {136,781,1016}.

Clinical VHL gene testing is performed with Southern blot analysis to identify large deletions and sequence analysis to identify intragenic mutations. This combined approach is estimated to detect the underlying mutation in greater than 95% of individuals with VHL {2137}. Once the mutation or deletion has been identified in the affected individual, other blood relatives can undergo targeted genetic testing which will reveal that the familial DNA alteration is either present (yielding a positive result) or absent (a true negative result).

First-degree relatives of an affected individual should be offered genetic testing. More distant relatives can also be offered testing if the intervening relative declines testing or is not available. Because

screening for VHL-associated tumours begins in childhood, it is reasonable to offer predictive genetic testing to individuals under age 18 (usually from age 5 years) {4}. Couples at risk for having a child with VHL can elect to have prenatal testing, but uptake of prenatal testing is low. Preimplantation testing for VHL has also been reported {1799}.

Preventive measures

Because of the diverse organs at risk, coordination of clinical care is challenging for individuals with VHL. At-risk individuals should be entered into a comprehensive screening programme in childhood (unless VHL is excluded by molecular genetic testing) {1308,1380}. Recommendations for detection of specific tumours are outlined below {1308, 1380,1972}.

Screening for renal cell carcinoma
Individuals at risk for VHL-associated tumours should have ultrasound examinations or MRI scans of the abdomen every 12 months beginning in adolescence.

Screening for retinal angioma
At-risk individuals should undergo careful ophthalmic examinations every 12 months beginning in infancy or early childhood.

Screening for haemangioblastoma
It is suggested that individuals at risk for VHL-associated tumours should have MRI scans of the head (+spine) every 12-36 months beginning in adolescence.

Screening for phaechromocytoma
At-risk individuals should undergo yearly screening for phaeochromocytoma beginning in early childhood. This consists of blood pressure monitoring and 24-hour urine studies to measure catecholamine metabolites. Measurement of plasma normetanephrine levels is reported to be the most sensitive test for detecting phaeochromocytoma in VHL disease {551}, but is not yet in widespread use.

Familial paraganglioma-phaeochromocytoma syndromes caused by *SDHB*, *SDHC* and *SDHD* mutations

K. Nathanson
B.E. Baysal
C. Drovdlic
P. Komminoth
H.P. Neumann

Definition
Syndromes characterised by susceptibility to phaeochromocytoma and paraganglioma resulting from germline mutations in *SDHB*, *SDHC* and *SDHD*.

MIM Numbers
MIM numbers were assigned according to location prior to gene identification. Therefore, both the locus and gene names and their MIM numbers are given. *See:* http://www.ncbi.nlm.nih.gov/omim {1468}.
Paragangliomas, familial nonchromaffin,1 (*SDHD*)   168000 (602690)
Paragangliomas, familial nonchromaffin, 3 (*SDHC*)   605373 (602413)
Carotid body tumours and multiple extra-adrenal phaeochromocytomas (*SDHB*)   115310 (185460)

Synonyms
Hereditary paraganglioma syndrome; hereditary phaeochromocytoma-paraganglioma syndrome.

Incidence / prevalence
The overall incidence of tumours of the autonomic nervous system including phaeochromocytomas, and sympathetic and parasympathetic paraganglioma has been estimated at ~1/300,000 {138}. The proportion of those tumours due to familial paraganglioma/phaeochromocytoma varies depending both on tumour type and population of ascertainment. The best estimate for isolated phaeochromocytoma comes from a population based study in Germany and Poland and in which 8.5% of patients without family history or other syndromic features had mutations in *SDHD* or *SDHB* {1585}. The rate of *SDHX* mutations in patients with parasympathetic paraganglioma is higher, ranging from 20% in a US clinic based population to over 50% in a Dutch clinic population {142,455}.

Diagnostic criteria
The finding of a mutation in *SDHB*, *SDHC*, or *SDHD* confirms the molecular diagnosis of a hereditary paraganglioma/phaeochromocytoma syndrome. Currently, there are no clinical criteria for the diagnosis.

Age distribution and penetrance
Males and females are affected equally. Age at diagnosis is known only from a limited member of germline mutation carriers. Mean age of diagnosis of phaeochromocytomas and paragangliomas for *SDHB* and *SDHD* mutation carriers in the population based study of phaeochromocytoma was 26 (range, 12-48) and 29 (range, 5-59) years, respectively {1585}. The mean age at diagnosis is, thus, 15-20 years younger than that for sporadic phaeochromocytoma and paraganglioma.

Sympathetic paraganglioma

Sympathetic paragangliomas are derived from the sympathetic chain, and usually located in the chest, abdomen or pelvis.

Clinical features
As described for phaeochromocytoma, the clinical features of sympathetic paraganglioma are a consequence of either the secretion of catecholamines or the size of the tumours with consequent impingement on other structures.

Pathology
The morphology of adrenal phaeochromocytomas and extra-adrenal paragangliomas is usually very similar and there is no reliable pattern to discriminate between them. Finding an attached adrenal remnant or an uninvolved adrenal may be helpful. It can be difficult to separate metastasising paragangliomas from multicentric paragangliomas. As in the adrenal medulla, there are no reliable criteria for predicting malignancy. However, the frequency of malignancy is significantly higher in sympathetic tumours with extra-adrenal location. Indicators of malignancy are the same as described for phaeochromocytomas in the adrenal.

Parasympathetic paragangliomas of head and neck

Parasympathetic paragangliomas are tumours of the parasympathetic ganglia, usually found in the head and neck region, arising from the cell nests located adjacent to blood vessels such as the carotid body or the ganglion jugulare, vestibulare and aortae. Various terms have been used in the past to describe paragangliomas of the head and neck region, including glomus tumours, chemodectomas, carotid body tumours, and nonchromaffin tumours. As glomus tumour is not a specific term and is more often used to describe a histologically different, benign, nonendocrine cutaneous tumour arising from neuromyoepithelial cells surrounding the cutaneous arteriovenous anastomosis {203}, it is best to define these tumours as paraganglioma based on the anatomical location (e.g. carotid paraganglioma, jugulotympanic paraganglioma or vagal paraganglioma).

Clinical features
The symptoms and signs in head and neck paragangliomas (HNP) depend on the anatomical locations of the tumours {2478}. The carotid body is the most common location of the HNPs followed by vagal, jugular, tympanic and laryngeal paragangliomas. The most common presentation of HNPs is a slow-growing painless mass in the neck and a visible bulge in the oropharynx. The neck mass in carotid body paragangliomas is movable from side to side but not up and down and may also have a pulsatile character. A thorough examination for a primary tumour of thyroid, oropharynx, and nasopharynx is necessary, since metastasis to a cervical node is a much more frequent cause of a neck mass than HNPs. The HNPs may cause cranial nerve defects that may present as weakness of tongue and as shoulder drop. Vocal cord paralysis is a common presenting sign of laryngeal paragangliomas. Jugular paragangliomas may

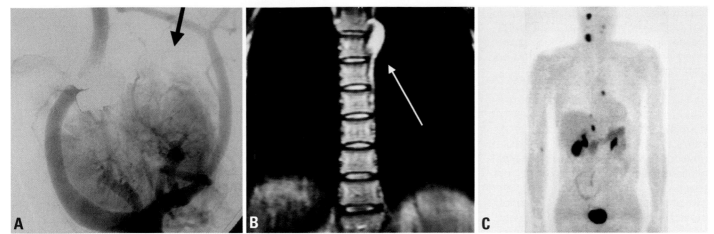

Fig. 5.27 SDHX. **A** MRI angiography demonstrating an intercarotid well vascularized tumour (carotid parasympathetic paraganglioma or glomus carotid tumour) in a carrier of a SDHD mutation. **B** Coronal thoracic MRI demonstrating a tumour of the upper thoracic part of the sympathetic trunk. **C** 18-Fluoro DOPA positron emission tomography (DOPA PET) of a carrier of SDHD mutation. Uptake is visible in the left skull base, the right carotid body, after parasympathetic paraganglioma resection in remnant of the contralateral carotid body, in projection of the cardiac atria, and the right adrenal gland. Uptake in all locations has been confirmed by MRI.

cause defects in cranial nerves IX, X and XI and may lead to hearing loss, tinnitus and balance abnormalities. Intracranial involvement is also possible and may lead to signs of increased intracranial pressure {1565}. Unlike paragangliomas in the abdomen, the HNPs are usually biochemically silent. Malignancy as indicated by local invasion or metastases is seen in less than 10% of the cases {1193}. The number and location of the tumours can be reliably identified using computerised tomography (CT) and magnetic resonance imaging (MRI). Conventional angiography or MR angiography can be of confirmatory value in the differential diagnosis because HNPs are extremely vascular. Similar to phaeochromocytoma, 18-fluoro dopa PET is highly sensitive for the diagnosis of HNPs and an ideal method for documentation of PGL syndromes with multiple tumours in more than one region of the body. Multiple HNPs strongly suggest a genetic predisposition.

Pathology

Morphologically, all paragangliomas are closely related to one another and to phaeochromocytomas of the adrenal gland. Hereditary paragangliomas are frequently bilateral/multicentric, exhibit an equal sex ratio and occur in a slightly younger age group than sporadic tumours {1584}. The rate of multifocal disease in patients with familial paragangliomas was reported to be about 40-50% reaching 78% in vagal paragangliomas {455,1583}. The most frequently

occurring familial paragangliomas are carotid body paragangliomas, followed by jugular and vagal paragangliomas {455,2288}. Furthermore, sympathetic paragangliomas also can occur in association with familial paragangliomas of the head and neck region {1379}.

Grossly, paragangliomas are fairly well circumscribed, rubbery-firm tumours with a fibrous pseudocapsule and tan to purple colour. The histological and immunohistochemical features of familial paragangliomas are similar to those of sporadically occurring tumours and as described for sympathetic tumours {994,1249}. However, in general, parasympathetic paragangliomas usually exhibit a pronounced „Zellballen" appearance and sheets of cells or spindle cell patterns are less commonly seen. Furthermore, intracytoplasmic hyaline globules are rare and some tumours may show prominent perivascular sclerosis or fibrosis. In other cases, marked dilation of the tumour vessels creates an angiomatous appearance. Nuclear pleomorphism and cellular hyperchromatism may be seen and should not be considered evidence of malignancy.

Several malignant parasympathetic paragangliomas in patients with inherited tumour forms have been reported {460, 1249,1499,1999}. As with tumours of the sympathetic paraganglia, there are no reliable histological criteria for predicting malignant behaviour. The malignant potential of the tumour is determined by the presence of local, regional or distant metastases. Numerous mitoses, exten-

sive vascular invasion and central necrosis of cell nests have been associated with malignancy.

Prognosis and prognostic factors

The head and neck paragangliomas grow slowly, metastasise rarely and may remain asymptomatic in certain individuals; the autopsy incidence of HNPs is much higher than their clinical incidence {138}. Surgery is the main mode of clinical management for symptomatic HNPs and leads to a complete cure if there is no metastasis or residual disease. However, surgical management of HNPs can result in mortality in less than 2% of the cases and in morbidity in approximately 40% of the cases, which is often caused by cranial nerve injury and cerebral ischaemic events. The benefits of pre-operative embolisation to reduce blood loss during surgery and the irradiation therapy are controversial {1702}.

Phaeochromocytoma

Clinical features

Patients with germline mutations of the *SDHB*, *SDHC*, or *SDHD* gene may develop one or multiple tumours in the abdomen or the thorax in addition to paragangliomas of the neck and skull base. Additional types of tumours have not been reported to be associated with *SDHX* mutations at this point. As mutations in these genes have been only recently identified as associated with cancer susceptibility, this may change in the future. The clinical features of phaeochromocytoma and paraganglioma are a consequence of their growth, along with the production, storage and release of catecholamines.

Phaeochromocytoma (including paraganglioma) has been called the 'great actor', as the presenting symptoms can be misinterpreted as signs of other diseases. The three classic symptoms of phaeochromocytoma are headache, palpitations and sweating {1400}. Hypertension is the major finding associated with phaeochromocytoma, and the blood pressure can be permanently elevated. However, more typical of phaeochromocytomas, and diagnostic, is intermittent hypertension. Hypertensive crises can occur and may result in intracranial haemorrhage or left ventricular failure. Episodes of catecholamine release lead to the sensation of palpitations resulting from paroxysmal tachycardia. During the periods of catecholamine release, patients often complain of headaches. The third classic symptom is increased perspiration, which may result in profuse sweating attacks without a clear etiology. Symptoms can vary and rarely give hints to tumour location; crises that happen after micturition can be due to paraganglioma of the urinary bladder {1705}.

Endocrine diagnosis

The release of catecholamines into the circulation and excretion of catecholamines and their metabolites can be used to make the diagnosis of phaeochromocytoma. Epinephrine, norepinephrine, vanillylmandelic acid, metanephrines and normetanephrines can be assayed in the plasma or the urine. It has been demonstrated that plasma free metanephrines are the single best test for detecting phaeochromocytoma {1277}. For hereditary cases of phaeochromocytoma, urinary fractionated metanephrines provide similar sensitivity (96% vs. 97%) but decreased specificity (82% vs. 96%).

Imaging

Conventional CT scan, MR imaging and MIBG scintigraphy are the classical diagnostic tools for the diagnosis of phaeochromocytomas and paragangliomas. Recently 18-fluoro dopa (or dopamine) positron emission tomography (PET) has been shown to be highly sensitive for abdominal phaeochromocytoma and neck paragangliomas {900, 1668}.

Location

Carriers of germline mutations of the SDHB and SDHD genes can develop tumours of the sympathetic trunk, including the adrenal medulla, as well as of the parasympathetic ganglia. In contrast, a SDHC germline mutation has so far only been found in one small family with paragangliomas of the neck {1599}. SDHB and SDHD germline mutations have been identified both in patients who have only one adrenal or extra-adrenal tumour and in patients with multiple tumours either in one or several parts of the body, e.g. abdomen, thorax, and neck {139, 717,746}.

The tumours can be multicentric and/or bilateral and may be associated with extra-adrenal chromaffin tumours (sympathetic paragangliomas). In a recent study of sporadic phaeochromocytoma patients with no family history or features of associated syndromes, carriers of SDHD and SDHB mutations were found to present with isolated adrenal phaeochromocytoma (60% with SDHD germline mutations and 50% with SDHB germline mutations) {1585}.

Histopathology

The histological structure of paragangliomas occurring in patients with familial paraganglioma syndromes is similar to that of sporadic counterpart tumours. However, no detailed comparative studies addressing this subject are available. Phaeochromocytomas usually are not demarcated by a fibrous capsule and exhibit a prominent vascular network. They show a mixture of alveolar („Zellballen") and trabecular patterns and may contain areas of spindle cells or a diffuse growth pattern. Nests of tumour cells may vary considerably in size and are surrounded by sustentacular cells that probably play a paracrine role. Tumour cells are usually polygonal with sharply defined cell borders, the cytoplasm is finely granular and may be lightly eosinophilic, amphophilic or basophilic and intracytoplasmic. PAS-positive, diastase-resistant hyaline globules may be observed. Tumour cell nuclei may be vesicular with prominent nucleoli and occasionally contain nuclear pseudoinclusions. Some tumours contain cells with moderate to marked nuclear enlargement and hyperchromasia as well as occasional mitotic figures, features which have no impact on prognosis.

Immunohistochemistry

Neuroendocrine cells of paraganglioma are negative for cytokeratins, express general neuroendocrine markers such as chromogranin A, PGP9.5 and synaptophysin and occasionally neurofilaments, neuropeptides such as enkephalins, neuropeptide Y and peptides derived from proopiomelanocortin. Synaptophysin is not an ideal marker to

Table 5.07
Summary of 14 different germline mutations of the SDHB gene as published in literature or found in the Freiburg Phaeochromocytoma Study

Mutation (cDNA Nucleotide)	Exon	Consequence (Amino Acid)	Adrenal PHEO	Abdominal Sympathetic Paraganglioma	Head/Neck Parasympathetic Paraganglioma	Reference
213 C/T	2	R27X		+		{746}
221 ins CAG	2	Ins Q30	+			{746}
270 C/G	2	R46G		+	+	{746}
309 C/T	2	Q59X			+	{138}
345-347 ins C	3	M71 frameshift			+	{138}
402 C/T	3	R90X		+	+	{97}
436 G/A	4	C101Y		+		{746}
526 C/G	4	P131R			+	{138}
708 T/C	6	C192R	+			{746}
721 G/A	6	C196Y		+		{746}
724 C/G	6	P197R		+		{97}
847/849 del TCTC	7	F238 frameshift	+	+		{746}
859 G/A	7	R242H		+		{746}
881 C/A	7	C249X	+			{746}

separate adrenocortical from medullary tumours since focal immunoreactivity for synaptophysin may also be seen in the normal and neoplastic adrenal cortex. Furthermore, enzymes involved in the synthesis of catecholamines such as tyrosine hydroxylase (TH), phenyletha-nolamine N-methyltransferase (PNMT) and dopamine-beta-hydroxylase (DBH) can be localized in the tumour cells. Sustentacular cells are immunoreactive for S100 protein and sometimes for glial fibrillary acidic protein (GFAP).

Similar to sporadically occurring counter-part tumours, there are no reliable criteria to predict clinical tumour behaviour. However, in general, malignant tumours are larger, exhibit a higher mitotic count, local or vascular invasion, coarse nodularity, confluent necrosis and absence of hyaline globules. They also contain a smaller number of sustentacular cells and express fewer neuropeptides on immunohistochemical study than benign tumours {1307}.

Precursor lesions. The precursor lesions of paragangliomas in the setting of para-ganglioma syndromes have not been as well characterised as those in MEN 2.

Prognosis and prognostic factors

Prognosis of phaeochromocytoma and paraganglioma depends on timely performed diagnostic imaging and measurement of catecholamines. The vast majority of these tumours are benign. The accepted criterion for malignancy is distant metastases, as local invasion is not always a sign of malignant phaeochromocytoma. In particular, the multi-focal nature of the tumours associated with the SDHX syndromes may be confusing and may lead to these separate primary tumours being misinterpreted as metastases and hence, malignant. Whether carriers of mutations in *SDHB* have a different aggressive disease and prognosis compared to *SDHD* is unknown. Truly malignant phaeochromocytoma has been observed in a few *SDHB* mutation carriers but not in *SDHD* mutation carriers (Neumann et al, unpublished data).

Genetics

Chromosomal location

SDHB maps to chromosome 1p35-36.1 {1260}, *SDHC* maps to chromosome 1q21-23 {555} and *SDHD* maps to chromosome 11q23 {890}. Pseudogenes also have been identified for each gene.

Gene structure

SDHB, *SDHC* and *SDHD* genes are composed of eight, six and four exons, respectively and span approximately 40 kilobases (kb), 50 kb and 8 kb of genomic distances, respectively {99,555,889}.

Gene expression

SDHB, *SDHC* and *SDHD* are housekeeping genes with TATA-less promoters. Their expression of the SDH subunits may be coordinated by transcription factors, such as the nuclear respiratory factors NRF-1 and NRF-2 {1955}. NRF-1 binding sites have been found upstream of *SDHB*, *SDHC* and *SDHD* {100,555,

889}. NRF-2 binding sites have also been found upstream of these genes. Promoter analysis of the *SDHB* gene indicates that both NRF-1 and NRF-2 are required for normal gene expression. This suggests that NRF-1 and, to a lesser extent, NRF-2 coordinate the expression of the complex II genes.

Gene function

SDHB, *SDHC* and *SDHD* encode three of the four distinct subunits of mitochondrial complex II (succinate dehydrogenase; succinate-ubiquinone oxidoreductase). *SDHB*, *SDHC* and *SDHD* encode 280 amino acids (aa), 159 aa and 169 aa and correspond to 30 kDa, 15kDa and12 kDa proteins, respectively. *SDHA* and *SDHB* gene products constitute the hydrophilic catalytic part of the complex. *SDHC* and

Table 5.08

Summary of 29 different germline mutations of the *SDHD* gene as published in literature or found in the Freiburg Phaeochromocytoma (PCC) Study

Mutation (cDNA nucleotide)	Exon	Consequence (Amino acid change)	Adrenal PCC	Abdominal Sympathetic Paraganglioma	Thoarcic Sypathetic Paraganglioma	Head/Neck Parasympathetic Paraganglioma	Reference
3 G/C	1	M1I				+	{107}
14 G/A	1	W5X	+		+	+	{746}
33 C/A	1	C11X	+		+	+	{746}
36,37 del T	1	Frameshift	+	+		+	{746}
52+2 T/G (IVS1+2)	Intron	Splice defect	+			+	{139,746}
54 ins C	2	Frameshift				+	{2201}
64 C/T	2	R22X				+	{715}
94 del TC	2	Frameshift	+	+			{97}
95 C/G or 95 C/A	2	S32X				+	{1504}
106 C/T	2	Q36X				+	{139}
112 C/T	2	R38X	+		+	+	{139,717,746}
120 ins C	2	Frameshift				+	{2201}
129 G/A	2	W43X				+	{325}
191,192 del TC	3	Frameshift				+	{107}
208 A/G	3	R70G				+	{2201}
242 C/T	3	P81L				+	{139}
274 G/T	3	D92Y	+	+		+	{139,455,746}
277 del TAT	3	del Y93				+	{107}
284 T/C	3	L95P				+	{455,2201}
305 A/T	3	H102L				+	{139}
325 C/T	4	Q109X				+	{138}
337 ins T	4	Frameshift				+	{1504}
337-340 del GACT	4	Frameshift				+	{325}
341 A/G	4	Y114C				+	{1504}
361 C/T	4	Q121X	+		+		{746}
381-383 del G	4	Frameshift				+	{139}
416 T/C	4	L139P				+	{455,2201}
443 del G	4	Frameshift				+	{1504}

SDHD gene products are hydrophobic integral membrane proteins, which form the cytochrome b and link the catalytic subunits to the mitochondrial inner membrane. Complex II is involved both in the Krebs (tricarboxylic acid) cycle and in aerobic electron transport chain {140}. Succinate dehydrogenase catalyzes the oxidation of succinate to fumarate in the Krebs cycle. The extracted electrons are transferred via FAD (Flavin adenine dinucleotide) and iron-sulfur clusters in the catalytic subunits to ubiquinone and enters the electron transport chain {1958}. The mechanism of tumourigenesis in PGL is unknown. Because sporadic carotid body paragangliomas develop in increased frequency among high altitude dwellers, it has been hypothesised that mitochondrial complex II may play an important role in oxygen sensing. This hypothesis is partly supported by the finding of increased expression of hypoxia-inducible genes in a phaeochromocytoma tumour with an SDHD mutation {715}.

Mutation spectrum

Germline heterozygous, inactivating mutations in SDHB, SDHC and SDHD genes cause hereditary paraganglioma (PGL) {97,107,139,325,1504,1599}. Mutations in these three genes account for at least 70% of familial, 8% of non-familial HNPs and 8% of non-syndromic, non-familial adrenal phaeochromocytomas and extra-adrenal paragangliomas {142}. Amongst mutations in the three genes, SDHD mutations are the leading cause of HNPs, whereas SDHD and SDHB mutations may contribute equally to the adrenal phaeochromocytomas and extra-adrenal paragangliomas. Only one SDHC coding region mutation has been reported. Paragangliomas are transmitted only through fathers in PGL1 (SDHD) families suggesting a role for genomic imprinting in the regulation of SDHD gene expression {2293}. SDHB and SDHC genes do not display parent of origin effects. There are strong founder effects in the etiology of HNPs in the Netherlands, where three SDHD mutations account for nearly all of their heritable HNPs {455,2201}. Currently, there is no evidence for an increased risk of developing other tumour types in individuals with SDHB, SDHC and SDHD mutations.

In SDHD, mutations are observed throughout the four exons, whereas in

Table 5.09
Cancer susceptibility syndromes associated with the pathogenesis of phaeochromocytoma and paragangliomas.

Syndrome	Gene	Chromosome	Adrenal Pheo	Abdominal Sympathetic Paraganglioma	Thoracic Sympathetic Paraganglioma	Head/Neck Parasympathetic Paraganglioma
PGL 1	SDHD	11q23	++	++	+	++
PGL 2	Unknown	11q13				++
PGL 3	SDHC	1q21-23				++
PGL 4	SDHB	1p36	++	++	++	++
VHL	VHL	3p25-26	++	++	+	ER
MEN 2	RET	10q11.2	++	ER		ER
NF 1	NF1	17q11	+			
Carney triad	Unknown	unknown				+

++/+: Observed in normal/decreased frequency, ER: exceptionally rare in association with this syndrome.

SDHB, mutations have been identified in exons 2, 3, 4, 6 and 7, but not in exons 1, 5, and 8. The data are currently too scarce to make inferences about possible hot spots and genotype-phenotype correlations.

Genetic counselling and preventive measures

In the absence of clinical or molecular features of MEN 2, neurofibromatosis type 1 or von Hippel-Lindau syndrome, the presence of a mutation in the SDHX genes should be considered upon presentation of isolated or familial paraganglioma or phaeochromocytoma {717, 1585}. In other words, based on the population-based study on apparently isolated phaeochromocytoma {1585}, all presentations of phaeochromocytoma or paraganglioma, irrespective of syndromic features of family history, should be offered genetic testing for the SDHX, VHL and RET genes.

Clinical testing is currently available for mutations in the SDHD and SDHB genes and should start with an individual who has had a phaeochromocytoma or paraganglioma in order to identify the familial mutation (See GeneTests for a list of laboratories http://www.genetests.org/-servlet/access). A negative test result does not rule out a hereditary syndrome and family members may still be at risk. Once a familial mutation is identified, subsequent predictive testing is possible

with high accuracy. Development of paragangliomas occurs primarily in adulthood, however, there are published reports of individuals diagnosed as young as age 5, indicating that testing of minors is reasonable {197,1453,1585, 2288}.

Because phenotypic expression of the SDHB gene does not demonstrate parent-of-origin effect, families can be counselled regarding classic autosomal dominant inheritance {97}. Families with SDHD mutations must be counselled regarding autosomal dominant inheritance of the mutant allele, but that individuals who inherit the allele from their mother are unlikely to develop tumours {2293}. It must be stressed that the children of men who have inherited the mutant allele from their mother are at 50% risk of carrying the mutant allele and at risk for tumour development. The exact penetrance of mutations in SDHD and SHDB is not known.

Neurofibromatosis type 1

D.G.R. Evans
P. Komminoth
B.W. Scheithauer
J. Peltonen

Definition

Type 1 neurofibromatosis (NF1) makes up 90% of the genetic disorders known clinically as the neurofibromatoses. NF1 is inherited in an autosomal dominant manner and gene penetrance is such that almost all cases show sufficient evidence of the disorder to allow diagnosis in childhood {945}. The condition is characterised by tumour and pigmentary involvement of the neural crest and bony dysplasia. Neurofibromas occur widely throughout the body, but characteristically in the skin. Café au lait patches and axillary/groin freckling are near constant. Other tumours include optic nerve and other brain stem gliomas, phaeochromocytoma, carcinoid and malignant peripheral nerve sheath tumours.

MIM No.
162200
See: http://www.ncbi.nlm.nih.gov/omim {1468}.

Synonyms
Von Recklinghausen disease, peripheral neurofibromatosis, NF1

Incidence/prevalence

NF1 has a birth incidence of 1 in 2,500-3,300 {434,945} and a prevalence of 1 in 4,150-4,950 {945}. Several major studies have addressed this. A study in South Wales (UK) found the above frequency in a population of 280,000 people. A large US study by Crowe and colleagues esti-

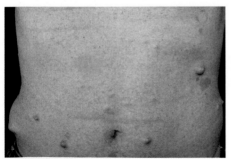

Fig. 5.28 Café au lait spots and subcutaneous neurofibromas in a 44 year old man with neurofibromatosis type 1 who had a benign adrenal phaeochromocytoma.

mated incidence at 1 in 2,500 {434}, but this was contaminated with NF2 patients. The highest frequency was reported in an Israeli study of military recruits with a prevalence of around 1 per thousand {794}.

Diagnostic criteria

The diagnostic criteria for NF1 (see table 5.10) are unlikely to lead to misdiagnosis or confusion {2}. They were originally laid out at the 1986 National Institutes of Health (NIH) consensus conference and have since been ratified by the National Neurofibromatosis Foundation (NNFF) working party. Patients with segmental neurofibromatosis can fulfil these criteria and clinicians should note any segmental involvement. Our own use of these criteria in over 740 patients and in a large North American database has lent further support for them {474,1462}.

Skin lesions

Age distribution and penetrance

Skin lesions are critical in the diagnosis of NF1, with café au lait patches being present from birth and nearly every affected child has 6 or more by 5 or 6 years of age {947,1462}. Cafe au lait patches are usually the first feature of NF1 in most affected patients. They are usually seen in the first year of life and increase in number and size until the early teens {947,1462}. Axillary and inguinal freckling usually follows some time afterwards although it may be present as early as 3 years of age. Around 90% of patients show freckling by adulthood {1462}. Plexiform tumours are often visible from birth with diffuse involvement of the skin and underlying structures. Externally visible plexiform neurofibromas occur in approximately 25% of cases {947,1462}. Cutaneous tumours typically start to occur at puberty but may well be present before that, and are present in >95% of adult patients. Subcutaneous tumours are less frequent, but show a similar age-dependent progression to their cutaneous counterparts.

Clinical features

In childhood, café au lait patches are smaller, as reflected in the diagnostic criteria, but they become larger and may merge with one another. They have a straight rather than ragged border, the so called "coast of California" as opposed to "Coast of Maine" seen in McCune-Albright syndrome. They often fade in later life against the generally darker "dirtier" looking skin and may be less easy to recognise. They are flat and not associated with hair or malignant transformation. Freckling occurs in non-sun exposed skin typically in the axilla more frequently than the groin, and this usually appears later than the café au lait spots. Neurofibromas on and under the skin are the characteristic feature of NF1. Plexiform tumours are often visible from birth with diffuse involvement of the skin and underlying structures. About 2-3% of patients have unsightly plexiform tumours affecting the head and neck. The overlying skin is often hyperpigmented and loses its elasticity. Cutaneous tumours usually start as soft, often purplish coloured areas on the skin, but can

Table 5.10
Diagnostic criteria for NF1. Two or more must be present.

1. Six or more *cafe au lait* macules, the greatest diameter of which is more than 5 mm in prepubertal patients and more than 15 mm in postpubertal patients.
2. Two or more neurofibromas of any type, or one plexiform neurofibroma.
3. Axillary or inguinal freckling.
4. Optic glioma.
5. Two or more Lisch nodules.
6. A distinctive osseous lesion such as sphenoid dysplasia or pseudarthrosis.
7. A first-degree relative with NF1 according to the preceding criteria.

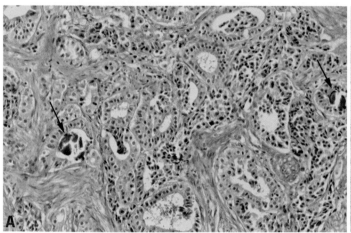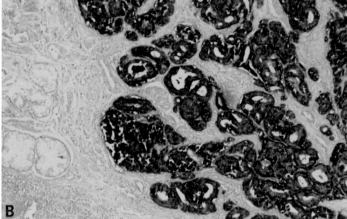

Fig. 5.29 Type 1 neurofibromatosis. **A** Somatostatinoma in a patient with neurofibromatosis type 1. Note the glandular structure of the tumour and the psammoma-like bodies (arrows). PAS stain. **B** Same tumour as illustrated in A stained for somatostatin.

evolve into unsightly warty outgrowths. Subcutaneous tumours occur as fusiform swellings on more major nerve routes and can be painful to touch. The deeper fusiform subcutaneous and plexiform tumours may undergo malignant change to malignant peripheral nerve sheath tumour (MPNST). Lifetime risk could be as high as 10% {1360,1462}. About 5% of patients develop xanthogranulomas aged 2-5 years, and these are associated with an increased risk of juvenile chronic myeloid leukaemia. Although the risk of malignant change in visible cutaneous tumours is probably small, it likely warrants monitoring of skin lesions. Although not strictly skin lesions, iris Lisch nodules (benign hamartomas) occur early in childhood and usually precede the appearance of cutaneous neurofibromas {587}. Ophthalmic slit lamp examination is therefore a useful diagnostic aid in equivocal cases.

Pathology
Café au lait macule
Macroscopically, *café au lait* macules vary greatly in size, millimetres to many centimetres. Flat and smooth bordered, they vary in colour from light to dark brown. *Café au lait* macules spots are not diagnostic of neurofibromatosis. Solitary examples are common in normal individuals. Histologically, they feature basilar hyperpigmentation with or without super-basilar melanosis. A minor degree of melanocytic hyperplasia may be seen. The macules are characterized by the presence of giant (2-6 micron) melanosomes within the melanocytes and at times in keratinocytes as well. Such

melanosomes are not limited to neurofibromatosis but may also be seen in Albright syndrome, in occasional examples of lentigo simplex and nevus spilus as well as in dysplastic nevi. Microscopically, they appear as markedly pigmented, rounded cytoplasmic bodies derived by fusion of primary melanosomes or secondary lysosomal residual bodies {1005}.

Neurofibroma
Neurofibromas are benign nerve sheath tumours composed largely of Schwann cells in the various neurofibroma types. All can be seen in NF1 including localized cutaneous, diffuse cutaneous, localized intraneural, plexiform, massive soft tissue, and visceral examples. Their clinicopathologic features have recently been summarized {1968}.
Localised cutaneous neurofibromas are common in NF1 and affect the dermis and subcutis and show no site predilection. Nodular or polypoid and unencapsulated, they infrequently exceed 2 cm. Whether sporadic or syndrome-associated, the microscopic features are similar. They consist mainly of uniform, spindle-shaped Schwann cells with barely discernible processes and delicate elongate or sinuous nuclei. Such neurofibroma show no tendency to malignant change.

Diffuse cutaneous neurofibroma.
This uncommon variant presents in children, and 10% are NF1 associated. They consist of sizable, diffuse plaque-like thickenings of dermis and subcutaneous tissue often of the head and neck region. They tend to nondestructively infiltrate

the dermis with extention into subcutaneous tissue. Pseudo-Meissnerian corpuscles are commonly seen as are minor plexiform components. Such tumours rarely undergo malignant change.
Localized intraneural neurofibroma infrequently involve skin. They affect spinal, cranial, or autonomic nerves. The neurofibroma cells grow within the nerve, transforming it into a fusiform mass. Such neurofibromas infrequently undergo malignant change.

Plexiform neurofibroma.
This characteristic tumour occurs almost exclusively in NF1 and generally affects sizable nerves. Cutaneous lesions are often part of diffuse neurofibromas, but they may occur in pure form. Occasional, usually small, tumours lack an NF1 association; these presumably result from a local mutation. Involvement of branching nerves often form worm-like tangles. Approximately 2-5% of plexiform neurofibromas undergo malignant change.
Neurofibromas vary in cellularity and in content of stromal mucin. The cells feature ovoid to elongate, often curved nuclei, scant cytoplasm and indiscernible processes. Accompanying mast cells are commonly seen. Melanin-containing cells are rare. Variations in the cell pattern include structures resembling Wagner-Meissner corpuscles or Pacinian corpuscles. Nodules of pure Schwann cells may be seen in plexiform tumours. Neurofibromas are generally diploid {1912}. All neurofibromas are S-100 protein immunoreactive. Leu-7 and collagen IV or laminin staining is frequent. As a rule, MIB-1 labelling indices are low,

often less than 1% {1087}. Ultrastructurally, the neoplastic Schwann cells are well-differentiated {578}.

Malignant peripheral nerve sheath tumour

Malignant peripheral nerve sheath tumours (MPNST) are uncommon tumours varying greatly in clinicopathologic features {1968}, about 50% are NF1-associated. Cutaneous MPNST is very rare {444,698,1510}; skin involvement is usually secondary to larger underlying tumours. Grossly, MPNST as a whole form globoid or fusiform masses, not all of which are nerve-associated. Approximately half of the tumours originate in neurofibromas of intraneural or plexiform type. Pathologically, they show a broad spectrum. Most are high grade, poorly differentiated and aneuploid. Only half can be shown to exhibit schwannian differentiation by immunohistochemical methods. The minority show perineurial features {893}. The epithelioid subtype shows no NF1 association. Particularly associated with NF1, however, are tumours exhibiting mesenchymal primarily rhabdomyosarcomatous differentiation ("Triton tumour") {2416} or differentiation toward mucinous, squamous, or neuroendocrine epithelium ("glandular MPNST") {2416}. As a rule, MPNSTs are highly aggressive tumours with a poor prognosis.

Prognosis and prognostic factors

Life expectancy in NF1 is reduced by an average of around 15 years partly due to excess deaths due to MPNST {1798, 2102}. Early detection and complete excision of MPNST is essential. They usually present with rapid growth or pain. The vast majority of skin tumours remain benign and usually become dormant after a period of fairly rapid evolution. Excision of tumours is often undertaken for cosmetic reasons, but is particularly problematic for plexiform tumours due to the indistinct borders and poor healing of the involved skin.

Duodenal endocrine lesions (carcinoid)

Age distribution and penetrance

Carcinoid tumours occur in NF1 with a frequency of around 1% {947}. A series of 27 patients with NF1 and duodenal carcinoids showed a peak incidence in the fourth and fifth decades {777}. Many patients with carcinoid and NF1 have a co-existent phaeochromocytoma.

Clinical features

Carcinoid tumours while predominantly occurring in the duodenum in NF1 very rarely also occur in other organs derived from the embryonic foregut such as the stomach, pancreas, thyroid and bronchus as well as elsewhere in the small intestine. Carcinoid or "somatostatinoma" syndromes are extremely rare. Duodenal tumours may present with obstructive jaundice, intestinal obstruction and or bleeding. As many as 50% of all duodenal somatostatinomas occur in the context of NF1 {464} and an association with NF1 is especially observed when the tumour is located in the ampullary region.

Pathology

Neuroendocrine tumours of the duodenum in NF1 patients are usually solitary and are located in the periampullary region. They may display a polypoid growth but infiltration of the sphincter of Oddi, the duodenal wall or head of the pancreas may also occur {464,2115}. The tumours have a mean diameter of 2 cm.

Histologically, they typically exhibit well-formed tubulo-glandular structures with some evidence of luminal secretion {776} and contain characteristic PAS-positive psammoma bodies composed of calcium apatite crystals in 66% of cases {34}. Immunohistochemically, they express neuroendocrine markers (but in 50% are negative for chromogranin A), cytokeratins and label strongly with somatostatin (representing non-functioning "pure" somatostatinomas) with rare single cells expressing other hormones (e.g. calcitonin, pancreatic polypeptide, ACTH, insulin) {2115}. This is in contrast to sporadically occurring somatostatinomas, which frequently display a multihormonal expression pattern {264}.

By electron microscopy, the neoplastic cells show signs of intestinal differentiation (microvilli, glycocalyceal bodies, filamentous core rootlets) as well as of neuroendocrine differentiation (D-type secretory granules, whorls of neurofilaments). These tumours are seldom associated with a recognisable "somatostatin syndrome" (diabetes, diarrhoea and biliary lithiasis) {768}, but often present with obstructive jaundice, duodenal obstruction, weight loss or gastrointestinal bleeding.

A genomic examination of a single resected somatostatinoma of a NF1 patient showed neither KRAS nor TP53 gene mutations {1019}.

Other tumours which may be encountered in the duodenum of NF1 patients include gastrointestinal stromal tumours, gangliocytic paragangliomas and ampullary adenocarcinomas {329,400, 421, 1039,1900,2124}.

Prognosis and prognostic factors

The endocrine tumours in the duodenum mostly remain localised but do metastasize in 27% of cases mainly to lymph nodes (88%) or the liver. However, they appear to be less aggressive than their pancreatic and sporadically occurring duodenal counterpart tumours which frequently exhibit a malignant clinical behaviour {813,2091}. The risk of metastasis significantly increases with tumours larger than 2.0 cm {2190}.

Phaeochromocytoma

Age distribution and penetrance

Phaeochromocytomas occur in <1% of NF1 patients, predominantly in the fourth and fifth decades, similar to carcinoids. About 5% of phaeochromocytoma patients have NF1 and inherited forms of these tumours are more frequently associated with MEN type 2 or VHL disease.

Clinical features

Headache is the most common presenting feature of phaeochromocytoma occurring in about 60% of patients. The headaches are usually frontal or occipital start suddenly and usually last about 15 minutes. Associated nausea, vomiting and neck ache are common if there is associated paroxysmal hypertension. Blurred vision and other visual features such as homonymous hemianopia occur in about 10% of patients. Visual scotomata scintillating in time with the heartbeat may also occur. Seizures and transient loss of consciousness due to cerebral ischaemia are later features. About a third of patients suffer from anxiety attacks, tremor and a feeling of impending doom. Cardiac complications due to catecholamine cardiomyopathy are the most serious complication and account for 58% of deaths {1868}. Palpitations due to arrythmias and chest pain due to cardiac ischaemia are manifestations of this. Night or constant sweats often confined to the upper body occur in around 50% of patients and weight loss is a less common accompanying sign {619}. Other vascular effects include claudication and gangrene of limbs. Unusual sites of phaeochromocytoma may cause unusual symptoms such as haematuria from bladder neck tumours. Clinically sustained or paroxysmal hypertension may be detectable with actively secreting tumours, but this is not a totally reliable sign. Any NF1 patient with persistent hypertension refractive to treatment, especially if there is a narrow pulse pressure or where beta- blockers actually increase blood pressure should be actively assessed for phaeochromocytoma {1868}. Most NF1 specialists do not screen their patients with regular abdominal ultrasound and 24-hour urine catecholamines due to the very low yield annually. However, an annual check of blood pressure and suggestive symptoms should prompt a more complete search including MRI or CT {619}.

Pathology
There is no evidence that NF1 related phaeochromocytoma differs significantly from other sporadic or syndrome related tumours from a histologic point of view.

Prognosis and prognostic factors
Hypertensive crisis especially during pregnancy is a life-threatening complication in NF1 patients with phaeochromocytomas. The majority of phaeochromocytomas are benign {392}. Malignant tumours have been described in single case reports {1782,2181} including composite tumours {1573,1949}. Compiled data indicate a malignancy rate of 11.5%, which is somewat higher than in sporadically occurring phaeochromocytomas {2345}. As for sporadic tumours it is difficult to predict malignant behaviour by histology when no gross invasion or metastases are present {2229}.

CNS lesions

Age distribution and penetrance
Large studies where children with NF1 have been screened with MRI or CT

scans indicate that around 15% have at least a unilateral optic glioma {898,1310}. It is unclear how many children who have a scan-detected glioma will ever develop symptoms as studies which have not specifically screened with imaging find much lower rates of between 0.7-5% {947,2062}. Tumours usually present between birth and 6 years of age peaking at around 3-4 years, but adult onset of symptoms does occur. Other brain stem gliomas are less frequent, affecting around 1-2% of patients, but are more frequent in those with optic gliomas {929}. Other CNS lesions include macrocephaly (45% above 97th centile), aqueduct stenosis (<1%) and "Unidentified Bright Objects" (UBOs) on T2-weighted MRI (33%). About 3% of NF1 patients have epilepsy.

Clinical features
Perhaps the most worrysome complication in NF1 is that of CNS tumours and malignancy. The area over which there is most current controversy is in the occurrence rate of optic gliomas and how or whether they should be screened for. The tumours themselves are often benign and vision may not deteriorate at all from presentation. Other features of optic glioma include precocious puberty with a rapid growth spurt or appearance of secondary sexual characteristics and ocular proptosis. It is also unclear whether treatment of even symptomatic cases is warranted {1311,1736}, although radiotherapy and chemotherapy have been shown to be beneficial in several series {1736}. The situation is made more confused by the appearance of focal hyperintensity or unidentified bright objects (UBOs) in many asymptomatic individuals on MRI scanning {249}. The full significance of these is not yet known, as even their association with learning disorders is controversial. Other CNS gliomas do occur but their frequency is probably below 5% even in neurological-based series {225}. Symptoms from these tumours will depend on their position in the brain stem or cerebellum, but signs of increased intracranial pressure may be the first manifestation. Meningiomas and vestibular Schwannomas probably do not occur in excess frequency in NF1 {474,947}. However, the old literature is littered with NF2 cases included in series with NF1. Spinal neurofibromas may cause weakness and wasting, paraes-

thesia or nerve root pain, but symptomatic tumours occur in only 1-2% {474, 947}. Nonetheless, MRI scans reveal evidence of spinal nerve root involvement in up to 60% of patients. A significant proportion of children with NF1 have learning difficulties particularly with reading and or minimal intellectual handicap. Although some studies have shown a large proportion (8-11%) with an IQ<70 indicating mental handicap {620,946, 1819}, population-based studies suggest that fewer children have moderate or severe handicap (3%) or need special schooling {620}. Learning difficulties improve with extra education and IQ in adulthood is better {620,946}.

Pathology
The medical literature describing gliomas in NF1 does so largely in topographic (optic nerve, chiasmal or visual pathway glioma, cerebellar astrocytoma, brainstem glioma) and radiologic, rather than histologic terms. Many reports of optic glioma are of small series and, as in the case of brainstem tumours, draw conclusions without the benefit of biopsy. Thus, it is difficult to critically discuss the pathology of NF1 associated CNS tumours and to meaningfully contrast them with sporadic lesions. Nevertheless, certain distinguishing features emerge.

Pilocytic astrocytoma, the common glioma in NF1, occurs in 15% of cases. It arises at any of the typical loci for this tumour type, but is especially prone to affect the optic nerve as a diffuse enlargement without cystic change. Bilateral involvement is typical. Optic pathway pilocytic astrocytomas in non-NF1 patients, on the other hand, are more likely to be cystic and situated more posteriorly, i.e. in the chiasm {355}. While it has been claimed that the NF1-associated optic nerve gliomas are more prone to massive leptomeningeal extension {2125}, this has not been the general experience. Pilocytic astrocytomas of the optic nerves in NF1 are notoriously indolent. At this location and others, NF1 and even sporadic pilocytic astrocytomas sometimes regress {1694}.

Gliomas of the brain stem in NF1 include focal contrast-enhancing masses consistent with classic pilocytic astrocytomas, but also radiologically diffuse lesions whose histological correlates are unclear. In spite of the similarity to the most common form of brain stem glioma, infiltrating or "diffuse" astrocytoma, this NF1-associated process is unusually indolent {1527,1757}.

With respect to cerebellar astrocytomas in NF1, it has been suggested they may be more aggressive than those occurring sporadically {954}. Whether this is due to inability to clearly distinguish pilocytic from diffuse astrocytomas in all cases is unclear, but some NF-1 associated astrocytic tumours do show indeterminate histologic features.

Rare among other astrocytic tumours occurring in NF1 is pleomorphic xanthoastrocytoma {1642}.

Although there is little literature on the subject, diffuse astrocytomas, in some cases high grade, also occur in the setting of NF1.The same is true of rare cases of gliomatosis {1648}.

The genetic underpinnings of NF1 suggest that abnormalities in the NF1 tumour suppressor gene are likely to be critical in the genesis of pilocytic astrocytomas that arise within the syndrome, and possibly in the much more common counterparts that arise sporadically in the non-NF1 patient. Loss of NF1 alleles occurs in the syndrome-associated astrocytomas, although not the pilocytic neoplasms arising in patients without NF1 {1119}. Loss of staining for the product of the NF1 gene, neurofibromin, has been found in an NF1 associated pilocytic astrocytoma, but not in surrounding parenchyma {1244}.

Unidentified Bright Objects (UBO) are a frequent abnormality in NF1 patients in the brain stem, as well as in the cerebellum and deep cerebral grey matter. They are often multiple, bilateral, foci on MRI. While they are often referred to as hamartomas, they are evanescent in some patients. Little is known about their histological features. One study suggested a form of spongiosis, whose water content explains the brightness in T2-weighted images {500}.

Prognosis and prognostic factors

Prognosis of CNS lesions depends on type, age of onset and location. Simple megalencephaly is common and usually harmless but can lead to increased skull circumference. Hydrocephalus with or without associated tumours may present at any age and can become symptomatic. Nerve root and spinal cord neurofibromas can lead to deficits depend-

ing on location. Gliomas and meningiomas may compromise surrounding structures or nerves causing neurological symptoms. Optic nerve gliomas may lead to visual loss. Pilocytic astrocytomas are relatively benign while half of fibrillary astrocytomas exhibit malignant behaviour. Some gliomas may progress to anaplastic tumours which have a poor prognosis.

Overall, the prognosis of CNS tumours in NF1 patients appears to be slightly better than those of sporadic tumours {2322}, In a retrospective study on 104 NF1 patients with CNS tumours, the overall survival rate was 90% at 5 years. Extra-optic location, tumour diagnosis in adulthood and symptomatic tumours are independent factors associated with shorter survival time {786}. UBOs which commonly occur in children usually regress with age and seem to be benign, however, young children with a large number and volume of UBO should be followed closely with regular MR examinations because of an increased risk of proliferative change {778}.

Bone and other lesions

Age distribution and penetrance

Bony abnormalities are frequently present from birth. While scoliosis typically advances at puberty, there are often underlying congenital bony abnormalities of the vertebrae. Scoliosis occurs in about 5-9% of cases, with about half requiring surgery {947}. Pseudoarthrosis of the tibia/fibula occurs congenitally in around 1-2% {474,947}. Sphenoid wing dysplasia and lamboid suture defects occur in about 1%. Less common non-bony lesions include gastrointestinal neurofibromas (2%), renal artery stenosis (1%) and congenital glaucoma in <1% {947,1462}.

Clinical features

Pseudoarthrosis is the development of a false joint in a long bone or the failure of a fracture to unite after 6 months to a year. It typically occurs in the upper tibia or fibula where 50-90% of such cases are due to NF1 {1541,1561}. However, it may occur in all other long bones. The tibial condition often presents with anterior bowing, and an hourglass appearance may be present at birth. Spontaneous fracture or fracture with minor trauma

often occurs by 2 years of age. Pseudoarthrosis may occur in relation to a bone cyst, sclerotic bone or even rarely, an intramedullary neurofibroma. Pseudoarthrosis can be managed with brace treatment {1768}, electrical stimulation {956} or free vascularised bone grafts {246}. The spine may be affected with scalloping of the posterior margins or dysplasia of vertebral bodies, enlargement of foramina, and defective pedicles. The above abnormalities give rise to a dystrophic scoliosis although idiopathic scoliosis is probably more common. Dystrophic scoliosis is relentlessly progressive involving a sequence of 4-6 vertebrae and cannot be managed by bracing. Surgical treatment with spinal fusion has a risk of paraplegia and pseudoarthrosis. Idiopathic scoliosis can be managed similarly to its sporadic counterpart. However, even in this form pseudoarthrosis may occur after surgery {2370}. Sphenoid wing dysplasia often presents with proptosis and can be associated with an orbital plexiform tumour.

Pathology

Although bony lesions are common in NF1, they show non-specific changes.

Prognosis and prognostic factors

Bony abnormalities may be clinically silent and only evident on x-ray. Congenital pseudarthrosis may be present at birth, with bowing of the tibia being the most typical presentation. Long bone abnormalities may be treated with limb-sparing procedures but sometimes necessitate amputation. Scoliosis in NF1 is often mild, but a subset of children younger than 10 years (especially young girls) develop a more rapidly progressive form of (kypho) scoliosis that requires aggressive intervention to prevent paraparesis. Scoliosis detected during adolescence is much less likely to require orthopedic intervention {428}. Sphenoid bone dysplasia is usually asymptomatic but occasionally can be associated with herniation through the bony defect. Massive osseous and soft tissue overgrowth may lead to facial deformity and disfigurement.

Stenosis of the renal artery (secondary to fibromuscular dysplasia) or coarctation of the aorta may lead to arterial hypertension. Vascular disease and cardiac involvement can cause early and sudden death.

Genetics

Chromosomal location

The *NF1* gene was mapped to 17q11.2 by family linkage studies {2003} and the gene was eventually cloned by the identification of 2 patients with balanced translocations involving the 17q locus.

Gene structure

The *NF1* gene was cloned in 1990 {2325}. It is a massive gene containing over 300 kilobases of DNA divided into more than 50 exons. The gene transcribes for a 327 kd GAP protein containing 2818 amino acids. It is unusual in having 3 embedded genes in one intron, which transcribe in the reverse direction.

Gene expression

The *NF1* gene is ubiquitously expressed in almost all tissues but most intensely in central and peripheral nervous systems {461,2421}. Mutations of the *NF1* gene lead to reduced levels of functional protein, which may not be sufficient for the proper function of the cell. Regulation of the *NF1* gene takes place at multiple levels: transcription, mRNA and protein stability, and mRNA targeting. The levels of *NF1* mRNA and protein, neurofibromin, can undergo rapid changes, and mRNA level may not always directly correlate with the protein level {242,775,894,2455}. During fetal development, the *NF1* gene is transiently expressed in many tissues and is needed for proper histogenesis. Mice homozygous for a mutation in the *Nf1* gene fail to develop the normal structure of heart and various neural crest derived tissues, and die *in utero* {984, 2421,2454}. Selected growth factors, such as basic fibroblast growth factor (bFGF), platelet derived growth factor (PDGF), and transforming growth factor β1 (TGFβ1) have been identified as up-regulators of NF1 *in vitro* {894,1270}.

Gene function

The function of the gene encoding neurofibromin is not fully understood but it seems likely that the gene encodes a multifunctional protein. Neurofibromin has been referred to as a tumour suppressor since cells of malignant peripheral nerve sheath tumours of neurofibromatosis patients may display loss of heterozygosity of markers in and around the *NF1* gene {52}. Somatic mutations of *NF1* have also been found in malignant tissues of persons who do not have neurofibromatosis {98,495,1009,1292,2224}. In addition to playing a role in foetal development, expression of the *NF1* gene has been associated with normal tissue repair in man and mouse {1270, 2431}.

Neurofibromin contains a domain that is related to the GTPase activating protein (GAP). This domain accelerates the switch of active Ras-GTP to inactive Ras-GDP in various cell types {131,209, 475,2431}. However, GAP activity alone is apparently not sufficient to explain the entire function of neurofibromin. Interaction of neurofibromin with cytoskeletal microtubules, actin microfilaments, and intermediate filaments has been demonstrated {210,770,1127,1289, 2432}. For instance, neurofibromin associates with intermediate type cytoskeleton in differentiating keratinocytes during the short period of formation of cell junctions {1127}. Furthermore, a bipartite interaction takes place between neurofibromin and syndecan transmembrane heparan sulfate proteoglycans {932}. Mutations of the *NF1* gene can also lead to altered calcium-mediated cell signalling between cells {1149}.

Mutation spectrum

Mutations have been identified throughout the *NF1* gene. There was an initial concentration on the RAS-GAP domain and reports of the predominance of mutations at this site are self-fulfilling. Most mutations are protein truncating consisting of nonsense, frameshift and splice site mutations. However, some pathogenic missense mutations have been described. 5-10% of patients have large deletions, often involving the whole gene that are easily detectable with FISH. While initial reports of fairly extensive testing using a single technique such as SSCP identified a relatively small proportion (10-20%) of mutations {9}, newer techniques such as DHPLC have boosted detection to 68% {814} and exhaustive screening including a deletion strategy boosts this to 95% {1487}.

Genotype-phenotype correlations

The search for a link between mutation type or location and disease features was initially elusive due to the poor identification rate in most surveys. However, large deletions have now been correlated with a greater neurofibroma burden, as well as dysmorphic features and more mental retardation {1059,1352}. There is also emerging evidence for an elevated risk of MPNST in those patients with *NF1* deletions {2425}. No clear correlation exists for other mutation type or site, although segmental disease has now been shown to be due to somatic mutation {403}.

Genetic counselling and preventive measures

NF1 can nearly always be diagnosed clinically using the NIH criteria. An individual fulfilling these criteria will have a 50% risk of transmitting the disease to their offspring, unless they show segmental involvement {403}, in which case, offspring risks may be substantially below this. Disease severity varies a great deal within families and it is not possible to predict the disease course in an affected offspring unless they have a large deletion. It is likely that there are significant genetic modifiers for NF1 {538}. There are unfortunately no real preventive measures that can be taken in NF1, but early detection of hypertension by regular blood pressure checks may detect complications such as renal artery stenosis and phaeochromocytoma and regular skin checks could detect early malignant change in a plexiform.

Carney complex

C.A. Stratakis
J.A. Carney

Definition

Carney complex (CNC) is a multiple neoplasia syndrome featuring cardiac, endocrine, cutaneous and neural tumours, and a variety of mucocutaneous pigmented lesions {318}. CNC is inherited as an autosomal dominant trait {314} and may involve several endocrine glands simultaneously (adrenal cortex, gonads, pituitary and thyroid, but not the parathyroid glands, the adrenal medulla or the endocrine pancreas), as in the classic multiple endocrine neoplasia (MEN) syndromes {312}. CNC also has some similarities to McCune-Albright syndrome and shares skin abnormalities and some non-endocrine tumours with the lentiginoses and/or the hamartomatoses, including Peutz-Jeghers syndrome in particular, but also Cowden syndrome, Bannayan-Riley-Ruvalcaba syndrome (Bannayan-Zonana; Bannayan-Myhre-Smith), Birt-Hogg-Dubé and neurofibromatosis syndromes {589, 2139,2141}.

MIM Number   160980

See: http://www.ncbi.nlm.nih.gov/omim {1468}.

Epidemiology

Approximately four hundred patients with CNC from all races and with equal distribution between the sexes are listed in the National Institutes of Health (NIH)-Mayo Clinic (MC) Registry {2146}. Most of the patients (more than two-thirds) belong to families in which the disease is inherited in an autosomal dominant fashion. The number of affected members in the majority of these families is small: in the NIH-MC registry, the maximum number of affected generations in a family was 5. CNC is a developmental disorder, occasionally diagnosed at birth {1468,2146}. Most commonly, however, the disease is diagnosed in late adolescence or young adulthood. Abnormal skin pigmentation may be present at birth and is usually the first manifestion of the disease; lentigines, however, do not assume their characteristic distribution, density and intensity until around and shortly after puberty. Heart myxomas or Cushing syndrome due to primary pigmented adrenocortical nodular disease (PPNAD) are the clinical conditions with which most CNC patients present {311,313,1468,2033}. Lentigines and other pigmented lesions, acromegaly, thyroid nodules, gonadal tumours and Schwannomas may be present at the time of diagnosis but are rarely the reason for which most patients seek medical attention initially {2146}.

Sites of involvement

Mucocutaneous involvement in CNC is extensive: lentigines and other pigmented lesions, including blue naevi, café-au-lait spots may be present at birth, and referred to as "birthmarks"; more frequently, however, these lesions develop in the early childhood years. The rare café-au-lait spots in CNC are usually smaller and less pigmented than those in McCune-Albright syndrome; they also tend to fade with time. Their shape is more reminiscent of the neurofibromatosis (NF) syndromes; however, unlike those of NF, café-au-lait spots in CNC do not usually enlarge or merge with time. Depigmented lesions, often mimicking vitiligo, may also be present in patients with CNC. The skin and the mucosal myxomas may also develop at any age; characteristic locations include the eyelids, the external ear canal, the nipples, the external female genitalia. When the myxoma includes an epithelial element (as it occasionally does), it is reminiscent of tumours of the hair follicle in Cowden syndrome and Birt-Hogg-Dubé syndrome. The heart and the breast are the next two most common locations for myxomas in CNC. The cardiac tumours may occur in any of the chambers of the heart, at any age and without any gender predilection, unlike sporadic cardiac myxoma that usually occurs in the left atrium, and in older females. Breast myxomatosis may be extensive and rarely accompanied by another, unusual, benign tumour of the mammary gland: ductal adenoma {317,423}. The adrenal cortex almost always has histologic changes consistent with PPNAD, and commonly the testis and ovary feature lesions, large-cell calcifying Sertoli cell tumours (LCCSCT) and cysts, respectively {1769,2147}. Non-functioning nodules, and occasionally, follicular or papillary carcinoma may be present in the thyroid {1625,2144}. All of these tumours are easily detectable by ultrasonography: LCCSCT appear as micro-calcifications

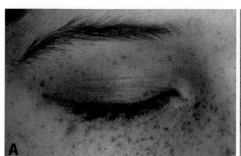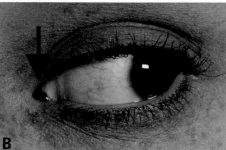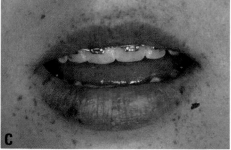

Fig. 5.30 Carney complex (CNC). **A** Characteristic distribution of pigmented skin lesions in CNC: around the eyes, **B** around the inner canthus, and **C** on the vermilion border of the lips.

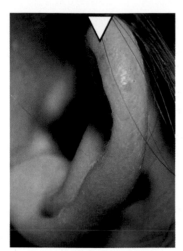

Fig. 5.31 Carney complex. Characteristic distribution of pigmented skin lesions on the helix (arrow) of the ear.

{1769}, and ovarian cysts and thyroid nodules as multiple hypoechoic lesions, the latter often within the first two decades of life {2144,2147}. The pituitary gland is affected in most patients with CNC; however, only 10% develop clinically significant acromegaly due to a growth hormone (GH)-producing adenoma {2146}. Finally, approximately 10% of patients with CNC develop a unique tumour of the peripheral nervous system, psammomatous melanotic schwannoma (PMS), which is often multicentric and may be found along the spine, in the esophagus or stomach, the mediastinum, the retroperitoneal space, and the pelvis {308, 2359}. PMS is one of the few tumours associated with CNC that may assume an aggressive clinical behaviour and metastasize to distant sites, primarily the lungs.

Clinical features

At least two of the classic manifestations of CNC need to be present to make the diagnosis of CNC {2146}. Most patients with CNC present with spotty mucocutaneous pigmentation on the face, vermilion border of the lips, the bridge of the nose, the inner canthi and around the eyes, and elsewhere, particularly the female external genitalia, and one of the two most common types of tumours: myxoma or PPNAD. Heart myxoma may present with symptoms of cardiac insufficiency or embolisation {313}. Skin myxomas resemble neurofibromas clinically and are often misdiagnosed as such histologically. They often present in the form of simple skin tags or they may grow over

several years to a large size and become tender, fixed subcutaneous nodules or masses affecting the trunk and gluteal region.

In the "classic" patient with spotty skin pigmentation (in the characteristic distribution), skin myxoma(s) and symptoms of Cushing syndrome (facial plethora, central obesity, striae), the diagnosis of CNC is easily made {2146}. In a patient with skin pigmentation suggestive of CNC but without a heart tumour or Cushing syndrome, echocardiogarphy or biochemical screening by a dexamethasone-stimulation test may reveal a myxoma or PPNAD, respectively. Ultrasonography has been used to detect some of the other tumours associated with the complex: LCCSCT (multicentric, bilateral testicular microcalcifications), Leydig cell and adrenal rest tumours (these rare tumours may also be present in CNC and almost always are found together with LCCSCT), thyroid nodules and ovarian cysts (multiple, bilateral, hypoechoic lesions) {1769, 2144,2147}. LCCSCT in CNC, as in Peutz-Jeghers syndrome, may be hormone-producing, and cause gynaecomastia in prepubertal and peripubertal boys {1769}. Clinically evident acromegaly occurs in about 10% of patients with CNC {1671,2359}. However, asymptomatic elevated levels of GH and insulin-like growth factor type-1 (IGF-1) and/or subtle hyperprolactinemia may be present in up to 75% of the patients {1671,1788}. Biochemical acromegaly is often unmasked by abnormal results of oral glucose tolerance test (oGTT) or paradoxical responses to thyrotropin-releasing hormone (TRH) administration {2146, 2359}. Somatomammotropic hyperplasia, a putative precursor of GH-producing adenoma, may explain the insidious and protracted period of establishment of clinical acromegaly in CNC patients {1671}. CNC is the only genetic condition other than the NF syndromes and familial isolated schwannomatosis that is associated with schwannomas, the rare and characteristic psammomatous melanotic schwannoma (PMS) {308}. Depending on its location, this tumour may cause pain or neurologic deficits or be asymptomatic. Metastatic PMS to the lungs or brain may cause obstructive lung disease or increased cerebrospinal fluid pressure and death, respectively. Imaging of the brain, spine, chest, abdomen (in particular the

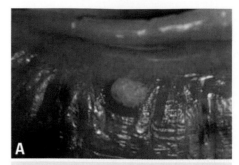
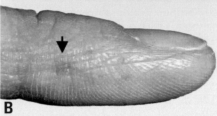

Fig. 5.32 Carney complex. **A** Lesions from a single patient with CNC at presentation: a myxoma on the lip, and **B** pigmented spots on the index finger (arrow).

retroperitoneum), and the pelvis, may be necessary for the detection of PMS, if there are suggestive symptoms. The most recently described tumour that is probably associated with the complex is osteochondromyxoma {310}. The tumour has occurred in the nasal sinuses and long bones, causing painless swelling; it may also be congenital. Rarely, a patient may be diagnosed with CNC at autopsy, usually after a fatal embolus or stroke due to a heart myxoma or, infrequently, due to complications of hypercortisolemia or metastatic PMS {2146}.

Histopathology

Lentigines

A spectrum of abnormalities is seen in the pigmented cutaneous macules {312}, ranging from localised hyperpigmentation of the basal epidermal layer, with or without an increase in melanocytes, to localised presence of coarse melanin granules throughout the epidermal layers, to hyperplasia of the epidermis with elongation of the rete pegs.

Blue naevi

Two types of blue naevi are seen {311}, the usual Jadassohn-Tièche type and the rare epithelioid type that was first described in connection with CNC. The usual blue naevus features elongated, melanin-laden, dendritic melanocytes located among the dermal collagen bundles. The cells have spindle nuclei and inconspicuous nucleoli. The melanocytes of the epithelioid blue nevus are similarly located but differ cytologically from those of the usual blue naevus; they are large and polygonal (epithelioid), and have large vesicular nuclei with a clear chromatin pattern and a prominent nucleolus. The pigmented lesions are often combined naevi, that is, composed of two different melanocytic pigmented lesions that occur side-by-side or are intermingled.

Electron microscopy. The epithelioid blue naevus features cells that are heavily laden with type III and type IV melanosomes and cells in which these organelles are sparse {311}. Nuclei are mostly round and occasionally have indentations. Collagen bundles separate the cells.

Myxoma

The variously located myxoid lesions in CNC (skin, heart, breast and other) show sufficient histologic similarity to suggest that these apparently distinct tumours are the result of a widespread, specific abnomality of an as yet unidentified population of mesenchymal cells {313}. Histologically, the myxomas are typically hypocellular lesions. They feature scattered polygonal, stellate and spindle cells in pools of ground substance. Capillaries are usually prominent. The cutaneous lesions when in contact with the epidermis may induce downward proliferation of the epidermis, which becomes incorporated in the myxoma, resulting in a tumour with mesenchymal and epithelial components.

Electron microscopy. The cutaneous tumour features widely separated polygonal and spindle cells set in a pale-staining matrix containing scattered collagen bundles {313 The nuclei are oval or spindle and deeply indented with pale or peripherally condensed heterochromatin. Some nuclei contain a huge vacuole. The plasmalemma often has microvilli. A basal lamina is not present.

Primary pigmented nodular adrenocortical disease

The gross findings of this remarkable pathology, PPNAD, include 1) decreased, normal, or slightly increased total adrenal gland weight, 2) studding of the cut surface by small (less than 4 mm) black or brown, rarely yellow, nodules

and 3) atrophy of the cortex and loss of normal zonation between the nodules {2033}. Microscopically, the nodules are composed of enlarged, globular cortical cells with granular eosinophilic cytoplasm that contains lipochrome pigment.

Large-cell calcifying Sertoli cell tumour

This tumour ranges in size from microscopic to a mass that may replace the entire testis. It is usually bilateral, multicentric and calcified {1772}. Microscopically, it tends to be ill-defined peripherally. The tumour cells assume a number of patterns but usually have a trabecular or solid element. An intratubular (*in situ*) component may be present. The tumour cells are large and have abundant granular eosinophilic cytoplasm. Mitotic figures are rare. Laminated calcospherites, few to many, often with confluence are a characteristic feature. Two other tumours, Leydig cell tumour and adrenocortical rest tumour, may also be present {312}.

Electron microscopy. The cortical nodules are composed of polygonal cells that have a straight or interdigitating plasmalemma {2033}. Junctional complexes are uncommon. The most prominent organelles in the cells are smooth endoplasmic reticulum, mitochondria, lysosomes and lipid vacuoles. Pigment bodies are prominent in most cells.

Pituitary adenoma

Lesions in the pituitary gland range from invasive macroadenoma to multiple minute but grossly visible zones of abnormality evident at surgery, to microscopic foci of pituitary cell (somatomammotroph) hyperplasia {1671}. Microscopically, the usual adenoma has a diffuse (solid) growth pattern and features round and polygonal cells with a variable amount of granular eosinophilic cytoplasm and a round or oval nucleus. Growth hormone or prolactin or both may be detected immunohistochemically in the tumours.

Electron microscopy. The pituitary adenoma features large, tightly packed somewhat irregular cells with complex interdigitations {1184}. Rough endoplasmic reticulum is abundant and may be disposed in parallel arrays and in short profiles. The Golgi apparatus is conspicuous. Secretory granules, ranging from 200 to 250 nm in diameter, are present in variable numbers.

Psammomatous melanotic schwannoma

This rare peripheral nerve sheath tumour was first recognised when it was found to be a component of CNC {308}. The neoplasm affects posterior spinal nerve roots, the alimentary tract (particularly esophagus and stomach), bone and skin. It is usually black grossly and may be multiple, and occur simultaneously or asynchronously at different sites. Microscopically, the tumour features spindle and epithelioid cells, melanin, psammoma bodies and fat. About 10% of the tumours are malignant and metastasize.

Electron microscopy. The fusiform, oval or stellate cells have long cell processes {308}. A continuous basal lamina that is sometimes reduplicated surrounds the cells. Scattered simple cell junctions may be present. Nuclei are round or oval and deeply indented. Premelanosomes and melanosomes in various stages of maturation are seen. There is long spacing collagen between the cells.

Genetics

Tumour studies have shown extensive genomic instability in CNC component tumour cells, an unusual finding among benign tumours {2145}. Linkage analysis in CNC families has shown genetic heterogeneity, with at least two main loci for candidate genes {326,2145}; others are likely to be found in the future.

2p15-16

A chromosome 2 (2p15-p16) locus was identified first {2142}, but the gene responsible for CNC in that region remains unknown. The most closely linked region on chromosome 2 centers around locus CA2/D2S123 {2142}.

17q22-24 / PRKAR1A

At the second locus, on chromosome 17 (17q22-24), mutations of the *PRKARIA* gene were recently identified {1094}. The *PRKARIA* gene encodes the regulatory 1-alpha (R1alpha) subunit of the protein kinase A (PKA), the main mediator of cAMP signaling in mammals. PRKAR1A is the most abundant subunit of the PKA tetramer {232,2143}.

The predominant type of PKA isoform (type-I versus type-II) in a cell depends on the differentiation and proliferation stage; hence, cellular PKA responses to cAMP can differ significantly depending on the predominant type of the PKA present {2143}. The expression of PRKARIA has been shown to be altered in several sporadically occurring tumours and tumour-derived cell lines from non-CNC patients and the gene was a likely candidate for endocrine and non-endocrine tumourigenesis in CNC. Among the kindreds registered at NIH-MC, about half carried *PRKAR1A* mutations {1095}, although this percentage may be higher among patients presenting with PPNAD only {784}. In almost all mutations, the sequence change is predicted to lead to a premature stop codon {1095}. Both the mutant transcript and the predicted mutant *PRKAR1A* protein products were absent in these cells. The most frequent *PRKAR1A* mutation in CNC is a deletion in exon 4B that results in a frameshift, 578delTG; other frequent mutations are present in exons 2 and 6 {1094,1095}. Nonsense-mediated decay (NMD), in which the cells degrade the mRNA containing a deleterious, premature stop codon mutation prior to its translation, is apparently responsible for destruction of the abnormal mRNA in mutant *PRKAR1A*-carrying cells.

Preliminary data suggested that *PRKAR1A* functions as a tumour suppressor gene in CNC: tumours showed LOH of 17q22-24, and the wild-type allele was lost in associated tumours {1094,1095}. As a result of NMD of the pathogenic allele and LOH of the normal allele, the PRKAR1A protein was not present in CNC tumour cells {1094,1095}. This loss of the most important regulatory subunit of the PKA tetramer was associated with a greater PKA response to cAMP than in non-CNC tumours. Additional data indicate that the loss of PRKAR1A in CNC tumours leads to compensatory increases in the other PKA subunits, type I (PRKAR1B) and type II (PRKAR2A and PRKAR2B) depending on the tissue, the cell cycle stage, and perhaps other factors. This is not unlike the situation in mouse models in which one of the PKA subunits is knocked out {50}. Thus, it appears that the increased cAMP response of PKA activity in CNC tumours is due to the up-regulation of other possible components of the PKA tetramer, type-II regulatory subunits, in particular {2140}. Supportive of this notion also are data indicating that the presence of an abnormal PRKAR1A (complete loss may not be necessary) in CNC tumours is associated with increased PKA signalling in response to cAMP {785}. Interestingly,

in most tumours from the kindred that had this mutation, there was no LOH, indicating that even in the presence of haplo-insufficiency, tumours may develop, presumably due to the imbalance between type I and type II PKA in the affected cells {785}. It remains to be seen how these abnormalities fit in what is known about the effects of cAMP and PKA on growth and proliferation, and whether, indeed, in functional studies, PRKAR1A directly suppresses tumourigenesis, or has a more complicated role in the regulation of other signaling pathways, the cell cycle or, perhaps, chromosomal stability {1865,2143}.

Prognostic factors

Most tumours associated with CNC are characterised by slow growth and show no malignant potential. However, lifespan is decreased in patients with CNC, due to an increased incidence of sudden death caused by heart myxoma or its complications. Other causes of early death in patients with CNC include complications of severe or chronic Cushing syndrome, malignant PMS, and metastatic pancreatic, ovarian and thyroid carcinoma.

Genetic counselling and preventive measures

Clinical and biochemical screening for CNC and medical surveillance for affected patients remain the gold standard for the care of patients with CNC {2146}. While the diagnosis of CNC can be made clinically in classic presentations, mutation analysis for *PRKAR1A* may be used as a molecular diagnostic adjunct when clinical diagnosis is difficult. Further, once a family-specific mutation is established in a known affected, it is advised that other family members be offered testing for that mutation so that relatives who are truly non-carriers can avoid unnecessary medical intervention {2140, 2146}.

In brief, for post-pubertal paediatric and for adult patients of both sexes with established CNC, the following annual studies are recommended: echochardiogram, measurement of urinary free cortisol levels (which may be supplemented by diurnal cortisol or the overnight 1 mg dexamethasone testing) and serum IGF-1 levels {2146}. Male patients should also have testicular ultrasonography at the initial evaluation; microscopic LCCSCT

may be followed by annual ultrasound thereafter {1769}. Thyroid ultrasonography should be obtained at the initial evaluation, and may be repeated, as needed {2144}. Transabdominal ultrasonography in female patients is recommended during the first evaluation but need not be repeated, unless there is a detectable abnormality, because of the relatively low risk of ovarian malignancy {2147}. More elaborate clinical and imaging studies may be necessary for the detection of PPNAD and pituitary tumours in affected patients who do not have overt clinical manifestations of Cushing syndrome or acromegaly {1671,2148}. For the former, a dexamethasone-stimulation test {784} is recommended, in addition to adrenal computed tomography and diurnal cortisol levels {1940,2148}. For the latter, oGTT may be obtained in addition to IGF-1 levels and pituitary magnetic resonance imaging {1671,2359}. Paediatric patients with CNC should have echocardiography during their first six months of life and annually thereafter; bi-annual echocardiographic evaluation may be necessary for patients with history of an excised myxoma {318,2146}. Most endocrine tumours in CNC do not become clinically significant until the second decade in life (although they might be detectable at a much earlier age) and imaging or biochemical screening in young, prepubertal children are not considered necessary, except for diagnostic purposes. However, paediatric patients with LCCSCT (or a microcalcification upon testicular ultrasonography) should have growth rate and pubertal status closely monitored; some might need bone age determination and further laboratory studies {2146}.

McCune-Albright syndrome (MAS)

L.S. Weinstein
M.A. Aldred

Definition

McCune-Albright syndrome (MAS) is defined by the triad of polyostotic fibrous dysplasia (POFD), *café-au-lait* skin lesions, and sexual precocity., caused by activating mutations in the complex *GNAS* locus at 20q13.2-13.3. MAS patients may also develop nodular hyperplasia or adenomas of endocrine glands with associated endocrinopathies or other, nonendocrine manifestations. Some MAS patients only develop a subset of the full syndrome. Mazabraud syndrome is the co-occurrence of POFD and intramuscular myxomas.

MIM No.   174800 {1468}

Synonyms

McCune-Albright syndrome, Albright syndrome, fibrous dysplasia (polyostotic and monostotic); Mazabraud syndrome.

Diagnostic criteria

The diagnosis of MAS is usually clinically obvious and is confirmed by excess circulating levels of one or more hormones (thyroid hormone, cortisol, growth hormone, or estrogen) in the absence of the respective stimulating hormones. FD is usually diagnosed by its characteristic ground glass (but occasionally sclerotic) appearance on X-ray, although it can be confused with osteofibrous dysplasia {1390,1902} or hyperparathyroid-jaw tumour syndrome {319,549,632,809}. In Mazabraud syndrome, FD is associated with intramuscular (but not juxtaarticular) myxomas {1643}.

Endocrine hyperfunction

Age distribution/penetrance

MAS/FD generally is diagnosed within the first decade of life. Penetrance is high but is primarily affected by the specific extent and distribution of mutant cells in each individual.

Clinical features

The classical clinical triad, which has generally defined the syndrome, is the co-occurrence of sexual precocity, POFD, and areas of skin hyperpigmentation (*café-au-lait* spots). However, multiple other endocrine and nonendocrine abnormalities may be present or patients may present with only 1 or 2 manifestations. In girls, sexual precocity usually presents as premature menses followed by breast development and is associated with gonadotropin-independent secretion of estrogen from large ovarian follicles {406,623,642,1442,1827}. Usually, females undergo normal development during adolescence and show normal reproductive function in adult life. Boys present with precocious puberty less commonly than girls. Testicular enlargement often results from maturation and growth of seminiferous tubules {424, 722}. MAS patients can develop nodular or multinodular thyroid disease detectable by ultrasound associated with increased radioiodine uptake and often associated with suppressed thyrotropin levels and varying levels of hyperthyroxinemia {625,1202,1426}. Acromegaly due to growth hormone-secreting pituitary adenomas may occur in 20% of MAS patients and is often associated with hyperprolactinemia {21}. Another less common endocrine manifestation is adrenocorticotropin-independent hypercortisolism, which can lead to decreased growth rate and many other severe problems in young children {457,1442}. Hyperphosphaturic hypophosphatemic rickets or osteomalacia can also occur in MAS and POFD patients and is usually associated with a more general renal tubulopathy {402}. This may result from a phosphaturic factor secreted from FD lesions {402,2441}.

A few severely affected patients (often with extensive POFD and hypercortisolism) also develop other nonendocrine manifestations. Liver abnormalities include severe neonatal jaundice and elevated liver enzymes {2032,2052}. Cardiac abnormalities, which may be associated with MAS include cardiomegaly, persistent tachycardia and unexplained sudden death in young patients. Other abnormalities, which are rarely associated with MAS include thymic hyperplasia, myelofibrosis with extramedullary haematopoiesis, gastrointestinal polyps, pancreatitis, breast and endometrial cancers, microcephaly and other neurological abnormalities {35, 457,1375,1459,2032}.

Pathology

Affected endocrine tissues generally have nodular hyperplasia or in some cases, adenomas that are hormone-secreting {457,1442,2371}. The ovaries have large follicular cysts with no evidence of ovulation. Acromegaly is associated with pituitary adenomas, which may be small {21}, or nodular hyperplasia {1158}. Hypercortisolism is generally associated with macronodular adrenal cortical hyperplasia although adrenal adenoma has also been reported {165,1093}. In some patients the liver shows atypical cholestatic and biliary abnormalities and the heart shows atypical myocyte hypertrophy {2032,2052}. Other pathological findings that have been found in MAS include hypertrophy of the thymus and spleen, myeloid metaplasia with extramedullary haematopoiesis, subtle brain abnormalities, gastrointestinal polyps, and breast and endometrial cancer {457,2032}.

Prognosis

While the vast majority of MAS patients have an excellent prognosis {457,837, 1267}, there are a small number of severely affected patients (often with extensive POFD and hypercortisolism) who present with one or more nonendocrine abnormalities which may lead to markedly increased morbidity and mortality {2032}. These patients may die of sudden death during surgery or illness, perhaps secondary to cardiomyopathy and arrythmia {2032}. MAS patients have the same morbidity from bone disease as those with POFD alone. Often, the endocrine abnormalities are treated medically or by surgical removal of the enlarged endocrine glands. Cyproheptadine, testolactone, tamoxifen, and ketoconazole have been used for sexual precocity with mixed success {581, 623,624,2165} Thyroid disease can be managed with surgery, antithyroid medications, or radioiodine therapy. Hypercortisolism is usually treated with bilateral adrenalectomy. Pituitary tumours are treated with surgery if possible, but can often be managed with a dopamine agonist, long-acting somatostatin analogue, or both {21}. Surgery may be impossible if FD is present in the base of the skull. Radiotherapy in these cases may increase of risk of malignancy in the surrounding bone.

Fibrous dysplasia

Fibrous dysplasia (FD) is a benign focal bone lesion composed of fibrous connective tissue, immature woven bone and, occasionally, cartilaginous tissue. FD may occur in multiple bones (polyostotic FD; POFD) or at a single site (monostotic fibrous dysplasia; MOFD).

Clinical features

MOFD is a common disorder that is often a clinically silent, incidental radiological finding. One study suggested the relative incidence among FD patients to be 70% MOFD, 30% POFD and less than 3% MAS {1570}.

FD lesions are most commonly found in the femur (femoral neck and intertrochanteric region), tibia, humerus, ribs, and craniofacial bones (most often the maxilla) {837,1570,1973}. Other long bones such as the radius, ulna and fibula are involved less frequently while the bones of the hands, feet and spine are usually spared. MOFD is often clinically silent and diagnosed as an incidental radiological finding, which does not require follow-up. More extensive FD can lead to deformities (often producing a limp), pathological fractures, pain and nerve compression {457,837,1973}. Deformities may include leg length discrepancy, outward bowing of the proximal femur (shepherd's-crook deformity), facial asymmetry, orbital displacement and visible or palpable bony enlargement. Deformity of the chest wall may lead to restrictive pulmonary disease {1570,1973}. Pathologic fractures occur frequently and are often recurrent. Pain can result from pathological fractures and

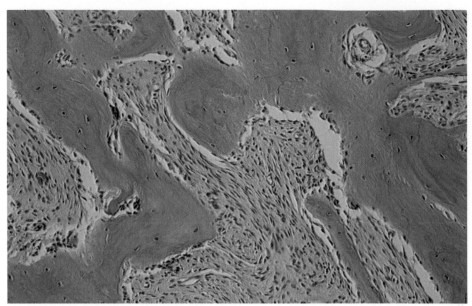

Fig. 5.33 McCune-Albright syndrome. An iliac crest biopsy showing the characteristic 'Chinese writing' pattern of fibrous dysplasia containing whirls of fibrous tissue interspersed with spicules of immature woven bone. Courtesy of Dr. Michael Collins, NIDCR/NIH.

secondary arthritic changes in nearby joints. The most common neurological complications include blindness, deafness and equilibrium disturbances due to compression of the occipital and auditory nerves. High output cardiac failure due to arteriovenous shunting through bone lesions has also been reported {633}. FD lesions occur in the metaphysis or diaphysis and on radiographs appear as radiolucent cysts expanding from the medullary cavity with thinning of the surrounding cortex. Often, there is a ground glass appearance but sclerosis and calcifications may also be present {1361}. Nuclear bone scanning and magnetic resonance imaging {732,964,998} are also useful for determining extent of disease. Active disease is associated with increased serum alkaline phosphatase and other biochemical markers of bone turnover. Extensive POFD may also be associated with hypophosphatemia and renal tubulopathy {402}. Coexistent intramuscular myxomas in Mazabraud syndrome tend to be large and are often located in the vicinity of the FD, usually in the thigh.

Histopathology

FD lesions are thought to be secondary to increased proliferation and decreased osteoblastic differentiation of bone marrow stromal cells resulting from elevated intracellular cAMP levels. FD lesions are primarily composed of fibrous tissue that expands concentrically from the medullary cavity to the cortical bone. Long, spindle-shaped fibroblasts are arranged in parallel arrays or in whirls {767}. These cells are of the osteoblastic lineage, as they express proteins associated with osteoblast differentiation {1832}. The matrix is composed of parallel collagen fibres and in some areas is more myxomatous. Spicules of immature woven bone are embedded within the fibrous tissue. These spicules are surrounded by flat lining cells with retracted cell bodies, forming pseudo-lacunar spaces {1832, 1833}. This retraction is probably due to increased intracellular cAMP, as cAMP produces similar changes in cultured osteoblasts. Unlike normal woven bone, the collagen fibrils at the surface are arranged perpendicular to the bone-forming surface (so-called Sharpey's fibres) {186,1832,1833}. The osseous components in FD contain osteonectin, but not osteopontin or bone sialoprotein, proteins that are present in the matrix of normal woven bone {1832}. The osteocytic lacunae are large with each containing multiple osteocytes (hyperosteocytic bone) {1832}. Changes consistent with osteomalacia may or may not be present within the bony component of FD lesions {186,2213}. The border between FD and normal bone is usually sharp and well demarcated.

The histology of FD lesions varies depending on the location of the affected bone {1833}. Lesions in the axial and appendicular skeleton have a 'Chinese writing' pattern, characterised by thin and disconnected bone trabeculae with interspersed fibrous tissue. Cranial bone lesions generally have a 'sclerotic/ Pagetoid' pattern, with dense, sclerotic trabecular bone forming an uninterrupted network and the presence of cement/ arrest lines similar to those observed in Pagetic bone. Gnathic bone lesions have a 'sclerotic/hypercellular' pattern, characterised by large trabeculae arranged in a parallel array with osteoblasts lining one side of the trabeculae. However, all FD lesions have retracted osteoblasts and Sharpey's fibers, which appear to be hallmarks for FD.

Occasionally, islands of hyaline cartilage are present in FD, probably due to a metaplastic process {767}. Rarely, the cartilaginous component may be a dominant feature (fibrocartilaginous dysplasia {968}). The cartilage may undergo endochondral ossification and, if prominent, may result in the presence of stippled or ring-like calcifications on radiographs. Some lesions of FD contain calcified spherules, a typical feature of cemento-ossifying fibroma. Other lesions, which appear histologically similar to FD, are osteofibrous dysplasia, osteitis fibrosa cystica (which is usually associated with hyperparathyroidism or chronic renal failure), and Paget disease (which develops in older adults). In osteitis fibrosa cystica and Paget disease, there is more active osteoclastic bone resorption within the lesions and no evidence of cartiginous islands.

FD often invades the outer cortical bone through the action of increased numbers of surrounding multinucleated osteoclasts {1832,2442}, resulting in cortical thinning and in some cases, concentric bulging of the cortex. Osteoclast activation is most likely the result of increased interleukin 6 secretion from FD cells. Rarely, these lesions are more aggressive, resulting in exophytic protuberances {524} or soft tissue invasion {1240}. FD is benign and does not metastasize. Rarely, it undergoes malignant progression, most often to osteosarcoma and less commonly to chondrosarcoma, fibrosarcoma or malignant fibrohistiosarcoma {1055,1883, 2435}.

Prognosis

POFD is usually diagnosed in the first decade of life, either due to symptoms or the presence of other MAS manifestations. It usually progresses in early life and then becomes quiescent after the third decade {457,837}, although in some cases FD continues to progress or may be initially diagnosed during puberty, pregnancy or the use of oral contraceptives {1973,2128}. FD rarely undergoes malignant degeneration, most often to osteosarcoma and occasionally to chondrosarcoma, fibrosarcomas or other types of sarcoma {1055,1883,2197, 2435}. Radiotherapy may increase the risk of malignant transformation. Generally, fractures heal well with conservative management {837} although surgery may be required for nonhealing fractures, severe pain or deformity, particularly on weight-bearing bones, or imminent signs of nerve compression {545,756,837,1062,1378,1570}. A recent study concluded that orbital decompression is not required in patients who do not have clinical symptoms due to optic nerve compression {1266}. Bisphosphonates, such as pamidronate, can also lead to clinical and radiological improvement of FD in some patients {352,967,1203,1299,2473}.

Skin lesions

Clinical features

Café-au-lait lesions in MAS are hyperpigmented flat macules that can be extensive but generally do not cross the midline and follow a segmental pattern following the distribution of the developmental lines of Blaschko {818}. Often, these lesions are on the same side affected by POFD. The borders of these lesions tend to be very irregular, as opposed to the *café-au-lait* lesions associated with neurofibromatosis {35}. The pigmentation becomes more obvious with age and may darken after sun exposure. These lesions likely result from Gsα activating mutations and increased intracellular cAMP in melanocytes, which leads to increased melanin production {1077}. Alopecia is rarely associated with MAS {1991}.

Histopathology

The skin lesions in MAS histologically appear similar to those in neurofibromatosis, with no change in the number of melanocytes but an increase in the number of melanin-containing pigment granules. Melanocytes cultured from these lesions have increased numbers of dendrites and melanosomes and increased levels of tyrosinase, the rate-limiting enzyme for the production of melanin {1077}.

Prognosis

The hyperpigmentation lesions in MAS are totally benign and do not lead to any complications beyond their cosmetic effect.

Genetics

Chromosomal location and gene structure

MAS/FD results from activating mutations of Gsα, one of several transcripts encoded by the complex GNAS locus at 20q13.2-q13.3. GNAS was originally described as a gene comprising only the 13 exons that encode Gsα, {1161}, but more recently, additional upstream exons have been described, designated 1A (or A/B), XLαs and NESP55 {848,849,1313}. Transcription of Gsα, XLαs, NESP55, and exon 1A mRNAs is initiated from distinct promoters and first exons that share a common set of downstream exons (exons 2-13). NESP55 contains a stop codon in its first exon and so exons 2-13 are not translated, whereas XLαs is identical to Gsα except at their amino-termini, which are encoded by their unique first exons. Exon 1A mRNAs are untranslated.

Mutation spectrum

Like all heterotrimeric G proteins, Gsα is activated by ligand-bound receptors through the release of bound GDP and binding of ambient GTP, which allows Gsα to bind to and activate the cAMP-generating enzyme adenylyl cyclase. The turn-off mechanism is an intrinsic GTPase activity that hydrolyzes bound GTP to GDP. Residues Arg201 and Gln227 are catalytically important for the GTPase reaction and therefore missense mutations leading to their substitution lead to constitutive activation of Gsα and its downstream effectors. MAS/FD and Mazabraud syndrome are associated with Arg201 mutations (most commonly R201H and R201C, more rarely R201G, R201L, and R201S. {186,290,1520,1644,

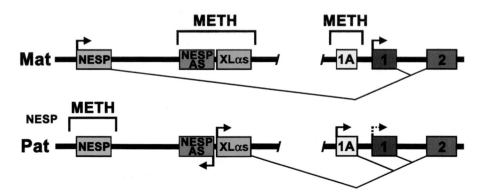

Fig. 5.34 Organization and imprinting of *GNAS*. The maternal (Mat) and paternal (Pat) alleles of *GNAS* are depicted with alternative first exons for NESP55, XLαs, 1A (untranslated), and Gsα (exon 1) mRNAs splicing to a common exon (exon 2). Exons 3-13 are not shown. Differentially methylated regions (METH) are shown above and splicing patterns are shown below each panel. Horizontal arrows show direction of transcription of active promoters. Transcription from the paternal Gsα (exon 1) promoter is suppressed in some tissues (indicated with dashed arrow). The first exon of antisense transcripts (NESPAS) is also shown.

1831,1992,2371}). The mutations arise post-zygotically and affected individuals are therefore somatic mosaics, which accounts for the significant variability observed in the extent and severity of clinical presentation. Germ-line transmission of these activating mutations has not been observed, suggesting they are embryonic lethal if present in non-mosaic form. Somatic Arg201 (R201H, R201C, R201S, R201L) or Gln227 (Q227H, Q227R) mutations are also in some sporadic hyperfunctioning endocrine tumours, including pituitary adenomas, thyroid adenomas, thyroid carcinomas, parathyroid adenomas and phaeochromocytomas {748,1224,1373, 2446} and in isolated intramuscular myxomas {1644}. Inactivating *Gsα* mutations lead to Albright hereditary osteodystrophy (with or without multihormone resistance) and progressive osseous heteroplasia.

Gene expression

Gsα is expressed in virtually all tissues while XLαs and NESP55 expression is restricted to neuroendocrine tissues. All products are subject to genomic imprinting as described below.

Gene function

Gsα is the heterotrimeric G protein α-subunit that couples seven-transmembrane receptors to the cAMP-generating enzyme adenylyl cyclase, and is, therefore, required for the intracellular cAMP response to hormones and other extracellular signals. Activating *Gsα* mutations lead to their pleiotrophic effects primarily by raising cAMP levels in affected tissues. XLαs is a Gsα isoform that has also been shown to be capable of coupling receptors to cAMP generation while NESP55 is a chromogranin-like neurosecretory protein. The biological functions of both of these latter proteins are presently unknown.

Imprinting

GNAS is subject to a complex pattern of imprinting. NESP55 is expressed only from the maternal allele while XLαs and the exon 1A transcripts are expressed only from the paternal allele {848,849, 1313}. Loss of exon 1A imprinting causes pseudohypoparathyroidism type Ib {1313}. *Gsα* is biallelically expressed in most human tissues, but shows exclusive or preferential expression from the mater-

nal allele in some tissues, including pituitary, thyroid and ovary {699,847,1403}. In pituitary tumours that harbour an activating *Gsα* mutation, the mutation almost always occurs on the maternal allele {847}. Therefore, the clinical manifestations observed in each MAS patient might possibly be affected by which parental allele harbours the *Gsα* mutation.

Genetic counselling and preventive measures

MAS and FD both result from somatic, rather than germline, *GNAS* mutations. These disorders are virtually never inherited, presumably due to the fact that the mutations are lethal in the germline. There are no known measures that can prevent their occurrence. Patients with FD should not be treated with radiation, as it is ineffective and may increase the risk for malignant transformation. POFD patients should be screened for endocrine manifestations of MAS.

Familial non-medullary thyroid cancer

W.D. Foulkes
R.T. Kloos
H.R. Harach
V. LiVolsi

Definition

There is no widely accepted definition for familial non-medullary thyroid cancer (FNMTC), but its existence is now accepted, mainly as a result of single-kindred linkage studies, which have identified several candidate regions. No 'site-specific' genes have yet been identified, but autosomal dominant inheritance is presumed for most of the currently identified loci. Under a broad classification of FNMTC, one could also include inherited thyroid-specific syndromes where non-medullary thyroid cancer (NMTC) is an occasional feature, such as familial multinodular goiter. Other syndromes that feature NMTC include Cowden syndrome, familial adenomatous polyposis (FAP), Carney complex and Werner syndrome.

MIM Numbers

See: http://www.ncbi.nlm.nih.gov/omim {1468}.
Multinodular goiter
    MNG1:   *138800
    MNG2:   *300273
Familial non-medullary thyroid cancer
    NMTC1:   *606240
Familial non-medullary thyroid cancer with cell oxyphilia: *603386
Papillary thyroid carcinoma with papillary renal neoplasia: *605642
Cowden Syndrome: #15830
    PTEN :   *601728
Familial adenomatous polyposis (FAP)
                *175100
Carney Complex
    Type 1:   #16980
    Type 2:   *605244
Werner syndrome   #277700

Synonyms

Familial site-specific non-medullary thyroid cancer (FNMTC); Familial papillary thyroid cancer (FPTC); Familial micropapillary thyroid cancer; Familial non-medullary thyroid cancer with cell oxyphilia (TCO); Familial Adenomatous Polyposis (FAP) / Gardner syndrome; Cowden syndrome / Multiple hamartoma syndrome

Incidence / prevalence

The annual incidence of thyroid cancer is between 0.9 and 5.2 per 100,000 people, with a ratio of women to men of 2-3:1 {380,656,864,1011,1854}. In 1955, twins with FNMTC were described {1845}. Approximately 4% of patients with PTC have at least one affected first degree relative {380,783,930,1146,1278,1344, 1676,2276}. A 4.2-10.3 fold excess risk of NMTC is seen in first relatives of patients with NMTC and this cancer risk among relatives is one of highest recorded {738,863,1676,1854}.

Like most known inherited cancer syndromes, there is age-related penetrance for Familial Papillary Thyroid Cancer (FPTC) {1344,1393}. Also similar to other inherited syndromes, an earlier age at diagnosis of NMTC (usually PTC) is more likely to be associated with potential genetic etiology {862}. It is unknown if penetrance is different between the sexes, and thus, if the sex ratio in FPTC is different from sporadic PTC. Some have suggested an unaltered sex ratio {1278,1345,2176,2276} while others have reported low penetrance in men {1676}, while others have suggested that it is high {783,862,930}.

Diagnostic criteria

Non-medullary thyroid cancer (NMTC) refers to primary thyroid malignancies derived from the thyroid follicular cells. A familial predisposition to NMTC is a component of several familial tumour syndromes. Diagnosis of familial NMTC (FNMTC) requires familial inheritance, including a first degree relative (parent, sibling, or offspring) {930} with papillary thyroid cancer (FPTC) or follicular thyroid cancer (FFTC) outside of a tumour syndrome where NMTC is an infrequent component. It is estimated that 47% of FNMTC patients from families with 2 affected members, and 99.9% of patients from families with 3 or more affected members, have an inherited form of the disease {353}. Around 90% of FNMTC is FPTC {1278}. The existence of familial follicular thyroid cancer (FFTC)

outside of an associated familial tumour syndrome is not established, but there are several case reports (see FFTC section). It can be appreciated from this that there are no universally accepted diagnostic criteria for FNMTC. Many families are rather small, and sometimes contain only 2 affected sibs, nonetheless, they have been counted as FNMTC. Operationally, two affected first-degree relatives could be regarded as sufficient to consider FNMTC. Common exposures, such as ionising radiation, could mimic a Mendelian genetic effect, particularly if there is a strong temporal relationship to a putative common exposure. The diagnostic criteria for Cowden syndrome includes follicular thyroid cancer as a major, but not pathognomonic criterion {561}. Any thyroid lesion, such as adenoma or goiter, is accepted as a minor criterion. NMTC is not regarded as a cardinal feature of familial adenomatous polyposis (FAP) as it is seen in less than 3% of all individuals with FAP {260}. Similarly, it is not a part of the diagnostic features of either Carney complex (see section on Carney complex) or Werner syndrome, but does occur at increased frequency in these syndromes, at least in some geographical areas (suggesting that environmental factors may be triggering a latent susceptibility {971,972, 1528,2144}.

Papillary thyroid cancer

Age distribution/penetrance

The penetrance of FPTC is high, although even in large kindreds used for linkage studies, there were unaffected obligate carriers. Similarly, the kindreds have been selected for early-onset cases, as these are more likely to be sampled than late-onset cases. Until specific genes have been identified and tested in the population, it will not be possible to accurately assess the penetrance of FPTC-related alleles. The situation for *PTEN* and *APC* is much clearer. The lifetime risk for thyroid cancer in

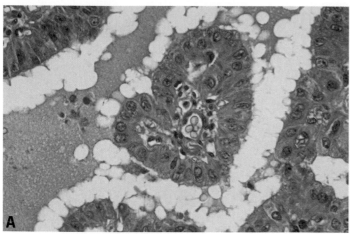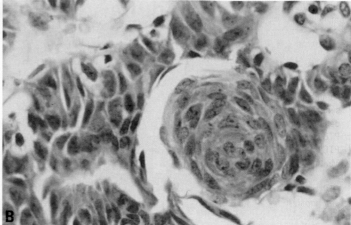

Fig. 5.35 Familial non-medullary thyroid cancer. **A** Oncocytic papillary carcinoma linked to chromosome 19p13.2. Papillae lined by oncocytic cells with abundant eosinophilic granular cytoplasm containing irregular grooved overlapping nuclei with prominent nucleoli. **B** Familial adenomatous polyposis associated thyroid carcinoma. Tumour cells show whorling and a trabecular growth pattern.

Cowden syndrome, caused by germline mutations in *PTEN*, has been estimated at approximately 10%. It is thought to be 1-3% in FAP. The average age of onset of thyroid cancer in Cowden syndrome is 26 years (range 9-43 years) {1879}, and in FAP, it is also 26 years (range 9-69 years) {337}, with the vast majority of the latter cases occurring in women {1879}. In Werner syndrome occurring in Japanese, the average age of onset has been reported to be 39 years (range 27-60) with an approximately 2:1 F:M ratio {971}. The lifetime risk is not known. Incidence of PTC in Carney complex is greater than expected, but the precise lifetime risks are unknown.

Clinical features
The age of diagnosis in FPTC may not be different from sporadic PTC {656,783, 930,1186,1676,2276}, while others have reported a peak incidence in the 4th decade of life, possibly a decade earlier than for sporadic PTC {1344,1368}. No given phenotype for FNMTC has been identified {1278,2276}, although an increased rate of intrathyroidal tumour multifocality, and an association with multiple benign nodules is reported {2276}. The onset of FPTC may be related to both genetics and an increased susceptibility to environmental factors such as radiation exposure {600,1391,1719,2134}. Women with FPTC may be at increased risk of breast cancer {930,2305}. Patients of both sexes with FPTC may be at increased risk of kidney cancer and CNS tumours {930}. An increased number of benign thyroid conditions, including nod-

ules, may be present in affected families {261,924,1278,1394,2134}, but this has not been a universal finding {1344,1676}. Members of families with FNMTC may be at increased risk of leukemia {738} and hormone-related cancers {1676}, although this has not been confirmed by others {656,862,930}. Specifically, the risks of breast and prostate cancer are uncertain {656,680,738,783,862,930, 1676,1854}.

Pathology of site-specific FPTC
In families with cellular oxyphilia
Both sporadic and familial NMTC with cell oxyphilia have been studied pathologically. In familial cases, there was a mixture of features, in particular a characteristic multiple adenomatous goiter, with or without PTC with oxyphilic features. Other affected individuals have only oxyphil PTC. Essentially, this is a variant form of multinodular goiter susceptibility, with prominent oxyphilic features. Multicentricity is a common feature and these adenomas are often encapsulated structures with variable oxyphilia. The oxyphil papillary carcinomas are characterised by irregular, grooved nuclei, occasional nuclear cytoplasmic inclusions and conspicuous nucleoli {293,827,1051}.

In families linked to 2q
Recently, linkage to chromosome 2q21 has been identified in one large Tasmanian family with FPTC and multinodular goiter (MNG) {261}. Interestingly, linkage to 2q21 was only obtained when it was observed that 7 of 8 family mem-

bers with PTC shared the same haplotype on 2q21 {1465}. The pathology of these PTCs was interesting: on review, 4 of the 8 PTC-affected individuals had the follicular variant of PTC (fvPTC). This variant accounts for less than 10% of all PTC's. Other families with at least one case of fvPTC appear also to be linked to this region.

In families with the papillary microcarcinoma
Microscopic papillary thyroid cancer is defined as a PTC that is 1 cm or less in size. It has been reported that, when familial, these cancers behave more aggressively {1368,1879}. The papillary microcarcinoma is common in the general population: nearly one quarter of those aged 45 years have papillary thyroid microcarcinoma {652}.

FPTC and papillary renal neoplasia
One large single pedigree has been reported with FPTC and papillary renal neoplasia. Linkage to 1q has been obtained {1393}. The PTC that occurs in this family appears to be "typical" PTC with no special features. Some individuals have thyroid nodules.

Pathology of syndromic FPTC
PTEN-related FPTC
Thyroid cancer in Cowden syndrome is usually follicular, rather than papillary in type (see section below). However, these carcinomas can often have an important papillary component {1028}. However, in these cases, classical features of PTC, such as psammoma bodies, are absent.

Table 5.11
Familial tumour syndromes predisposing to non-medullary thyroid cancer.

Syndrome	Gene or chromosomal location	Thyroid cancer histology and incidence (%)
Cowden	PTEN	FTC and PTC(3-21%) {924,1412,2116}
Familial adenomatous polyposis, (also Gardner syndrome, Turcot syndrome, hereditary desmoid disease)	APC	PTC (2%) {160,706}
PTC with cell oxyphilia	TCO, 19p13.2	Oncocytic PTC {293}
PTC without oxyphilia	19p13.2	PTC {183}
Multinodular goiter	MNG1, 14q31 MNG2, Xp22	2 PTC-like lesions in the MNG1 kindred, none in the MNG2 kindred {189,298}
PTC, nodular thyroid disease, and papillary renal cell carcinoma	1q21	PTC {1393}
PTC and clear cell renal cell carcinoma	t(3;8)(p14.2;q24.1)	PTC {397,560}
Carney complex	PRKAR1A	FTC (2%) and PTC (2%) {1625,2144}
Werner syndrome	WRN	PTC, FTC, anaplastic {972}
FNMTC	NMTC1, 2q21	fvPTC {1465} [such as CK 5/6])

FAP-related FNMTC

Thyroid tumours associated with familial adenomatous polyposis are detected in 2% of affected individuals by palpation alone and up to 25% in selected series by ultrasonography {979,1879}. While traditionally classified as a papillary thyroid carcinoma or a cribriform subtype, a growing number of pathologists and thyroidologists believe that FAP-related thyroid carcinomas are histologically distinct {343,830}. Distinct histological patterns of growth include cribriform, morular (squamoid whorling) and short fascicles of spindle cells. Other frequent cytoarchitectural patterns include eosinophilic to amphophilic cuboidal to columnar sometimes stratified epithelium lining papillae and follicles with angular or tubular shapes, as well as trabecular or solid structures with occasional adamantinomatous and hyalinizing trabecular adenoma – like features. Microscopic hypercellular foci with similar cytoarchitecture to large tumours may occur admixed with normal looking background thyroid parenchyma. The tumours are usually well circumscribed and/or encapsulated, fibrosis is often prominent in the tumour capsule or stroma, and evidence of capsular, lymphatic or vascular invasion may not be present. Notably, FAP associated thyroid tumours, in contrast to classic papillary carcinoma, do not show the typical fir tree branching papillary pattern, psammoma bodies are rare or non-existent, nuclei lack the pale dusty 'ground glass' chromatin, show inconstant grooving and occasional, if any, cytoplasmic inclu-

sions. Only 5% show regional lymph node metastasis {830,1727,1879}. It should be noted that the distinct architecture seen in FAP-related thyroid carcinomas is very unusual in sporadic PTC {343}.

Carney complex-related FPTC

There has been no systematic analysis of thyroid lesions in Carney complex, but up to 11% may have some form of thyroid disease {2144}. Case reports of PTC have suggested that the fvPTC (see above) and FTC (see below) may be seen. The lesions are usually multifocal.

Werner syndrome-related FPTC

No increase in PTC has been seen in non-Asian kindreds with Werner syndrome. It is not clear whether the incidence of thyroid cancer in Japanese affected by WRN is due to differences in mutation spectrum {971,972}, or reflects differences in iodine levels, and hence is more related to environmental factors than any observed differences in mutation spectrum {1528}. In Japanese kindreds, PTC (35%), FTC (48%) and anaplastic carcinoma (13%) have all been reported {971}. Detailed pathological description of these cases is awaited.

Prognosis and prognostic factors

The performance of prognostic factors that predict outcome in sporadic PTC is unknown in FPTC. The overall prognosis of FPTC is not well established, but may be the same as for sporadic tumours {1146,1186,1278,1344,1391}. Some have suggested a more aggressive tumour

behaviour in FPTC {783,1355,1666,2176, 2276}, perhaps surprisingly, including those with microcarcinoma (< 1 cm) {1368}. Thyroid cancer occurring as a part of FAP seems to have a favourable prognosis {1879}.

Follicular thyroid carcinoma

Clinical features

Familial FTC may be inherited as part of a syndrome with additional associated phenotypic features such as Cowden Syndrome, Carney Complex or Werner Syndrome {1879}. Inheritance of isolated FTC outside of a well-defined syndrome has not been clearly established {656, 863,1392,1854}, especially given the possibilities of chance occurrence and misclassification of PTC as FTC. FTC comprises approximately 6% of thyroid cancer cases from FNMTC series {1344}.

Pathology
PTEN-related FTC

Thyroid cancer is an important aspect of Cowden syndrome {561}. Up to 10% of Cowden individuals develop non-medullary thyroid (usually follicular) carcinoma. The lesions seen in this syndrome are usually multicentric and follicular, rather than papillary. The follicular adenomas tend to have classic follicular architecture. Follicular carcinomas that are seen in Cowden syndrome are believed to progress from pre-existing follicular adenomas {1879}.

Werner syndrome-related FTC

FTC is more common in Japanese Werner syndrome patients than is PTC. Detailed comparisons of FTC occurring in Werner syndrome and in the general Japanese population would be of interest.

Other FFTC

One study reported an African American family with congenital goiter in which two children with goiter also developed metastatic FTC {411}. The metastatic thyroid cancer occurred many years after subtotal thyroidectomy without thyroid hormone replacement therapy. This family has not been studied from a molecular standpoint. Another study described a small Ashkenazi Jewish family with MNG, FTC and alveolar rhabdomyosarcoma. The pathology of the thyroid glands did not reveal any special features {530}. A positive LOD score was obtained for chromosome 14q markers {189}.

Follicular neoplasms, and classic thyroid papillary carcinoma and microcarcinoma (1.0 cm or less in diameter) have been occasionally described in FAP patients {830,1727,1879}. This is probably due to chance occurrence since, for instance, small papillary cancers show a prevalence of up to 22%/24% in subjects aged 16-30/45 years, respectively {1879}.

Prognosis and prognostic factors

It appears that FTC has a slightly worse prognosis than PTC {763}, but this is largely due to the higher percentage of cases with FTC who present with metastatic disease, and when these are excluded, there are no differences {1451}. As FFTC is somewhat rarer than FTPC, there have been no systematic studies of outcome, but is not thought to be a common cause of death in Cowden syndrome (C. Eng, personal communication).

Multinodular goiter

Familial euthyroid multinodular goiter (MNG) occurs with or without intrathyroid calcification.

Clinical features

Several families have been reported where the dominant feature is multinodular goiter, and thyroid cancer either occurs rarely, or not at all {422,1562, 1591}. In other families, PTC has been reported, but the relationship between the linked locus and MNG is much less clear in these cases, particularly as goiter may be endemic in countries with high iodine exposure {261,1465}. It may be that the MNG is attributable to another locus. In most of the families reported, the age of onset of MNG was adolescence or earlier.

Pathology

In general, the MNG seen in these families is typical (multiple nodules, epithelial hyperplasia, calcification and haemorrhage) and by definition, there is no evidence of altered thyroid function. The pathological description of the MNG does not provide evidence for a different etiology of the goiter in these families {298,422,1591}. In a Scottish family, a notable feature was the extensive calcification, but this probably results from the haemorrhage, infarction, necrosis and subsequent fibrosis {1562}.

Prognosis and prognostic factors

The prognosis in those with MNG is usually excellent. If PTC arises in a MNG, then the prognosis will be determined by the PTC. Death related to the thyroid gland disorder has very rarely, if ever, been reported in euthyroid MNG kindreds.

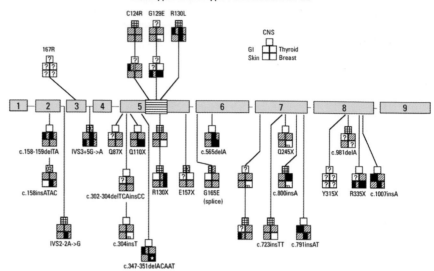

Fig. 5.36 Familial non-medullary thyroid cancer. Genotype-phaenotype correlations of *PTEN* mutations, the cause of Cowden syndrome (CS), Bannayan-Ruvalcaba-Riley-Smith syndrome and related hamartomatous conditions.

Genetics

Chromosomal locations

Multinodular goiter

MNG1:	*138800	14q
MNG2:	*300273	Xp22

Familial non-medullary thyroid cancer

NMTC1:	*606240	2q

Familial non-medullary thyroid cancer with cell oxyphilia: *603386 19p

Cowden Syndrome: #15830 10q

PTEN:	*601728	10q

Familial adenomatous polyposis

*175100 5q

Carney Complex

Type 1:	#16980	17q
Type 2:	*605244	2p

Werner syndrome #277700 8p

Gene structure, expression and function

PTEN

This tumour suppressor gene encodes a lipid and protein phosphatase that lies in the Protein Kinase B (PKB, Akt) and PI3K pathways, and is therefore implicated in many cytoplasmic signaling pathways. Of note, loss of PTEN function results in escape from programmed cell death and G1 arrest. *PTEN* is composed of 9 coding exons, and mutations are spread across the exons {563}. Cowden syndrome is inherited in an autosomal dominant fashion.

APC

This tumour suppressor gene which has multiple functions, but is mainly implicated in the Wnt pathway. The Armadillo region is of particular interest as it is also present in B-catenin, and interacts with protein phosphatase 2A, which in turn binds axin. B-catenin can accumulate when APC is inactivated, and translocation of B-catenin to the nucleus can activate the Tcf/Lef system. *APC* has 15 coding exons, the last of which occupies more than three-quarters of the coding region. The site of mutations can have functional significance (see below) {611,643}. FAP is inherited in as an autosomal dominant trait.

PRKAR1A

This is probably a tumour suppressor gene. It encodes a protein kinase A type 1a regulatory subunit, and therefore, like PTEN, has a crucial role in intracellular signalling pathways. It is placed downstream of cAMP, and its presence is a vital component of cAMP-dependent signalling. *PRKAR1A* has 10 coding exons {2140}. Carney complex is an autosomal dominant trait.

WRN

This gene is a member of the RecQ-type DNA helicase family, which includes *BLM*. It encodes a protein whose role is to assist in the control of the unwinding of intermediates of recombination. Loss of *WRN* results in elevated levels of recombination, and results in the characteristic cancer and premature ageing phenotype of Werner syndrome. It is a large gene with 35 exons {1438,1575}. Werner syndrome is an autosomal recessive trait.

Mutation spectrum and genotype / phenotype correlations
PTEN
Germline mutations have been reported throughout *PTEN*, although there is a paucity of mutations in exons 1, 4 and 9

{1412}. Classic Cowden probands found to have intragenic germline *PTEN* mutations may have a higher likelihood of developing breast cancer compared to those without mutation {1412}. Mutations within and 5' of the PTPase, core motif may be associated with multi-organ involvement. The relatively large number of missense mutations in the PTPase core motif suggests its biological importance, and these mutations likely act in a dominant negative manner {1412}. With regard to NMTC, mutations in families associated with this cancer site have been reported in most exons and are not limited to missense mutations.

APC

Most disease-associated mutations in *APC* are predicted to truncate the protein. There are fairly clear genotype-phenotype associations but their clinical usefulness is fairly limited {705}. The cribriform type of thyroid carcinoma is seen in FAP {830}. A large European study showed that mutations 5' of codon 1220 were significantly more likely to be associated with thyroid cancer than were mutations 3' of this point (P = .005) {336} but this requires confirmation.

PRKAR1A

As Carney complex is rare, and NMTC is not common in this syndrome, there are no reliable data on the role of mutations in this gene and thyroid cancer risk.

WRN

It is debatable whether there truly is an excess of thyroid cancer in Werner syndrome {1528}. The Japanese group has argued for a genotype-phenotype correlation between mutation position and thyroid cancer, in that all the affected individuals had mutations that were outside the helicase domain, and all 4 FTC cases were seen in those with 3' mutations, but the numbers are too small to make more definitive statements {971}.

Genetic counseling and preventive measures

Genetic counselling for non-syndromic FNMTC is not widely practised, partly because such families are rare, but also because they may not come to the attention of medical geneticists. Often, affected individuals from FNMTC families are seen only by their treating endocrinologist or surgeon.

Unlike the situation in medullary thyroid cancer, preventive thyroidectomy is rarely, if ever, recommended in FNMTC. This is partly because in the absence of identified genes, it can be difficult to identify individuals at risk. Individuals with adenomas, multinodular goiters or other possible pre-cancerous lesions may elect to have thyroidectomies for relatively minor symptoms because of the known family history and the possibility of malignant transformation. The discovery of specific susceptibility genes for FNMTC may lead to a change in counselling practice. An illustration is from Cowden syndrome where germline *PTEN* mutations have been identified. Because benign thyroid disease, e.g. multinodular goiter, is quite common (approximately 70%) and thyroid carcinoma, a true component in Cowden syndrome, thyroid surveillance is recommended starting in the teens {561,563}. Similarly, if thyroidectomy is to be performed for either benign or malignant conditions, a total thyroidectomy is recommended because of the high likelihood of developing further benign and malignant disease in the thyroid.

Contributors

Dr. Susan L. ABBONDANZO
Department of Haematopathology
Armed Forces Institute of Pathology
6825, 16th Street NW, Rm 2051
Washington, DC 20306-6000
USA
Tel. +1 202 782 1723
Fax. +1 202 782 9157
abbondan@afip.osd.mil

Dr. Göran ÅKERSTRÖM
Department of Surgical Sciences
Uppsala University Hospital
Akademiska sjukhuset
SE-751 85 Uppsala
SWEDEN
Tel. +46 18 611 46 24
Fax. +46 18 50 44 14
goran.akerstrom@kirurgi.uu.se

Dr. Lars Andreas AKSLEN
Department of Pathology
The Gade Institute
Haukeland University Hospital
N-5021 Bergen
NORWAY
Tel. +47 55 97 31 82
Fax. +47 55 97 31 58
lars.akslen@gades.uib.no

Dr. Jorge ALBORES-SAAVEDRA*
Anatomic Pathology
LSU Health Sciences Center
School of Medicine
1501 Kings Highway
Shreveport, LA 71130, USA
Tel. +1 318 675 7732
Fax. +1 318 675 7662
jalbor@lsuhsc.edu

Dr. Micheala A. ALDRED
Human Cancer Genetics Program
The Ohio State University
420 West 12th Avenue
Columbus, OH 43210
USA
Tel. +1 614 688 4493
Fax. +1 614 688 4245
maldred@hgmp.mrc.ac.uk

Dr. Katsuyki AOZASA
Department of Pathology (C3)
Osaka University Medical School
2-2 Yamadaoka Suita
Osaka 565-0871
JAPAN
Tel. +81 6 6879 3711
Fax. +81 6 6879 3719
aozasa@molpath.med.osaka-u.ac.jp

---

* The asterisk indicates participation
in the Working Group Meeting on the
WHO Classification of Tumours of
Endocrine Organs that was held in
Lyon, France, April 23-26, 2003.

Dr. Andrew ARNOLD
Division of Endocrinology / Metabolism
Center for Molecular Medicine
Univ. Connecticut Medical School
263 Farmington Avenue
Farmington, CT 06030-3101, USA
Tel. +1 860 679 7640
Fax. +1 860 679 7639
molecularmedicine@uchc.edu

Dr. Sylvia L. ASA*
Dept. of Laboratory Medicine and
Pathobiology, University of Toronto
University Health Network and Toronto
Medical Laboratories
610 University Avenue, Rm. 4-302
Toronto, Ontario M5G 2M9, CANADA
Tel. +1 416 946 2099 / Fax. +1 416 946 6579
sylvia.asa@uhn.on.ca

Dr. Zubair W. BALOCH
Department of Pathology and Laboratory
Medicine, Cytopathology
University of Pennsylvania Medical Center
3400 Spruce Street
Philadelphia, PA 19104, USA
Tel. +1 215 898 8001
Fax. +1 215 349 8994
baloch@mail.med.upenn.edu

Dr. Ariel L. BARKAN
Div. of Endocrinology and Metabolism
University of Michigan Medical Center
3920 Taubman Center, Box 0354
Ann Arbor, MI 48109
USA
Tel. +1 734 615 6964
Fax. +1 734 936 9240
abarkan@umich.edu

Dr. Bora E. BAYSAL
Department of Obstetrics, Gynecology and
Reproductive Sciences
Magee-Womens Research Institute
204 Craft Street, R330
Pittsburgh, PA 15213, USA
Tel. +1 412 641 6093
Fax. +1 412 641 5373
baysalb@mwri.magee.edu

Dr. Gazanfer BELGE
Center for Human Genetics and
Genetic Counseling
University of Bremen
Leobenerstr. ZHG
D-28359 Bremen, GERMANY
Tel. +49 421 218 2907
Fax. +49 421 218 4239
belge@uni-bremen.de

Dr. Xavier BERTAGNA
Endocrinologie et Maladies Métaboliques
27, rue du Faubourg Saint Jacques
75679 Paris cedex 14
FRANCE
Tel. +33 1 58 41 17 91
Fax. +33 1 46 33 80 60
xavier.bertagna@cch.ap-hop-paris.fr

Dr. Wojciech BIERNAT
Department of Tumour Pathology
Medical University of Lodz
4 Paderewski Street
93-509 Lodz
POLAND
Tel. +48 42 6895783
Fax. +48 42 6895422
biernat@csk.am.lodz.pl

Dr. John P. BILEZIKIAN
Department of Endocrinology - PH 8 WEST - 864
College of Physicians and Surgeons
Columbia University
630 West 168th Street
New York, NY 10032, USA
Tel. +1 212 305 6238
Fax. +1 212 305 6486
jpb2@columbia.edu

Dr. Scott BOERNER
Cytopathology, University Health Network
Princess Margaret Hospital 4-206A
610 University Avenue
Toronto, Ontario M5G 2M9
CANADA
Tel. +416 946 4597
Fax. +416 946 6579
scott.boerner@uhn.on.ca

Dr. Tom BÖHLING
Department of Pathology
University of Helsinki and HUSLAB
POB 21
FIN-00014 Helsinki
FINLAND
Tel. +358 50 427 1900
Fax. +358 9 19126700
tom.bohling@helsinki.fi

Dr. Lennart BONDESON*
Department of Pathology and Cytology
Malmö University Hospital
SE-20502 Malmö
SWEDEN
Tel. +46 40 33 14 58
Fax. +46 40 33 62 46
lennart.bondeson@skane.se

Dr. Cesare BORDI*
Department of Pathology and
Laboratory Medicine
University of Parma
Via Gramsci 14
I-43100 Parma, ITALY
Tel. +390 521 702621
Fax. +390 521 292710
cesare.bordi@unipr.it

Dr. Gianni BUSSOLATI
Department of Biomedical Sciences
and Oncology
Sezione di Anatomia Patologica
University of Turin
Via Santena 7
I-10126 Torino, ITALY
Tel. +39 011 6706505 / Fax. +39 011 6635267
gianni.bussolati@unito.it

Dr. Blake CADY
Rhode Island Hospital
Department of Surgery
593 Eddy Street APC 435
Providence, RI 02903
USA
Tel. +1 401 444 6158
Fax. +1 401 444 6681
bcady@usasurg.org

Dr. Alain CALENDER*
Unité Fonctionnelle de Génétique UF 29437
Hôpital Edouard Herriot
Place d'Arsonval
69437 Lyon Cedex 03
FRANCE
Tel. +33 4 72 11 73 80 secr.
Fax. +33 4 72 11 73 81 secr.
alain.calender@chu-lyon.fr

Dr. José CAMESELLE-TEIJEIRO
Department of Pathology
Hospital Clinico Universitario
15706 Santiago de Compostela
SPAIN
Tel. +34 981 950858
Fax. +34 981 950889
apjocame@usc.es

Dr. Carlo CAPELLA
Servizio di Anatomia Patologica
Ospedale di Circolo
Università Dell' Insubria
Viale Borri 57
I-21100 Varese, ITALY
Tel. +390 332 264 557
Fax. +390 332 262 313
carlo.capella@ospedale.varese.it

Dr. Maria Luisa CARCANGIU
Dipartimento di Patologia
Anatomia Patologica A
National Cancer Institute
Via Giacomo Venezian 1
I-20133 Milano, ITALY
Tel. +39 02 23902264
Fax. +39 02 23902877
carcangiu@istitutotumori.mi.it

Dr. J. Aidan CARNEY
Department of Laboratory Medicine
and Pathology
Mayo Clinic and Mayo Foundation
200 First Street SW
Rochester, MN 55905, USA
Tel. +1 507 284 2691
Fax. +1 507 284 5036
carney.aidan@mayo.edu

Dr. Paul CARUSO
Department of Radiology
Massachusetts Eye and Ear Infirmary
243 Charles Street
Boston, MA 02114
USA
Tel. +1 617 573 3555
Fax. +1 617 573 3490
alweber1@aol.com

Dr. Barbara Ann CENTENO
H. Lee Moffitt Cancer Center and
Research Institute
12902 Magnolia Drive.
Tampa, FL 33612
USA
Tel. +1 813 979 3001
Fax. +1 813 632 1708
centenba@moffitt.usf.edu

Dr. John K. C. CHAN
Department of Pathology
Queen Elizabeth Hospital
Wylie Road,
Kowloon, Hong Kong
SAR CHINA
Tel. +852 2958 6830
Fax. +852 2385 2455
jkcchan@ha.org.hk

Dr. Liang CHENG
Department of Pathology
Indiana University School of Medicine
550 N. University Boulevard, Room 3465
Indianapolis, IN 46202, USA
Tel. +1 317 274 1756
+1 554 0000 ext 2859
Fax. +1 317 274 5346
lcheng@iupui.edu

Dr. Runjan CHETTY
Department of Pathology
University Health Network
The Princess Hospital
610 University Avenue, 4th Fl. Rm. 302
Toronto, Ontario M5G 2M9 , CANADA
Tel. +1 416 946 2876
Fax. +1 416 946 6579
runjan.chetty@uhn.on.ca

Dr. Wah CHEUK
Department of Pathology
Queen Elizabeth Hospital
Wylie Road
Kowloon Hong Kong
SAR CHINA
Tel. +852 2958 6835
Fax. +852 2385 2455
cheuk_wah@hotmail.com

Dr. George P. CHROUSOS
Pediatric and Reproductive Endocrinology
Branch
NIH, Rm.10/ 9D42
10 Center Drive, MSC 1583
Bethesda, MD 20892, USA
Tel. +1 301 496 5800
Fax. +1 301 402 0884
chrousog@mail.nih.gov

Dr. Orlo H. CLARK
Department of Surgery
UCSF/Mt. Zion Medical Center
1600 Divisadero Street
San Francisco, CA 94143-1674
USA
Tel. +1 415 353 7789 clin.
Fax. +1 415 885 7617
clarko@surgery.ucsf.edu

Dr. Randall D. CRAVER
Department of Pathology
Louisiana State University
Health Sciences Center
1901 Perdido Street
New Orleans, LA 70112, USA
Tel. +1 504 896 9815
Fax. +1 504 894 5119
rcrave@lsuhsc.edu

Dr. Yogeshwar DAYAL*
Department of Pathology
New England Medical Center Hospital
750 Washington Street
Boston, MA 02111
USA
Tel. +1 617 636 5829
Fax. +1 617 636 8302
ydayal@tufts-nemc.org.

Dr. Ronald R. DE KRIJGER
Department of Pathology, Rm. Be 222
Erasmus Medical Center
PO BOX 1738
3000 DR Rotterdam
THE NETHERLANDS
Tel. +31 10 408 7900
Fax. +31 10 408 9487
r.dekrijger@erasmusmc.nl

Dr. Ronald A. DELELLIS*
Department of Pathology and
Laboratory Medicine
Rhode Island Hospital
593 Eddy Street
Providence, Rhode Island 02903, USA
Tel. +1 401 444 5154/5011
Fax. +1 401 444 9038
rdelellis@lifespan.org

Dr. Karl-Michael DERWAHL
Department of Medicine
St. Hedwig Hospital and
Humboldt University Berlin
Grosse Hamburger Str. 5-11
D-10115 Berlin, GERMANY
Tel. +49 30 23 11 25 03
Fax. +49 30 23 11 23 24
m.derwahl@alexius.de

Dr. David M. DORFMAN
Department of Pathology
Brigham and Women's Hospital and
Harvard Medical School
75 Francis Street
Boston, MA 02115, USA
Tel. +1 617 732 7518
Fax. +1 617 731 4872
ddorfman@partners.org

Carrie Melvin DROVDLIC
The Arthur G. James Cancer Hospital and
Richard J. Solove Research Institute,
Clinical Cancer Genetics Program
The Ohio State University
2050 Kenny Rd., 8th Fl. Tower
Columbus, OH 43221, USA
Tel. +1 614 293 6694 / Fax. +1 614 293 2314
drovdlic-1@medctr.osu.edu

Dr. Damian E. DUPUY
Department of Diagnostic Imaging
Rhode Island Hospital
Brown Medical School
593 Eddy Street
Providence, RI 02903, USA
Tel. +1 444 5184
Fax. +1 444 5017
d.dupuy@lifespan.org

Dr. Charis ENG*
Division of Human Genetics
Department of Internal Medicine
Clinical Cancer Genetics Program
The Ohio State University
420 W. 12th Ave., Ste 690 TMRF
Columbus, OH 43210, USA
Tel. +1 614 292 2347 / Fax. +1 614 688 3582
eng-1@medctr.osu.edu

Dr. Vincenzo EUSEBI*
Department of Pathology
University of Bologna
Ospedale Bellaria, Via Altura 3
I-40139 Bologna
ITALY
Tel. +39 051 622 5750/5523
Fax. +39 051 622 5759
vincenzo.eusebi@ausl.bologna.it

Dr. Harry L. EVANS
Division of Anatomic Pathology,
Dept. of Surgical Pathology, Box 0085
University of Texas MD Anderson
Cancer Center
1515 Holcombe Boulevard
Houston, TX 77030, USA
Tel. +1 713 792 3152 / Fax. +1 713 745 3356
hlevans@mdanderson.org

Dr. D. Gareth EVANS
Academic Unit of Medical Genetics
and Regional Genetics Service
St Mary's Hospital
Hathersage Road
Manchester M13 0JH
UNITED KINGDOM
Tel. +44 161 276 6206 / Fax. +44 161 276 6145
gareth.evans@CMMC.nhs.uk

Dr. Shereen EZZAT
Department of Medicine,
University Health Network
Mount Sinai Hospital
The University of Toronto
600 University Avenue
Toronto Ontario M5G 1X5, CANADA
Tel. +1 416 586 8505 / Fax. +1 416 586 8834
sezzat@mtsinai.on.ca

Dr. James A. FAGIN
Division of Endocrinology and Metabolism
Internal Medicine
University of Cincinnati College of
Medicine
3125 Bethesda Avenue Rm. 1331
Cincinnati, OH 45267-0547 , USA
Tel. +1 513 558 4444 / Fax. +1 513 558 8581
james.fagin@uc.edu

Dr. William Clay FAQUIN
Department of Pathology
Massachusets General Hospital
55 Fruit Street, Warren 219
Boston, MA 02114
USA
Tel. +1 617 573 3159
Fax. +1 617 573 3389
wfaquin@partners.org

Dr. Nadir R. FARID
Osancor Biotech. Inc.
31 Woodland Drive
Watford, Herts WD17 3BY
UNITED KINGDOM
Tel. +44 1923 800 034
Fax. +44 208 423 1501
farid@osancor96.fsnet.co.uk

Dr. P. FARID
1st Institute of Pathology and
Experimental Cancer Research
Semmelweis University
Üllöi ut 26
H-1085 Budapest
HUNGARY
Tel/Fax. +36 1 266 0451
farid9@mail.datanet.hu

Dr. William E. FARRELL
Centre for Cell and Molecular Medicine
University of Keele
North Staffordshire Hospital
Thornburon Drive, Hartshill
Stoke-on-Trent, ST4 7QB
UNITED KINGDOM
Tel. +44 1782 555225 / Fax. +44 1782 747319
w.e.farrell@keele.ac.uk

Dr. William FOULKES
Departments of Oncology & Human
Genetics
McGill University
546 Pine Avenue West
Montreal, Quebec H2W 1S6
CANADA
Tel. +1 514 934 1934 / Fax. +1 514 934 8273
william.foulkes@mcgill.ca

Dr. Kaarle O. FRANSSILA
Department of Pathology
Medix Laboratories
Nihtisillankuja 1
FIN-02630 Espoo
FINLAND
Tel. +358 9 884 9480
Fax. +358 9 525 6263
kaarle.franssila@kolumbus.fi

Dr. Robert F. GAGEL
Department of Endocrine Neoplasia
and Hormonal Disorders
University of Texas MD Anderson
Cancer Center
1515 Holcombe Boulevard, Box 0433
Houston, TX 77030, USA
Tel. +1 713 792 6517 / Fax. +1 713 794 1818
rgagel@mdanderson.org

Dr. Kim R. GEISINGER
Dept. of Pathology
Surgical Pathology and Cytopathology
Wake Forest University and the North
Carolina Baptist Hospital Medical Center
Medical Center Boulevard
Winston-Salem, NC 27157-1072, USA
Tel. +1 336 716 2608 / Fax. +1 336 716 7595
kgeis@wfubmc.edu

Dr. Ronald A. GHOSSEIN
Department of Pathology
Memorial Sloan Kettering Cancer Center
1275 York Avenue
New York, NY 10021
USA
Tel. +1 212 639 2701/5914
Fax. +1 212 717 3203
ghosseir@mskcc.org

Dr. Oliver GIMM*
Department of General, Visceral and
Vascular Surgery
Martin-Luther-University Halle-Wittenberg
Ernst-Grube-Str. 40
D-06097 Halle, GERMANY
Tel. +49 345 557 2314
Fax. +49 345 557 2551
oliver.gimm@medizin.uni-halle.de

Dr. Thomas J. GIORDANO
Pathology Department, Rm 2G332/0054
University of Michigan Hospital
1500 East Medical Center Drive
Ann Arbor, MI 48109-0054
USA
Tel. +1 734 936 6776
Fax. +1 734 763 4095
giordano@umich.edu

Dr. Dario GIUFFRIDA
Division of Medical Oncology
Istituto Oncologico del Mediterraneo
Viagrande
I-95125 Catania
ITALY
Tel. +390 957895000
Fax. +390 957901320
dariogiuffrida@netscape.net

Dr. Lars GRIMELIUS*
Department of Genetics and Pathology
Uppsala University Hospital
Dag Hammarskjölds väg 20, Office 315
Rudbeck Laboratory
SE-751 85 Uppsala, SWEDEN
Tel. +46 18 611 38 37
Fax. +46 18 50 21 72
lars.grimelius@genpat.uu.se

Dr. Gerardo Esteban GUITER
Rhode Island Hospital
Dept. of Pathology. APC-12
593 Eddy Street
Providence, RI 02903
USA
Tel. +1 401 444 2780
Fax. +1 401 444 8514
gguiter@lifespan.org

Dr. Philip I. HAIGH
Oncologic and Endocrine Surgery
Department of Surgery
Kaiser Permanente Los Angeles Medical
Center
4760 Sunset Boulevard
Los Angeles, CA 90027, USA
Tel. +1 323 783 7510 / Fax. +1 323 783 8747
philip.i.haigh@kp.org

Dr. Héctor Rubén HARACH
Service of Pathology
Dr. A. Oñativia Endocrinology and
Metabolism Hospital
E. Paz Chain 36
4400 Salta, ARGENTINA
Tel. +54 387 431 5245
Fax. +54 387 421 2629
rubenharach@ciudad.com.ar

Dr. Ian D. HAY
Division of Endocrinology
Mayo Clinic
200 First Street SW
Rochester, MN 55905-0001
USA
Tel. +1 507 284 3915
Fax. +1 507 284 5745
hay.ian@mayo.edu

Dr. Philipp U. HEITZ*
Department of Pathology
University Hospital
Schmelzbergstr. 12
CH-8091 Zurich
SWITZERLAND
puh@heitz.net

Dr. Geoffrey N. HENDY
Calcium Research Laboratory, Rm. H4.67
Department of Royal Victoria Hospital
687 Pine Avenue West
Montreal, Quebec H3A 1A1
CANADA
Tel. +1 514 843 1632
Fax. +1 514 843 1712
geoffrey.hendy@mcgill.ca

Dr. Mitsuyoshi HIROKAWA
Department of Pathology
University of Tokushima School of
Medicine
3-18-15 Kuramoto-cho
770-8503 Tokushima
JAPAN
Tel. +81 88 6337064 / Fax. +81 88 6339423
hirokawa@basic.med.tokushima-u.ac.jp

Dr. Eva HORVATH
Department of Pathology
St. Michaels Hospital
30 Bond Street
Toronto, Ontario M5B 1W8
CANADA
Tel. +1 416 864 5858/5851
Fax. +1 416 864 5648
kovacsk@smh.toronto.on.ca

Dr. Leonard B. KAHN
Department of Pathology,
Long Island Jewish Medical Center
Albert Einstein College of Medicine
270-05, 76th Avenue
New Hyde Park, NY 11040, USA
Tel. +1 718 470 7491
Fax. +1 718 470 4431
kahn@lij.edu

Dr. Klaus KASERER
Klinisches Institut für Pathologie
Allgemeines Krankenhaus
Medizinische Universität Wien
Währinger Gürtel 18-20
A-1090 Wien, AUSTRIA
Tel. +43 1 40400 3650
Fax. +43 1 40400 3707
klaus.kaserer@meduniwien.ac.at

Dr. Akira KAWASHIMA
Department of Radiology
Mayo Clinic
200 First Street SW
Rochester, MN 55905
USA
Tel. +1 507 284 3908
Fax. +1 507 264 4735
kawashima.akira@mayo.edu

Dr. Noriko KIMURA*
Pathology and Laboratory Medicine
Tohoku Rosai Hospital, Japan Labor Health
and Welfare Organization
21-3-4 Dainohara Aoba-ku
981-8563 Sendai, JAPAN
Tel. +81 22 275 1111 / Fax. +81 22 275 7541
nkimura-path@tohokuh.rofuku.go.jp

Dr. Yutuka KITAMURA
Department of Surgery
Yugawara Kosei-Nenkin Hospital
438, Miyakami, Yugawara
Kanagawa 259-0396
JAPAN
Tel. +81 465 63 2211
Fax. +81 465 62 3704
yutakakit@msn.com

Dr. Paul KLEIHUES*
Department of Pathology
University Hospital
Schmelzbergstr.12
CH-8091 Zurich
SWITZERLAND
Tel. +41 1 255 3516
Fax. +41 1 255 2525
paul.kleihues@usz.ch

Dr. David S. KLIMSTRA*
Department of Pathology
Memorial Sloan-Kettering Cancer Center
1275 York Avenue
New York, NY 10021, USA
Tel. +1 212 639 2410
Fax. +1 212 717 3203
klimstrd@mskcc.org

Dr. Richard T. KLOOS
Departments of Internal Medicine and
Radiology, Divisions of Endocrinology and
Nuclear Medicine
The Ohio State University
1581 Dodd Drive
Columbus, OH 43210-1296, USA
Tel. +1 614 292 3800 / Fax. +1 614 292 1550
kloos-1@medctr.osu.edu

Dr. Günter KLÖPPEL*
Department of Pathology
University of Kiel
Michaelistrasse 11
D-24105 Kiel
GERMANY
Tel. +49 431 5973400
Fax. +49 431 5973462
gkloeppel@path.uni-kiel.de

Dr. Christian A. KOCH
Division of Endocrinology and Nephrology,
University of Leipzig
Philipp-Rosenthalstr. 27
D-04103 Leipzig
GERMANY
Tel. +49 341 971 3270
Fax. +49 341 971 3277
kochc@exchange.nih.gov

Dr. Paul KOMMINOTH*
Institute of Pathology
Kantonsspital Baden
CH-5404 Baden
SWITZERLAND
Tel. +41 56 486 3901
Fax. +41 56 486 3919
paul.komminoth@ksb.ch

Dr. George KONTOGEORGOS*
Department of Pathology,
KOFKA Building, 1st floor
G. Gennimatas Athens General Hospital
154 Messogion Avenue
11527 Athens, GREECE
Tel. +302 1077 84302 / Fax. +302 1077 05980
gkonto@med.uoa.gr

Dr. Kalman KOVACS*
Department of Laboratory Medicine
and Pathobiology
St. Michaels Hospital
30 Bond Street
Toronto, Ontario M5B 1W8, CANADA
Tel. +1 416 864 5858
Fax. +1 416 864 5648
kovacsk@smh.toronto.on.ca

Dr. Todd Gerard KROLL
Department of Pathology
University of Chicago Hospitals
P-323, MC 1089
5841 S. Maryland Avenue
Chicago, IL 60637, USA
Tel. +1 773 702 3017
Fax. +1 773 834 5251
tkroll@bsd.uchicago.edu

Dr. Alfred King Yin LAM*
Molecular Pathology
Griffith Medical School
Gold Coast Campus
Griffith University
PMB 50 GCMC
Bundall QLD 4217, AUSTRALIA
Tel. +61 75552 9217 / Fax. + 61 75552 9197
a.lam@griffith.edu.au

Dr. Catharina LARSSON
Department of Molecular Medicine
Karolinska University Hospital, Solna
CMM L8:01
SE-171 76 Stockholm
SWEDEN
Tel. +46 8 517 73930/73616
Fax. +46 8 517 76180
catharina.larsson@cmm.ki.se

Dr. Juan LECHAGO*
Department of Pathology and
Laboratory Medicine
Cedars - Sinai Medical Center
8700 Beverly Boulevard, Room 8740
Los Angeles, CA 90048, USA
Tel. +1 310 423 6604
Fax. +1 310 423 0122
lechagoj@cshs.org

Dr. E. Paul LINDELL
Department of Radiology
Division of Neuroradiology
Mayo Clinic
200 First Street SW
Rochester MN, USA
Tel. +1 507 255 6598
Fax. +1 507 266 1657
lindell.edward@mayo.edu

Dr. Virginia LIVOLSI
Department of Pathology and
Laboratory Medicine
University of Pennsylvania Medical Center
3400 Spruce Street, Founders 6-039
Philadelphia, PA 19104, USA
Tel. +1 215 662 6544
Fax. +1 215 349 5910
linus@mail.med.upenn.edu

Dr. Ricardo V. LLOYD*
Laboratory Medicine and Pathology
Mayo Clinic
200 First Street SW
Rochester, MN 55905, USA
Tel. +1 507 284 4022
Fax. +1 507 284 1875
lloyd.ricardo@mayo.edu
busciglio.Mary@mayo.edu

Dr. M. Beatriz S. LOPES
Dept. of Pathology (Neuropathology)
Box 800214 - HSC
University of Virginia Health System
Charlottesville, VA 22908-0214
USA
Tel. +1 434 924 9175
Fax. +1 434 924 9177
msl2e@virginia.edu

Dr. Eamonn R. MAHER
Section of Medical andMolecular Genetics
Department of Paediatrics and Child Health
The Medical School, Edgbaston
The University of Birmingham
B15 2TT Birmingham
UNITED KINGDOM
Tel. +44 121 627 2741 / Fax. +44 121 627 2618
e.r.maher@bham.ac.uk

Dr. Xavier MATIAS-GUIU*
Department of Pathology and
Molecular Genetics
Hospital Universitari Arnau de Vilanova
Universitat de Lleida
Av Alcalde Rovira Roure 80
25198 Lleida, SPAIN
Tel. +34 973 705340 / Fax. +34 973 248754
xmatias@arnau.scs.es

Dr. Ernest L. MAZZAFERRI
University of Florida
4020 SW 93rd Drive
Gainesville, FL 32608-4653
USA
Tel. +1 352 331 5192
Fax. +1 352 331 3192
mazz01@bellsouth.net

Dr. Anne Marie MCNICOL*
Department of Pathology
Glasgow Royal Infirmary
84 Castle Street
G4 0SF Glasgow
United Kingdom
Tel. +44 141 211 4764
Fax. +44 141 211 4884
a.m.mcnicol@clinmed.gla.ac.uk

Dr. L. Jeffrey MEDEIROS
Department of Hematopathology
University of Texas MD Anderson
Cancer Center
1515 Holcombe Boulevard, Box 0072
Houston, TX 77030, USA
Tel. +1 713 794 5446
Fax. +1 713 745 0736
jmedeiro@mdanderson.org

Dr. Maria J. MERINO
Surgical Pathology Section
National Cancer Institute
Bldg. 10, Rm. 2N212
9000 Rockville Pike
Bethesda, MD 20892, USA
Tel. +1 301 496 2441
Fax. +1 301 480 9488
mjmerino@box-m.nih.gov

Dr. Jeffrey F. MOLEY
Washington University School of Medicine
660 S. Euclid Avenue
Campus Box 8109
St. Louis, MO 63110
USA
Tel. +1 314 747 0064
Fax. +1 314 747 1310
moleyj@wustl.edu

Dr. Carl D. MORRISON
Research Histology Core Facility
University Hospitals
Department of Pathology
M-418 Starling Loving Hall
320 West 10th Avenue
Columbus, OH 43210, USA
Tel. +1 614 293 6628 / Fax. +1 614 293 7626
morrison-4@medctr.osu.edu

Dr. Lois MULLIGAN
Departments of Paediatrics and Pathology
Lab: Botterell Hall, Rm. 319
Queens University
20 Barrie Street
Kingston, Ontario K7L 3N6, CANADA
Tel. +1 613 533 6310 / Fax. +1 613 548 1348
mulligal@post.queensu.ca

Dr. Katherine L. NATHANSON
Division of Medical Genetics, Department
of Medicine
University of Pennsylvania School of
Medicine
513 BRB 2/3, 421 Curie Boulevard
Philadelphia, PA 19104, USA
Tel. +1 215 573 9840 / Fax. +1 215 573 2486
knathans@mail.med.upenn.edu

Dr. Hartmut P. NEUMANN
Department of Nephrology and
Hypertension
Albert-Ludwigs-University
Hugstetterstr. 55
D-79106 Freiburg, GERMANY
Tel. +49 761 270 3578
Fax. +49 761 270 3778
neumann@med1.ukl.uni-freiburg.de

Dr. Yuri E. NIKIFOROV
Department of Pathology and
Laboratory Medicine
University of Cincinnati College of
Medicine
231 Albert Sabin Way
Cincinnati, OH 45267-0529, USA
Tel. +1 513 558 5798 / Fax. +1 513 558 2289
yuri.nikiforov@uc.edu

Dr. Shiro NOGUCHI
Noguchi Thyroid Clinic and
Hospital Foundation
6-33 Noguchi-Nakamachi
Beppu, Oita 874-0932
JAPAN
Tel. +81 977 21 2151
Fax. +81 977 21 2176
noguchi@noguchi-med.or.jp

Dr. Vania NOSE
Department of Pathology
Brigham and Women's Hospital
75 Francis Street
Boston MA 02115
USA
Tel. +1 617 732 6772
Fax. +1 617 566 3897
v.nose@partners.org

Professor Kjell ÖBERG
Uppsala University
Akademiska sjukhuset
SE-751 85 Uppsala
SWEDEN
Tel. +46 18 6114917
Fax. +46 18 507268
kjell.oberg@medsci.uu.se

Dr. Nelson G. ORDÓÑEZ
Department of Pathology and Laboratory
Medicine
The University of Texas MD Anderson
Cancer Center
1515 Holcombe Boulevard, Box 0085
Houston, TX 77030, USA
Tel. +1 713 792 3167 / Fax. +1 713 792 3696
nordonez1@houston.rr.com

Dr. Josep ORIOLA
Department of Hormonology/
Molecular Biology
escalera 7, piso 5.
Hospital Clinic
C/ Villarroel no.170
08036 Barcelona, SPAIN
Tel. +34 932275510 / Fax. +34 932275454
joriola@clinic.ub.es

Dr. Robert Yoshiyuki OSAMURA*
Department of Pathology
Tokai University School of Medicine
Bohseidai Isehara City
259-1193 Kanagawa
JAPAN
Tel. +81 463 93 1121 (ext. 3171)
Fax. +81 463 911370
osamura@is.icc.u-tokai.ac.jp

Dr. Mauro PAPOTTI*
Department of Biomedical Sciences
and Oncology
University of Turin
Via Santena 7
I-10126 Torino, ITALY
Tel. +390 011 6706504/6691
Fax. +390 011 6635267
mauro.papotti@unito.it

Dr. Ralf PASCHKE
Medizinische Klinik und Poliklinik III
Universitätsklinikum Leipzig
Philipp-Rosenthal-Str. 27
D-04103 Leipzig
GERMANY
Tel. +49 341 97 13200
Fax. +49 341 97 13209
pasr@medizin.uni-leipzig.de

Dr. Juha PELTONEN
Department of Anatomy and Cell Biology
University of Oulu
Aapistie 7 (PB 5000)
FIN-90014 Oulu
FINLAND
Tel. +358 8 5375186
Fax. +358 8 5375172
juha.peltonen@oulu.fi

Dr. Aurel PERREN*
Departement Pathologie
Institut für Klinische Pathologie
Labor für Endokrinopathologie
Schmelzbergstrasse 12
CH-8091 Zurich
SWITZERLAND
Tel. +41 1 255 11 11 / Fax. +41 1 255 44 40
aurel.perren@usz.ch

Dr. Silvana PILOTTI
Dipartimento di Patologia
Anatomia Patologica C
Istituto Nazionale per lo Studio e la Cura
dei Tumori, Via G. Venezian, 1
I-20133 Milano
ITALY
Tel. +39 02 23902293 / Fax. +39 02 23902756
silvana.pilotti@istitutotumori.mi.it

Dr. Karl H. PLATE
Neurologisches Institute (Edinger Institut)
Der Johann Wolfgang Goethe-Universität
Deutschordenstr. 46
D-60528 Frankfurt/Main
GERMANY
Tel. +49 69 63016042
Fax. +49 69 679487
karl-heinz.plate@kgu.de

Dr. Hartmut M. RABES
Institute of Pathology
Ludwig Maximilians University of Munich
Thalkirchner Strasse 36
D-80337 Munich
GERMANY
Tel. +49 89 5160 4081
Fax. +49 89 5160 4083
hm.rabes@lrz.uni-muenchen.de

Dr. Guido RINDI
Dipartimento di Patologia Umana e
Medicina di Laboratorio
Sezione di Anatomia Patologica, Università
degli Studi
Via A. Gramsci, 14
I-43100 Parma, ITALY
Tel. +390 521 290 386 / Fax. +390 521 292710
guido.rindi@unipr.it

Dr. Federico RONCAROLI
Department of Neuropathology
Imperial College, Faculty of Medicine
Charing Cross Hospital
Fulham Palace Rd.
London W6 8RF, UNITED KINGDOM
Tel. +44 208 846 7178
Fax. +44 208 846 7794
f.roncaroli@imperial.ac.uk

Dr. Wolfgang SAEGER
Institut für Pathologie
Marienkrankenhaus
Alfredstrasse 9
D-22087 Hamburg
GERMANY
Tel. +49 40 2546 2701
Fax. +49 40 2546 2730
wolfgangsaeger.hh@t-online.de

Dr. Atsuhiko SAKAMOTO
Department of Pathology
Kyorin University School of Medicine
6-20-2 Shinkawa, Mitaka-shi
Tokyo 181-8611
JAPAN
Tel. +81 422 47 5511
Fax. +81 422 40 7093
sakamoto@kyorin-u.ac.jp

Dr. Toshiaki SANO*
Department of Pathology
University of Tokushima
School of Medicine
3-18-15 Kuramoto-cho
770-8503 Tokushima, JAPAN
Tel. +81 88 633 7063
Fax. +81 88 633 9423
sano@basic.med.tokushima-u.ac.jp

Dr. Massimo SANTORO
Dipartimento di Biologia e
Patologia Cellulare e Molecolare
Universita di Napoli Federico II
Via S. Pansini 5
I-80131 Naples, ITALY
Tel. +39 081 746 3056
Fax. +39 081 746 3037
masantor@unina.it

Dr. Hironobu SASANO*
Department of Pathology
Tohoku University School of Medicine
2-1 Seiryou-machi, Aoba-ku
Sendai-Shi, Miyagi-Ken 980-8575
JAPAN
Tel. +81 22 717 8050
Fax. +81 22 273 5976
hsasano@patholo2.med.tohoku.ac.jp

Dr. Bernd W. SCHEITHAUER
Department of Laboratory Medicine
and Pathology
200 First Street SW
Rochester, MN 55905
USA
Tel. +1 507 284 8350
Fax. +1 507 284 1599
scheithauer.bernd@mayo.edu

Dr. Katherine A. SCHNEIDER
Dana-Farber Cancer Institute SM331
44 Binney Street
Boston, MA 02115
USA
Tel. +1 617 632 3480
Fax. +1 617 632 681/3161
katherine_schneider@dfci.harvard.edu

Dr. Arthur B. SCHNEIDER
Section of Endocrinology
University of Illinois at Chicago
1819 W. Polk Street (M/C 640)
Chicago, IL 60612-7333
USA
Tel. +1 312 996 6062
Fax. +1 312 413 0437
abschnei@uic.edu

Dr. Jean Yves SCOAZEC
Department of Pathology
Hôpital Edouard Herriot
F-69437 LYON Cedex 03
France
Tel. +33 4 72 11 07 50
Fax. +33 4 72 11 69 81
jean-yves.scoazec@chu-lyon.fr

Dr. Elizabeth SHANE
Division of Endocrinology
Columbia University College of Physicians
and Surgeons
PH 8 West 864, 630 West 168th Street
New York, NY 10032, USA
Tel. +1 212 305 6238
Fax. +1 212 305 6486
es54@columbia.edu

Dr. Leslie H. SOBIN
Hepatic and Gastrointestinal Pathology
Armed Forces Institute of Pathology
14th Street and Alaska Avenue
Washington, DC 20306
USA
Tel. +1 202 782 2880
Fax. +1 202 782 9020
sobin@afip.osd.mil

Dr. Manuel SOBRINHO-SIMOES*
IPATIMUP
Rua Roberto Frias, S/N
P-4200-465 Porto
PORTUGAL
Tel. +351 22 5570700
Fax. +351 22 5570799/03940
sobrinho.simoes@ipatimup.pt

Dr. Ernst J. M. SPEEL
Department of Molecular Cell Biology
University of Maastricht
Research Institute Growth
and Development
6200 MD Maastricht, THE NETHERLANDS
Tel. +31 43 3881361
Fax. +31 43 3884151
ernstjan.speel@molcelb.unimaas.nl

Dr. Constantine A. STRATAKIS
Section on Endocrinology & Genetics/
DEB & Heritable Disorders Branch
NICHD, NIH, Bldg. 10, Rm. 10N262,
10 Center Drive
Bethesda, MD 20892-1862, USA
Tel. +1 301 496 4686
Fax. +1 301 402 0574
stratakc@mail.nih.gov

Dr. Hugo STUDER
Breichtenstrasse 13
CH-3074 Muri
SWITZERLAND
Tel. +41 31 951 39 89
Fax. +41 31 951 08 80
h.studer@bgb.ch

Dr. Iwao SUGITANI
Division of Head and Neck
Cancer Institute Hospital
1-37-1 Kami-ikebukuro, Toshima-ku
170-8455 Tokyo
JAPAN
Tel. +81 3 3918 0111
Fax. +81 3 3918 0167
isugitani@jfcr.or.jp

Dr. Saul SUSTER
Department of Pathology
The Ohio State University
E411 Doan Hall, 410 W 10th Avenue
Columbus, OH 43210
USA
Tel. +1 614 293 7625/5905
Fax. +1 614 293 7626
suster.3@osu.edu

Mr. Kevin M. SWEET
Division of Human Genetics,
Department of Internal Medicine
The Ohio State University
2050 Kenny Road, 8th Fl. Tower
Columbus, OH 43221, USA
Tel. +1 614 293 6694
Fax. +1 614 293 2314
sweet-3@medctr.osu.edu

Dr. Giovanni TALLINI
Department of Pathology
University of Bologna School of Medicine
Ospedale Bellaria
Via Altura 3
40139 Bologna, ITALY
Tel. +39 051 622 5757
Fax. +39 051 622 5759
giovanni.tallini@ausl.bo.it

Dr. Bin Tean TEH
Van Andel Research Institute
333 Bostwick NE
Grand Rapids, MI 49503
USA
Tel. +1 616 234 5296
Fax. +1 616 234 5297
bin.teh@vai.org

Dr. Lester D.R. THOMPSON*
Southern California Permanente
Medical Group
Department of Pathology
Woodland Hills Medical Center
5601 De Soto Avenue
Woodland Hills, CA 91365, USA
Tel. +1 818 719 2613 / Fax. +1 818 719 2309
lester.d.thompson@kp.org

Dr. Arthur S. TISCHLER*
Department of Pathology
Tufts New England Medical Center
750 Washington Street, Box 802
Boston, MA 02111
USA
Tel. +1 617 636 1038
Fax. +1 617 636 8302
atischler@tufts-nemc.org

Dr. Jacqueline TROUILLAS*
Unite INSERM U433 - Laboratoire
d'Histologie et Embryologie moleculaires
Faculté de Medecine Laennec
Rue Guillaume Paradin
69372 Lyon Cedex 8, FRANCE
Tel. +33 4 78 77 86 55
Fax. +33 4 78 77 86 16
lhem@laennec.univ-lyon1.fr

Dr. Thomas M. ULBRIGHT
Department of Pathology and Laboratory
Medicine, Rm. 3465
Indiana University Hospital
550 N. University Boulevard
Indianapolis, IN 46202-5280, USA
Tel. +1 317 274 5786/2498
Fax. +1 317 274 5346
tulbrigh@iupui.edu

Dr. Sergio VIDAL RUIBAL (deceased)
Department of Anatomy
Laboratory of Histology
University of Santiago de Compostela
27002 Lugo
SPAIN
Tel. +34 9 82 252231
Fax. +34 9 82 252195

Dr. M. VOLANTE
Department of Biomedical Sciences
and Oncology
University of Turin
Via Santena 7
I-10126 Torino, ITALY
Tel. +390 11 670 6504/6691/6514
Fax. +390 11 663 5267
marco.volante@unito.it

Dr. Petri E. VOUTILAINEN
Selkämeri Hospital
Lapväärtintie 8
FIN-64100 Kristiinankaupunki
FINLAND
Tel. +358 40 7478678/0763318
Fax. +358 62 218364
petri.voutilainen@vshp.fi

Dr. Robert WATSON
Division of Neuroradiology,
Department of Diagnostic Radiology,
Mayo Clinic
200 First Street SW
Rochester, MN 55905, USA
Tel. +1 507 266 1206
Fax. +1 507 266 1657
watson.robert16@mayo.edu

Dr. A.L. WEBER
Department of Radiology
Massachusetts Eye and Ear Infirmary
243 Charles Street
Boston, MA 02114
USA
Tel. +1 617 573 3563
Fax. +1 617 573 3490
alweber1@aol.com

Dr. Lee S. WEINSTEIN
Metabolic Diseases Branch
National Institute of Diabetes, Digestive
and Kidney Diseases
National Institutes of Health
Bldg. 10/Rm. 8C101
Bethesda, MD 20892-1752, USA
Tel. +1 301 402 2923 / Fax. +1 301 402 0374
leew@amb.niddk.nih.gov

Dr. Lawrence M. WEISS
Division of Pathology,
Main Medical Building NW 2250
City of Hope National Medical Center
1500 East Duarte Road
Duarte, CA 91010, USA
Tel. +1 626 256 4673 (ext.62583)
Fax. +1 626 301 8842
lweiss@coh.org

Dr. Bruce M. WENIG
Department of Pathology
Beth Israel Medical Center
1st Avenue at 16th Street
11 Silver Rm. 10
New York, NY 10543, USA
Tel. +1 212 420 4031
Fax. +1 212 420 3449
bwenig@bethisraelny.org

Dr. E. Dillwyn WILLIAMS*
Thyroid Carcinogenesis Group
Strangeways Research Laboratory
Worts Causeway
CB1 8RN Cambridge
UNITED KINGDOM
Tel. +44 1223 740180
Fax. +44 1223 411609
dillwyn@srl.cam.ac.uk

Dr. Shozo YAMADA
Department of Neurosurgery
Toranomon Hospital
2-2-2 Toranomon, Minato-Ku
Tokyo 105
JAPAN
Tel. +81 3 3588 1111
Fax. +81 3 3582 7068
syamadays11@hotmail.com

Dr. William F. YOUNG JR*
Division of Endocrinology
Mayo Clinic
200 First Street SW
Rochester, MN 55905
USA
Tel. +1 507 284 2191
Fax. +1 507 284 5745
young.william@mayo.edu

Dr. Maureen ZAKOWSKI
Department of Pathology
Memorial Sloan-Kettering
Cancer Center
1275 York Avenue
New York, NY 10021
Tel. +1 212 639 5946
Fax. +1 212 639 6318
zakowskm@mskcc.org

Source of charts and photographs

1.

1.01A-D	Dr. R. Watson/ Dr. E.P. Lindell
1.02A-C	Dr. S.L. Asa
1.02D	Dr. T. Sano
1.03A-D	Dr. S.L. Asa
1.04A-1.05	Dr. C. Stratakis
1.06A,B	Dr. W.E. Farrell
1.07 A-1.08	Dr. T. Sano
1.09A,B	Dr. K. Kovacs
1.10A-C	Dr. V. Nose'
1.11A	D. T. Sano
1.11B	Dr. K. Kovacs
1.12A,B	Dr. R. Watson/ Dr. E.P. Lindell
1.13A,C	Dr. T. Sano
1.13B	Dr. J. Trouillas
1.13D	Dr. R.V. Lloyd
1.14A	Dr. J. Trouillas
1.14B	Dr. K. Kovacs
1.15A-1.17-D	Dr. S.L. Asa
1.18	Dr. R. Watson/ Dr. E.P. Lindell
1.19A,B	Dr. T. Sano
1.20A	Dr. K. Kovacs
1.20B	Dr. T. Sano
1.21	Dr. R. Watson/ Dr. E.P. Lindell
1.22A-1.23A	Dr. R. Lloyd
1.23B-1.23D	Dr. V. Nose'
1.24A,B	Dr. R.V. Lloyd
1.25-1.26	Dr. M.B.S. Lopes
1.27A,B	Dr. M.B.S. Lopes
1.28	Dr. R. Watson/ Dr. E.P. Lindell
1.29-1.30C	Dr. K. Kovacs

2.

2.001A,B	J. Ferlay, IARC, Lyon, France
2.002	Dr. Y.E. Demichik Belarussian Medical University, Minsk, Belarus
2.003A,B	Dr. L.D.R. Thompson

The copyright remains with the authors. Requests for permission to reproduce figures or charts should be directed to the respective contributor. For addresses see Contributors List.

2.003C	Dr. D. Dupuy
2.004A	Dr. X. Matias-Guiu
2.004B,C	Dr. J. Albores-Saavedra
2.004D	Dr. L. Bondeson
2.005A,B	Dr. J. Cameselle-Teijeiro
2.006A	Dr. R.A. DeLellis
2.006B	Dr. S. Boerner
2.006C	Dr. Z. Baloch Dept. of Pathology, University of Pennsylvania Medical Ctr. Philadelphia, PA 19104, USA
2.006D	Dr. S. Boerner
2.007	Dr. J. Cameselle-Teijeiro
2.008A,B	Dr. L.D.R. Thompson
2.009A-2.011D	Dr. R.A. DeLellis
2.012A	Dr. X. Matias-Guiu
2.012B	Dr. S. Boerner
2.012C	Dr. R.A. DeLellis
2.013	Dr. J. Albores-Saavedra
2.014A	Dr. L. Bondeson
2.014B	Dr. J. Albores-Saavedra
2.015A	Dr. R.A. DeLellis
2.015B	Dr. J. Cameselle-Teijeiro
2.015C	Dr. L.D.R. Thompson
2.016A,C	Dr. S.L. Asa
2.016B	Dr. J. Albores-Saavedra
2.017A,B	Dr. X. Matias-Guiu
2.017C,D	Dr. L.D.R. Thompson
2.018	S.L. Asa
2.019A	Dr. R.A. Delellis
2.019B,C	Dr. L.D.R. Thompson
2.019D-2.020	Dr. R.A. DeLellis
2.021-2.022	Dr. L.D.R. Thompson
2.023	Dr. J. Cameselle-Teijeiro
2.024A	Dr. Z. Baloch
2.024B	Dr. R.A. DeLellis
2.025A	Dr. L.D.R. Thompson
2.025B	Dr. R.A. DeLellis
2.025C-2.026A	Dr. M. Sobrinho-Simoes
2.026B-2.027	Dr. R.A. DeLellis
2.028	Dr. X. Matias-Guiu
2.029-2.030D	Dr. R.A. DeLellis

2.031A-2.032	Dr. T.G. Kroll
2.033	Dr. X. Matias-Guiu
2.034	Dr. M.F. Zakowski
2.035A	Dr. X. Matias-Guiu
2.035B	Dr. M. Papotti
2.035C	Dr. M. Sobrinho-Simoes
2.035D	Dr. R.A. DeLellis
2.036A,B	Dr. M. Sobrinho-Simoes
2.037	Dr. R.V. Lloyd
2.038	Dr. J. Cameselle-Teijeiro
2.039A	Dr. S. Boerner
2.039B	Dr. R.A. DeLellis
2.039C	Dr. X. Matias-Guiu
2.040A,B	Dr. R.A. DeLellis
2.041A	Dr. L.D.R. Thompson
2.041B-2.042A	Dr. X. Matias-Guiu
2.042B-2.043A	Dr. L.D.R. Thompson
2.043B	Dr. R.A. DeLellis
2.044	Dr. A.K.Y. Lam
2.045	Dr. J.K.C. Chan
2.046	Dr. M. Sobrinho-Simoes
2.047A,B	Dr. B.M. Wenig
2.048A	Dr. L.D.R. Thompson
2.048B	Dr. B.M. Wenig
2.049A	Dr. L. Bondeson
2.049B	Dr. J.K.C. Chan
2.049C	Dr. L.D.R. Thompson
2.050-2.052	Dr. M. Sobrinho-Simoes
2.053A,B	Dr. X. Matias-Guiu
2.054A-C	Dr. L. Bondeson
2.055A,B	Dr. R.A. DeLellis
2.056A	Dr. L.D.R. Thompson
2.056B-2.059D	Dr. R.A. DeLellis
2.060-2.061	Dr. M. Papotti
2.062A-2.063	Dr. R.A. DeLellis
2.064A-C	Dr. X. Matias-Guiu
2.065A-2.066C	Dr. J.K.C. Chan
2.066D	Dr. L.D.R. Thompson
2.067A-2.068C	Dr. J.K.C. Chan
2.069	Dr. L.D.R. Thompson
2.070	Dr. D. Dupuy
2.071	Dr. L. Bondeson
2.072A-2.073C	Dr. J.K.C. Chan
2.074A-2.075C	Dr. R.A. DeLellis
2.076A	Dr. J.K.C. Chan
2.076B	Dr. L.D.R. Thompson
2.077A-2.078B	Dr. J.K.C. Chan
2.078C	Dr. M. Hirokawa

2.078D-2.079B	Dr. J.K.C. Chan
2.080A	Dr. M. Papotti
2.080B-2.081	Dr. R.A. DeLellis
2.082A	Dr. M. Papotti
2.082B	Dr. S.L. Asa
2.083A	Dr. L.D.R. Thompson
2.083B,C	Dr. S.L. Asa
2.084-2.088	Dr. L.D.R. Thompson
2.089A,B	Dr. S. Boerner
2.090A-2.091C	Dr. L.D.R. Thompson
2.092A,B	Dr. J.K.C. Chan
2.093-2.095B	Dr. V. Eusebi
2.096A-2.098B	Dr. L.D.R. Thompson
2.099	Dr. R.A. DeLellis
2.100	Dr. X. Matias-Guiu
2.101A	Dr. M. Sobrinho-Simoes
2.101B	Dr. J. Cameselle-Teijeiro
2.101C	Dr. M. Sobrinho-Simoes
2.102	Dr. J. Cameselle-Teijeiro
2.103A,B	Dr. L.B. Kahn
2.104	Dr. R.A. DeLellis
2.105	Dr. L.D.R. Thompson
2.106A	Dr. R.A. DeLellis
2.106B,C	Dr. L.D.R. Thompson
2.106D	Dr. R.A. DeLellis
2.107A	Dr. J. Cameselle-Teijeiro
2.107B	Dr. L.D.R. Thompson
2.108	Dr. S. Asa
2.109A-2.110	Dr. R.A. DeLellis
2.111A,B	Dr. L. Bondeson
2.111C,D	Dr. R.A. DeLellis
2.111E	Dr. L. Bondeson
2.111F-2.112B	Dr. R.A. DeLellis
2.112C,D	Dr. L. Bondeson
2.113A-C	Dr. D. Dupuy
2.114A	Dr. R.V. Lloyd
2.114B,C	Dr. L. Bondeson
2.115A	Dr. L. Grimelius
2.115B,2.116A	Dr. R.A. DeLellis
2.116B,C	Dr. L. Grimelius
2.116D	Dr. R.A. DeLellis
2.117A,B	Dr. L. Grimelius
2.117B	Dr. L. Grimelius
2.118	Dr. R.A. Delellis
2.119	Dr. L. Grimelius
2.120	Dr. R.A. DeLellis

3.

3.01	Dr. X. Bertagna
3.02A	Dr. D.S. Klimstra
3.02B	Dr. R. V. Lloyd
3.02C	Dr. L.D.R. Thompson
3.03A	Dr. A. Perren
3.03B	Dr. L.D.R. Thompson
3.04	Dr. W.F. Young
3.05A	Dr. H. Sasano
3.05B,C	Dr. A.S. Tischler
3.06A	Dr. H. Sasano
3.06B	Dr. A.K.Y. Lam
3.06C,D	Dr. A.S. Tischler
3.07A,B	Dr. L.D.R. Thompson
3.08A-C	Dr. W.F. Young
3.09A	Dr. A. McNicol
3.09B-3.13B	Dr. L.D.R. Thompson
3.14A-D	Dr. W.F. Young
3.15A	Dr. A.S. Tischler
3.15B,C	Dr. R.V. Lloyd
3.16A,D	Dr. A. Perren
3.16B,C	Dr. L.D.R. Thompson
3.17	Dr. P. Komminoth
3.18A-3.19C	Dr. A.S. Tischler
3.20	Dr. W.F. Young
3.21	Dr. J. Albores-Saavedra
3.22A-3.22D	Dr. N. Kimura
3.23A,B	Dr. R.V. Lloyd
3.24A-C	Dr. J. Albores-Saavedra
3.25A	Dr. N. Kimura
3.25B	Dr. A.K.Y. Lam
3.25C	Dr. R.V. Lloyd
3.26A	Dr. F.W. Abdul-Karim, Deptm. Pathology, University Hospitals of Cleveland, Cleveland, OH 44106 USA
3.26B-3.27A	Dr. L.D.R. Thompson
3.27B,C	Dr. A.K.Y. Lam
3.28A,B	Dr. R.V. Lloyd
3.29A,B	Dr. A.S. Tischler
3.29C-3.30B	Dr. L.D.R. Thompson
3.31A,C	Dr. R.V. Lloyd
3.31B,D	Dr. L.D.R. Thompson
3.32A,B	Dr. R.V. Lloyd

4.

4.01	Dr. Ph.U. Heitz
4.02A-4.02F	Dr. D.S. Klimstra
4.03	Dr. B. Centeno
4.04A,B	Dr. Ph.U. Heitz
4.05	Dr. D.S. Klimstra
4.06A	Dr. G. Klöppel
4.06B-4.07	Dr. A. Perren
4.08	Dr. P. Komminoth
4.09	Dr. Ph.U. Heitz
4.10	Dr. B. Marincek, Institute of Diagnostic Radiology, University Hospital, 8091 Zurich, Switzerland
4.11	Dr. D.T. Schmid Division of Nuclear Medicine, University Hospital , 8091 Zurich, Switzerland.
4.12A	Dr. A. Perren
4.12B	Dr. G. Klöppel
4.13-4.14A	Dr. A. Perren
4.14B,C	Dr. G. Klöppel
4.14D-F	Dr. A. Perren
4.14G	Dr. P. Komminoth
4.14H,I	Dr. Ph.U. Heitz
4.15,4.16	Dr. A. Perren
4.17,4.18	Dr. G. Klöppel
4.19A	Dr. A. Perren
4.19B	Dr. Ph.U. Heitz
4.20	Dr. A. Perren
4.21	Dr. Y. Dayal
4.22A	Dr. A. Perren
4.22B	Dr. Y. Dayal
4.23A,B	Dr. A. Perren
4.24	Dr. R.Y. Osamura
4.25A-C	Dr. A. Perren
4.25D	Dr. G. Klöppel
4.26	Dr. A. Perren
4.27A-4.29B	Dr. Ph.U. Heitz
4.30	Dr. A. Perren
4.31	Dr. H. Miwa Juntendo University, 113 8421 School of Medicine, Tokyo, Japan.
4.32	Dr. R.Y. Osamura
4.33	Dr. H. Miwa
4.34	Dr. G. Klöppel
4.35A	Dr. Y. Hirata Dept. of Clinical and Mol. Endocrinology, Tokyo Medical and Dental University, Tokyo 113-8519, Japan.
4.35B	Dr. G. Klöppel
4.36-4.37B	Dr. Ph.U. Heitz
4.38A	Dr. D.S. Klimstra
4.38B	Dr. Ph.U. Heitz
4.38C,D	Dr. D.S. Klimstra
4.39A	Dr. Ph.U. Heitz
4.39B	Dr. A. Perren
4.40-4.42B	Dr. D.S. Klimstra
4.43	Dr. A. Perren
4.44A	Dr. D.S. Klimstra
4.44B-4.46A	Dr. C. Capella
4.46B	Dr. G. Klöppel

5.

5.01A-5.07	Dr. P. Komminoth
5.08	Dr. F.B. Chazot, Service d'Endocrinologie, Hôpital de l'Antiquaille, 69005 Lyon, France
5.09A	Dr. P. Komminoth
5.09B-5.10B	Dr. G. Klöppel
5.10C-5.11A	Dr. P. Komminoth
5.11B-5.12	Dr. G. Klöppel
5.13A,B	Dr. P. Komminoth
5.13C	Dr. G. Klöppel
5.14A-5.16	Dr. P. Komminoth
5.17- 5.19	Dr. A. Calender
5.20A,B	Dr. B.T. Teh
5.21A-C	Dr. H.P.H. Neumann
5.22-5.25	Dr. P. Komminoth
5.26	Dr. A. Perren
5.27A-C	Dr. K.L. Nathanson
5.28	Dr. W.F. Young
5.29A,B	Dr. P. Komminoth
5.30A-5.32B	Dr. C.A. Stratakis
5.33	Dr. M. Collins, Natl. Inst. of Diabetes, Digestive and Kidney Diseases, NIH, Bethesda, MD 20892-1752, USA
5.34	Dr. L.S. Weinstein
5.35A,B	Dr. H.R. Harach
5.36	Dr. W. Foulkes

References

1. Anon. (1979). Gastrointestinal hormones in clinical disease: recent developments. Ann Intern Med 90: 817-828.
2. Anon. (1988). Neurofibromatosis. Conference statement. National Institutes of Health Consensus Development Conference. Arch Neurol 45: 575-578.
3. Anon. (1991). NIH conference. Diagnosis and management of asymptomatic primary hyperparathyroidism: consensus development conference statement. Ann Intern Med 114: 593-597.
4. Anon. (1995). Points to consider: ethical, legal, and psychosocial implications of genetic testing in children and adolescents. American Society of Human Genetics Board of Directors, American College of Medical Genetics Board of Directors. Am J Hum Genet 57: 1233-1241.
5. Anon. (2001). Case records of the Massachusetts General Hospital. Weekly clinicopathological exercises. Case 13-2001. A 19-year-old man with bouts of hypertension and severe headaches. N Engl J Med 344: 1314-1320.
6. Abbass SA, Asa SL, Ezzat S (1997). Altered expression of fibroblast growth factor receptors in human pituitary adenomas. J Clin Endocrinol Metab 82: 1160-1166.
7. Abe T, Matsuda H, Shindo J, Nonomura K, Koyanagi T (2000). Ectopic pheochromocytoma arising in the spermatic cord 5 years after removal of bilateral carotid body tumors and adrenal pheochromocytomas. Int J Urol 7: 110-111.
8. Abe T, Matsumoto K, Iida M, Hayashi M, Sanno N, Osamura RY (1997). Malignant carcinoid tumor of the anterior mediastinum metastasis to a prolactin-secreting pituitary adenoma: a case report. Surg Neurol 48: 389-394.
9. Abernathy CR, Rasmussen SA, Stalker HJ, Zori R, Driscoll DJ, Williams CA, Kousseff BG, Wallace MR (1997). NF1 mutation analysis using a combined heteroduplex/SSCP approach. Hum Mutat 9: 548-554.
10. Abrams HL, Spiro R, Goldstein N (1950). Metastases in carcinoma. Analysis of 1000 autopsied cases. Cancer 3: 74-85.
11. Adamson AR, Grahame-Smith DG, Bogomoletz V, Maw DS, Rothnie NG (1971). Malignant argentaffinoma with carcinoid syndrome and hypoglycaemia. Br Med J 3: 93-94.
12. Agarwal SK, Guru SC, Heppner C, Erdos MR, Collins RM, Park SY, Saggar S, Chandrasekharappa SC, Collins FS, Spiegel AM, Marx SJ, Burns AL (1999). Menin interacts with the AP1 transcription factor JunD and represses JunD-activated transcription. Cell 96: 143-152.
13. Agarwal SK, Kester MB, Debelenko LV, Heppner C, Emmert-Buck MR, Skarulis MC, Doppman JL, Kim YS, Lubensky IA, Zhuang Z, Green JS, Guru SC, Manickam P, Olufemi SE, Liotta LA, Chandrasekharappa SC, Collins FS, Spiegel AM, Burns AL, Marx SJ (1997). Germline mutations of the MEN1 gene in familial multiple endocrine neoplasia type 1 and related states. Hum Mol Genet 6: 1169-1175.
14. Agarwal SK, Schrock E, Kester MB, Burns AL, Heffess CS, Ried T, Marx SJ (1998). Comparative genomic hybridization analysis of human parathyroid tumors. Cancer Genet Cytogenet 106: 30-36.
15. Aghakhani N, George B, Parker F (1999). Paraganglioma of the cauda equina region—report of two cases and review of the literature. Acta Neurochir (Wien) 141: 81-87.
16. Aguiar RC, Cox G, Pomeroy SL, Dahia PL (2001). Analysis of the SDHD gene, the susceptibility gene for familial paraganglioma syndrome (PGL1), in pheochromocytomas. J Clin Endocrinol Metab 86: 2890-2894.
17. Aguiar RC, Dahia PL, Sill H, Toledo SP, Goldman JM, Cross NC (1996). Deletion analysis of the p16 tumour suppressor gene in phaeochromocytomas. Clin Endocrinol (Oxf) 45: 93-96.
18. Akerstrom G, Rudberg C, Grimelius L, Bergstrom R, Johansson H, Ljunghall S, Rastad J (1986). Histologic parathyroid abnormalities in an autopsy series. Hum Pathol 17: 520-527.
19. Akerstrom G, Rudberg C, Grimelius L, Rastad J (1988). Recurrent hyperparathyroidism due to peroperative seeding of neoplastic or hyperplastic parathyroid tissue. Case report. Acta Chir Scand 154: 549-552.
20. Akin MR, Nguyen GK (1999). Fine-needle aspiration biopsy cytology of hyalinizing trabecular adenomas of the thyroid. Diagn Cytopathol 20: 90-94.
21. Akintoye SO, Chebli C, Booher S, Feuillan P, Kushner H, Leroith D, Cherman N, Bianco P, Wientroub S, Robey PG, Collins MT (2002). Characterization of gsp-mediated growth hormone excess in the context of McCune-Albright syndrome. J Clin Endocrinol Metab 87: 5104-5112.
22. Akoojee SB (1980). Teratoma of the thyroid gland. S Afr Med J 57: 93-94.
23. Akslen LA, LiVolsi VA (2000). Prognostic significance of histologic grading compared with subclassification of papillary thyroid carcinoma. Cancer 88: 1902-1908.
23A. Albareda M, Puig-Domingo M, Wengrowicz S, Soldevila J, Matias-Guiu X, Caballero A, Chico A, De Leiva A (1998). Clinical forms of presentation and evolution of diffuse sclerosing variant of papillary carcinoma and insular variant of follicular carcinoma of the thyroid. Thyroid 8(5): 385-391.
24. Al Ghamdi S, Fageeh N, Dewan M (2000). Malignant schwannoma of the thyroid gland. Otolaryngol Head Neck Surg 122: 143-144.
25. al Kaisi N, Weaver MG, Abdul-Karim FW, Siegler E (1992). Fine needle aspiration cytology of neuroendocrine tumors of the pancreas. A cytologic, immunocytochemical and electron microscopic study. Acta Cytol 36: 655-660.
26. Albores-Saavedra J, Gorraez de la Mora T, Torre-Rendon F, Gould E (1990). Mixed medullary-papillary carcinoma of the thyroid: a previously unrecognized variant of thyroid carcinoma. Hum Pathol 21: 1151-1155.
27. Albores-Saavedra J, Gould E, Vardaman C, Vuitch F (1991). The macrofollicular variant of papillary thyroid carcinoma: a study of 17 cases. Hum Pathol 22: 1195-1205.
28. Albores-Saavedra J, Housini I, Vuitch F, Snyder WHI (1997). Macrofollicular variant of papillary thyroid carcinoma with minor insular component. Cancer 80: 1110-1116.
29. Albores-Saavedra J, LiVolsi VA, Williams ED (1985). Medullary carcinoma. Semin Diagn Pathol 2: 137-146.
30. Albores-Saavedra J, Monforte H, Nadji M, Morales AR (1988). C-cell hyperplasia in thyroid tissue adjacent to follicular cell tumors. Hum Pathol 19: 795-799.
31. Albores-Saavedra J, Sharma S (2001). Poorly differentiated follicular thyroid carcinoma with rhabdoid phenotype: a clinicopathologic, immunohistochemical and electron microscopic study of two cases. Mod Pathol 14: 98-104.
32. Albores-Saavedra JA, Krueger JE (2001). C-cell hyperplasia and medullary thyroid microcarcinoma. Endocr Pathol 12: 365-377.
33. Albrecht S, Bilbao JM, Kovacs K (2002). Non-pituitary tumors of the sellar region. In: The Pituitary, Melmed S, ed., 2nd ed. Blackwell Science Inc.: Malden , pp. 592-609.
34. Albrecht S, Gardiner GW, Kovacs K, Ilse G, Kaiser U (1989). Duodenal somatostatinoma with psammoma bodies. Arch Pathol Lab Med 113: 517-520.
35. Albright F, Butler AM, Hampton AO, Smith PH (1937). Syndrome characterized by osteitis fibrosa disseminata, areas of pigmentation and endocrine dysfunction, with precocious puberty in females. N Engl J Med 216: 727-746.
36. Aldinger KA, Samaan NA, Ibanez M, Hill CSJr (1978). Anaplastic carcinoma of the thyroid: a review of 84 cases of spindle and giant cell carcinoma of the thyroid. Cancer 41: 2267-2275.
37. Aleotti A, Cervellati F, Bovolenta MR, Zago S, Orvieto E, Caramori G, Bezzi T (1998). Birbeck granules: contribution to the comprehension of intracytoplasmic evolution. J Submicrosc Cytol Pathol 30: 295-298.
38. Alexander JM, Jameson JL, Bikkal HA, Schwall RH, Klibanski A (1991). The effects of activin on follicle-stimulating hormone secretion and biosynthesis in human glycoprotein hormone-producing pituitary adenomas. J Clin Endocrinol Metab 72: 1261-1267.
39. Alpers CE, Clark OH (1989). Atypical spindle cell pattern (?carcinoma) arising in a parathyroid adenoma. Surg Pathol 2: 157-161.
40. Alsop JE, Yerbury PJ, O'Donnell PJ, Heyderman E (1986). Signet-ring cell microfollicular adenoma arising in a nodular ectopic thyroid. A case report. J Oral Pathol 15: 518-519.
41. Altavilla G, Chiarelli S, Fassina A (2001). Duodenal periampullary gangliocytic paraganglioma: report of two cases with immunohistochemical and ultrastructural study. Ultrastruct Pathol 25: 137-145.
42. Alumets J, Ekelund G, Hakanson R, Ljungberg O, Ljungqvist U, Sundler F, Tibblin S (1978). Jejunal endocrine tumor composed of somatostatin and gastrin cells and associated with duodenal ulcer disease. Virchows Arch A Pathol Anat Histol 378: 17-22.
43. Alvaro V, Levy L, Dubray C, Roche A, Peillon F, Querat B, Joubert D (1993). Invasive human pituitary tumors express a point-mutated a-protein kinase-C. J Clin Endocrinol Metab 77: 1125-1129.
44. Alvaro V, Touraine P, Raisman Vozari R, Bai-Grenier F, Birman P, Joubert D (1992). Protein kinase C activity and expression in normal and adenomatous human pituitaries. Int J Cancer 50: 724-730.
45. Alves P, Soares P, Fonseca E, Sobrinho-Simoes M (1999). Papillary Thyroid Carcinoma Overexpresses Fully and Underglycosylated Mucins Together with Native and Sialylated Simple Mucin Antigens and Histo-Blood Group Antigens. Endocr Pathol 10: 315-324.
46. Alves P, Soares P, Rossi S, Fonseca E, Sobrinho-Simoes M (1999). Clinicopathologic and Prognostic Significance of the Expression of Mucins, Simple Mucin Antigens and Histo-Blood Group Antigens in Papillary Thyroid Carcinoma. Endocr Pathol 10: 305-313.
47. Amar AP, Hinton DR, Krieger MD, Weiss MH (1999). Invasive pituitary adenomas: significance of proliferation parameters. Pituitary 2: 117-122.
48. Ambros IM, Amann G, Ambros PF (2002). Correspondence re: J. Mora et al., Neuroblastic and Schwannian stromal cells of neuroblastoma are derived from a tumoral progenitor cell. Cancer Res., 61: 6892-6898, 2001. Cancer Res 62: 2986-2987.
49. Ambros IM, Attarbaschi A, Rumpler S, Luegmayr A, Turkof E, Gadner H, Ambros PF (2001). Neuroblastoma cells provoke Schwann cell proliferation in vitro. Med Pediatr Oncol 36: 163-168.
50. Amieux PS, McKnight GS (2002). The essential role of RI alpha in the maintenance of regulated PKA activity. Ann N Y Acad Sci 968: 75-95.
51. Andersen DK (1989). Current diagnosis and management of Zollinger-Ellison syndrome. Ann Surg 210: 685-703.
52. Andersen LB, Fountain JW, Gutmann DH, Tarle SA, Glover TW, Dracopoli NC, Housman DE, Collins FS (1993). Mutations in the neurofibromatosis 1 gene in sporadic malignant melanoma cell lines. Nat Genet 3: 118-121.
53. Anderson MA, Carpenter S, Thompson NW, Nostrant TT, Elta GH, Scheiman JM (2000). Endoscopic ultrasound is highly accurate and directs man-

agement in patients with neuroendocrine tumors of the pancreas. Am J Gastroenterol 95: 2271-2277.

54. Anderson TJ, Ewen SW (1974). Amyloid in normal and pathological parathyroid glands. J Clin Pathol 27: 656-663.

55. Anderson WR, Cameron JD, Tsai SH (1980). Primary intracranial leiomyosarcoma. Case report with ultrastructural study. J Neurosurg 53: 401-405.

56. Ando S, Sarlis NJ, Krishnan J, Feng X, Refetoff S, Zhang MQ, Oldfield EH, Yen PM (2001). Aberrant alternative splicing of thyroid hormone receptor in a TSH-secreting pituitary tumor is a mechanism for hormone resistance. Mol Endocrinol 15: 1529-1538.

57. Andrion A, Bellis D, Delsedime L, Bussolati G, Mazzucco G (1988). Leiomyoma and neurilemoma: report of two unusual non-epithelial tumours of the thyroid gland. Virchows Arch A Pathol Anat Histopathol 413: 367-372.

58. Ang SO, Chen H, Hirota K, Gordeuk VR, Jelinek J, Guan Y, Liu E, Sergueeva AI, Miasnikova GY, Mole D, Maxwell PH, Stockton DW, Semenza GL, Prchal JT (2002). Disruption of oxygen homeostasis underlies congenital Chuvash polycythemia. Nat Genet 32: 614-621.

59. Angeles-Angeles A, Reyes E, Munoz-Fernandez L, Angritt P (1997). Adenomatoid Tumor of the Right Adrenal Gland in a Patient with AIDS. Endocr Pathol 8: 59-64.

60. Anscombe AM, Wright DH (1985). Primary malignant lymphoma of the thyroid—a tumour of mucosa-associated lymphoid tissue: review of seventy-six cases. Histopathology 9: 81-97.

61. Ansell SM, Grant CS, Habermann TM (1999). Primary thyroid lymphoma. Semin Oncol 26: 316-323.

62. Antonioli DA, Dayal Y, Dvorak AM, Banks PA (1987). Zollinger-Ellison syndrome. Cure by surgical resection of a jejunal gastrinoma containing growth hormone releasing factor. Gastroenterology 92: 814-823.

63. Aozasa K, Inoue A, Katagiri S, Matsuzuka F, Katayama S, Yonezawa T (1986). Plasmacytoma and follicular lymphoma in a case of Hashimoto's thyroiditis. Histopathology 10: 735-740.

64. Aozasa K, Inoue A, Tajima K, Miyauchi A, Matsuzuka F, Kuma K (1986). Malignant lymphomas of the thyroid gland. Analysis of 79 patients with emphasis on histologic prognostic factors. Cancer 58: 100-104.

65. Aozasa K, Tsujimoto M, Sakurai M, Honda M, Yamashita K, Hanada M, Sugimoto A (1985). Non-Hodgkin's lymphomas in Osaka, Japan. Eur J Cancer Clin Oncol 21: 487-492.

66. Apel RL, Alpert LC, Rizzo A, LiVolsi VA, Asa SL (1994). A metastasizing composite carcinoma of the thyroid with distinct medullary and papillary components. Arch Pathol Lab Med 118: 1143-1147.

67. Apel RL, Asa SL, LiVolsi VA (1995). Papillary Hurthle cell carcinoma with lymphocytic stroma. "Warthin-like tumor" of the thyroid. Am J Surg Pathol 19: 810-814.

68. Apel RL, Ezzat S, Bapat BV, Pan N, LiVolsi VA, Asa SL (1995). Clonality of thyroid nodules in sporadic goiter. Diagn Mol Pathol 4: 113-121.

69. Arafah BM, Nasrallah MP (2001). Pituitary tumors: pathophysiology, clinical manifestations and management. Endocr Relat Cancer 8: 287-305.

70. Arber DA, Weiss LM, Chang KL (1998). Detection of Epstein-Barr Virus in inflammatory pseudotumor. Semin Diagn Pathol 15: 155-160.

71. Arceci RJ, Brenner MK, Pritchard J (1998). Controversies and new approaches to treatment of Langerhans cell histiocytosis. Hematol Oncol Clin North Am 12: 339-357.

72. Archer KF, Hurwitz JJ, Balogh JM, Fernandes BJ (1989). Orbital nonchromaffin paraganglioma. A case report and review of the literature. Ophthalmology 96: 1659-1666.

73. Arezzo A, Patetta R, Ceppa P, Borgonovo G, Torre G, Mattioli FP (1998). Mucoepidermoid carcinoma of the thyroid gland arising from a papillary epithelial neoplasm. Am Surg 64: 307-311.

74. Arnaldi G, Masini AM, Giacchetti G, Taccaliti A, Faloia E, Mantero F (2000). Adrenal incidentaloma. Braz J Med Biol Res 33: 1177-1189.

75. Arnold A, Shattuck TM, Mallya SM, Krebs LJ, Costa J, Gallagher J, Wild Y, Saucier K (2002). Molecular pathogenesis of primary hyperparathyroidism. J Bone Miner Res 17 Suppl 2: N30-N36.

76. Aron DC, Findling JW, Fitzgerald PA, Forsham PH, Wilson CB, Tyrrell JB (1982). Cushing's syndrome: problems in management. Endocr Rev 3: 229-244.

77. Aron DC, Howlett TA (2000). Pituitary incidentalomas. Endocrinol Metab Clin North Am 29: 205-221.

78. Arps H, Dietel M, Schulz A, Janzarik H, Kloppel G (1986). Pancreatic endocrine carcinoma with ectopic PTH-production and paraneoplastic hypercalcaemia. Virchows Arch A Pathol Anat Histopathol 408: 497-503.

79. Asa SL (1998). Tumors of the Pituitary Gland. 3rd ed. Armed Forces Institute of Pathology: Washington, DC.

80. Asa SL, Bamberger AM, Cao B, Wong M, Parker KL, Ezzat S (1996). The transcription activator steroidogenic factor-1 is preferentially expressed in the human pituitary gonadotroph. J Clin Endocrinol Metab 81: 2165-2170.

81. Asa SL, Bilbao JM, Kovacs K, Linfoot JA (1980). Hypothalamic neuronal hamartoma associated with pituitary growth hormone cell adenoma and acromegaly. Acta Neuropathol (Berl) 52: 231-234.

82. Asa SL, Dardick I, van Nostrand AW, Bailey DJ, Gullane PJ (1988). Primary thyroid thymoma: a distinct clinicopathologic entity. Hum Pathol 19: 1463-1467.

83. Asa SL, Ezzat S (1998). The cytogenesis and pathogenesis of pituitary adenomas. Endocr Rev 19: 798-827.

84. Asa SL, Ezzat S (2002). The pathogenesis of pituitary tumours. Nat Rev Cancer 2: 836-849.

85. Asa SL, Kovacs K, Horvath E, Ezrin C, Weiss MH (1984). Sellar glomangioma. Ultrastruct Pathol 7: 49-54.

86. Asa SL, Kovacs K, Horvath E, Losinski NE, Laszlo FA, Domokos I, Halliday WC (1988). Human fetal adenohypophysis. Electron microscopic and ultrastructural immunocytochemical analysis. Neuroendocrinology 48: 423-431.

87. Asa SL, Kovacs K, Killinger DW, Marcon N, Platts M (1980). Pancreatic islet cell carcinoma producing gastrin, ACTH, alpha-endorphin, somatostatin and calcitonin. Am J Gastroenterol 74: 30-35.

88. Asa SL, Kovacs K, Stefaneanu L, Horvath E, Billestrup N, Gonzalez-Manchon C, Vale W (1992). Pituitary adenomas in mice transgenic for growth hormone-releasing hormone. Endocrinology 131: 2083-2089.

89. Asa SL, Kovacs K, Tindall GT, Barrow DL, Horvath E, Vecsei P (1984). Cushing's disease associated with an intrasellar gangliocytoma producing corticotrophin-releasing factor. Ann Intern Med 101: 789-793.

90. Asa SL, Puy LA, Lew AM, Sundmark VC, Elsholtz HP (1993). Cell type-specific expression of the pituitary transcription activator pit-1 in the human pituitary and pituitary adenomas. J Clin Endocrinol Metab 77: 1275-1280.

91. Asa SL, Scheithauer BW, Bilbao JM, Horvath E, Ryan N, Kovacs K, Randall RV, Laws ERJr, Singer W, Linfoot JA, Thorner MO, Vale W (1984). A case for hypothalamic acromegaly: a clinicopathological study of six patients with hypothalamic gangliocytomas producing growth hormone-releasing factor. J Clin Endocrinol Metab 58: 796-803.

92. Asa SL, Somers K, Ezzat S (1998). The MEN-1 gene is rarely down-regulated in pituitary adenomas. J Clin Endocrinol Metab 83: 3210-3212.

93. Asai N, Iwashita T, Matsuyama M, Takahashi M (1995). Mechanism of activation of the ret proto-oncogene by multiple endocrine neoplasia 2A mutations. Mol Cell Biol 15: 1613-1619.

94. Ashfaq R, Vuitch F, Delgado R, Albores-Saavedra J (1994). Papillary and follicular thyroid carcinomas with an insular component. Cancer 73: 416-423.

95. Asteria C, Anagni M, Fugazzola L, Faglia G, Vezzadini P, Beck-Peccoz P (2002). MEN1 gene mutations are a rare event in patients with sporadic neuroendocrine tumors. Eur J Intern Med 13: 319-323.

96. Astuti D, Douglas F, Lennard TW, Aligianis IA, Woodward ER, Evans DG, Eng C, Latif F, Maher ER (2001). Germline SDHD mutation in familial phaeochromocytoma. Lancet 357: 1181-1182.

97. Astuti D, Latif F, Dallol A, Dahia PL, Douglas F, George E, Skoldberg F, Husebye ES, Eng C, Maher ER (2001). Gene mutations in the succinate dehydrogenase subunit SDHB cause susceptibility to familial pheochromocytoma and to familial paraganglioma. Am J Hum Genet 69: 49-54.

98. Atit RP, Crowe MJ, Greenhalgh DG, Wenstrup RJ, Ratner N (1999). The Nf1 tumor suppressor regulates mouse skin wound healing, fibroblast proliferation, and collagen deposited by fibroblasts. J Invest Dermatol 112: 835-842.

99. Au HC, Ream-Robinson D, Bellew LA, Broomfield PL, Saghbini M, Scheffler IE (1995). Structural organization of the gene encoding the human iron-sulfur subunit of succinate dehydrogenase. Gene 159: 249-253.

100. Au HC, Scheffler IE (1998). Promoter analysis of the human succinate dehydrogenase iron-protein gene—both nuclear respiratory factors NRF-1 and NRF-2 are required. Eur J Biochem 251: 164-174.

101. Aubert S, Wacrenier A, Leroy X, Devos P, Carnaille B, Proye C, Wemeau JL, Lecomte-Houcke M, Leteurtre E (2002). Weiss system revisited: a clinicopathologic and immunohistochemical study of 49 adrenocortical tumors. Am J Surg Pathol 26: 1612-1619.

102. Avantaggiato V, Dathan NA, Grieco M, Fabien N, Lazzaro D, Fusco A, Simeone A, Santoro M (1994). Developmental expression of the RET protooncogene. Cell

Growth Differ 5: 305-311.

103. Avery AK, Beckstead J, Renshaw AA, Corless CL (2000). Use of antibodies to RCC and CD10 in the differential diagnosis of renal neoplasms. Am J Surg Pathol 24: 203-210.

104. Avsare SS, Prabhu SR, Vengsarkar US, Manghani DK, Dastur DK (1982). Von Recklinghausen's disease with a malignant meningeal, cerebral and optic nerve tumour and bilateral vagal schwannomas. Possible mesenchymal histogenesis on light and electron microscopy. J Neurol Sci 54: 427-443.

105. Axelrod L, Bush MA, Hirsch HJ, Loo SW (1981). Malignant somatostatinoma: clinical features and metabolic studies. J Clin Endocrinol Metab 52: 886-896.

106. Ayabe H, Tsuji H, Hara S, Tagawa Y, Kawahara K, Tomita M (1995). Surgical management of adrenal metastasis from bronchogenic carcinoma. J Surg Oncol 58: 149-154.

107. Badenhop RF, Cherian S, Lord RS, Baysal BE, Taschner PE, Schofield PR (2001). Novel mutations in the SDHD gene in pedigrees with familial carotid body paraganglioma and sensorineural hearing loss. Genes Chromosomes Cancer 31: 255-263.

108. Baghai M, Thompson GB, Young WFJr, Grant CS, Michels VV, van Heerden JA (2002). Pheochromocytomas and paragangliomas in von Hippel-Lindau disease: a role for laparoscopic and cortical-sparing surgery. Arch Surg 137: 682-688.

109. Baker BL (1974). Functional cytology of the hypophyseal pars distalis and pars intermedia. In: Handbook of Physiology, Section 7, Greep R, Astwood E, Kaobil E, eds., American Physiological Society: Washington, DC, pp. 45-80.

110. Bale GF (1950). Teratoma of the neck in the region of the thyroid gland: a review of the literature and report of four cases. Am J Pathol 26: 565-579.

111. Ballard HS, Frame B, Hartsock RJ (1991). Familial multiple endocrine adenoma-peptic ulcer complex. 1964. Medicine (Baltimore) 70: 281-283.

112. Baloch ZW, Abraham S, Roberts S, LiVolsi VA (1999). Differential expression of cytokeratins in follicular variant of papillary carcinoma: an immunohistochemical study and its diagnostic utility. Hum Pathol 30: 1166-1171.

113. Baloch ZW, LiVolsi VA (1999). Tumor-to-tumor metastasis to follicular variant of papillary carcinoma of thyroid. Arch Pathol Lab Med 123: 703-706.

114. Baloch ZW, LiVolsi VA (2000). Encapsulated follicular variant of papillary thyroid carcinoma with bone metastases. Mod Pathol 13: 861-865.

115. Baloch ZW, Solomon AC, LiVolsi VA (2000). Primary mucoepidermoid carcinoma and sclerosing mucoepidermoid carcinoma with eosinophilia of the thyroid gland: a report of nine cases. Mod Pathol 13: 802-807.

116. Baloch ZW, Wu H, LiVolsi VA (1999). Post-fine-needle aspiration spindle cell nodules of the thyroid (PSCNT). Am J Clin Pathol 111: 70-74.

117. Bamberger CM, Fehn M, Bamberger AM, Ludecke DK, Beil FU, Saeger W, Schulte HM (1999). Reduced expression levels of the cell-cycle inhibitor p27Kip1 in human pituitary adenomas. Eur J Endocrinol 140: 250-255.

118. Banerjee SS, Faragher B, Hasleton PS (1983). Nuclear diameter in parathyroid disease. J Clin Pathol 36: 143-148.

119. Bar M, Friedman E, Jakobovitz O, Leibowitz G, Lerer I, Abeliovich D, Gross DJ (1997). Sporadic phaeochromocytomas are rarely associated with germline mutations in the von Hippel-Lindau and RET genes. Clin Endocrinol (Oxf) 47: 707-712.

120. Barghorn A, Komminoth P, Bachmann D, Rutimann K, Saremaslani P, Muletta-Feurer S, Perren A, Roth J, Heitz PU, Speel EJ (2001). Deletion at 3p25.3-p23 is frequently encountered in endocrine pancreatic tumours and is associated with metastatic progression. J Pathol 194: 451-458.

121. Barghorn A, Speel EJ, Farspour B, Saremaslani P, Schmid S, Perren A, Roth J, Heitz PU, Komminoth P (2001). Putative tumor suppressor loci at 6q22 and 6q23-q24 are involved in the malignant progression of sporadic endocrine pancreatic tumors. Am J Pathol 158: 1903-1911.

122. Barksdale SK, Marincola FM, Jaffe G (1993). Carcinosarcoma of the adrenal cortex presenting with mineralocorticoid excess. Am J Surg Pathol 17: 941-945.

123. Barnes L (1991). Paraganglioma of the larynx. A critical review of the literature. ORL J Otorhinolaryngol Relat Spec 53: 220-234.

124. Barnett CCJr, Varma DG, el Naggar AK, Dackiw AP, Porter GA, Pearson AS, Kudelka AP, Gagel RF, Evans DB, Lee JE (2000). Limitations of size as a criterion in the evaluation of adrenal tumors. Surgery 128: 973-982.

125. Barrou Z, Abecassis JP, Guilhaume B, Thomopoulos P, Bertagna X, Derome P, Bonnin A, Luton JP (1997). [Magnetic resonance imaging in Cushing disease. Prediction of surgical results]. Presse Med 26: 7-11.

126. Bartolazzi A, Gasbarri A, Papotti M, Bussolati G, Lucante T, Khan A, Inohara H, Marandino F, Orlandi F, Nardi F, Vecchione A, Tecce R, Larsson O (2001). Application of an immunodiagnostic method for improving preoperative diagnosis of nodular thyroid lesions. Lancet 357: 1644-1650.

127. Barzon L, Chilosi M, Fallo F, Martignoni G, Montagna L, Palu G, Boscaro M (2001). Molecular analysis of CDKN1C and TP53 in sporadic adrenal tumors. Eur J Endocrinol 145: 207-212.

128. Basolo F, Giannini R, Monaco C, Melillo RM, Carlomagno F, Pancrazi M, Salvatore G, Chiappetta G, Pacini F, Elisei R, Miccoli P, Pinchera A, Fusco A, Santoro M (2002). Potent mitogenicity of the RET/PTC3 oncogene correlates with its prevalence in tall-cell variant of papillary thyroid carcinoma. Am J Pathol 160: 247-254.

129. Basolo F, Pisaturo F, Pollina LE, Fontanini G, Elisei R, Molinaro E, Iacconi P, Miccoli P, Pacini F (2000). N-ras mutation in poorly differentiated thyroid carcinomas: correlation with bone metastases and inverse correlation to thyroglobulin expression. Thyroid 10: 19-23.

130. Bassett JH, Forbes SA, Pannett AA, Lloyd SE, Christie PT, Wooding C, Harding B, Besser GM, Edwards CR, Monson JP, Sampson J, Wass JA, Wheeler MH, Thakker RV (1998). Characterization of mutations in patients with multiple endocrine neoplasia type 1. Am J Hum Genet 62: 232-244.

131. Basu TN, Gutmann DH, Fletcher JA, Glover TW, Collins FS, Downward J (1992). Aberrant regulation of ras proteins in malignant tumour cells from type 1 neurofibromatosis patients. Nature 356: 713-715.

132. Bates AS, Buckley N, Boggild MD, Bicknell EJ, Perrett CW, Broome JC, Clayton RN (1995). Clinical and genetic changes in a case of a Cushing's carcinoma. Clin Endocrinol (Oxf) 42: 663-670.

133. Bates AS, Farrell WE, Bicknell EJ, McNicol AM, Talbot AJ, Broome JC, Perrett CW, Thakker RV, Clayton RN (1997). Allelic deletion in pituitary adenomas reflects aggressive biological activity and has potential value as a prognostic marker. J Clin Endocrinol Metab 82: 818-824.

134. Batsakis JG, Littler ER, Oberman HA (1964). Teratomas of the neck. A clinicopathologic appraisal. Arch Otolaryngol 79: 619-624.

135. Baudin E, Bidart JM, Bachelot A, Ducreux M, Elias D, Ruffie P, Schlumberger M (2001). Impact of chromogranin A measurement in the work-up of neuroendocrine tumors. Ann Oncol 12 Suppl 2: S79-S82.

136. Baum A, Friedman AL, Zakowski SG (1997). Stress and genetic testing for disease risk. Health Psychol 16: 8-19.

137. Baumgartner I, von Hochstetter A, Baumert B, Luetolf U, Follath F (1997). Langerhans'-cell histiocytosis in adults. Med Pediatr Oncol 28: 9-14.

138. Baysal BE (2002). Hereditary paraganglioma targets diverse paraganglia. J Med Genet 39: 617-622.

139. Baysal BE, Ferrell RE, Willett-Brozick JE, Lawrence EC, Myssiorek D, Bosch A, van der Mey A, Taschner PE, Rubinstein WS, Myers EN, Richard CWI, Cornelisse CJ, Devilee P, Devlin B (2000). Mutations in SDHD, a mitochondrial complex II gene, in hereditary paraganglioma. Science 287: 848-851.

140. Baysal BE, Rubinstein WS, Taschner PE (2001). Phenotypic dichotomy in mitochondrial complex II genetic disorders. J Mol Med 79: 495-503.

141. Baysal BE, van Schothorst EM, Farr JE, James MR, Devilee P, Richard CWI (1997). A high-resolution STS, EST, and gene-based physical map of the hereditary paraganglioma region on chromosome 11q23. Genomics 44: 214-221.

142. Baysal BE, Willett-Brozick JE, Lawrence EC, Drovdlic CM, Savul SA, McLeod DR, Yee HA, Brackmann DE, Slattery WHI, Myers EN, Ferrell RE, Rubinstein WS (2002). Prevalence of SDHB, SDHC, and SDHD germline mutations in clinic patients with head and neck paragangliomas. J Med Genet 39: 178-183.

143. Beard CM, Sheps SG, Kurland LT, Carney JA, Lie JT (1983). Occurrence of pheochromocytoma in Rochester, Minnesota, 1950 through 1979. Mayo Clin Proc 58: 802-804.

144. Beauchesne P, Trouillas J, Barral F, Brunon J (1995). Gonadotropic pituitary carcinoma: case report. Neurosurgery 37: 810-815.

145. Becherer A, Vierhapper H, Potzi C, Karanikas G, Kurtaran A, Schmaljohann J, Staudenherz A, Dudczak R, Kletter K (2001). FDG-PET in adrenocortical carcinoma. Cancer Biother Radiopharm 16: 289-295.

146. Beck-Peccoz P, Brucker-Davis F, Persani L, Smallridge RC, Weintraub BD (1996). Thyrotropin-secreting pituitary tumors. Endocr Rev 17: 610-638.

147. Beckers A, Abs R, Mahler C, Vandalem JL, Pirens G, Hennen G, Stevenaert A (1991). Thyrotropin-secreting pituitary adenomas: report of seven cases. J Clin Endocrinol Metab 72: 477-483.

148. Beckers A, Abs R, Willems PJ, van der Auwera B, Kovacs K, Reznik M, Stevenaert A (1992). Aldosterone-secreting adrenal adenoma as part of multiple

endocrine neoplasia type 1 (MEN1): loss of heterozygosity for polymorphic chromosome 11 deoxyribonucleic acid markers, including the MEN1 locus. J Clin Endocrinol Metab 75: 564-570.

149. Bedetti CD, Dekker A, Watson CG (1984). Functioning oxyphil cell adenoma of the parathyroid gland: a clinicopathologic study of ten patients with hyperparathyroidism. Hum Pathol 15: 1121-1126.

150. Bednar MM, Trainer TD, Aitken PA, Grenko R, Dorwart R, Duckworth J, Gross CE, Pendlebury WW (1992). Orbital paraganglioma: case report and review of the literature. Br J Ophthalmol 76: 183-185.

151. Bedri S, Erfanian K, Schwaitzberg S, Tischler AS (2002). Mature cystic teratoma involving adrenal gland. Endocr Pathol 13: 59-64.

152. Beer TW (1992). Malignant thyroid haemangioendothelioma in a non-endemic goitrous region, with immunohistochemical evidence of a vascular origin. Histopathology 20: 539-541.

153. Behrens RJ, Levi AW, Westra WH, Dutta D, Cooper DS (2001). Langerhans cell histiocytosis of the thyroid: a report of two cases and review of the literature. Thyroid 11: 697-705.

154. Beimfohr C, Klugbauer S, Demidchik EP, Lengfelder E, Rabes HM (1999). NTRK1 re-arrangement in papillary thyroid carcinomas of children after the Chernobyl reactor accident. Int J Cancer 80: 842-847.

155. Bejarano PA, Nikiforov YE, Swenson ES, Biddinger PW (2000). Thyroid transcription factor-1, thyroglobulin, cytokeratin 7, and cytokeratin 20 in thyroid neoplasms. Appl Immunohistochem Mol Morphol 8: 189-194.

156. Beldjord C, Desclaux-Arramond F, Raffin-Sanson M, Corvol JC, de Keyzer Y, Luton JP, Plouin PF, Bertagna X (1995). The RET protooncogene in sporadic pheochromocytomas: frequent MEN 2-like mutations and new molecular defects. J Clin Endocrinol Metab 80: 2063-2068.

157. Belfiore A, La Rosa GL, La Porta GA, Giuffrida D, Milazzo G, Lupo L, Regalbuto C, Vigneri R (1992). Cancer risk in patients with cold thyroid nodules: relevance of iodine intake, sex, age, and multinodularity. Am J Med 93: 363-369.

158. Belge G, Rippe V, Meiboom M, Drieschner N, Garcia E, Bullerdiek J (2001). Delineation of a 150-kb breakpoint cluster in benign thyroid tumors with 19q13.4 aberrations. Cytogenet Cell Genet 93: 48-51.

159. Belge G, Roque L, Soares J, Bruckmann S, Thode B, Fonseca E, Clode A, Bartnitzke S, Castedo S, Bullerdiek J (1998). Cytogenetic investigations of 340 thyroid hyperplasias and adenomas revealing correlations between cytogenetic findings and histology. Cancer Genet Cytogenet 101: 42-48.

160. Bell B, Mazzaferri EL (1993). Familial adenomatous polyposis (Gardner's syndrome) and thyroid carcinoma. A case report and review of the literature. Dig Dis Sci 38: 185-190.

161. Bell DA (1987). Cytologic features of islet-cell tumors. Acta Cytol 31: 485-492.

162. Bender BU, Altehofer C, Januszewicz A, Gartner R, Schmidt H, Hoffmann MM, Heidemann PH, Neumann HP (1997). Functioning thoracic paraganglioma: association with Von Hippel-Lindau syndrome. J Clin Endocrinol Metab 82: 3356-3360.

163. Bender BU, Eng C, Olschewski M, Berger DP, Laubenberger J, Altehofer C,

Kirste G, Orszagh M, van Velthoven V, Miosczka H, Schmidt D, Neumann HP (2001). VHL c.505 T>C mutation confers a high age related penetrance but no increased overall mortality. J Med Genet 38: 508-514.

164. Bender BU, Gutsche M, Glasker S, Muller B, Kirste G, Eng C, Neumann HP (2000). Differential genetic alterations in von Hippel-Lindau syndrome-associated and sporadic pheochromocytomas. J Clin Endocrinol Metab 85: 4568-4574.

165. Benjamin DR, McRoberts JW (1973). Polyostotic fibrous dysplasia associated with Cushing syndrome. Arch Pathol 96: 175-178.

166. Benn DE, Dwight T, Richardson AL, Delbridge L, Bambach CP, Stowasser M, Gordon RD, Marsh DJ, Robinson BG (2000). Sporadic and familial pheochromocytomas are associated with loss of at least two discrete intervals on chromosome 1p. Cancer Res 60: 7048-7051.

167. Bennedbaek FN, Hegedus L (2000). Management of the solitary thyroid nodule: results of a North American survey. J Clin Endocrinol Metab 85: 2493-2498.

168. Beressi N, Campos JM, Beressi JP, Franc B, Niccoli-Sire P, Conte-Devolx B, Murat A, Caron P, Baldet L, Kraimps JL, Cohen R, Bigorgne JC, Chabre O, Lecomte P, Modigliani E (1998). Sporadic medullary microcarcinoma of the thyroid: a retrospective analysis of eighty cases. Thyroid 8: 1039-1044.

169. Berezin M, Karasik A (1995). Familial prolactinoma. Clin Endocrinol (Oxf) 42: 483-486.

170. Berezin M, Shimon I, Hadani M (1995). Prolactinoma in 53 men: clinical characteristics and modes of treatment (male prolactinoma). J Endocrinol Invest 18: 436-441.

171. Berezowski K, Grimes MM, Gal A, Kornstein MJ (1996). CD5 immunoreactivity of epithelial cells in thymic carcinoma and CASTLE using paraffin-embedded tissue. Am J Clin Pathol 106: 483-486.

172. Berg KK, Scheithauer BW, Felix I, Kovacs K, Horvath E, Klee GG, Laws ERJr (1990). Pituitary adenomas that produce adrenocorticotropic hormone and alpha-subunit: clinicopathological, immunohistochemical, ultrastructural, and immunoelectron microscopic studies in nine cases. Neurosurgery 26: 397-403.

173. Berger G, Trouillas J, Bloch B, Sassolas G, Berger F, Partensky C, Chayvialle JA, Brazeau P, Claustrat B, Lesbros F, Girod C (1984). Multihormonal carcinoid tumor of the pancreas. Secreting growth hormone-releasing factor as a cause of acromegaly. Cancer 54: 2097-2108.

174. Berger M, Bordi C, Cuppers HJ, Berchtold P, Gries FA, Munterfering H, Sailer R, Zimmermann H, Orci L (1983). Functional and morphologic characterization of human insulinomas. Diabetes 32: 921-931.

175. Bergholm U, Adami HO, Auer G, Bergstrom R, Backdahl M, Grimelius L, Hansson G, Ljungberg O, Wilander E (1989). Histopathologic characteristics and nuclear DNA content as prognostic factors in medullary thyroid carcinoma. A nationwide study in Sweden. The Swedish MTC Study Group. Cancer 64: 135-142.

176. Bergholm U, Adami HO, Bergstrom R, Johansson H, Lundell G, Telenius-Berg M, Akerstrom G (1989). Clinical characteristics in sporadic and familial medullary thyroid carcinoma. A nationwide study of

249 patients in Sweden from 1959 through 1981. Cancer 63: 1196-1204.

177. Bergholm U, Bergstrom R, Ekbom A (1997). Long-term follow-up of patients with medullary carcinoma of the thyroid. Cancer 79: 132-138.

178. Berho M, Suster S (1997). The oncocytic variant of papillary carcinoma of the thyroid: a clinicopathologic study of 15 cases. Hum Pathol 28: 47-53.

179. Berndt I, Reuter M, Saller B, Frank-Raue K, Groth P, Grussendorf M, Raue F, Ritter MM, Hoppner W (1998). A new hot spot for mutations in the ret protooncogene causing familial medullary thyroid carcinoma and multiple endocrine neoplasia type 2A. J Clin Endocrinol Metab 83: 770-774.

180. Berry CL, Keeling J, Hilton C (1969). Teratomata in infancy and childhood: a review of 91 cases. J Pathol 98: 241-252.

181. Bertherat J, Chanson P, Montminy M (1995). The cyclic adenosine 3′,5′-monophosphate-responsive factor CREB is constitutively activated in human somatotroph adenomas. Mol Endocrinol 9: 777-783.

182. Bertholon-Gregoire M, Trouillas J, Guigard MP, Loras B, Tourniaire J (1999). Mono- and plurihormonal thyrotropic pituitary adenomas: pathological, hormonal and clinical studies in 12 patients. Eur J Endocrinol 140: 519-527.

183. Bevan S, Pal T, Greenberg CR, Green H, Wixey J, Bignell G, Narod SA, Foulkes WD, Stratton MR, Houlston RS (2001). A comprehensive analysis of MNG1, TCO1, fPTC, PTEN, TSHR, and TRKA in familial nonmedullary thyroid cancer: confirmation of linkage to TCO1. J Clin Endocrinol Metab 86: 3701-3704.

184. Bhagavan BS, Slavin RE, Goldberg J, Rao RN (1986). Ectopic gastrinoma and Zollinger-Ellison syndrome. Hum Pathol 17: 584-592.

185. Bhattacharyya N (2003). A population-based analysis of survival factors in differentiated and medullary thyroid carcinoma. Otolaryngol Head Neck Surg 128: 115-123.

186. Bianco P, Riminucci M, Majolagbe A, Kuznetsov SA, Collins MT, Mankani MH, Corsi A, Bone HG, Wientroub S, Spiegel AM, Fisher LW, Robey PG (2000). Mutations of the GNAS1 gene, stromal cell dysfunction, and osteomalacic changes in non-McCune-Albright fibrous dysplasia of bone. J Bone Miner Res 15: 120-128.

187. Biankin SA, Cachia AR (1999). Leiomyoma of the thyroid gland. Pathology 31: 64-66.

188. Biddle DA, Ro JY, Yoon GS, Yong YW, Ayala AG, Ordonez NG, Ro J (2002). Extranodal follicular dendritic cell sarcoma of the head and neck region: three new cases, with a review of the literature. Mod Pathol 15: 50-58.

189. Bignell GR, Canzian F, Shayeghi M, Stark M, Shugart YY, Biggs P, Mangion J, Hamoudi R, Rosenblatt J, Buu P, Sun S, Stoffer SS, Goldgar DE, Romeo G, Houlston RS, Narod SA, Stratton MR, Foulkes WD (1997). Familial nontoxic multinodular thyroid goiter locus maps to chromosome 14q but does not account for familial nonmedullary thyroid cancer. Am J Hum Genet 61: 1123-1130.

190. Bigner SH, Cox EB, Mendelsohn G, Baylin SB, Wells SAJr, Eggleston JC (1981). Medullary carcinoma of the thyroid in the multiple endocrine neoplasia IIA syndrome. Am J Surg Pathol 5: 459-472.

191. Bikhazi PH, Messina L, Mhatre AN,

Goldstein JA, Lalwani AK (2000). Molecular pathogenesis in sporadic head and neck paraganglioma. Laryngoscope 110: 1346-1348.

192. Bilimoria MM (2002). Prophylactic surgery in hereditary cancer syndromes: an ounce of prevention may be the only cure. J Surg Oncol 79: 131-133.

193. Biller BM (1994). Pathogenesis of pituitary Cushing's syndrome. Pituitary versus hypothalamic. Endocrinol Metab Clin North Am 23: 547-554.

194. Bindra RS, Vasselli JR, Stearman R, Linehan WM, Klausner RD (2002). VHL-mediated hypoxia regulation of cyclin D1 in renal carcinoma cells. Cancer Res 62: 3014-3019.

195. Black BK, Ackerman LV (1950). Tumors of the parathyroid gland. A review of 23 cases. Cancer 3: 415-444.

196. Black WC, Haff RC (1970). The surgical pathology of parathyroid chief cell hyperplasia. Am J Clin Pathol 53: 565-579.

197. Blasius S, Brinkschmidt C, Poremba C, Terpe HJ, Halm H, Schleef J, Ritter J, Wortler K, Bocker W, Dockhorn-Dworniczak B (1998). Metastatic retroperitoneal paraganglioma in a 16-year-old girl. Case report, molecular pathological and cytogenetic findings. Pathol Res Pract 194: 439-444.

198. Bleistein M, Geiger K, Franz K, Stoldt P, Schlote W (2000). Transthyretin and transferrin in hemangioblastoma stromal cells. Pathol Res Pract 196: 675-681.

199. Blevins LS, Shore D, Weinstein J, Isaacs S (1998). Clinical presentation of pituitary tumors. In: Pituitary Disorders, Krisht AF, Tindall GT, eds., Lippincott Williams & Wilkins: Baltimore , pp. 145-163.

200. Block MA, Jackson CE, Greenawald KA, Yott JB, Tashjian AHJr (1980). Clinical characteristics distinguishing hereditary from sporadic medullary thyroid carcinoma. Treatment implications. Arch Surg 115: 142-148.

201. Bloom SR, Polak JM (1987). Glucagonoma syndrome. Am J Med 82: 25-36.

202. Bloom SR, Yiangou Y, Polak JM (1988). Vasoactive intestinal peptide secreting tumors. Pathophysiological and clinical correlations. Ann N Y Acad Sci 527: 518-527.

203. Blume-Peytavi U, Adler YD, Geilen CC, Ahmad W, Christiano A, Goerdt S, Orfanos CE (2000). Multiple familial cutaneous glomangioma: a pedigree of 4 generations and critical analysis of histologic and genetic differences of glomus tumors. J Am Acad Dermatol 42: 633-639.

204. Boccato P, Mannara GM, La Rosa F, Rinaldo A, Ferlito A (2000). Hyalinizing trabecular adenoma of the thyroid diagnosed by fine-needle aspiration biopsy. Ann Otol Rhinol Laryngol 109: 235-238.

205. Boecher-Schwarz HG, Fries G, Bornemann A, Ludwig B, Perneczky A (1992). Suprasellar granular cell tumor. Neurosurgery 31: 751-754.

206. Boggild MD, Jenkinson S, Pistorello M, Boscaro M, Scanarini M, McTernan P, Perrett CW, Thakker RV, Clayton RN (1994). Molecular genetic studies of sporadic pituitary tumors. J Clin Endocrinol Metab 78: 387-392.

207. Bohling T, Turunen O, Jaaskelainen J, Carpen O, Sainio M, Wahlstrom T, Vaheri A, Haltia M (1996). Ezrin expression in stromal cells of capillary hemangioblastoma. An immunohistochemical survey of brain tumors. Am J Pathol 148: 367-373.

208. Bolino A, Schuffenecker I, Luo Y, Seri M, Silengo M, Tocco T, Chabrier G, Houdent C, Murat A, Schlumberger M (1995). RET mutations in exons 13 and 14 of FMTC patients. Oncogene 10: 2415-2419.

209. Bollag G, McCormick F (1992). Ras regulation. NF is enough of GAP. Nature 356: 663-664.

210. Bollag G, McCormick F, Clark R (1993). Characterization of full-length neurofibromin: tubulin inhibits Ras GAP activity. EMBO J 12: 1923-1927.

211. Bollen EC, Lamers CB, Jansen JB, Larsson LI, Joosten HJ (1981). Zollinger-Ellison syndrome due to a gastrin-producing ovarian cystadenocarcinoma. Br J Surg 68: 776-777.

212. Bondeson AG, Bondeson L, Ljungberg O, Tibblin S (1985). Fat staining in parathyroid disease—diagnostic value and impact on surgical strategy: clinicopathologic analysis of 191 cases. Hum Pathol 16: 1255-1263.

213. Bondeson AG, Bondeson L, Thompson NW (1989). Hyperparathyroidism after treatment with radioactive iodine: not only a coincidence? Surgery 106: 1025-1027.

214. Bondeson AG, Bondeson L, Thompson NW (1993). Clinicopathological peculiarities in parathyroid disease with hypercalcaemic crisis. Eur J Surg 159: 613-617.

215. Bondeson L, Bondeson AG (1994). Clue helping to distinguish hyalinizing trabecular adenoma from carcinoma of the thyroid in fine-needle aspirates. Diagn Cytopathol 10: 25-29.

216. Bondeson L, Bondeson AG (1996). Cytologic features in fine-needle aspirates from a sclerosing mucoepidermoid thyroid carcinoma with eosinophilia. Diagn Cytopathol 15: 301-305.

217. Bondeson L, Bondeson AG, Nissborg A, Thompson NW (1997). Cytopathological variables in parathyroid lesions: a study based on 1,600 cases of hyperparathyroidism. Diagn Cytopathol 16: 476-482.

218. Bondeson L, Bondeson AG, Thompson NW (1991). Papillary carcinoma of the thyroid with mucoepidermoid features. Am J Clin Pathol 95: 175-179.

219. Bondeson L, Sandelin K, Grimelius L (1993). Histopathological variables and DNA cytometry in parathyroid carcinoma. Am J Surg Pathol 17: 820-829.

220. Bonfils S, Landor JH, Mignon M, Hervoir P (1981). Results of surgical management in 92 consecutive patients with Zollinger-Ellison syndrome. Ann Surg 194: 692-697.

221. Bongarzone I, Butti MG, Coronelli S, Borrello MG, Santoro M, Mondellini P, Pilotti S, Fusco A, Della Porta G, Pierotti MA (1994). Frequent activation of ret protooncogene by fusion with a new activating gene in papillary thyroid carcinomas. Cancer Res 54: 2979-2985.

222. Bongarzone I, Fugazzola L, Vigneri P, Mariani L, Mondellini P, Pacini F, Basolo F, Pinchera A, Pilotti S, Pierotti MA (1996). Age-related activation of the tyrosine kinase receptor protooncogenes RET and NTRK1 in papillary thyroid carcinoma. J Clin Endocrinol Metab 81: 2006-2009.

223. Bongarzone I, Monzini N, Borrello MG, Carcano C, Ferraresi G, Arighi E, Mondellini P, Della Porta G, Pierotti MA (1993). Molecular characterization of a thyroid tumor-specific transforming sequence formed by the fusion of ret tyrosine kinase

and the regulatory subunit RI alpha of cyclic AMP-dependent protein kinase A. Mol Cell Biol 13: 358-366.

224. Bongarzone I, Vigneri P, Mariani L, Collini P, Pilotti S, Pierotti MA (1998). RET/NTRK1 rearrangements in thyroid gland tumors of the papillary carcinoma family: correlation with clinicopathological features. Clin Cancer Res 4: 223-228.

225. Borberg A (1951). Clinical and genetic investigations into tuberous sclerosis and Recklinghausen's neurofibromatosis: contribution to elucidation of interrelationship and eugenics of the syndromes. Acta Psychiat Neurol Scand 71 (Suppl.): 1-239.

226. Bordeaux MC, Forcet C, Granger L, Corset V, Bidaud C, Billaud M, Bredesen DE, Edery P, Mehlen P (2000). The RET proto-oncogene induces apoptosis: a novel mechanism for Hirschsprung disease. EMBO J 19: 4056-4063.

227. Bordi C, Corleto VD, Azzoni C, Pizzi S, Ferraro G, Gibril F, Delle Fave G, Jensen RT (2001). The antral mucosa as a new site for endocrine tumors in multiple endocrine neoplasia type 1 and Zollinger-Ellison syndromes. J Clin Endocrinol Metab 86: 2236-2242.

228. Bordi C, D'Adda T, Azzoni C, Ferraro G (1998). Pathogenesis of ECL cell tumors in humans. Yale J Biol Med 71: 273-284.

229. Bordi C, De Vita O, Pilato FP, Carfagna G, D'Adda T, Missale G, Peracchia A (1987). Multiple islet cell tumors with predominance of glucagon-producing cells and ulcer disease. Am J Clin Pathol 88: 153-161.

230. Bordi C, Ravazzola M, Baetens D, Gorden P, Unger RH, Orci L (1979). A study of glucagonomas by light and electron microscopy and immunofluorescence. Diabetes 28: 925-936.

231. Borrello MG, Smith DP, Pasini B, Bongarzone I, Greco A, Lorenzo MJ, Arighi E, Miranda C, Eng C, Alberti L, Bocciardi R, Mondellini P, Scopsi L, Romeo G, Ponder BA, Pierotti MA (1995). RET activation by germline MEN2A and MEN2B mutations. Oncogene 11: 2419-2427.

232. Bossis I, Voutetakis A, Matyakhina L, Pack S, Abu-Asab M, Bourdeau I, Griffin KJ, Courcoutsakis N, Stergiopoulos S, Batista D, Tsokos M, Stratakis CA (2004). A pleiomorphic GH pituitary adenoma from a Carney complex patient displays universal allelic loss at the protein kinase A regulatory subunit 1A (PRKARIA) locus. J Med Genet 41: 596-600.

233. Bots GT, Tijssen CC, Wijnalda D, Teepen JL (1988). Alveolar soft part sarcoma of the pituitary gland with secondary involvement of the right cerebral ventricle. Br J Neurosurg 2: 101-107.

234. Bounacer A, Wicker R, Caillou B, Cailleux AF, Sarasin A, Schlumberger M, Suarez HG (1997). High prevalence of activating ret proto-oncogene rearrangements, in thyroid tumors from patients who had received external radiation. Oncogene 15: 1263-1273.

235. Bourcigaux N, Gaston V, Logie A, Bertagna X, Le Bouc Y, Gicquel C (2000). High expression of cyclin E and G1 CDK and loss of function of p57KIP2 are involved in proliferation of malignant sporadic adrenocortical tumors. J Clin Endocrinol Metab 85: 322-330.

236. Brada M, Rajan B, Traish D, Ashley S, Holmes-Sellors PJ, Nussey S, Uttley D (1993). The long-term efficacy of conservative surgery and radiotherapy in the control of pituitary adenomas. Clin Endocrinol (Oxf) 38: 571-578.

237. Bradford CR, Devaney KO, Lee JI (1999). Spindle epithelial tumor with thymus-like differentiation: a case report and review of the literature. Otolaryngol Head Neck Surg 120: 603-606.

238. Brady S, Lechan RM, Schwaitzberg SD, Dayal Y, Ziar J, Tischler AS (1997). Composite pheochromocytoma/ganglioneuroma of the adrenal gland associated with multiple endocrine neoplasia 2A: case report with immunohistochemical analysis. Am J Surg Pathol 21: 102-108.

239. Branch CLJr, Laws ERJr (1987). Metastatic tumors of the sella turcica masquerading as primary pituitary tumors. J Clin Endocrinol Metab 65: 469-474.

240. Brand SJ, Babyatsky M, Bachwich D, Demediuk B, Tillotson L, Wang TC (1993). Regulation of gastrin gene transcription. In: Gastrin, Walsh JH, ed., Raven Press: New York , pp. 73-89.

241. Brandi ML, Gagel RF, Angeli A, Bilezikian JP, Beck-Peccoz P, Bordi C, Conte-Devolx B, Falchetti A, Gheri RG, Libroia A, Lips CJ, Lombardi G, Mannelli M, Pacini F, Ponder BA, Raue F, Skogseid B, Tamburrano G, Thakker RV, Thompson NW, Tomassetti P, Tonelli F, Wells SAJr, Marx SJ (2001). Guidelines for diagnosis and therapy of MEN type 1 and type 2. J Clin Endocrinol Metab 86: 5658-5671.

242. Brannan CI, Perkins AS, Vogel KS, Ratner N, Nordlund ML, Reid SW, Buchberg AM, Jenkins NA, Parada LF, Copeland NG (1994). Targeted disruption of the neurofibromatosis type-1 gene leads to developmental abnormalities in heart and various neural crest-derived tissues. Genes Dev 8: 1019-1029.

243. Branum GD, Epstein RE, Leight GS, Seigler HF (1991). The role of resection in the management of melanoma metastatic to the adrenal gland. Surgery 109: 127-131.

244. Brauch H, Hoeppner W, Jahnig H, Wohl T, Engelhardt D, Spelsberg F, Ritter MM (1997). Sporadic pheochromocytomas are rarely associated with germline mutations in the vhl tumor suppressor gene or the ret protooncogene. J Clin Endocrinol Metab 82: 4101-4104.

245. Brauch H, Kishida T, Glavac D, Chen F, Pausch F, Hofler H, Latif F, Lerman MI, Zbar B, Neumann HP (1995). Von Hippel-Lindau (VHL) disease with pheochromocytoma in the Black Forest region of Germany: evidence for a founder effect. Hum Genet 95: 551-556.

246. Brighton CT, Friedenberg ZB, Zemsky LM, Pollis PR (1975). Direct-current stimulation of non-union and congenital pseudarthrosis. Exploration of its clinical application. J Bone Joint Surg Am 57: 368-377.

247. Bronner MP, LiVolsi VA, Jennings TA (1988). FPlat: paraganglioma-like adenomas of the thyroid. Surg Pathol 1: 383-389.

248. Broughan TA, Leslie JD, Soto JM, Hermann RE (1986). Pancreatic islet cell tumors. Surgery 99: 671-678.

249. Brown EW, Riccardi VM, Mawad M, Handel S, Goldman A, Bryan RN (1987). MR imaging of optic pathways in patients with neurofibromatosis. AJNR Am J Neuroradiol 8: 1031-1036.

250. Brown FM, Gaffey TA, Wold LE, Lloyd RV (2000). Myxoid neoplasms of the adrenal cortex: a rare histologic variant. Am J Surg Pathol 24: 396-401.

251. Brown HM, Komorowski RA, Wilson SD, Demeure MJ, Zhu YR (1999). Predicting metastasis of pheochromocytomas using DNA flow cytometry and immunohistochemical markers of cell proliferation: A positive correlation between MIB-1 staining and malignant tumor behavior. Cancer 86: 1583-1589.

252. Brown JA, Segura JW (1996). A symptomatic testicular cyst in a patient with von Hippel-Lindau disease. Urology 48: 494-495.

253. Brunnemann RB, Ro JY, Ordonez NG, Mooney J, el Naggar AK, Ayala AG (1999). Extrapleural solitary fibrous tumor: a clinicopathologic study of 24 cases. Mod Pathol 12: 1034-1042.

254. Bubl R, Hugo HH, Hempelmann RG, Barth H, Mehdorn HM (2001). Granular-cell tumour: a rare suprasellar mass. Neuroradiology 43: 309-312.

255. Buchanan KD, Johnston CF, O'Hare MM, Ardill JE, Shaw C, Collins JS, Watson RG, Atkinson AB, Hadden DR, Kennedy TL, Sloan JM (1986). Neuroendocrine tumors. A European view. Am J Med 81: 14-22.

256. Buckley N, Bates AS, Broome JC, Strange RC, Perrett CW, Burke CW, Clayton RN (1995). P53 protein accumulates in Cushings adenomas and invasive non-functional adenomas. J Clin Endocrinol Metab 80: 4.

257. Buckley NJ, Burch WM, Leight GS (1986). Malignant teratoma in the thyroid gland of an adult: a case report and a review of the literature. Surgery 100: 932-937.

258. Buetow PC, Levine MS, Buck JL, Pantongrag-Brown L, Emory TS (1997). Duodenal gangliocytic paraganglioma: CT, MR imaging, and US findings. Radiology 204: 745-747.

259. Bulow B, Ahren B (2002). Adrenal incidentaloma—experience of a standardized diagnostic programme in the Swedish prospective study. J Intern Med 252: 239-246.

260. Bulow C, Bulow S (1997). Is screening for thyroid carcinoma indicated in familial adenomatous polyposis? The Leeds Castle Polyposis Group. Int J Colorectal Dis 12: 240-242.

261. Burgess JR, Duffield A, Wilkinson SJ, Ware R, Greenaway TM, Percival J, Hoffman L (1997). Two families with an autosomal dominant inheritance pattern for papillary carcinoma of the thyroid. J Clin Endocrinol Metab 82: 345-348.

262. Burgess JR, Nord B, David R, Greenaway TM, Parameswaran V, Larsson C, Shepherd JJ, Teh BT (2000). Phenotype and phenocopy: the relationship between genotype and clinical phenotype in a single large family with multiple endocrine neoplasia type 1 (MEN 1). Clin Endocrinol (Oxf) 53: 205-211.

263. Burgess JR, Shepherd JJ, Greenaway TM (1994). Thyrotropinomas in multiple endocrine neoplasia type 1 (MEN-1). Aust N Z J Med 24: 740-741.

264. Burke AP, Federspiel BH, Sobin LH, Shekitka KM, Helwig EB (1989). Carcinoids of the duodenum. A histologic and immunohistochemical study of 65 tumors. Am J Surg Pathol 13: 828-837.

265. Burke AP, Helwig EB (1989). Gangliocytic paraganglioma. Am J Clin Pathol 92: 1-9.

266. Burke AP, Sobin LH, Federspiel BH, Shekitka KM, Helwig EB (1990). Carcinoid tumors of the duodenum. A clinicopathologic study of 99 cases. Arch Pathol Lab Med 114: 700-704.

267. Burke BA, Johnson D, Gilbert EF, Drut RM, Ludwig J, Wick MR (1987). Thyrocalcitonin-containing cells in the Di George anomaly. Hum Pathol 18: 355-360.

268. Burrow GN, Wortzman G, Rewcastle NB, Holgate RC, Kovacs K (1981). Microadenomas of the pituitary and abnormal sellar tomograms in an unselected autopsy series. N Engl J Med 304: 156-158.

269. Burton EM, Schellhammer PF, Weaver DL, Woolfitt RA (1986). Paraganglioma of urinary bladder in patient with neurofibromatosis. Urology 27: 550-552.

270. Busam KJ, Iversen K, Coplan KA, Old LJ, Stockert E, Chen YT, McGregor D, Jungbluth A (1998). Immunoreactivity for A103, an antibody to melan-A (Mart-1), in adrenocortical and other steroid tumors. Am J Surg Pathol 22: 57-63.

271. Bussolati G, Foster GV, Clark MB, Pearse AG (1969). Immunofluorescent localisation of calcitonin in medullary C-cell thyroid carcinoma, using antibody to the pure porcine hormone. Virchows Arch B Cell Pathol 2: 234-238.

272. Bystrom C, Larsson C, Blomberg C, Sandelin K, Falkmer U, Skogseid B, Oberg K, Werner S, Nordenskjold M (1990). Localization of the MEN1 gene to a small region within chromosome 11q13 by deletion mapping in tumors. Proc Natl Acad Sci U S A 87: 1968-1972.

273. Cabanne F, Gerard-Marchant R, Heimann R, Williams ED (1974). [Malignant tumors of the thyroid gland. Problems of histopathologic diagnosis. Apropos of 692 lesions collected by the thyroid cancer Cooperative Group of the O.E.R.T.C]. Ann Anat Pathol (Paris) 19: 129-148.

274. Cadiot G, Cattan D, Mignon M (1998). Diagnosis and treatment of ECL cell tumors. Yale J Biol Med 71: 311-323.

275. Cady B (2003). Risk group analysis for differentiated thyroid carcinoma. In: Surgery of the Thyroid and Parathyroid Glands., Randolph GW, ed., Saunders Publishing: Philadelphia , pp. 219-225.

276. Cai WY, Alexander JM, Hedley-Whyte ET, Scheithauer BW, Jameson JL, Zervas NT, Klibanski A (1994). ras mutations in human prolactinomas and pituitary carcinomas. J Clin Endocrinol Metab 78: 89-93.

277. Calender A, Giraud S, Porchet N, Gaudray P, Cadiot G, Mignon M (1998). [Clinicogenetic study of MEN1: recent physiopathological data and clinical applications. Study Group of Multiple Endocrine Neoplasia (GENEM)]. Ann Endocrinol (Paris) 59: 444-451.

278. Calender A, Vercherat C, Gaudray P, Chayvialle JA (2001). Deregulation of genetic pathways in neuroendocrine tumors. Ann Oncol 12 Suppl 2: S3-11.

279. Calmettes C, Caillou B, Moukhtar MS, Milhaud G, Gerard-Marchant R (1982). Calcitonin and carcinoembryonic antigen in poorly differentiated follicular carcinoma. Cancer 49: 2342-2348.

280. Calmettes C, Rosenberg-Gourgin M, Caron J, Feingold N (1992). Pheochromocytoma: a frequent indicator for MEN 2. Henry Ford Hosp Med J 40: 276-277.

281. Cameron AJ, Hoffman HN (1974). Zollinger-Ellison syndrome. Clinical features and long-term follow-up. Mayo Clin Proc 49: 44-51.

282. Cameselle-Teijeiro J, Chan JK (1999). Cribriform-morular variant of papillary carcinoma: a distinctive variant representing the sporadic counterpart of familial adenomatous polyposis-associated thyroid carcinoma? Mod Pathol 12: 400-411.

283. Cameselle-Teijeiro J, Febles-Perez C, Sobrinho-Simoes M (1995). Papillary and mucoepidermoid carcinoma of the thyroid with anaplastic transformation: a case report with histologic and immunohistochemical findings that support a provocative histogenetic hypothesis. Pathol Res Pract 191: 1214-1221.

284. Cameselle-Teijeiro J, Febles-Perez C, Sobrinho-Simoes M (1997). Cytologic features of fine needle aspirates of papillary and mucoepidermoid carcinoma of the thyroid with anaplastic transformation. A case report. Acta Cytol 41: 1356-1360.

285. Cameselle-Teijeiro J, Lopes JM, Villanueva JP, Gil-Gil P, Sobrinho-Simoes M (2002). Lipomatous hemangiopericytoma of the thyroid. Pathologica 94: 74.

285A. Cameselle-Teijeiro J, Ruiz-Ponte C, Loidi L, Suarez-Penaranda J, Baltar J, Sobrinho-Simoes M (2001). Somatic but not germline mutation of the APC gene in a case of cribriform-morular variant of papillary thyroid carcinoma. Am J Clin Pathol 115: 486-493.

286. Cameselle-Teijeiro J, Sobrinho-Simoes M (1999). Cytomorphologic features of mucoepidermoid carcinoma of the thyroid. Am J Clin Pathol 111: 134-136.

287. Cameselle-Teijeiro J, Varela-Duran J (1995). CD34 and thyroid fibrous tumor. Am J Surg Pathol 19: 1096.

288. Cameselle-Teijeiro J, Varela-Duran J, Fonseca E, Villanueva JP, Sobrinho-Simoes M (1994). Solitary fibrous tumor of the thyroid. Am J Clin Pathol 101: 535-538.

289. Candanedo-Gonzalez FA, Alvarado-Cabrero I, Gamboa-Dominguez A, Cerbulo-Vazquez A, Lopez-Romero R, Bornstein-Quevedo L, Salcedo-Vargas M (2001). Sporadic type composite pheochromocytoma with neuroblastoma: clinicomorphologic, DNA content and ret gene analysis. Endocr Pathol 12: 343-350.

290. Candeliere GA, Roughley PJ, Glorieux FH (1997). Polymerase chain reaction-based technique for the selective enrichment and analysis of mosaic arg201 mutations in G alpha s from patients with fibrous dysplasia of bone. Bone 21: 201-206.

291. Canos JC, Serrano A, Matias-Guiu X (2001). Paucicellular variant of anaplastic thyroid carcinoma: report of two cases. Endocr Pathol 12: 157-161.

292. Cantor AM, Rigby CC, Beck PR, Mangion D (1982). Neurofibromatosis, phaeochromocytoma, and somatostatinoma. Br Med J (Clin Res Ed) 285: 1618-1619.

293. Canzian F, Amati P, Harach HR, Kraimps JL, Lesueur F, Barbier J, Levillain P, Romeo G, Bonneau D (1998). A gene predisposing to familial thyroid tumors with cell oxyphilia maps to chromosome 19p13.2. Am J Hum Genet 63: 1743-1748.

294. Capella C, Polak JM, Buffa R, Tapia FJ, Heitz PU, Usellini L, Bloom SR, Solcia E (1983). Morphologic patterns and diagnostic criteria of VIP-producing endocrine tumors. A histologic, histochemical, ultrastructural, and biochemical study of 32 cases. Cancer 52: 1860-1874.

295. Capella C, Riva C, Leutner M, La Rosa S (1995). Pituitary lesions in multiple endocrine neoplasia syndrome (MENS) type 1. Pathol Res Pract 191: 345-347.

296. Capella G, Matias-Guiu X, Ampudia X, De Leiva A, Perucho M, Prat J (1996). Ras oncogene mutations in thyroid tumors: polymerase chain reaction-restriction-fragment-length polymorphism analysis from paraffin-embedded tissues. Diagn Mol Pathol 5: 45-52.

297. Caplan RH, Abellera RM, Kisken WA (1984). Hurthle cell tumors of the thyroid

gland. A clinicopathologic review and long-term follow-up. JAMA 251: 3114-3117.
298. Capon F, Tacconelli A, Giardina E, Sciacchitano S, Bruno R, Tassi V, Trischitta V, Filetti S, Dallapiccola B, Novelli G (2000). Mapping a dominant form of multinodular goiter to chromosome Xp22. Am J Hum Genet 67: 1004-1007.
299. Cappabianca P, Cirillo S, Alfieri A, D'Amico A, Maiuri F, Mariniello G, Caranci F, de Divitiis E (1999). Pituitary macroadenoma and diaphragma sellae meningioma: differential diagnosis on MRI. Neuroradiology 41: 22-26.
300. Carcangiu ML, Bianchi S (1989). Diffuse sclerosing variant of papillary thyroid carcinoma. Clinicopathologic study of 15 cases. Am J Surg Pathol 13: 1041-1049.
301. Carcangiu ML, Bianchi S, Savino D, Voynick IM, Rosai J (1991). Follicular Hurthle cell tumors of the thyroid gland. Cancer 68: 1944-1953.
302. Carcangiu ML, Sibley RK, Rosai J (1985). Clear cell change in primary thyroid tumors. A study of 38 cases. Am J Surg Pathol 9: 705-722.
303. Carcangiu ML, Steeper T, Zampi G, Rosai J (1985). Anaplastic thyroid carcinoma. A study of 70 cases. Am J Clin Pathol 83: 135-158.
304. Carcangiu ML, Zampi G, Rosai J (1984). Poorly differentiated ("insular") thyroid carcinoma. A reinterpretation of Langhans' "wuchernde Struma". Am J Surg Pathol 8: 655-668.
305. Carling T, Correa P, Hessman O, Hedberg J, Skogseid B, Lindberg D, Rastad J, Westin G, Akerstrom G (1998). Parathyroid MEN1 gene mutations in relation to clinical characteristics of nonfamilial primary hyperparathyroidism. J Clin Endocrinol Metab 83: 2960-2963.
306. Carlson KM, Dou S, Chi D, Scavarda N, Toshima K, Jackson CE, Wells SAJr, Goodfellow PJ, Donis-Keller H (1994). Single missense mutation in the tyrosine kinase catalytic domain of the RET protooncogene is associated with multiple endocrine neoplasia type 2B. Proc Natl Acad Sci U S A 91: 1579-1583.
307. Carney JA (1979). The triad of gastric epithelioid leiomyosarcoma, functioning extra-adrenal paraganglioma, and pulmonary chondroma. Cancer 43: 374-382.
308. Carney JA (1990). Psammomatous melanotic schwannoma. A distinctive, heritable tumor with special associations, including cardiac myxoma and the Cushing syndrome. Am J Surg Pathol 14: 206-222.
309. Carney JA (1999). Gastric stromal sarcoma, pulmonary chondroma, and extra-adrenal paraganglioma (Carney Triad): natural history, adrenocortical component, and possible familial occurrence. Mayo Clin Proc 74: 543-552.
310. Carney JA, Boccon-Gibod L, Jarka DE, Tanaka Y, Swee RG, Unni KK, Stratakis CA (2001). Osteochondromyxoma of bone: a congenital tumor associated with lentigines and other unusual disorders. Am J Surg Pathol 25: 164-176.
311. Carney JA, Ferreiro JA (1996). The epithelioid blue nevus. A multicentric familial tumor with important associations, including cardiac myxoma and psammomatous melanotic schwannoma. Am J Surg Pathol 20: 259-272.
312. Carney JA, Gordon H, Carpenter PC, Shenoy BV, Go VL (1985). The complex of myxomas, spotty pigmentation, and endocrine overactivity. Medicine (Baltimore) 64: 270-283.
313. Carney JA, Headington JT, Su WP (1986). Cutaneous myxomas. A major component of the complex of myxomas, spotty pigmentation, and endocrine overactivity. Arch Dermatol 122: 790-798.
314. Carney JA, Hruska LS, Beauchamp GD, Gordon H (1986). Dominant inheritance of the complex of myxomas, spotty pigmentation, and endocrine overactivity. Mayo Clin Proc 61: 165-172.
315. Carney JA, Ryan J, Goellner JR (1987). Hyalinizing trabecular adenoma of the thyroid gland. Am J Surg Pathol 11: 583-591.
316. Carney JA, Sizemore GW, Sheps SG (1976). Adrenal medullary disease in multiple endocrine neoplasia, type 2: pheochromocytoma and its precursors. Am J Clin Pathol 66: 279-290.
317. Carney JA, Stratakis CA (1996). Ductal adenoma of the breast and the Carney complex. Am J Surg Pathol 20: 1154-1155.
318. Carney JA, Young WF (1992). Primary pigmented nodular adrenocortical disease and its associated conditions. Endocrinologist 2: 6-21.
319. Carpten JD, Robbins CM, Villablanca A, Forsberg L, Presciuttini S, Bailey-Wilson J, Simonds WF, Gillanders EM, Kennedy AM, Chen JD, Agarwal SK, Sood R, Jones MP, Moses TY, Haven C, Petillo D, Leotlela PD, Harding B, Cameron D, Pannett AA, Hoog A, Heath HI, James-Newton LA, Robinson B, Zarbo RJ, Cavaco BM, Wassif W, Perrier ND, Rosen IB, Kristoffersson U, Turnpenny PD, Farnebo LO, Besser GM, Jackson CE, Morreau H, Trent JM, Thakker RV, Marx SJ, Teh BT, Larsson C, Hobbs MR (2002). HRPT2, encoding parafibromin, is mutated in hyperparathyroidism-jaw tumor syndrome. Nat Genet 32: 676-680.
320. Carstens PH, Cressman FKJr (1989). Malignant oncocytic carcinoid of the pancreas. Ultrastruct Pathol 13: 69-75.
321. Carstens PH, Kuhns JG, Ghazi C (1984). Primary malignant melanomas of the lung and adrenal. Hum Pathol 15: 910-914.
322. Carty SE, Helm AK, Amico JA, Clarke MR, Foley TP, Watson CG, Mulvihill JJ (1998). The variable penetrance and spectrum of manifestations of multiple endocrine neoplasia type 1. Surgery 124: 1106-1113.
323. Caruso M, Shaw E, Davis D, Scheithauer B, Abboud C, Speed J, Ilstrup D, Root L, Schleck C (1991). Radiation treatment of growth secreting pituitary adenomas. Int J Radiat Oncol Biol Phys 21: 121-122.
324. Casanova S, Rosenberg-Bourgin M, Farkas D, Calmettes C, Feingold N, Heshmati HM, Cohen R, Conte-Devolx B, Guillausseau PJ, Houdent C, Bigorgne JC, Boiteau V, Caron J, Modigliani E (1993). Phaeochromocytoma in multiple endocrine neoplasia type 2 A: survey of 100 cases. Clin Endocrinol (Oxf) 38: 531-537.
325. Cascon A, Ruiz-Llorente S, Cebrian A, Telleria D, Rivero JC, Diez JJ, Lopez-Ibarra PJ, Jaunsolo MA, Benitez J, Robledo M (2002). Identification of novel SDHD mutations in patients with phaeochromocytoma and/or paraganglioma. Eur J Hum Genet 10: 457-461.
326. Casey M, Mah C, Merliss AD, Kirschner LS, Taymans SE, Denio AE, Korf B, Irvine AD, Hughes A, Carney JA, Stratakis CA, Basson CT (1998). Identification of a novel genetic locus for familial cardiac myxomas and Carney complex. Circulation 98: 2560-2566.
327. Casey M, Vaughan CJ, He J, Hatcher CJ, Winter JM, Weremowicz S, Montgomery K, Kucherlapati R, Morton CC, Basson CT (2000). Mutations in the protein kinase A R1alpha regulatory subunit cause familial cardiac myxomas and Carney complex. J Clin Invest 106: R31-R38.
328. Castleman B, Mallory TB (1935). The pathology of the parathyroid glands in hyperparathyroidism. A study of 25 cases. Am J Pathol 11: 1-72.
329. Castoldi L, De Rai P, Marini A, Ferrero S, De Luca VM, Tiberio G (2001). Neurofibromatosis-1 and ampullary gangliocytic paraganglioma causing biliary and pancreatic obstruction. Int J Pancreatol 29: 93-97.
330. Castro P, Sansonetty F, Soares P, Dias A, Sobrinho-Simoes M (2001). Fetal adenomas and minimally invasive follicular carcinomas of the thyroid frequently display a triploid or near triploid DNA pattern. Virchows Arch 438: 336-342.
331. Cavaco BM, Barros L, Pannett AA, Ruas L, Carvalheiro M, Ruas MM, Krausz T, Santos MA, Sobrinho LG, Leite V, Thakker RV (2001). The hyperparathyroidism-jaw tumour syndrome in a Portuguese kindred. QJM 94: 213-222.
332. Cavallaro A, De Toma G, Mingazzini PL, Cavallaro G, Mosiello G, Marchetti G, Memeo L, La Fauci M (2001). Cysts of the adrenal gland: revision of a 15-year experience. Anticancer Res 21: 1401-1406.
333. Cavallo-Perin P, De Paoli M, Guiso G, Sapino A, Papotti M, Coda R, Pagano G (1988). A combined glucagonoma and VIPoma syndrome. First pathologic and clinical report. Cancer 62: 2576-2579.
334. Cavazza A, Toschi E, Valcavi R, Piana S, Scotti R, Carlinfante G, Gardini G (1999). [Sclerosing mucoepidermoid carcinoma with eosinophilia of the thyroid: description of a case]. Pathologica 91: 31-35.
335. Cetani F, Pinchera A, Pardi E, Cianferotti L, Vignali E, Picone A, Miccoli P, Viacava P, Marcocci C (1999). No evidence for mutations in the calcium-sensing receptor gene in sporadic parathyroid adenomas. J Bone Miner Res 14: 878-882.
336. Cetta F, Montalto G, Gori M, Curia MC, Cama A, Olschwang S (2000). Germline mutations of the APC gene in patients with familial adenomatous polyposis-associated thyroid carcinoma: results from a European cooperative study. J Clin Endocrinol Metab 85: 286-292.
337. Cetta F, Pelizzo MR, Curia MC, Barbarisi A (1999). Genetics and clinicopathological findings in thyroid carcinomas associated with familial adenomatous polyposis. Am J Pathol 155: 7-9.
338. Chaidarun SS, Klibanski A, Alexander JM (1997). Tumor-specific expression of alternatively spliced estrogen receptor messenger ribonucleic acid variants in human pituitary adenomas. J Clin Endocrinol Metab 82: 1058-1065.
339. Chambers EF, Turski PA, LaMasters D, Newton TH (1982). Regions of low density in the contrast-enhanced pituitary gland: normal and pathologic processes. Radiology 144: 109-113.
340. Chambers TP, Fishman EK, Hruban RH (1997). Pancreatic metastases from renal cell carcinoma in von Hippel-Lindau disease. Clin Imaging 21: 40-42.
341. Chan JK, Albores-Saavedra J, Battifora H, Carcangiu ML, Rosai J (1991). Sclerosing mucoepidermoid thyroid carcinoma with eosinophilia. A distinctive low-grade malignancy arising from the metaplastic follicles of Hashimoto's thyroiditis. Am J Surg Pathol 15: 438-448.
342. Chan JK, Fletcher CD, Nayler SJ, Cooper K (1997). Follicular dendritic cell sarcoma. Clinicopathologic analysis of 17 cases suggesting a malignant potential higher than currently recognized. Cancer 79: 294-313.
343. Chan JK, Loo KT (1990). Cribriform variant of papillary thyroid carcinoma. Arch Pathol Lab Med 114: 622-624.
344. Chan JK, Rosai J (1991). Tumors of the neck showing thymic or related branchial pouch differentiation: a unifying concept. Hum Pathol 22: 349-367.
345. Chan JK, Tse CC (1989). Solid cell nest-associated C-cells: another possible explanation for "C-cell hyperplasia" adjacent to follicular cell tumors. Hum Pathol 20: 498-499.
346. Chan JK, Tse CC, Chiu HS (1990). Hyalinizing trabecular adenoma-like lesion in multinodular goitre. Histopathology 16: 611-614.
347. Chan TJ, Libutti SK, McCart JA, Chen C, Khan A, Skarulis MK, Weinstein LS, Doppman JL, Marx SJ, Alexander HR (2003). Persistent primary hyperparathyroidism caused by adenomas identified in pharyngeal or adjacent structures. World J Surg 27: 675-679.
348. Chan YF, Ma L, Boey JH, Yeung HY (1986). Angiosarcoma of the thyroid. An immunohistochemical and ultrastructural study of a case in a Chinese patient. Cancer 57: 2381-2388.
349. Chandler WF (1991). Sellar and parasellar lesions. Clin Neurosurg 37: 514-527.
350. Chandrasekharappa S, Teh B (2001). Clinical and molecular aspects of multiple endocrine neoplasia type 1. In: Genetic Disorders of Endocrine Neoplasia, Dahia PLM, Eng C, eds., Karger: Basel , pp. 50-80.
351. Chandrasekharappa SC, Guru SC, Manickam P, Olufemi SE, Collins FS, Emmert-Buck MR, Debelenko LV, Zhuang Z, Lubensky IA, Liotta LA, Crabtree JS, Wang Y, Roe BA, Weisemann J, Boguski MS, Agarwal SK, Kester MB, Kim YS, Heppner C, Dong Q, Spiegel AM, Burns AL, Marx SJ (1997). Positional cloning of the gene for multiple endocrine neoplasia-type 1. Science 276: 404-407.
352. Chapurlat RD, Delmas PD, Liens D, Meunier PJ (1997). Long-term effects of intravenous pamidronate in fibrous dysplasia of bone. J Bone Miner Res 12: 1746-1752.
353. Charkes ND (1998). On the prevalence of familial nonmedullary thyroid cancer. Thyroid 8: 857-858.
354. Chastain MA (2001). The glucagonoma syndrome: a review of its features and discussion of new perspectives. Am J Med Sci 321: 306-320.
355. Chateil JF, Soussotte C, Pedespan JM, Brun M, Le Manh C, Diard F (2001). MRI and clinical differences between optic pathway tumours in children with and without neurofibromatosis. Br J Radiol 74: 24-31.
356. Chaudhary RK, Barnes EL, Myers EN (1994). Squamous cell carcinoma arising in Hashimoto's thyroiditis. Head Neck 16: 582-585.
357. Chauveau D, Duvic C, Chretien Y, Paraf F, Droz D, Melki P, Helenon O, Richard S, Grunfeld JP (1996). Renal involvement in von Hippel-Lindau disease. Kidney Int 50: 944-951.
358. Chen F, Kishida T, Yao M, Hustad T, Glavac D, Dean M, Gnarra JR, Orcutt ML, Duh FM, Glenn G, Green J, Hsia YE, Lamiell

J, Li H, Wei MH, Schmidt L, Tory K, Kuzmin I, Stackhouse T, Latif F, Linehan WM, Lerman M, Zbar B (1995). Germline mutations in the von Hippel-Lindau disease tumor suppressor gene: correlations with phenotype. Hum Mutat 5: 66-75.

359. Cheng L, Leibovich BC, Cheville JC, Ramnani DM, Sebo TJ, Neumann RM, Nascimento AG, Zincke H, Bostwick DG (2000). Paraganglioma of the urinary bladder: can biologic potential be predicted? Cancer 88: 844-852.

360. Chesyln-Curtis S, Akosa AB (1990). Primary plasmacytoma of the thyroid. Postgrad Med J 66: 477-478.

361. Chetty R (1990). Hurthle cell medullary carcinomas of the thyroid gland. S Afr J Surg 28: 95-97.

362. Chetty R, Clark SP, Dowling JP (1993). Leiomyosarcoma of the thyroid: immunohistochemical and ultrastructural study. Pathology 25: 203-205.

363. Chetty R, Clark SP, Pitson GA (1993). Primary small cell carcinoma of the pancreas. Pathology 25: 240-242.

364. Chetty R, Duhig JD (1993). Bilateral pheochromocytoma-ganglioneuroma of the adrenal in type 1 neurofibromatosis. Am J Surg Pathol 17: 837-841.

365. Chetty R, Goetsch S, Nayler S, Cooper K (1998). Spindle epithelial tumour with thymus-like element (SETTLE): the predominantly monophasic variant. Histopathology 33: 71-74.

366. Cheuk W, Jacobson AA, Chan JK (2000). Spindle epithelial tumor with thymus-like differentiation (SETTLE): a distinctive malignant thyroid neoplasm with significant metastatic potential. Mod Pathol 13: 1150-1155.

367. Cheung CC, Boerner SL, MacMillan CM, Ramyar L, Asa SL (2000). Hyalinizing trabecular tumor of the thyroid: a variant of papillary carcinoma proved by molecular genetics. Am J Surg Pathol 24: 1622-1626.

368. Cheung CC, Ezzat S, Freeman JL, Rosen IB, Asa SL (2001). Immunohistochemical diagnosis of papillary thyroid carcinoma. Mod Pathol 14: 338-342.

369. Cheung CC, Ezzat S, Ramyar L, Freeman JL, Asa SL (2000). Molecular basis off hurthle cell papillary thyroid carcinoma. J Clin Endocrinol Metab 85: 878-882.

370. Chevinsky AH, Minton JP, Falko JM (1990). Metastatic pheochromocytoma associated with multiple endocrine neoplasia syndrome type II. Arch Surg 125: 935-938.

371. Chew SL (1994). Phaeochromocytoma and familial tumour syndromes. Clin Endocrinol (Oxf) 40: 715-716.

372. Chiang MF, Brock M, Patt S (1990). Pituitary metastases. Neurochirurgia (Stuttg) 33: 127-131.

373. Chiappetta G, Toti P, Cetta F, Giuliano A, Pentimalli F, Amendola I, Lazzi S, Monaco M, Mazzuchelli L, Tosi P, Santoro M, Fusco A (2002). The RET/PTC oncogene is frequently activated in oncocytic thyroid tumors (Hurthle cell adenomas and carcinomas), but not in oncocytic hyperplastic lesions. J Clin Endocrinol Metab 87: 364-369.

374. Chien RN, Chen TC, Chiu CT, Tsai SL, Jen LB, Liaw YF (2001). Primary calcified gastrinoma of the liver. Dig Dis Sci 46: 370-375.

375. Choi PC, To KF, Lai FM, Lee TW, Yim AP, Chan JK (2000). Follicular dendritic cell sarcoma of the neck: report of two cases complicated by pulmonary metastases. Cancer 89: 664-672.

376. Chong BW, Kucharczyk W, Singer W, George S (1994). Pituitary gland MR: a comparative study of healthy volunteers and patients with microadenomas. AJNR Am J Neuroradiol 15: 675-679.

377. Choutet P, Benatre A, Cosnay P, Huten N, Alison D, Ginies G, Perrotin D, Lamisse F (1981). [Tumor of the adrenal gland associating pheochromocytoma and ganglioneuroma (author's transl)]. Sem Hop 57: 590-592.

378. Choyke PL, Glenn GM, Wagner JP, Lubensky IA, Thakore K, Zbar B, Linehan WM, Walther MM (1997). Epididymal cystadenomas in von Hippel-Lindau disease. Urology 49: 926-931.

379. Choyke PL, Glenn GM, Walther MM, Zbar B, Weiss GH, Alexander RB, Hayes WS, Long JP, Thakore KN, Linehan WM (1992). The natural history of renal lesions in von Hippel-Lindau disease: a serial CT study in 28 patients. AJR Am J Roentgenol 159: 1229-1234.

380. Christensen SB, Ljungberg O, Tibblin S (1984). A clinical epidemiologic study of thyroid carcinoma in Malmo, Sweden. Curr Probl Cancer 8: 1-49.

381. Chu T, Jaffe E (1994). The normal Langerhans cell and the LCH cell. Br J Cancer Suppl 23: S4-10.

382. Chung DC, Smith AP, Louis DN, Graeme-Cook F, Warshaw AL, Arnold A (1997). A novel pancreatic endocrine tumor suppressor gene locus on chromosome 3p with clinical prognostic implications. J Clin Invest 100: 404-410.

383. Chung DH, Kang GH, Kim WH, Ro JY (1999). Clonal analysis of a solitary follicular nodule of the thyroid with the polymerase chain reaction method. Mod Pathol 12: 265-271.

384. Chung J, Lee SK, Gong G, Kang DY, Park JH, Kim SB, Ro JY (1999). Sclerosing Mucoepidermoid carcinoma with eosinophilia of the thyroid glands: a case report with clinical manifestation of recurrent neck mass. J Korean Med Sci 14: 338-341.

385. Cibas ES, Medeiros LJ, Weinberg DS, Gelb AB, Weiss LM (1990). Cellular DNA profiles of benign and malignant adrenocortical tumors. Am J Surg Pathol 14: 948-955.

386. Ciccarelli E, Faccani G, Longo A, Dalle Ore G, Papotti M, Grottoli S, Razzore P, Ghe C, Muccioli G (1995). Prolactin receptors in human pituitary adenomas. Clin Endocrinol (Oxf) 42: 487-491.

387. Cifuentes N, Pickren JW (1979). Metastases from carcinoma of mammary gland: an autopsy study. J Surg Oncol 11: 193-205.

388. Cinti S, Colussi G, Minola E, Dickersin GR (1986). Parathyroid glands in primary hyperparathyroidism: an ultrastructural study of 50 cases. Hum Pathol 17: 1036-1046.

389. Civantos F, Albores-Saavedra J, Nadji M, Morales AR (1984). Clear cell variant of thyroid carcinoma. Am J Surg Pathol 8: 187-192.

390. Clark ES, Carney JA (1984). Pancreatic islet cell tumor associated with Cushing's syndrome. Am J Surg Pathol 8: 917-924.

391. Clarke MR, Baker EE, Weyant RJ, Hill L, Carty SE (1997). Proliferative Activity in Pancreatic Endocrine Tumors: Association with Function, Metastases, and Survival. Endocr Pathol 8: 181-187.

392. Clarke MR, Weyant RJ, Watson CG, Carty SE (1998). Prognostic markers in pheochromocytoma. Hum Pathol 29: 522-526.

393. Clifford SC, Cockman ME, Smallwood AC, Mole DR, Woodward ER, Maxwell PH, Ratcliffe PJ, Maher ER (2001). Contrasting effects on HIF-1alpha regulation by disease-causing pVHL mutations correlate with patterns of tumourigenesis in von Hippel-Lindau disease. Hum Mol Genet 10: 1029-1038.

394. Clifford SC, Maher ER (2001). Von Hippel-Lindau disease: clinical and molecular perspectives. Adv Cancer Res 82: 85-105.

395. Cocker RS, Kang J, Kahn LB (2003). Rosai-Dorfman disease. Report of a case presenting as a midline thyroid mass. Arch Pathol Lab Med 127: e197-e200.

396. Cockman ME, Masson N, Mole DR, Jaakkola P, Chang GW, Clifford SC, Maher ER, Pugh CW, Ratcliffe PJ, Maxwell PH (2000). Hypoxia inducible factor-alpha binding and ubiquitylation by the von Hippel-Lindau tumor suppressor protein. J Biol Chem 275: 25733-25741.

397. Cohen AJ, Li FP, Berg S, Marchetto DJ, Tsai S, Jacobs SC, Brown RS (1979). Hereditary renal-cell carcinoma associated with a chromosomal translocation. N Engl J Med 301: 592-595.

398. Cohen J, Gierlowski TC, Schneider AB (1990). A prospective study of hyperparathyroidism in individuals exposed to radiation in childhood. JAMA 264: 581-584.

399. Colao A, Loche S, Cappa M, Di Sarno A, Landi ML, Sarnacchiaro F, Facciolli G, Lombardi G (1998). Prolactinomas in children and adolescents. Clinical presentation and long-term follow-up. J Clin Endocrinol Metab 83: 2777-2780.

400. Colarian J, Pietruk T, LaFave L, Calzada R (1990). Adenocarcinoma of the ampulla of vater associated with neurofibromatosis. J Clin Gastroenterol 12: 118-119.

401. Collins BT, Cramer HM (1996). Fine-needle aspiration cytology of islet cell tumors. Diagn Cytopathol 15: 37-45.

402. Collins MT, Chebli C, Jones J, Kushner H, Consugar M, Rinaldo P, Wientroub S, Bianco P, Robey PG (2001). Renal phosphate wasting in fibrous dysplasia of bone is part of a generalized renal tubular dysfunction similar to that seen in tumor-induced osteomalacia. J Bone Miner Res 16: 806-813.

403. Colman SD, Rasmussen SA, Ho VT, Abernathy CR, Wallace MR (1996). Somatic mosaicism in a patient with neurofibromatosis type 1. Am J Hum Genet 58: 484-490.

404. Colombo N, Loli P, Vignati F, Scialfa G (1994). MR of corticotropin-secreting pituitary microadenomas. AJNR Am J Neuroradiol 15: 1591-1595.

405. Colton JJ, Batsakis JG, Work WP (1978). Teratomas of the neck in adults. Arch Otolaryngol 104: 271-272.

406. Comite F, Shawker TH, Pescovitz OH, Loriaux DL, Cutler GBJr (1984). Cyclical ovarian function resistant to treatment with an analogue of luteinizing hormone releasing hormone in McCune-Albright syndrome. N Engl J Med 311: 1032-1036.

407. Cone L, Srinivasan M, Romanul FC (1990). Granular cell tumor (choristoma) of the neurohypophysis: two cases and a review of the literature. AJNR Am J Neuroradiol 11: 403-406.

408. Constantini S, Soffer D, Siegel T, Shalit MN (1989). Paraganglioma of the thoracic spinal cord with cerebrospinal fluid metastasis. Spine 14: 643-645.

409. Contreras LN, Budd D, Yen TS, Thomas C, Tyrrell JB (1991). Adrenal ganglioneuroma-pheochromocytoma secreting vasoactive intestinal polypeptide. West J Med 154: 334-337.

410. Cook AM, Vini L, Harmer C (1999). Squamous cell carcinoma of the thyroid: outcome of treatment in 16 patients. Eur J Surg Oncol 25: 606-609.

411. Cooper DS, Axelrod L, DeGroot LJ, Vickery ALJr, Maloof F (1981). Congenital goiter and the development of metastatic follicular carcinoma with evidence for a leak of nonhormonal iodide: clinical, pathological, kinetic, and biochemical studies and a review of the literature. J Clin Endocrinol Metab 52: 294-306.

412. Cor A (1999). Proliferative activity of Hurthle cell thyroid tumours. Oncology 57: 17-22.

412A. Corbetta S, Pizzocaro A, Peracchi M, Beck-Peccoz P, Faglia G, Spada A (1997). Multiple endocrine neoplasia type 1 in patients with recognized pituitary tumours of different types. Clin Endocrinol (Oxf) 47: 507-512.

413. Cordeiro AC, Montenegro FL, Kulcsar MA, Dellanegra LA, Tavares MR, Michaluart PJr, Ferraz AR (1998). Parathyroid carcinoma. Am J Surg 175: 52-55.

414. Corenblum B, Donovan L (1993). The safety of physiological estrogen plus progestin replacement therapy and with oral contraceptive therapy in women with pathological hyperprolactinemia. Fertil Steril 59: 671-673.

415. Corless CL, Kibel AS, Iliopoulos O, Kaelin WGJr (1997). Immunostaining of the von Hippel-Lindau gene product in normal and neoplastic human tissues. Hum Pathol 28: 459-464.

416. Cornish D, Pont A, Minor D, Coombs JL, Bennington J (1984). Metastatic islet cell tumor in von Hippel-Lindau disease. Am J Med 77: 147-150.

417. Correa P, Chen VW (1995). Endocrine gland cancer. Cancer 75: 338-352.

418. Corrin B, Gilby ED, Jones NF, Patrick J (1973). Oat cell carcinoma of the pancreas with ectopic ACTH secretion. Cancer 31: 1523-1527.

419. Corvi R, Berger N, Balczon R, Romeo G (2000). RET/PCM-1: a novel fusion gene in papillary thyroid carcinoma. Oncogene 19: 4236-4242.

420. Costello RT (1936). Subclinical adenoma of the pituitary gland. Am J Pathol 12: 205-214.

421. Costi R, Caruana P, Sarli L, Violi V, Roncoroni L, Bordi C (2001). Ampullary adenocarcinoma in neurofibromatosis type 1. Case report and literature review. Mod Pathol 14: 1169-1174.

422. Couch RM, Hughes IA, DeSa DJ, Schiffrin A, Guyda H, Winter JS (1986). An autosomal dominant form of adolescent multinodular goiter. Am J Hum Genet 39: 811-816.

423. Courcoutsakis NA, Chow CK, Shawker TH, Carney JA, Stratakis CA (1997). Syndrome of spotty skin pigmentation, myxomas, endocrine overactivity, and schwannomas (Carney complex): breast imaging findings. Radiology 205: 221-227.

424. Coutant R, Lumbroso S, Rey R, Lahlou N, Venara M, Rouleau S, Sultan C, Limal JM (2001). Macroorchidism due to autonomous hyperfunction of Sertoli cells and G(s)alpha gene mutation: an unusual expression of McCune-Albright syndrome in a prepubertal boy. J Clin Endocrinol Metab 86: 1778-1781.

425. Crabtree JS, Scacheri PC, Ward JM, Garrett-Beal L, Emmert-Buck MR, Edgemon KA, Lorang D, Libutti SK, Chandrasekharappa SC, Marx SJ, Spiegel AM, Collins FS (2001). A mouse model of multiple endocrine neoplasia, type 1, develops multiple endocrine tumors. Proc Natl Acad Sci U S A 98: 1118-1123.
426. Crain EL, Thorn GW (1940). Functioning pancreatic islet cell adenomas: a review of the literature and presentation of two new differential tests. Medicine 28: 427-447.
427. Craver RD, Lipscomb JT, Suskind D, Velez MC (2001). Malignant teratoma of the thyroid with primitive neuroepithelial and mesenchymal sarcomatous components. Ann Diagn Pathol 5: 285-292.
428. Crawford AH (1989). Pitfalls of spinal deformities associated with neurofibromatosis in children. Clin Orthop 29-42.
429. Creutzfeldt W (1985). Endocrine tumors of the pancreas. In: The diabetic pancreas, Volk BW, Arquilla ER, eds., Plenum: New York , pp. 543-586.
430. Creutzfeldt W, Arnold R, Creutzfeldt C, Deuticke U, Frerichs H, Track NS (1973). Biochemical and morphological investigations of 30 human insulinomas. Correlation between the tumour content of insulin and proinsulin-like components and the histological and ultrastructural appearance. Diabetologia 9: 217-231.
431. Creutzfeldt W, Arnold R, Creutzfeldt C, Track NS (1975). Pathomorphologic, biochemical, and diagnostic aspects of gastrinomas (Zollinger-Ellison syndrome). Hum Pathol 6: 47-76.
432. Crooke AC (1935). A change in the basophile cells of the pituitary gland common to conditions which exhibit the syndrome attributed to basophile adenoma. Journal of Pathology 41: 339-349.
433. Crossey PA, Richards FM, Foster K, Green JS, Prowse A, Latif F, Lerman MI, Zbar B, Affara NA, Ferguson-Smith MA, Maher ER (1994). Identification of intragenic mutations in the von Hippel-Lindau disease tumour suppressor gene and correlation with disease phenotype. Hum Mol Genet 3: 1303-1308.
434. Crowe FW, Schull WJ, Neel JV (1956). A Clinical, Pathological, and Genetic Study of Multiple Neurofibromatosis. Charles C. Thomas: Springfield.
435. Crowley PF, Slavin JL, Rode J (1996). Massive amyloid deposition in pancreatic vipoma: a case report. Pathology 28: 377-379.
436. Cruz MC, Marques LP, Sambade C, Sobrinho-Simoes M (1991). Primary mucinous carcinoma of the thyroid. Surg Pathol 4: 266-273.
437. Cryns VL, Alexander JM, Klibanski A, Arnold A (1993). The retinoblastoma gene in human pituitary tumors. J Clin Endocrinol Metab 77: 644-646.
438. Cryns VL, Thor A, Xu HJ, Hu SX, Wierman ME, Vickery ALJr, Benedict WF, Arnold A (1994). Loss of the retinoblastoma tumor-suppressor gene in parathyroid carcinoma. N Engl J Med 330: 757-761.
439. Cubilla AL, Hajdu SI (1975). Islet cell carcinoma of the pancreas. Arch Pathol 99: 204-207.
440. Cudennec YF, Trannoy P, Briche T, Meyran M, Roguet E, Beautru R, Soubeyrand L (1992). [Thyroid teratoma in adults]. Rev Laryngol Otol Rhinol (Bord) 113: 213-215.
441. Cupisti K, Hoppner W, Dotzenrath C, Simon D, Berndt I, Roher HD, Goretzki PE (2000). Lack of MEN1 gene mutations in 27 sporadic insulinomas. Eur J Clin Invest 30: 325-329.
442. Cushing HW (1932). The basophil adenomas of the pituitary body and their clinical manifestations (pituitary basophilism). Bull John Hopkins Hosp 50: 137-195.
443. D'Adda T, Pizzi S, Azzoni C, Bottarelli L, Crafa P, Pasquali C, Davoli C, Corleto VD, Fave GD, Bordi C (2002). Different patterns of 11q allelic losses in digestive endocrine tumors. Hum Pathol 33: 322-329.
444. Dabski C, Reiman HMJr, Muller SA (1990). Neurofibrosarcoma of skin and subcutaneous tissues. Mayo Clin Proc 65: 164-172.
445. Dackiw AP, Cote GJ, Fleming JB, Schultz PN, Stanford P, Vassilopoulou-Sellin R, Evans DB, Gagel RF, Lee JE (1999). Screening for MEN1 mutations in patients with atypical endocrine neoplasia. Surgery 126: 1097-1103.
446. Dahia PL, Aguiar RC, Tsanaclis AM, Bendit I, Bydlowski SP, Abelin NM, Toledo SP (1995). Molecular and immunohistochemical analysis of P53 in phaeochromocytoma. Br J Cancer 72: 1211-1213.
447. Dahia PL, Marsh DJ, Zheng Z, Zedenius J, Komminoth P, Frisk T, Wallin G, Parsons R, Longy M, Larsson C, Eng C (1997). Somatic deletions and mutations in the Cowden disease gene, PTEN, in sporadic thyroid tumors. Cancer Res 57: 4710-4713.
448. Daneshdoost L, Gennarelli TA, Bashey HM, Savino PJ, Sergott RC, Bosley TM, Snyder PJ (1991). Recognition of gonadotroph adenomas in women. N Engl J Med 324: 589-594.
449. Danforth DNJr, Gorden P, Brennan MF (1984). Metastatic insulin-secreting carcinoma of the pancreas: clinical course and the role of surgery. Surgery 96: 1027-1037.
450. Daniely M, Aviram A, Adams EF, Buchfelder M, Barkai G, Fahlbusch R, Goldman B, Friedman E (1998). Comparative genomic hybridization analysis of nonfunctioning pituitary tumors. J Clin Endocrinol Metab 83: 1801-1805.
451. Danila DC, Haidar JN, Zhang X, Katznelson L, Culler MD, Klibanski A (2001). Somatostatin receptor-specific analogs: effects on cell proliferation and growth hormone secretion in human somatotroph tumors. J Clin Endocrinol Metab 86: 2976-2981.
452. Danilowicz K, Albiger N, Vanegas M, Gomez RM, Cross G, Bruno OD (2002). Androgen-secreting adrenal adenomas. Obstet Gynecol 100: 1099-1102.
453. Dannenberg H, de Krijger RR, van der Harst E, Abbou M, Ijzendoorn Y, Komminoth P, Dinjens WN (2003). Von Hippel-Lindau gene alterations in sporadic benign and malignant pheochromocytomas. Int J Cancer 105: 190-195.
454. Dannenberg H, de Krijger RR, Zhao J, Speel EJ, Saremaslani P, Dinjens WN, Mooi WJ, Roth J, Heitz PU, Komminoth P (2001). Differential loss of chromosome 11q in familial and sporadic parasympathetic paragangliomas detected by comparative genomic hybridization. Am J Pathol 158: 1937-1942.
455. Dannenberg H, Dinjens WN, Abbou M, Van Urk H, Pauw BK, Mouwen D, Mooi WJ, de Krijger RR (2002). Frequent germline succinate dehydrogenase subunit D gene mutations in patients with apparently sporadic parasympathetic paraganglioma. Clin Cancer Res 8: 2061-2066.
456. Dannenberg H, Speel EJ, Zhao J, Saremaslani P, van der Harst E, Roth J, Heitz PU, Bonjer HJ, Dinjens WN, Mooi WJ, Komminoth P, de Krijger RR (2000). Losses of chromosomes 1p and 3q are early genetic events in the development of sporadic pheochromocytomas. Am J Pathol 157: 353-359.
457. Danon M, Crawford JD (1987). The McCune-Albright syndrome. Ergeb Inn Med Kinderheilkd 55: 81-115.
458. Dao AH, Page DL, Reynolds VH, Adkins RBJr (1990). Primary malignant melanoma of the adrenal gland. A report of two cases and review of the literature. Am Surg 56: 199-203.
459. Darling TN, Skarulis MC, Steinberg SM, Marx SJ, Spiegel AM, Turner M (1997). Multiple facial angiofibromas and collagenomas in patients with multiple endocrine neoplasia type 1. Arch Dermatol 133: 853-857.
460. Darrouzet V, Rivel J, Deminiere C, Boissieras P, Verhust J, Bebear JP, Portmann M, Vital C (1982). [Familial malignant carotid body chemodectoma with lymph node metastases. Light and electron microscopy study (author's transl)]. Ann Pathol 2: 163-167.
461. Daston MM, Ratner N (1992). Neurofibromin, a predominantly neuronal GTPase activating protein in the adult, is ubiquitously expressed during development. Dev Dyn 195: 216-226.
462. Davaris P, Petraki K, Arvanitis D, Papacharalammpous N, Morakis A, Zorzos S (1986). Urinary bladder paraganglioma (U.B.P.). Pathol Res Pract 181: 101-106.
463. Dayal Y (1991). Pancreatic Endocrine Cells and Their Non-Neoplastic Proliferations. In: Endocrine Pathology of the Gut and Pancreas, Dayal Y, ed., CRC Press: Boca Raton , pp. 69-104.
464. Dayal Y, Tallberg KA, Nunnemacher G, DeLellis RA, Wolfe HJ (1986). Duodenal carcinoids in patients with and without neurofibromatosis. A comparative study. Am J Surg Pathol 10: 348-357.
465. De Graeff J, Horak BJV (1964). The incidence of phaeochromocytoma in the Netherlands. Acta Med Scand 176: 583-593.
466. de Keyzer Y, Rene P, Beldjord C, Lenne F, Bertagna X (1998). Overexpression of vasopressin (V3) and corticotrophin-releasing hormone receptor genes in corticotroph tumours. Clin Endocrinol (Oxf) 49: 475-482.
467. de Keyzer Y, Rene P, Lenne F, Auzan C, Clauser E, Bertagna X (1997). V3 vasopressin receptor and corticotropic phenotype in pituitary and nonpituitary tumors. Horm Res 47: 259-262.
468. de Krijger RR, van der Harst E, Muletta-Feurer S, Bruining HA, Lamberts SW, Dinjens WN, Roth J, Heitz PU, Komminoth P (2000). RET is expressed but not mutated in extra-adrenal paragangliomas. J Pathol 191: 264-268.
469. de Krijger RR, van der Harst E, van der Ham F, Stijnen T, Dinjens WN, Koper JW, Bruining HA, Lamberts SW, Bosman FT (1999). Prognostic value of p53, bcl-2, and c-erbB-2 protein expression in phaeochromocytomas. J Pathol 188: 51-55.
470. de la Monte SM, Hutchins GM, Moore GW (1984). Endocrine organ metastases from breast carcinoma. Am J Pathol 114: 131-136.
471. de Perrot M, Licker M, Robert JH, Spiliopoulos A (1999). Long-term survival after surgical resections of bronchogenic carcinoma and adrenal metastasis. Ann Thorac Surg 68: 1084-1085.
472. Dean DS, Hay ID (2000). Prognostic indicators in differentiated thyroid carcinoma. Cancer Control 7: 229-239.
473. Debas HT, Mulvihill SJ (1994). Neuroendocrine gut neoplasms. Important lessons from uncommon tumors. Arch Surg 129: 965-971.
474. DeBella K, Szudek J, Friedman JM (2000). Use of the national institutes of health criteria for diagnosis of neurofibromatosis 1 in children. Pediatrics 105: 608-614.
475. DeClue JE, Papageorge AG, Fletcher JA, Diehl SR, Ratner N, Vass WC, Lowy DR (1992). Abnormal regulation of mammalian p21ras contributes to malignant tumor growth in von Recklinghausen (type 1) neurofibromatosis. Cell 69: 265-273.
476. Decorato JW, Gruber H, Petti M, Levowitz BS (1990). Adrenal carcinosarcoma. J Surg Oncol 45: 134-136.
477. Delcore RJr, Cheung LY, Friesen SR (1988). Outcome of lymph node involvement in patients with the Zollinger-Ellison syndrome. Ann Surg 208: 291-298.
478. DeLellis RA (1993). Tumors of the Parathyroid Gland. 3rd ed. Armed Forces Institute of Pathology: Washington, DC.
479. DeLellis RA (1995). Multiple endocrine neoplasia syndromes revisited. Clinical, morphologic, and molecular features. Lab Invest 72: 494-505.
480. DeLellis RA, Nunnemacher G, Wolfe HJ (1977). C-cell hyperplasia. An ultrastructural analysis. Lab Invest 36: 237-248.
481. DeLellis RA, Rule AH, Spiler I, Nathanson L, Tashjian AHJr, Wolfe HJ (1978). Calcitonin and carcinoembryonic antigen as tumor markers in medullary thyroid carcinoma. Am J Clin Pathol 70: 587-594.
482. DeLellis RA, Suchow E, Wolfe HJ (1980). Ultrastructure of nuclear "inclusions" in pheochromocytoma and paraganglioma. Hum Pathol 11: 205-207.
483. DeLellis RA, Wolfe HJ, Gagel RF, Feldman ZT, Miller HH, Gang DL, Reichlin S (1976). Adrenal medullary hyperplasia. A morphometric analysis in patients with familial medullary thyroid carcinoma. Am J Pathol 83: 177-196.
484. Delgrange E, Trouillas J, Maiter D, Donckier J, Tourniaire J (1997). Sex-related difference in the growth of prolactinomas: a clinical and proliferation marker study. J Clin Endocrinol Metab 82: 2102-2107.
485. Deligdisch L, Subhani Z, Gordon RE (1980). Primary mucinous carcinoma of the thyroid gland: report of a case and ultrastructural study. Cancer 45: 2564-2567.
486. Demeter JG, De Jong SA, Lawrence AM, Paloyan E (1991). Anaplastic thyroid carcinoma: risk factors and outcome. Surgery 110: 956-961.
487. Derringer GA, Thompson LD, Frommelt RA, Bijwaard KE, Heffess CS, Abbondanzo SL (2000). Malignant lymphoma of the thyroid gland: a clinicopathologic study of 108 cases. Am J Surg Pathol 24: 623-639.
488. Derwahl M, Broecker M, Kraiem Z (1999). Clinical review 101: Thyrotropin may not be the dominant growth factor in benign and malignant thyroid tumors. J Clin Endocrinol Metab 84: 829-834.
489. Deshmukh NS, Mangham DC, Warfield AT, Watkinson JC (2001). Solitary fibrous tumour of the thyroid gland. J Laryngol Otol 115: 940-942.
490. Deshmukh RR, Kumar V, Kumbhani

D (2003). Sinus histiocytosis of the thyroid with massive lymphadenopathy (Rosai-Dorfman disease). J Indian Med Assoc 101: 597-598.

491. Deshpande V, Muzikansky A, Fernandez del Castillo C (2003). Cytokeratin 19 is a powerful predictor of survival in pancreatic endocrine tumors. Mod Pathol 16: 272A.

492. Devilee P, van Schothorst EM, Bardoel AF, Bonsing B, Kuipers-Dijkshoorn N, James MR, Fleuren G, van der Mey AG, Cornelisse CJ (1994). Allelotype of head and neck paragangliomas: allelic imbalance is confined to the long arm of chromosome 11, the site of the predisposing locus PGL. Genes Chromosomes Cancer 11: 71-78.

493. Dey P, Luthra UK, Sheikh ZA (1999). Fine needle aspiration cytology of Langerhans cell histiocytosis of the thyroid. A case report. Acta Cytol 43: 429-431.

494. Dial PF, Braasch JW, Rossi RL, Lee AK, Jin GL (1985). Management of nonfunctioning islet cell tumors of the pancreas. Surg Clin North Am 65: 291-299.

495. Diaz-Cano SJ, Blanes A, Rubio J, Matilla A, Wolfe HJ (2000). Molecular evolution and intratumor heterogeneity by topographic compartments in muscle-invasive transitional cell carcinoma of the urinary bladder. Lab Invest 80: 279-289.

496. Diaz-Cano SJ, de Miguel M, Blanes A, Tashjian R, Wolfe HJ (2001). Germline RET 634 mutation positive MEN 2A-related C-cell hyperplasias have genetic features consistent with intraepithelial neoplasia. J Clin Endocrinol Metab 86: 3948-3957.

497. Diaz-Perez R, Quiroz H, Nishiyama RH (1976). Primary mucinous adenocarcinoma of thyroid gland. Cancer 38: 1323-1325.

498. Dieterich KD, Gundelfinger ED, Ludecke DK, Lehnert H (1998). Mutation and expression analysis of corticotropin-releasing factor 1 receptor in adrenocorticotropin-secreting pituitary adenomas. J Clin Endocrinol Metab 83: 3327-3331.

499. Dietrich CU, Pandis N, Bjerre P, Schroder HD, Heim S (1993). Simple numerical chromosome aberrations in two pituitary adenomas. Cancer Genet Cytogenet 69: 118-121.

500. DiPaolo DP, Zimmerman RA, Rorke LB, Zackai EH, Bilaniuk LT, Yachnis AT (1995). Neurofibromatosis type 1: pathologic substrate of high-signal-intensity foci in the brain. Radiology 195: 721-724.

501. Djalilian HR, Linzie B, Maisel RH (2000). Malignant teratoma of the thyroid: review of literature and report of a case. Am J Otolaryngol 21: 112-115.

502. Dluhy RG (2003). Endocrine hypertension. In: Williams Textbook of Endocrinology, Larsen PR, Kronenberg HM, Melmed S, Polonsky KS, eds., 10th ed. Saunders: Philadelphia , pp. 552-585.

503. Dobashi Y, Sakamoto A, Sugimura H, Mernyei M, Mori M, Oyama T, Machinami R (1993). Overexpression of p53 as a possible prognostic factor in human thyroid carcinoma. Am J Surg Pathol 17: 375-381.

504. Dobashi Y, Sugimura H, Sakamoto A, Mernyei M, Mori M, Oyama T, Machinami R (1994). Stepwise participation of p53 gene mutation during dedifferentiation of human thyroid carcinomas. Diagn Mol Pathol 3: 9-14.

505. Dodd LG, Evans DB, Symmans F, Katz RL (1994). Fine-needle aspiration of pancreatic extramedullary plasmacytoma: possible confusion with islet cell tumor. Diagn Cytopathol 10: 371-374.

506. Dohna M, Reincke M, Mincheva A, Allolio B, Solinas-Toldo S, Lichter P (2000). Adrenocortical carcinoma is characterized by a high frequency of chromosomal gains and high-level amplifications. Genes Chromosomes Cancer 28: 145-152.

507. Doi M, Imai T, Shichiri M, Tateno T, Fukai N, Ozawa N, Sato R, Teramoto K, Hirata Y (2003). Octreotide-sensitive ectopic ACTH production by islet cell carcinoma with multiple liver metastases. Endocr J 50: 135-143.

508. Dollinger MR, Ratner LH, Shamoian CA, Blackbourne BD (1967). Carcinoid syndrome associated with pancreatic tumors. Arch Intern Med 120: 575-580.

509. Dominguez-Malagon H, Delgado-Chavez R, Torres-Najera M, Gould E, Albores-Saavedra J (1989). Oxyphil and squamous variants of medullary thyroid carcinoma. Cancer 63: 1183-1188.

510. Dominguez-Malagon H, Flores-Flores G, Vilchis JJ (2001). Lymphoepithelioma-like anaplastic thyroid carcinoma: report of a case not related to Epstein-Barr virus. Ann Diagn Pathol 5: 21-24.

511. Donghi R, Longoni A, Pilotti S, Michieli P, Della Porta G, Pierotti MA (1993). Gene p53 mutations are restricted to poorly differentiated and undifferentiated carcinomas of the thyroid gland. J Clin Invest 91: 1753-1760.

512. Donis-Keller H, Dou S, Chi D, Carlson KM, Toshima K, Lairmore TC, Howe JR, Moley JF, Goodfellow P, Wells SAJr (1993). Mutations in the RET proto-oncogene are associated with MEN 2A and FMTC. Hum Mol Genet 2: 851-856.

513. Donnell CA, Pollock WJ, Sybers WA (1987). Thyroid carcinosarcoma. Arch Pathol Lab Med 111: 1169-1172.

514. Donovan DT, Levy ML, Furst EJ, Alford BR, Wheeler T, Tschen JA, Gagel RF (1989). Familial cutaneous lichen amyloidosis in association with multiple endocrine neoplasia type 2A: a new variant. Henry Ford Hosp Med J 37: 147-150.

515. Donow C, Pipeleers-Marichal M, Schroder S, Stamm B, Heitz PU, Kloppel G (1991). Surgical pathology of gastrinoma. Site, size, multicentricity, association with multiple endocrine neoplasia type 1, and malignancy. Cancer 68: 1329-1334.

516. Donow C, Pipeleers-Marichal M, Stamm B, Heitz PU, Kloppel G (1990). [The pathology of insulinoma and gastrinoma. The location, size, multicentricity, association with multiple endocrine type-I neoplasms and malignancy]. Dtsch Med Wochenschr 115: 1386-1391.

517. Dookhan DB, Miettinen M, Finkel G, Gibas Z (1993). Recurrent duodenal gangliocytic paraganglioma with lymph node metastases. Histopathology 22: 399-401.

518. Doppman JL, Frank JA, Dwyer AJ, Oldfield EH, Miller DL, Nieman LK, Chrousos GP, Cutler GBJr, Loriaux DL (1988). Gadolinium DTPA enhanced MR imaging of ACTH-secreting microadenomas of the pituitary gland. J Comput Assist Tomogr 12: 728-735.

519. Doppman JL, Nieman LK, Cutler GBJr, Chrousos GP, Fraker DL, Norton JA, Jensen RT (1994). Adrenocorticotropic hormone—secreting islet cell tumors: are they always malignant? Radiology 190: 59-64.

520. Doppman JL, Shawker TH, Fraker DL, Alexander HR, Skarulis MC, Lack EE, Spiegel AM (1994). Parathyroid adenoma within the vagus nerve. AJR Am J Roentgenol 163: 943-945.

521. Dorfman DM, Shahsafaei A, Chan JK (1997). Thymic carcinomas, but not thymomas and carcinomas of other sites, show CD5 immunoreactivity. Am J Surg Pathol 21: 936-940.

522. Dorfman DM, Shahsafaei A, Miyauchi A (1998). Immunohistochemical staining for bcl-2 and mcl-1 in intrathyroidal epithelial thymoma (ITET)/carcinoma showing thymus-like differentiation (CASTLE) and cervical thymic carcinoma. Mod Pathol 11: 989-994.

523. Dorfman DM, Shahsafaei A, Miyauchi A (1998). Intrathyroidal epithelial thymoma (ITET)/carcinoma showing thymus-like differentiation (CASTLE) exhibits CD5 immunoreactivity: new evidence for thymic differentiation. Histopathology 32: 104-109.

524. Dorfman HD, Ishida T, Tsuneyoshi M (1994). Exophytic variant of fibrous dysplasia (fibrous dysplasia protuberans). Hum Pathol 25: 1234-1237.

525. Dottorini ME, Assi A, Sironi M, Sangalli G, Spreafico G, Colombo L (1996). Multivariate analysis of patients with medullary thyroid carcinoma. Prognostic significance and impact on treatment of clinical and pathologic variables. Cancer 77: 1556-1565.

526. Dralle H, Gimm O, Simon D, Frank-Raue K, Gortz G, Niederle B, Wahl RA, Koch B, Walgenbach S, Hampel R, Ritter MM, Spelsberg F, Heiss A, Hinze R, Hoppner W (1998). Prophylactic thyroidectomy in 75 children and adolescents with hereditary medullary thyroid carcinoma: German and Austrian experience. World J Surg 22: 744-750.

527. Drange MR, Fram NR, Herman-Bonert V, Melmed S (2000). Pituitary tumor registry: a novel clinical resource. J Clin Endocrinol Metab 85: 168-174.

528. Driman D, Murray D, Kovacs K, Stefaneanu L, Higgins HP (1991). Encapsulated medullary carcinoma of the thyroid. A morphologic study including immunocytochemistry, electron microscopy, flow cytometry, and in situ hybridization. Am J Surg Pathol 15: 1089-1095.

529. Drovdlic CM, Myers EN, Peters JA, Baysal BE, Brackmann DE, Slattery WHI, Rubinstein WS (2001). Proportion of heritable paraganglioma cases and associated clinical characteristics. Laryngoscope 111: 1822-1827.

530. Druker HA, Kasprzak L, Begin LR, Jothy S, Narod SA, Foulkes WD (1997). Family with Graves disease, multinodular goiter, nonmedullary thyroid carcinoma, and alveolar rhabdomyosarcoma. Am J Med Genet 72: 30-33.

531. Ducatman BS, Scheithauer BW, Piepgras DG, Reiman HM, Ilstrup DM (1986). Malignant peripheral nerve sheath tumors. A clinicopathologic study of 120 cases. Cancer 57: 2006-2021.

532. Duerr EM, Gimm O, Neuberg DS, Kum JB, Clifford SC, Toledo SP, Maher ER, Dahia PL, Eng C (1999). Differences in allelic distribution of two polymorphisms in the VHL-associated gene CUL2 in pheochromocytoma patients without somatic CUL2 mutations. J Clin Endocrinol Metab 84: 3207-3211.

533. Durbec PL, Larsson-Blomberg LB, Schuchardt A, Costantini F, Pachnis V (1996). Common origin and developmental dependence on c-ret of subsets of enteric and sympathetic neuroblasts. Development 122: 349-358.

534. Dwight T, Thoppe SR, Foukakis T, Lui WO, Wallin G, Hoog A, Frisk T, Larsson C, Zedenius J (2003). Involvement of PAX8/peroxisome proliferator-activated receptor gamma rearrangement in follicular thyroid tumors. J Clin Endocrinol Metab 88: 4440-4445.

535. Dwyer AJ, Frank JA, Doppman JL, Oldfield EH, Hickey AM, Cutler GB, Loriaux DL, Schiable TF (1987). Pituitary adenomas in patients with Cushing disease: initial experience with Gd-DTPA-enhanced MR imaging. Radiology 163: 421-426.

536. Dyer EH, Civit T, Abecassis JP, Derome PJ (1994). Functioning ectopic supradiaphragmatic pituitary adenomas. Neurosurgery 34: 529-532.

537. Earnest F, McCullough EC, Frank DA (1981). Fact or artifact: an analysis of artifact in high-resolution computed tomographic scanning of the sella. Radiology 140: 109-113.

538. Easton DF, Ponder MA, Huson SM, Ponder BA (1993). An analysis of variation in expression of neurofibromatosis (NF) type 1 (NF1): evidence for modifying genes. Am J Hum Genet 53: 305-313.

539. Ebersold MJ, Laws ERJr, Scheithauer BW, Randall RV (1983). Pituitary apoplexy treated by transsphenoidal surgery. A clinicopathological and immunocytochemical study. J Neurosurg 58: 315-320.

540. Ebersold MJ, Quast LM, Laws ERJr, Scheithauer B, Randall RV (1986). Long-term results in transsphenoidal removal of nonfunctioning pituitary adenomas. J Neurosurg 64: 713-719.

541. Ebrahimi SA, Wang EH, Wu A, Schreck RR, Passaro EJ, Sawicki MP (1999). Deletion of chromosome 1 predicts prognosis in pancreatic endocrine tumors. Cancer Res 59: 311-315.

542. Eckert F, Schmid U, Gloor F, Hedinger C (1986). Evidence of vascular differentiation in anaplastic tumours of the thyroid—an immunohistological study. Virchows Arch A Pathol Anat Histopathol 410: 203-215.

543. Eckhauser FE, Cheung PS, Vinik AI, Strodel WE, Lloyd RV, Thompson NW (1986). Nonfunctioning malignant neuroendocrine tumors of the pancreas. Surgery 100: 978-988.

544. Edery P, Lyonnet S, Mulligan LM, Pelet A, Dow E, Abel L, Holder S, Nihoul-Fekete C, Ponder BA, Munnich A (1994). Mutations of the RET proto-oncogene in Hirschsprung's disease. Nature 367: 378-380.

545. Edgerton MT, Persing JA, Jane JA (1985). The surgical treatment of fibrous dysplasia. With emphasis on recent contributions from cranio-maxillo-facial surgery. Ann Surg 202: 459-479.

546. Edstrom Elder E, Nord B, Carling T, Juhlin C, Backdahl M, Hoog A, Larsson C (2002). Loss of heterozygosity on the short arm of chromosome 1 in pheochromocytoma and abdominal paraganglioma. World J Surg 26: 965-971.

547. Edstrom E, Mahlamaki E, Nord B, Kjellman M, Karhu R, Hoog A, Goncharov N, Teh BT, Backdahl M, Larsson C (2000). Comparative genomic hybridization reveals frequent losses of chromosomes 1p and 3q in pheochromocytomas and abdominal paragangliomas, suggesting a common genetic etiology. Am J Pathol 156: 651-659.

548. Egloff B (1983). The hemangioendothelioma of the thyroid. Virchows Arch A

Pathol Anat Histopathol 400: 119-142.

549. Ehrig U, Wilson DR (1972). Fibrous dysplasia of bone and primary hyperparathyroidism. Ann Intern Med 77: 234-238.

550. Eisenhofer G, Lenders JW, Linehan WM, Walther MM, Goldstein DS, Keiser HR (1999). Plasma normetanephrine and metanephrine for detecting pheochromocytoma in von Hippel-Lindau disease and multiple endocrine neoplasia type 2. N Engl J Med 340: 1872-1879.

551. Eisenhofer G, Walther MM, Huynh TT, Li ST, Bornstein SR, Vortmeyer A, Mannelli M, Goldstein DS, Linehan WM, Lenders JW, Pacak K (2001). Pheochromocytomas in von Hippel-Lindau syndrome and multiple endocrine neoplasia type 2 display distinct biochemical and clinical phenotypes. J Clin Endocrinol Metab 86: 1999-2008.

552. Eissele R, Goke R, Weichardt U, Fehmann HC, Arnold R, Goke B (1994). Glucagon-like peptide 1 immunoreactivity in gastroentero-pancreatic endocrine tumors: a light- and electron-microscopic study. Cell Tissue Res 276: 571-579.

553. el Halabi DA, el Sayed M, Eskaf W, Anim JT, Dey P (2000). Langerhans cell histiocytosis of the thyroid gland. A case report. Acta Cytol 44: 805-808.

553A. Elisei R, Bottici V, Luchetti F, Di Coscio G, Romei C, Grasso L (2004). Impact of routine measurement of serum calcitonin on the diagnosis and outcome of medullary thyroid cancer: experience in 10,864 patients with nodular thyroid disorders. J Clin Endocrinol Metab 89: 163-168.

554. el Naggar AK, Evans DB, Mackay B (1991). Oncocytic adrenal cortical carcinoma. Ultrastruct Pathol 15: 549-556.

555. Elbehti-Green A, Au HC, Mascarello JT, Ream-Robinson D, Scheffler IE (1998). Characterization of the human SDHC gene encoding of the integral membrane proteins of succinate-quinone oxidoreductase in mitochondria. Gene 213: 133-140.

556. Ellison EH, Wilson SD (1964). The Zollinger-Ellison syndrome: reappraisal and evaluation of 260 registered cases. Ann Surg 160: 512-530.

557. Emery D, Kucharczyk W (2001). Imaging of pituitary tumors. In: Diagnosis and management of pituitary tumors, Thapar K, Kovacs K, Scheithauer BW, Lloyd RV, eds., Humana Press: Totowa , pp. 201-217.

558. Emmert-Buck MR, Lubensky IA, Dong Q, Manickam P, Guru SC, Kester MB, Olufemi SE, Agarwal S, Burns AL, Spiegel AM, Collins FS, Marx SJ, Zhuang Z, Liotta LA, Chandrasekharappa SC, Debelenko LV (1997). Localization of the multiple endocrine neoplasia type I (MEN1) gene based on tumor loss of heterozygosity analysis. Cancer Res 57: 1855-1858.

559. Eng C (1999). RET proto-oncogene in the development of human cancer. J Clin Oncol 17: 380-393.

560. Eng C (2000). Familial papillary thyroid cancer—many syndromes, too many genes? J Clin Endocrinol Metab 85: 1755-1757.

561. Eng C (2000). Will the real Cowden syndrome please stand up: revised diagnostic criteria. J Med Genet 37: 828-830.

562. Eng C (2001). Multiple endocrine neoplasia type 2. In: Molecular genetics of cancer, Cowell J, ed., 2nd ed. Bios Scientific: Oxford , pp. 171-194.

563. Eng C (2002). Role of PTEN, a lipid phosphatase upstream effector of protein kinase B, in epithelial thyroid carcinogenesis. Ann N Y Acad Sci 968: 213-221.

564. Eng C, Clayton D, Schuffenecker I, Lenoir G, Cote G, Gagel RF, van Amstel HK, Lips CJ, Nishisho I, Takai SI, Marsh DJ, Robinson BG, Frank-Raue K, Raue F, Xue F, Noll WW, Romei C, Pacini F, Fink M, Niederle B, Zedenius J, Nordenskjold M, Komminoth P, Hendy GN, Gharib H, Thibodeau SN, Lacroix A, Frilling A, Ponder BA, Mulligan LM (1996). The relationship between specific RET proto-oncogene mutations and disease phenotype in multiple endocrine neoplasia type 2. International RET mutation consortium analysis. JAMA 276: 1575-1579.

565. Eng C, Crossey PA, Mulligan LM, Healey CS, Houghton C, Prowse A, Chew SL, Dahia PL, O'Riordan JL, Toledo SP, Smith DP, Maher ER, Ponder BA (1995). Mutations in the RET proto-oncogene and the von Hippel-Lindau disease tumour suppressor gene in sporadic and syndromic phaeochromocytomas. J Med Genet 32: 934-937.

566. Eng C, Mulligan LM, Healey CS, Houghton C, Frilling A, Raue F, Thomas GA, Ponder BA (1996). Heterogeneous mutation of the RET proto-oncogene in subpopulations of medullary thyroid carcinoma. Cancer Res 56: 2167-2170.

567. Eng C, Mulligan LM, Smith DP, Healey CS, Frilling A, Raue F, Neumann HP, Ponder MA, Ponder BA (1995). Low frequency of germline mutations in the RET proto-oncogene in patients with apparently sporadic medullary thyroid carcinoma. Clin Endocrinol (Oxf) 43: 123-127.

568. Eng C, Smith DP, Mulligan LM, Nagai MA, Healey CS, Ponder MA, Gardner E, Scheumann GF, Jackson CE, Tunnacliffe A, Ponder BA (1994). Point mutation within the tyrosine kinase domain of the RET proto-oncogene in multiple endocrine neoplasia type 2B and related sporadic tumours. Hum Mol Genet 3: 237-241.

569. Erickson D, Kudva YC, Ebersold MJ, Thompson GB, Grant CS, van Heerden JA, Young WFJr (2001). Benign paragangliomas: clinical presentation and treatment outcomes in 236 patients. J Clin Endocrinol Metab 86: 5210 5216.

570. Erickson LA (2000). p27(kip1) and Other Cell-Cycle Protein Expression in Normal and Neoplastic Endocrine Tissues. Endocr Pathol 11: 109-122.

571. Erickson LA, Jalal SM, Goellner JR, Law ME, Harwood A, Jin L, Roche PC, Lloyd RV (2001). Analysis of Hurthle cell neoplasms of the thyroid by interphase fluorescence in situ hybridization. Am J Surg Pathol 25: 911-917.

572. Erickson LA, Jin L, Goellner JR, Lohse C, Pankratz VS, Zukerberg LR, Thompson GB, van Heerden JA, Grant CS, Lloyd RV (2000). Pathologic features, proliferative activity, and cyclin D1 expression in Hurthle cell neoplasms of the thyroid. Mod Pathol 13: 186-192.

573. Erickson LA, Jin L, Papotti M, Lloyd RV (2002). Oxyphil parathyroid carcinomas: a clinicopathologic and immunohistochemical study of 10 cases. Am J Surg Pathol 26: 344-349.

574. Erickson LA, Jin L, Sebo TJ, Lohse C, Pankratz VS, Kendrick ML, van Heerden JA, Thompson GB, Grant CS, Lloyd RV (2001). Pathologic features and expression of insulin-like growth factor-2 in adrenocortical neoplasms. Endocr Pathol 12: 429-435.

575. Erickson LA, Jin L, Wollan P, Thompson GB, van Heerden JA, Lloyd RV (1999). Parathyroid hyperplasia, adenomas, and carcinomas: differential expression of p27Kip1 protein. Am J Surg Pathol 23: 288-295.

576. Erickson LA, Jin L, Wollan PC, Thompson GB, van Heerden J, Lloyd RV (1998). Expression of p27kip1 and Ki-67 in benign and malignant thyroid tumors. Mod Pathol 11: 169-174.

577. Eriksson B, Oberg K, Skogseid B (1989). Neuroendocrine pancreatic tumors. Clinical findings in a prospective study of 84 patients. Acta Oncol 28: 373-377.

578. Erlandson RA (1994). Diagnostic Transmission Electron Microscopy of Tumors. Raven Press: New York.

579. Etxabe J, Vazquez JA (1994). Morbidity and mortality in Cushing's disease: an epidemiological approach. Clin Endocrinol (Oxf) 40: 479-484.

580. Eubanks PJ, Sawicki MP, Samara GJ, Wan YJ, Gatti RA, Hurwitz M, Passaro EJ (1997). Pancreatic endocrine tumors with loss of heterozygosity at the multiple endocrine neoplasia type I locus. Am J Surg 173: 518-520.

581. Eugster EA, Shankar R, Feezle LK, Pescovitz OH (1999). Tamoxifen treatment of progressive precocious puberty in a patient with McCune-Albright syndrome. J Pediatr Endocrinol Metab 12: 681-686.

582. Eusebi V, Capella C, Bondi A, Sessa F, Vezzadini P, Mancini AM (1981). Endocrine-paracrine cells in pancreatic exocrine carcinomas. Histopathology 5: 599-613.

583. Eusebi V, Carcangiu ML, Dina R, Rosai J (1990). Keratin-positive epithelioid angiosarcoma of thyroid. A report of four cases. Am J Surg Pathol 14: 737-747.

584. Eusebi V, Damiani S, Riva C, Lloyd RV, Capella C (1990). Calcitonin free oat-cell carcinoma of the thyroid gland. Virchows Arch A Pathol Anat Histopathol 417: 267-271.

585. Evans CO, Young AN, Brown MR, Brat DJ, Parks JS, Neish AS, Oyesiku NM (2001). Novel patterns of gene expression in pituitary adenomas identified by complementary deoxyribonucleic acid microarrays and quantitative reverse transcription-polymerase chain reaction. J Clin Endocrinol Metab 86: 3097-3107.

586. Evans CP, Vaccaro JA, Storrs BG, Christ PJ (1988). Suprarenal occurrence of an adenomatoid tumor. J Urol 139: 348-349.

587. Evans DG, Baser ME, McGaughran J, Sharif S, Howard E, Moran A (2002). Malignant peripheral nerve sheath tumours in neurofibromatosis 1. J Med Genet 39: 311-314.

588. Evans HL (1987). Encapsulated papillary neoplasms of the thyroid. A study of 14 cases followed for a minimum of 10 years. Am J Surg Pathol 11: 592-597.

589. Evans HL (1991). Criteria for diagnosis of parathyroid carcinoma. Surg Pathol 4: 244-265.

590. Evans HL, Vassilopoulou-Sellin R (1998). Follicular and Hurthle cell carcinomas of the thyroid: a comparative study. Am J Surg Pathol 22: 1512-1520.

591. Ezaki H, Ebihara S, Fujimoto Y, Iida F, Ito K, Kuma K, Izuo M, Makiuchi M, Oyamada H, Matoba N, Yagawa K (1992). Analysis of thyroid carcinoma based on material registered in Japan during 1977-1986 with special reference to predominance of papillary type. Cancer 70: 808-814.

592. Ezzat S, Ezrin C, Yamashita S, Melmed S (1993). Recurrent acromegaly resulting from ectopic growth hormone gene expression by a metastatic pancreatic tumor. Cancer 71: 66-70.

593. Ezzat S, Horvath E, Harris AG, Kovacs K (1994). Morphological effects of octreotide on growth hormone-producing pituitary adenomas. J Clin Endocrinol Metab 79: 113-118.

594. Ezzat S, Horvath E, Kovacs K, Smyth HS, Singer W, Asa SL (1995). Basic Fibroblast Growth Factor Expression by Two Prolactin and Thyrotropin-Producing Pituitary Adenomas. Endocr Pathol 6: 125-134.

595. Ezzat S, Melmed S (1991). Acromegaly: etiology, diagnosis and management. Compr Ther 17: 31-35.

596. Ezzat S, Smyth HS, Ramyar L, Asa SL (1995). Heterogenous in vivo and in vitro expression of basic fibroblast growth factor by human pituitary adenomas. J Clin Endocrinol Metab 80: 878-884.

597. Ezzat S, Zheng L, Kolenda J, Safarian A, Freeman JL, Asa SL (1996). Prevalence of activating ras mutations in morphologically characterized thyroid nodules. Thyroid 6: 409-416.

598. Ezzat S, Zheng L, Zhu XF, Wu GE, Asa SL (2002). Targeted expression of a human pituitary tumor-derived isoform of FGF receptor-4 recapitulates pituitary tumorigenesis. J Clin Invest 109: 69-78.

599. Fadda G, Fiorino MC, Mule A, LiVolsi VA (2002). Macrofollicular encapsulated variant of papillary thyroid carcinoma as a potential pitfall in histologic and cytologic diagnosis. A report of three cases. Acta Cytol 46: 555-559.

600. Fagin JA (1997). Familial non-medullary thyroid carcinoma—the case for genetic susceptibility. J Clin Endocrinol Metab 82: 342-344.

601. Fagin JA, Matsuo K, Karmakar A, Chen DL, Tang SH, Koeffler HP (1993). High prevalence of mutations of the p53 gene in poorly differentiated human thyroid carcinomas. J Clin Invest 91: 179-184.

602. Fahlbusch R, Schott W (2002). Pterional surgery of meningiomas of the tuberculum sellae and planum sphenoidale: surgical results with special consideration of ophthalmological and endocrinological outcomes. J Neurosurg 96: 235-243.

603. Fajans SS, Vinik AI (1989). Insulin-producing islet cell tumors. Endocrinol Metab Clin North Am 18: 45-74.

604. Fan X, Paetau A, Aalto Y, Valimaki M, Sane T, Poranen A, Castresana JS, Knuutila S (2001). Gain of chromosome 3 and loss of 13q are frequent alterations in pituitary adenomas. Cancer Genet Cytogenet 128: 97-103.

605. Farhi F, Dikman SH, Lawson W, Cobin RH, Zak FG (1976). Paragangliomatosis associated with multiple endocrine adenomas. Arch Pathol Lab Med 100: 495-498.

606. Farid NR (2001). P53 mutations in thyroid carcinoma: tidings from an old foe. J Endocrinol Invest 24: 536-545.

607. Farnebo F, Auer G, Farnebo LO, Teh BT, Twigg S, Aspenblad U, Thompson NW, Grimelius L, Larsson C, Sandelin K (1999). Evaluation of retinoblastoma and Ki-67 immunostaining as diagnostic markers of benign and malignant parathyroid disease. World J Surg 23: 68-74.

608. Farnebo F, Kytola S, Teh BT, Dwight T, Wong FK, Hoog A, Elvius M, Wassif WS, Thompson NW, Farnebo LO, Sandelin K, Larsson C (1999). Alternative genetic pathways in parathyroid tumorigenesis. J Clin

Endocrinol Metab 84: 3775-3780.

609.   Farnebo F, Teh BT, Kytola S, Svensson A, Phelan C, Sandelin K, Thompson NW, Hoog A, Weber G, Farnebo LO, Larsson C (1998). Alterations of the MEN1 gene in sporadic parathyroid tumors. J Clin Endocrinol Metab 83: 2627-2630.

610.   Farrell WE, Clayton RN (2000). Molecular pathogenesis of pituitary tumors. Front Neuroendocrinol 21: 174-198.

611.   Fearnhead NS, Britton MP, Bodmer WF (2001). The ABC of APC. Hum Mol Genet 10: 721-733.

612.   Feldman DE, Thulasiraman V, Ferreyra RG, Frydman J (1999). Formation of the VHL-elongin BC tumor suppressor complex is mediated by the chaperonin TRiC. Mol Cell 4: 1051-1061.

613.   Feldman GL, Edmonds MW, Ainsworth PJ, Schuffenecker I, Lenoir GM, Saxe AW, Talpos GB, Roberson J, Petrucelli N, Jackson CE (2000). Variable expressivity of familial medullary thyroid carcinoma (FMTC) due to a RET V804M (GTG—>ATG) mutation. Surgery 128: 93-98.

614.   Feldman JM (1987). Carcinoid tumors and syndrome. Semin Oncol 14: 237-246.

615.   Feldman JM, Moore J (1989). Biogenic amines in carcinoid tumors. Biogenic Amines 6: 247-252.

616.   Felix IA, Horvath E, Kovacs K (1981). Massive Crooke's hyalinization in corticotroph cell adenomas of the human pituitary. A histological, immunocytological, and electron microscopic study of three cases. Acta Neurochir (Wien) 58: 235-243.

617.   Fenton CL, Lukes Y, Nicholson D, Dinauer CA, Francis GL, Tuttle RM (2000). The ret/PTC mutations are common in sporadic papillary thyroid carcinoma of children and young adults. J Clin Endocrinol Metab 85: 1170-1175.

618.   Ferlay J, Bray F, Pisani P, Parkin DM (2001). GLOBOCAN 2000: Cancer Incidence, Mortality and Prevalence Worldwide. IARC Press: Lyon.

619.   Ferner R (1994). Medical complications of neurofibromatosis. In: The Neurofibromatoses: A Pathogenic and Clinical Overview, Huson SM, Hughes RAC, eds., Chapman and Hall: London , pp. 316-330.

620.   Ferner RE, Hughes RA, Weinman J (1996). Intellectual impairment in neurofibromatosis 1. J Neurol Sci 138: 125-133.

621.   Ferrozzi F, Tognini G, Bova D, Zuccoli G, Pavone P (2001). Hemangiosarcoma of the adrenal glands: CT findings in two cases. Abdom Imaging 26: 336-339.

622.   Fetsch PA, Powers CN, Zakowski MF, Abati A (1999). Anti-alpha-inhibin: marker of choice for the consistent distinction between adrenocortical carcinoma and renal cell carcinoma in fine-needle aspiration. Cancer 87: 168-172.

623.   Feuillan PP (1993). Treatment of sexual precocity in girls with the McCune-Albright syndrome. In: Sexual Precocity: Etiology, Diagnosis and Management, Grave GD, Cutler GB, eds., Raven Press: New York , pp. 243-251.

624.   Feuillan PP, Jones J, Cutler GBJr (1993). Long-term testolactone therapy for precocious puberty in girls with the McCune-Albright syndrome. J Clin Endocrinol Metab 77: 647-651.

625.   Feuillan PP, Shawker T, Rose SR, Jones J, Jeevanram RK, Nisula BC (1990). Thyroid abnormalities in the McCune-Albright syndrome: ultrasonography and hormonal studies. J Clin Endocrinol Metab

71: 1596-1601.

626.   Figueiredo BC, Stratakis CA, Sandrini R, DeLacerda L, Pianovsky MA, Giatzakis C, Young HM, Haddad BR (1999). Comparative genomic hybridization analysis of adrenocortical tumors of childhood. J Clin Endocrinol Metab 84: 1116-1121.

627.   Filipi CJ, Higgins GA (1973). Diagnosis and management of insulinoma. Am J Surg 125: 231-239.

628.   Finelli P, Giardino D, Rizzi N, Buiatiotis S, Virduci T, Franzin A, Losa M, Larizza L (2000). Non-random trisomies of chromosomes 5, 8 and 12 in the prolactinoma sub-type of pituitary adenomas: conventional cytogenetics and interphase FISH study. Int J Cancer 86: 344-350.

629.   Finelli P, Pierantoni GM, Giardino D, Losa M, Rodeschini O, Fedele M, Valtorta E, Mortini P, Croce CM, Larizza L, Fusco A (2002). The High Mobility Group A2 gene is amplified and overexpressed in human prolactinomas. Cancer Res 62: 2398-2405.

630.   Fink A, Tomlinson G, Freeman JL, Rosen IB, Asa SL (1996). Occult micropapillary carcinoma associated with benign follicular thyroid disease and unrelated thyroid neoplasms. Mod Pathol 9: 816-820.

631.   Fiocca R, Sessa F, Tenti P, Usellini L, Capella C, O'Hare MM, Solcia E (1983). Pancreatic polypeptide (PP) cells in the PP-rich lobe of the human pancreas are identified ultrastructurally and immunocytochemically as F cells. Histochemistry 77: 511-523.

632.   Firat D, Stutzman L (1968). Fibrous dysplasia of the bone. Review of twenty-four cases. Am J Med 44: 421-429.

633.   Fischer JA, Bollinger A, Lichtlen P, Wellauer J (1970). Fibrous dysplasia of the bone and high cardiac output. Am J Med 49: 140-146.

634.   Fischler DF, Nunez C, Levin HS, McMahon JT, Sheeler LR, Adelstein DJ (1992). Adrenal carcinosarcoma presenting in a woman with clinical signs of virilization. A case report with immunohistochemical and ultrastructural findings. Am J Surg Pathol 16: 626-631.

635.   Fishman EK, Deutch BM, Hartman DS, Goldman SM, Zerhouni EA, Siegelman SS (1987). Primary adrenocortical carcinoma: CT evaluation with clinical correlation. AJR Am J Roentgenol 148: 531-535.

636.   Flamme I, Krieg M, Plate KH (1998). Up-regulation of vascular endothelial growth factor in stromal cells of hemangioblastomas is correlated with up-regulation of the transcription factor HRF/HIF-2alpha. Am J Pathol 153: 25-29.

637.   Fleming MV, Oertel YC, Rodriguez ER, Fidler WJ (1993). Fine-needle aspiration of six carotid body paragangliomas. Diagn Cytopathol 9: 510-515.

638.   Fletcher CDM, Unni KK, Mertens F (2002). World Health Organization Classification of Tumours. Pathology and Genetics of Tumours of Soft Tissue and Bone. IARCPress : Lyon.

639.   Flickinger JC, Nelson PB, Martinez AJ, Deutsch M, Taylor F (1989). Radiotherapy of nonfunctional adenomas of the pituitary gland. Results with long-term follow-up. Cancer 63: 2409-2414.

640.   Fonseca E, Castanhas S, Sobrinho-Simoes M (1996). Expression of Simple Mucin Type Antigens and Lewis Type 1 and Type 2 Chain Antigens in the Thyroid Gland: An Immunohistochemical Study of Normal Thyroid Tissues, Benign Lesions, and Malignant Tumors. Endocr Pathol 7: 291-301.

641.   Fonseca E, Nesland JM, Sobrinho-Simoes M (1997). Expression of stratified epithelial-type cytokeratins in hyalinizing trabecular adenomas supports their relationship with papillary carcinomas of the thyroid. Histopathology 31: 330-335.

642.   Foster CM, Ross JL, Shawker T, Pescovitz OH, Loriaux DL, Cutler GBJr, Comite F (1984). Absence of pubertal gonadotropin secretion in girls with McCune-Albright syndrome. J Clin Endocrinol Metab 58: 1161-1165.

643.   Foulkes WD (1995). A tale of four syndromes: familial adenomatous polyposis, Gardner syndrome, attenuated APC and Turcot syndrome. QJM 88: 853-863.

644.   Fox PS, Hofmann JW, Wilson SD, DeCosse JJ (1974). Surgical management of the Zollinger-Ellison syndrome. Surg Clin North Am 54: 395-407.

645.   Fraker DL, Travis WD, Merendino JJJr, Zimering MB, Streeten EA, Weinstein LS, Marx SJ, Spiegel AM, Aurbach GD, Doppman JL, Norton JA (1991). Locally recurrent parathyroid neoplasms as a cause for recurrent and persistent primary hyperparathyroidism. Ann Surg 213: 58-65.

646.   Franc B, Rosenberg-Bourgin M, Caillou B, Dutrieux-Berger N, Floquet J, Houcke-Lecomte M, Justrabo E, Lange F, Labat-Moleur F, Le Bodic MF, Patey M, Beauchet A, Saint-Andre JP, Hejblum G, Viennet G (1998). Medullary thyroid carcinoma: search for histological predictors of survival (109 proband cases analysis). Hum Pathol 29: 1078-1084.

647.   Franceschi S, Preston-Martin S, Dal Maso L, Negri E, La Vecchia C, Mack WJ, McTiernan A, Kolonel L, Mark SD, Mabuchi K, Jin F, Wingren G, Galanti R, Hallquist A, Glattre E, Lund E, Levi F, Linos D, Ron E (1999). A pooled analysis of case-control studies of thyroid cancer. IV. Benign thyroid diseases. Cancer Causes Control 10: 583-595.

648.   Francis IR, Korobkin M (1996). Pheochromocytoma. Radiol Clin North Am 34: 1101-1112.

649.   Franks LM, Bollen A, Seeger RC, Stram DO, Matthay KK (1997). Neuroblastoma in adults and adolescents: an indolent course with poor survival. Cancer 79: 2028-2035.

650.   Franquemont DW, Mills SE, Lack EE (1994). Immunohistochemical detection of neuroblastomatous foci in composite adrenal pheochromocytoma-neuroblastoma. Am J Clin Pathol 102: 163-170.

651.   Franssila K (1971). Value of histologic classification of thyroid cancer. Acta Pathol Microbiol Scand [A] 225: Suppl-76.

652.   Franssila KO, Harach HR (1986). Occult papillary carcinoma of the thyroid in children and young adults. A systemic autopsy study in Finland. Cancer 58: 715-719.

653.   Franssila KO, Harach HR, Wasenius VM (1984). Mucoepidermoid carcinoma of the thyroid. Histopathology 8: 847-860.

654.   Freeman C, Berg JW, Cutler SJ (1972). Occurrence and prognosis of extranodal lymphomas. Cancer 29: 252-260.

655.   French CA, Alexander EK, Cibas ES, Nose V, Laguette J, Faquin W, Garber J, Moore FJ, Fletcher JA, Larsen PR, Kroll TG (2003). Genetic and biological subgroups of low-stage follicular thyroid cancer. Am J Pathol 162: 1053-1060.

656.   Frich L, Glattre E, Akslen LA (2001). Familial occurrence of nonmedullary thyroid cancer: a population-based study of 5673 first-degree relatives of thyroid can-

cer patients from Norway. Cancer Epidemiol Biomarkers Prev 10: 113-117.

657.   Friedman M, Shimaoka K, Lopez CA, Shedd DP (1983). Parathyroid adenoma diagnosed as papillary carcinoma of thyroid on needle aspiration smears. Acta Cytol 27: 337-340.

658.   Friedrich CA (2001). Genotype-phenotype correlation in von Hippel-Lindau syndrome. Hum Mol Genet 10: 763-767.

659.   Friend KE, Chiou YK, Lopes MB, Laws ERJr, Hughes KM, Shupnik MA (1994). Estrogen receptor expression in human pituitary: correlation with immunohistochemistry in normal tissue, and immunohistochemistry and morphology in macroadenomas. J Clin Endocrinol Metab 78: 1497-1504.

660.   Fries JG, Chamberlin JA (1968). Extra-adrenal pheochromocytoma: litterature review and report of a cervical pheochromocytoma. Surgery 63: 268-279.

661.   Frisk T, Foukakis T, Dwight T, Lundberg J, Hoog A, Wallin G, Eng C, Zedenius J, Larsson C (2002). Silencing of the PTEN tumor-suppressor gene in anaplastic thyroid cancer. Genes Chromosomes Cancer 35: 74-80.

662.   Frisk T, Kytola S, Wallin G, Zedenius J, Larsson C (1999). Low frequency of numerical chromosomal aberrations in follicular thyroid tumors detected by comparative genomic hybridization. Genes Chromosomes Cancer 25: 349-353.

663.   Frisk T, Zedenius J, Lundberg J, Wallin G, Kytola S, Larsson C (2001). CGH alterations in medullary thyroid carcinomas in relation to the RET M918T mutation and clinical outcome. Int J Oncol 18: 1219-1225.

664.   Fritz A, Percy C, Jack A, Shanmugaratnam K, Sobin LH, Parkin DM, Whelan S (2000). International Classification of Diseases for Oncology. 3rd. ed. WHO: Geneva.

665.   Froböse C (1923). Das aus markhaltigen nervenfasern bestehende ganlienzellenlose echte neurom in rankenform - zugleich ein beitrag zu den nervösengeschwulsten der zunge und des augenlides. Virchows Arch A Pathol Anat 240: 312-327.

666.   Frohnauer MK, Decker RA (2000). Update on the MEN 2A c804 RET mutation: is prophylactic thyroidectomy indicated? Surgery 128: 1052-1057.

667.   Frost AR, Tenner S, Tenner M, Rollhauser C, Tabbara SO (1995). ACTH-producing pituitary carcinoma presenting as the cauda equina syndrome. Arch Pathol Lab Med 119: 93-96.

668.   Frucht H, Howard JM, Slaff JI, Wank SA, McCarthy DM, Maton PN, Vinayek R, Gardner JD, Jensen RT (1989). Secretin and calcium provocative tests in the Zollinger-Ellison syndrome. A prospective study. Ann Intern Med 111: 713-722.

669.   Fujikawa M, Okamura K, Sato K, Mizokami T, Tamaki K, Yanagida T, Fujishima M (1998). Familial isolated hyperparathyroidism due to multiple adenomas associated with ossifying jaw fibroma and multiple uterine adenomyomatous polyps. Eur J Endocrinol 138: 557-561.

670.   Fujimoto Y, Obara T, Ito Y, Kodama T, Nobori M, Ebihara S (1986). Localization and surgical resection of metastatic parathyroid carcinoma. World J Surg 10: 539-547.

671.   Fujiwara T, Kawamura M, Sasou S, Hiramori K (2000). Results of surgery for a compound adrenal tumor consisting of pheochromocytoma and ganglioneuroblas-

toma in an adult: 5-year follow-up. Intern Med 39: 58-62.
672. Fung JW, Lam KS (1995). Neurofibromatosis and insulinoma. Postgrad Med J 71: 485-486.
673. Furihata M, Ohtsuki Y, Matsumoto M, Sonobe H, Okada Y, Watanabe R (2001). Immunohistochemical characterisation of a case of insular thyroid carcinoma. Pathology 33: 257-261.
674. Gadelha MR, Kineman RD, Frohman LA (1999). Familial somatotropinomas: clinical and genetic aspects. Endocrinologist 9: 277-285.
675. Gaffey MJ, Lack EE, Christ ML, Weiss LM (1991). Anaplastic thyroid carcinoma with osteoclast-like giant cells. A clinicopathologic, immunohistochemical, and ultrastructural study. Am J Surg Pathol 15: 160-168.
676. Gaffey MJ, Traweek ST, Mills SE, Travis WD, Lack EE, Medeiros LJ, Weiss LM (1992). Cytokeratin expression in adrenocortical neoplasia: an immunohistochemical and biochemical study with implications for the differential diagnosis of adrenocortical, hepatocellular, and renal cell carcinoma. Hum Pathol 23: 144-153.
677. Gaffey TA, Scheithauer BW, Lloyd RV, Burger PC, Robbins P, Fereidooni F, Horvath E, Kovacs K, Kuroki T, Young WFJr, Sebo TJ, Riehle DL, Belzberg AJ (2002). Corticotroph carcinoma of the pituitary: a clinicopathological study. Report of four cases. J Neurosurg 96: 352-360.
678. Gaffney RL, Carney JA, Sebo TJ, Erickson LA, Volante M, Papotti M, Lloyd RV (2003). Galectin-3 expression in hyalanizing trabecular tumors of the thyroid gland. Am J Surg Pathol 27: 494-498.
679. Gaitan D, Loosen PT, Orth DN (1993). Two patients with Cushing's disease in a kindred with multiple endocrine neoplasia type I. J Clin Endocrinol Metab 76: 1580-1582.
680. Galanti MR, Ekbom A, Grimelius L, Yuen J (1997). Parental cancer and risk of papillary and follicular thyroid carcinoma. Br J Cancer 75: 451-456.
681. Galati LT, Barnes EL, Myers EN (1999). Dendritic cell sarcoma of the thyroid. Head Neck 21: 273-275.
682. Galbut DL, Markowitz AM (1980). Insulinoma: diagnosis, surgical management and long-term follow-up. Review of 41 cases. Am J Surg 139: 682-690.
683. Gall RM, Witterick IJ, Noyek AM, Leslie WD (2003). Preoperative localization tests. In: Surgery of the Thyroid and Parathyroid Glands, Randolph GW, ed., Saunders: Philadelphia , pp. 498-506.
684. Gallay BJ, Ahmad S, Xu L, Toivola B, Davidson RC (2001). Screening for primary aldosteronism without discontinuing hypertensive medications: plasma aldosterone-renin ratio. Am J Kidney Dis 37: 699-705.
685. Gallivan MV, Chun B, Rowden G, Lack EE (1980). Intrathoracic paravertebral malignant paraganglioma. Arch Pathol Lab Med 104: 46-51.
686. Gallo A, Cuozzo C, Esposito I, Maggiolini M, Bonofiglio D, Vivacqua A, Garramone M, Weiss C, Bohmann D, Musti AM (2002). Menin uncouples Elk-1, JunD and c-Jun phosphorylation from MAP kinase activation. Oncogene 21: 6434-6445.
687. Ganda OP, Weir GC, Soeldner JS, Legg MA, Chick WL, Patel YC, Ebeid AM, Gabbay KH, Reichlin S (1977). "Somatostatinoma": a somatostatin-containing tumor of the endocrine pancreas. N Engl J Med 296: 963-967.
688. Garcia-Escudero A, Miguel-Rodriguez M, Moreno-Fernandez A, Navarro-Bustos G, Galera-Ruiz H, Galera-Davidson H (2001). Prognostic value of DNA flow cytometry in sympathoadrenal paragangliomas. Anal Quant Cytol Histol 23: 238-244.
689. Garcia-Rostan G, Camp RL, Herrero A, Carcangiu ML, Rimm DL, Tallini G (2001). Beta-catenin dysregulation in thyroid neoplasms: down-regulation, aberrant nuclear expression, and CTNNB1 exon 3 mutations are markers for aggressive tumor phenotypes and poor prognosis. Am J Pathol 158: 987-996.
690. Garcia-Rostan G, Tallini G, Herrero A, D'Aquila TG, Carcangiu ML, Rimm DL (1999). Frequent mutation and nuclear localization of beta-catenin in anaplastic thyroid carcinoma. Cancer Res 59: 1811-1815.
691. Garcia-Rostan G, Zhao H, Camp RL, Pollan M, Herrero A, Pardo J, Wu R, Carcangiu ML, Costa J, Tallini G (2003). Ras mutations are associated with aggressive tumor phenotypes and poor prognosis in thyroid cancer. J Clin Oncol 21: 3226-3235.
692. Gardner DF, Barlascini COJr, Downs RWJr, Sahni KS (1989). Cushing's disease in two sisters. Am J Med Sci 297: 387-389.
693. Gasque CR, Marti-Bonmati L, Dosda R, Martinez AG (1999). MR imaging of a case of adenomatoid tumor of the adrenal gland. Eur Radiol 9: 552-554.
694. Geelhoed GW (1982). Parathyroid adenolipoma: clinical and morphologic features. Surgery 92: 806-810.
695. Geisinger KR, Steffee CH, McGee RS, Woodruff RD, Buss DH (1998). The cytomorphologic features of sclerosing mucoepidermoid carcinoma of the thyroid gland with eosinophilia. Am J Clin Pathol 109: 294-301.
696. Geller G, Botkin JR, Green MJ, Press N, Biesecker BB, Wilfond B, Grana G, Daly MB, Schneider K, Kahn MJ (1997). Genetic testing for susceptibility to adult-onset cancer. The process and content of informed consent. JAMA 277: 1467-1474.
697. Gentile S, Rainero I, Savi L, Rivoiro C, Pinessi L (2001). Brain metastasis from pheochromocytoma in a patient with multiple endocrine neoplasia type 2A. Panminerva Med 43: 305-306.
698. George E, Swanson PE, Wick MR (1989). Malignant peripheral nerve sheath tumors of the skin. Am J Dermatopathol 11: 213-221.
699. Germain-Lee EL, Ding CL, Deng Z, Crane JL, Saji M, Ringel MD, Levine MA (2002). Paternal imprinting of Galpha(s) in the human thyroid as the basis of TSH resistance in pseudohypoparathyroidism type 1a. Biochem Biophys Res Commun 296: 67-72.
700. Gersell DJ, King TC (1988). Papillary cystadenoma of the mesosalpinx in von Hippel-Lindau disease. Am J Surg Pathol 12: 145-149.
701. Gharib H, Goellner JR, Johnson DA (1993). Fine-needle aspiration cytology of the thyroid. A 12-year experience with 11,000 biopsies. Clin Lab Med 13: 699-709.
702. Ghazanfar S, Quraishy MS, Essa K, Muzaffar S, Saeed MU, Sultan T (2002). Mucosa associated lymphoid tissue lymphoma (Maltoma) in patients with cold nodule thyroid. J Pak Med Assoc 52: 131-133.
703. Gherardi G (1987). Signet ring cell 'mucinous' thyroid adenoma: a follicle cell tumour with abnormal accumulation of thyroglobulin and a peculiar histochemical profile. Histopathology 11: 317-326.
704. Giannini C, Scheithauer BW, Hellbusch LC, Rasmussen AG, Fox MW, McCormick SR, Davis DH (1998). Peripheral nerve hemangioblastoma. Mod Pathol 11: 999-1004.
705. Giardiello FM, Krush AJ, Petersen GM, Booker SV, Kerr M, Tong LL, Hamilton SR (1994). Phenotypic variability of familial adenomatous polyposis in 11 unrelated families with identical APC gene mutation. Gastroenterology 106: 1542-1547.
706. Giardiello FM, Offerhaus GJ, Lee DH, Krush AJ, Tersmette AC, Booker SV, Kelley NC, Hamilton SR (1993). Increased risk of thyroid and pancreatic carcinoma in familial adenomatous polyposis. Gut 34: 1394-1396.
707. Gibbs MK, Carney JA, Hayles AB, Telander RL (1977). Simultaneous adrenal and cervical pheochromocytomas in childhood. Ann Surg 185: 273-278.
708. Gibril F, Chen YJ, Schrump DS, Vortmeyer A, Zhuang Z, Lubensky IA, Reynolds JC, Louie A, Entsuah LK, Huang K, Asgharian B, Jensen RT (2003). Prospective study of thymic carcinoids in patients with multiple endocrine neoplasia type 1. J Clin Endocrinol Metab 88: 1066-1081.
709. Gibril F, Curtis LT, Termanini B, Fritsch MK, Lubensky IA, Doppman JL, Jensen RT (1997). Primary cardiac gastrinoma causing Zollinger-Ellison syndrome. Gastroenterology 112: 567-574.
710. Gibril F, Venzon DJ, Ojeaburu JV, Bashir S, Jensen RT (2001). Prospective study of the natural history of gastrinoma in patients with MEN1: definition of an aggressive and a nonaggressive form. J Clin Endocrinol Metab 86: 5282-5293.
711. Gicquel C, Bertagna X, Gaston V, Coste J, Louvel A, Baudin E, Bertherat J, Chapuis Y, Duclos JM, Schlumberger M, Plouin PF, Luton JP, Le Bouc Y (2001). Molecular markers and long-term recurrences in a large cohort of patients with sporadic adrenocortical tumors. Cancer Res 61: 6762-6767.
712. Gicquel C, Bertagna X, Schneid H, Francillard-Leblond M, Luton JP, Girard F, Le Bouc Y (1994). Rearrangements at the 11p15 locus and overexpression of insulin-like growth factor-II gene in sporadic adrenocortical tumors. J Clin Endocrinol Metab 78: 1444-1453.
713. Gicquel C, Raffin-Sanson ML, Gaston V, Bertagna X, Plouin PF, Schlumberger M, Louvel A, Luton JP, Le Bouc Y (1997). Structural and functional abnormalities at 11p15 are associated with the malignant phenotype in sporadic adrenocortical tumors: study on a series of 82 tumors. J Clin Endocrinol Metab 82: 2559-2565.
714. Giercksky KE, Halse J, Mathisen W, Gjone E, Flatmark A (1980). Endocrine tumors of the pancreas. Scand J Gastroenterol 15: 129-135.
715. Gimenez-Roqueplo AP, Favier J, Rustin P, Mourad JJ, Plouin PF, Corvol P, Rotig A, Jeunemaitre X (2001). The R22X mutation of the SDHD gene in hereditary paraganglioma abolishes the enzymatic activity of complex II in the mitochondrial respiratory chain and activates the hypoxia pathway. Am J Hum Genet 69: 1186-1197.
716. Gimm O (2001). Multiple endocrine neoplasia type 2: clinical aspects. Front Horm Res 28: 103-130.
717. Gimm O, Armanios M, Dziema H, Neumann HP, Eng C (2000). Somatic and occult germ-line mutations in SDHD, a mitochondrial complex II gene, in nonfamilial pheochromocytoma. Cancer Res 60: 6822-6825.
718. Gimm O, Marsh DJ, Andrew SD, Frilling A, Dahia PL, Mulligan LM, Zajac JD, Robinson BG, Eng C (1997). Germline dinucleotide mutation in codon 883 of the RET proto-oncogene in multiple endocrine neoplasia type 2B without codon 918 mutation. J Clin Endocrinol Metab 82: 3902-3904.
719. Gimm O, Niederle BE, Weber T, Bockhorn M, Ukkat J, Brauckhoff M, Thanh PN, Frilling A, Klar E, Niederle B, Dralle H (2002). RET proto-oncogene mutations affecting codon 790/791: A mild form of multiple endocrine neoplasia type 2A syndrome? Surgery 132: 952-959.
720. Gimm O, Perren A, Weng LP, Marsh DJ, Yeh JJ, Ziebold U, Gil E, Hinze R, Delbridge L, Lees JA, Mutter GL, Robinson BG, Komminoth P, Dralle H, Eng C (2000). Differential nuclear and cytoplasmic expression of PTEN in normal thyroid tissue, and benign and malignant epithelial thyroid tumors. Am J Pathol 156: 1693-1700.
721. Giordano TJ, Thomas DG, Kuick R, Lizyness M, Misek DE, Smith AL, Sanders D, Aljundi RT, Gauger PG, Thompson NW, Taylor JM, Hanash SM (2003). Distinct transcriptional profiles of adrenocortical tumors uncovered by DNA microarray analysis. Am J Pathol 162: 521-531.
722. Giovannelli G, Bernasconi S, Banchini G (1978). McCune-Albright syndrome in a male child: a clinical and endocrinologic enigma. J Pediatr 92: 220-226.
723. Giraud S, Choplin H, Teh BT, Lespinasse J, Jouvet A, Labat-Moleur F, Lenoir G, Hamon B, Hamon P, Calender A (1997). A large multiple endocrine neoplasia type 1 family with clinical expression suggestive of anticipation. J Clin Endocrinol Metab 82: 3487-3492.
724. Girelli ME, Dotto S, Nacamulli D, Piccolo M, De Vido D, Russo T, Bernante P, Pelizzo MR, Busnardo B (1994). Prognostic value of early postoperative calcitonin level in medullary thyroid carcinoma. Tumori 80: 113-117.
725. Giuffrida D, Gharib H (2000). Anaplastic thyroid carcinoma: current diagnosis and treatment. Ann Oncol 11: 1083-1089.
726. Giuffrida D, Gharib H (2001). Cardiac metastasis from primary anaplastic thyroid carcinoma: report of three cases and a review of the literature. Endocr Relat Cancer 8: 71-73.
727. Glatz K, Wegmann W (2000). Papillary adenomatoid tumour of the adrenal gland. Histopathology 37: 376-377.
728. Glenner GG, Grimley PM (1974). Tumors of the Extra-Adrenal Paraganglion System (including Chemoreceptors). 2nd ed. Armed Forces Institute of Pathology: Washington, DC.
729. Glickman MH, Hart MJ, White TT (1980). Insulinoma in Seattle: 39 cases in 30 years. Am J Surg 140: 119-125.
730. Glomset DA (1938). The incidence of metastasis of malignant tumors to the adrenals. Am J Cancer 32: 57-61.
731. Gnarra JR, Zhou S, Merrill MJ, Wagner JR, Krumm A, Papavassiliou E, Oldfield EH, Klausner RD, Linehan WM (1996). Post-transcriptional regulation of vascular endothelial growth factor mRNA by the product of the VHL tumor suppressor

gene. Proc Natl Acad Sci U S A 93: 10589-10594.
732. Gober GA, Nicholas RW (1993). Case report 800: Skeletal fibrous dysplasia associated with intramuscular myxoma (Mazabraud's syndrome). Skeletal Radiol 22: 452-455.
733. Gobl AE, Berg M, Lopez-Egido JR, Oberg K, Skogseid B, Westin G (1999). Menin represses JunD-activated transcription by a histone deacetylase-dependent mechanism. Biochim Biophys Acta 1447: 51-56.
734. Goebel SU, Heppner C, Burns AL, Marx SJ, Spiegel AM, Zhuang Z, Lubensky IA, Gibril F, Jensen RT, Serrano J (2000). Genotype/phenotype correlation of multiple endocrine neoplasia type 1 gene mutations in sporadic gastrinomas. J Clin Endocrinol Metab 85: 116-123.
735. Goebel SU, Iwamoto M, Raffeld M, Gibril F, Hou W, Serrano J, Jensen RT (2002). Her-2/neu expression and gene amplification in gastrinomas: correlations with tumor biology, growth, and aggressiveness. Cancer Res 62: 3702-3710.
736. Gokalp HZ, Arasil E, Kanpolat Y, Balim T (1993). Meningiomas of the tuberculum sella. Neurosurg Rev 16: 111-114.
737. Goldfarb DA, Neumann HP, Penn I, Novick AC (1997). Results of renal transplantation in patients with renal cell carcinoma and von Hippel-Lindau disease. Transplantation 64: 1726-1729.
738. Goldgar DE, Easton DF, Cannon-Albright LA, Skolnick MH (1994). Systematic population-based assessment of cancer risk in first-degree relatives of cancer probands. J Natl Cancer Inst 86: 1600-1608.
739. Goldman RL (1961). Primary squamous cell carcinoma of the thyroid gland: a report of a case and a reveiw of the literature. Am Surg 30: 247-251.
740. Goldstein N, Layfield LJ (1991). Thyromegaly secondary to simultaneous papillary carcinoma and histiocytosis X. Report of a case and review of the literature. Acta Cytol 35: 422-426.
741. Golouh R, Us-Krasovec M, Auersperg M, Jancar J, Bondi A, Eusebi V (1985). Amphicrine—composite calcitonin and mucin-producing—carcinoma of the thyroid. Ultrastruct Pathol 8: 197-206.
742. Gomez JM, Biarnes J, Volpini V, Marti T (1998). Neuromas and prominent corneal nerves without MEN 2B. Ann Endocrinol (Paris) 59: 492-494.
743. Gonsky R, Herman V, Melmed S, Fagin J (1991). Transforming DNA sequences present in human prolactin-secreting pituitary tumors. Mol Endocrinol 5: 1687-1695.
744. Gonzalez-Campora R, Diaz-Cano S, Lerma-Puertas E, Rios Martin JJ, Salguero Villadiego M, Villar Rodriguez JL, Bibbo M, Davidson HG (1993). Paragangliomas. Static cytometric studies of nuclear DNA patterns. Cancer 71: 820-824.
745. Gonzalez-Campora R, Lopez-Garrido J, Martin-Lacave I, Miralles-Sanchez EJ, Villar JL (1992). Concurrence of a symptomatic encapsulated follicular carcinoma, an occult papillary carcinoma and a medullary carcinoma in the same patient. Histopathology 21: 380-382.
746. Gordon C, Majzoub JA, Marsh DJ, Mulliken JB, Ponder BA, Robinson BG, Eng C (1998). Four cases of mucosal neuroma syndrome: multiple endocrine neoplasm 2B or not 2B? J Clin Endocrinol Metab 83: 17-20.
747. Gordon DL, Lo MC, Schwartz MA (1971). Carcinoid of the pancreas. Am J Med 51: 412-415.
748. Gorelov VN, Dumon K, Barteneva NS, Palm D, Roher HD, Goretzki PE (1995). Overexpression of Gs alpha subunit in thyroid tumors bearing a mutated Gs alpha gene. J Cancer Res Clin Oncol 121: 219-224.
749. Goren E, Bensal D, Reif RM, Eidelman A (1986). Cavernous hemangioma of the adrenal gland. J Urol 135: 341-342.
750. Gortz B, Roth J, Krahenmann A, de Krijger RR, Muletta-Feurer S, Rutimann K, Saremaslani P, Speel EJ, Heitz PU, Komminoth P (1999). Mutations and allelic deletions of the MEN1 gene are associated with a subset of sporadic endocrine pancreatic and neuroendocrine tumors and not restricted to foregut neoplasms. Am J Pathol 154: 429-436.
751. Gosset P, Lecomte-Houcke M, Duhamel A, Labat-Moleur F, Patey M, Floquet J, Viennet G, Berger-Dutrieux N, Caillou B, Franc B (1999). [112 cases of sporadic and genetically determined pheochromocytoma: a comparative pathologic study]. Ann Pathol 19: 480-486.
752. Gossner W, Korting GW (1960). A case of pemphigus foliaceus with renal diabetes and alpha-cell islet carcinoma. Dtsch Med Wochenschr 85: 434-437.
753. Gotchall J, Traweek ST, Stenzel P (1987). Benign oncocytic endocrine tumor of the pancreas in a patient with polyarteritis nodosa. Hum Pathol 18: 967-969.
754. Gottfredsson M, Oury TD, Bernstein C, Carpenter C, Bartlett JA (1996). Lymphoma of the pituitary gland: an unusual presentation of central nervous system lymphoma in AIDS. Am J Med 101: 563-564.
755. Gottschalk D, Fehm M, Patt S, Saeger W, Kirchner T, Aigner T (2001). Matrix gene expression analysis and cellular phenotyping in chordoma reveals focal differentiation pattern of neoplastic cells mimicking nucleus pulposus development. Am J Pathol 158: 1571-1578.
756. Grabias SL, Campbell CJ (1977). Fibrous dysplasia. Orthop Clin North Am 8: 771-783.
757. Grama D, Skogseid B, Wilander E, Eriksson B, Martensson H, Cedermark B, Ahren B, Kristofferson A, Oberg K, Rastad J, Akerstrom G (1992). Pancreatic tumors in multiple endocrine neoplasia type 1: clinical presentation and surgical treatment. World J Surg 16: 611-618.
758. Granberg D, Stridsberg M, Seensalu R, Eriksson B, Lundqvist G, Oberg K, Skogseid B (1999). Plasma chromogranin A in patients with multiple endocrine neoplasia type 1. J Clin Endocrinol Metab 84: 2712-2717.
759. Grant CS (2003). Minimal access parathyroidectomy. In: Surgery of the Thyroid and Parathyroid Glands, Randolph GW, ed., Saunders: Philadelphia , pp. 549-556.
760. Granter SR, DiNisco S, Granados R (1995). Cytologic diagnosis of papillary cystic neoplasm of the pancreas. Diagn Cytopathol 12: 313-319.
761. Graziani N, Dufour H, Figarella-Branger D, Bouillot P, Grisoli F (1995). Suprasellar granular-cell tumour, presenting with intraventricular haemorrhage. Br J Neurosurg 9: 97-102.
762. Grebe SK, Hay ID (1995). Follicular thyroid cancer. Endocrinol Metab Clin North Am 24: 761-801.
763. Grebe SK, Hay ID (1997). Follicular cell-derived thyroid carcinomas. Cancer Treat Res 89: 91-140.
764. Grebe SK, McIver B, Hay ID, Wu PS, Maciel LM, Drabkin HA, Goellner JR, Grant CS, Jenkins RB, Eberhardt NL (1997). Frequent loss of heterozygosity on chromosomes 3p and 17p without VHL or p53 mutations suggests involvement of unidentified tumor suppressor genes in follicular thyroid carcinoma. J Clin Endocrinol Metab 82: 3684-3691.
765. Greco A, Mariani C, Miranda C, Lupas A, Pagliardini S, Pomati M, Pierotti MA (1995). The DNA rearrangement that generates the TRK-T3 oncogene involves a novel gene on chromosome 3 whose product has a potential coiled-coil domain. Mol Cell Biol 15: 6118-6127.
766. Greco A, Pierotti MA, Bongarzone I, Pagliardini S, Lanzi C, Della Porta G (1992). TRK-T1 is a novel oncogene formed by the fusion of TPR and TRK genes in human papillary thyroid carcinomas. Oncogene 7: 237-242.
767. Greco MA, Steiner GC (1986). Ultrastructure of fibrous dysplasia of bone: a study of its fibrous, osseous, and cartilaginous components. Ultrastruct Pathol 10: 55-66.
768. Green BT, Rockey DC (2001). Duodenal somatostatinoma presenting with complete somatostatinoma syndrome. J Clin Gastroenterol 33: 415-417.
769. Greene LF, Page DL, Fritz A, Batch M, Haller DG, Morrow M (2002). American Joint Committee on Cancer (AJCC). Cancer Staging Manual. 6th Edition.
770. Gregory PE, Gutmann DH, Mitchell A, Park S, Boguski M, Jacks T, Wood DL, Jove R, Collins FS (1993). Neurofibromatosis type 1 gene product (neurofibromin) associates with microtubules. Somat Cell Mol Genet 19: 265-274.
771. Gregory RA, Tracy HJ, French JM, Sircus W (1960). Extraction of a gastrin-like substance from a pancreatic tumor in a case of Zollinger-Ellison syndrome. Lancet 1: 1045-1048.
772. Greider MH, Elliott DW (1964). Electron microscopy of human pancreatic tumors of islet cell origin. Am J Pathol 44: 663-678.
773. Greider MH, Rosai J, McGuigan JE (1974). The human pancreatic islet cells and their tumors. II. Ulcerogenic and diarrheogenic tumors. Cancer 33: 1423-1443.
774. Grieco M, Santoro M, Berlingieri MT, Melillo RM, Donghi R, Bongarzone I, Pierotti MA, Della Porta G, Fusco A, Vecchio G (1990). PTC is a novel rearranged form of the ret proto-oncogene and is frequently detected in vivo in human thyroid papillary carcinomas. Cell 60: 557-563.
775. Griesser J, Kaufmann D, Maier B, Mailhammer R, Kuehl P, Krone W (1997). Post-transcriptional regulation of neurofibromin level in cultured human melanocytes in response to growth factors. J Invest Dermatol 108: 275-280.
776. Griffiths DF, Jasani B, Newman GR, Williams ED, Williams GT (1984). Glandular duodenal carcinoid—a somatostatin rich tumour with neuroendocrine associations. J Clin Pathol 37: 163-169.
777. Griffiths DF, Williams GT, Williams ED (1987). Duodenal carcinoid tumours, phaeochromocytoma and neurofibromatosis: islet cell tumour, phaeochromocytoma and the von Hippel-Lindau complex: two distinctive neuroendocrine syndromes. Q J Med 64: 769-782.
778. Griffiths PD, Blaser S, Mukonoweshuro W, Armstrong D, Milo-Mason G, Cheung S (1999). Neurofibromatosis bright objects in children with neurofibromatosis type 1: a proliferative potential? Pediatrics 104: e49.
779. Grimelius L, Hultquist GT, Stenkvist B (1975). Cytological differentiation of asymptomatic pancreatic islet cell tumours in autopsy material. Virchows Arch A Pathol Anat Histol 365: 275-288.
780. Grimelius L, Johansson H, Lindquist B (1972). A case of unusual stromal development in a parathyroid adenoma. Acta Chir Scand 138: 628-629.
781. Grosfeld FJM, Lips CJM, Beemer FA, ten Kroode HF (2000). Psychological distress in genetic testing programs for hereditary cancer disorders. J Genet Counseling 9: 253-466.
782. Grosfeld JL, Ballantine TV, Lowe D, Baehner RL (1976). Benign and malignant teratomas in children: analysis of 85 patients. Surgery 80: 297-305.
783. Grossman RF, Tu SH, Duh QY, Siperstein AE, Novosolov F, Clark OH (1995). Familial nonmedullary thyroid cancer. An emerging entity that warrants aggressive treatment. Arch Surg 130: 892-897.
784. Groussin L, Jullian E, Perlemoine K, Louvel A, Leheup B, Luton JP, Bertagna X, Bertherat J (2002). Mutations of the PRKAR1A gene in Cushing's syndrome due to sporadic primary pigmented nodular adrenocortical disease. J Clin Endocrinol Metab 87: 4324-4329.
785. Groussin L, Kirschner LS, Vincent-Dejean C, Perlemoine K, Jullian E, Delemer B, Zacharieva S, Pignatelli D, Carney JA, Luton JP, Bertagna X, Stratakis CA, Bertherat J (2002). Molecular analysis of the cyclic AMP-dependent protein kinase A (PKA) regulatory subunit 1A (PRKAR1A) gene in patients with Carney complex and primary pigmented nodular adrenocortical disease (PPNAD) reveals novel mutations and clues for pathophysiology: augmented PKA signaling is associated with adrenal tumorigenesis in PPNAD. Am J Hum Genet 71: 1433-1442.
786. Guillamo JS, Creange A, Kalifa C, Grill J, Rodriguez D, Doz F, Barbarot S, Zerah M, Sanson M, Bastuji-Garin S, Wolkenstein P (2003). Prognostic factors of CNS tumours in Neurofibromatosis 1 (NF1): a retrospective study of 104 patients. Brain 126: 152-160.
787. Guiter GE, Auger M, Ali SZ, Allen EA, Zakowski MF (1999). Cytopathology of insular carcinoma of the thyroid. Cancer 87: 196-202.
788. Gumbs AA, Moore PS, Falconi M, Bassi C, Beghelli S, Modlin I, Scarpa A (2002). Review of the clinical, histological, and molecular aspects of pancreatic endocrine neoplasms. J Surg Oncol 81: 45-53.
789. Gupta A, Horattas MC, Moattari AR, Shorten SD (2001). Disseminated brown tumors from hyperparathyroidism masquerading as metastatic cancer: a complication of parathyroid carcinoma. Am Surg 67: 951-955.
790. Gupta D, Shidham V, Holden J, Layfield L (2000). Prognostic value of immunohistochemical expression of topoisomerase alpha II, MIB-1, p53, E-cadherin, retinoblastoma gene protein product, and HER-2/neu in adrenal and extra-adrenal pheochromocytomas. Appl Immunohistochem Mol Morphol 8: 267-274.
791. Guru SC, Goldsmith PK, Burns AL,

Marx SJ, Spiegel AM, Collins FS, Chandrasekharappa SC (1998). Menin, the product of the MEN1 gene, is a nuclear protein. Proc Natl Acad Sci U S A 95: 1630-1634.

792. Guru SC, Prasad NB, Shin EJ, Hemavathy K, Lu J, Ip YT, Agarwal SK, Marx SJ, Spiegel AM, Collins FS, Oliver B, Chandrasekharappa SC (2001). Characterization of a MEN1 ortholog from Drosophila melanogaster. Gene 263: 31-38.

793. Gustafson LM, Liu JH, Rutter MJ, Stern Y, Cotton RT (2001). Primary neurilemoma of the thyroid gland: a case report. Am J Otolaryngol 22: 84-86.

794. Gutmann DH, Aylsworth A, Carey JC, Korf B, Marks J, Pyeritz RE, Rubenstein A, Viskochil D (1997). The diagnostic evaluation and multidisciplinary management of neurofibromatosis 1 and neurofibromatosis 2. JAMA 278: 51-57.

795. Gutmann DH, Geist RT, Rose K, Wallin G, Moley JF (1995). Loss of neurofibromatosis type I (NF1) gene expression in pheochromocytomas from patients without NF1. Genes Chromosomes Cancer 13: 104-109.

796. Guyetant S, Dupre F, Bigorgne JC, Franc B, Dutrieux-Berger N, Lecomte-Houcke M, Patey M, Caillou B, Viennet G, Guerin O, Saint-Andre JP (1999). Medullary thyroid microcarcinoma: a clinicopathologic retrospective study of 38 patients with no prior familial disease. Hum Pathol 30: 957-963.

797. Guyetant S, Wion-Barbot N, Rousselet MC, Franc B, Bigorgne JC, Saint-Andre JP (1994). C-cell hyperplasia associated with chronic lymphocytic thyroiditis: a retrospective quantitative study of 112 cases. Hum Pathol 25: 514-521.

798. Haddad G, Penabad JL, Bashey HM, Asa SL, Gennarelli TA, Cirullo R, Snyder PJ (1994). Expression of activin/inhibin subunit messenger ribonucleic acids by gonadotroph adenomas. J Clin Endocrinol Metab 79: 1399-1403.

799. Hage C, Willman CL, Favara BE, Isaacson PG (1993). Langerhans' cell histiocytosis (histiocytosis X): immunophenotype and growth fraction. Hum Pathol 24: 840-845.

800. Haigh PI, Ituarte PH, Wu HS, Treseler PA, Posner MD, Quivey JM, Duh QY, Clark OH (2001). Completely resected anaplastic thyroid carcinoma combined with adjuvant chemotherapy and irradiation is associated with prolonged survival. Cancer 91: 2335-2342.

801. Hakaim AG, Esselstyn CBJr (1993). Parathyroid carcinoma: 50-year experience at The Cleveland Clinic Foundation. Cleve Clin J Med 60: 331-335.

802. Halachmi N, Halachmi S, Evron E, Cairns P, Okami K, Saji M, Westra WH, Zeiger MA, Jen J, Sidransky D (1998). Somatic mutations of the PTEN tumor suppressor gene in sporadic follicular thyroid tumors. Genes Chromosomes Cancer 23: 239-243.

803. Hales M, Rosenau W, Okerlund MD, Galante M (1982). Carcinoma of the thyroid with a mixed medullary and follicular pattern: morphologic, immunohistochemical, and clinical laboratory studies. Cancer 50: 1352-1359.

804. Hall WA, Luciano MG, Doppman JL, Patronas NJ, Oldfield EH (1994). Pituitary magnetic resonance imaging in normal human volunteers: occult adenomas in the general population. Ann Intern Med 120: 817-820.

805. Hameed A, Coleman RL (2000). Fine-needle aspiration cytology of primary granulosa cell tumor of the adrenal gland: A case report. Diagn Cytopathol 22: 1107-1109.

806. Hamid QA, Bishop AE, Sikri KL, Varndell IM, Bloom SR, Polak JM (1986). Immunocytochemical characterization of 10 pancreatic tumours, associated with the glucagonoma syndrome, using antibodies to separate regions of the pro-glucagon molecule and other neuroendocrine markers. Histopathology 10: 119-133.

807. Hamill J, Maoate K, Beasley SW, Corbett R, Evans J (2002). Familial parathyroid carcinoma in a child. J Paediatr Child Health 38: 314-317.

808. Hamilton I, Reis L, Bilimoria S, Long RG (1980). A renal vipoma. Br Med J 281: 1323-1324.

809. Hammami MM, al Zahrani A, Butt A, Vencer LJ, Hussain SS (1997). Primary hyperparathyroidism-associated polyostotic fibrous dysplasia: absence of McCune-Albright syndrome mutations. J Endocrinol Invest 20: 552-558.

810. Hammel P, Beigelman C, Chauveau D, Resche F, Bougerolles E, Flejou JF, Bernades P, Delchier JC, Richard S (1995). [Variety of pancreatic lesions observed in von Hippel-Lindau disease. Apropos of 8 cases]. Gastroenterol Clin Biol 19: 1011-1017.

811. Hammel PR, Vilgrain V, Terris B, Penfornis A, Sauvanet A, Correas JM, Chauveau D, Balian A, Beigelman C, O'Toole D, Bernades P, Ruszniewski P, Richard S (2000). Pancreatic involvement in von Hippel-Lindau disease. The Groupe Francophone d'Etude de la Maladie de von Hippel-Lindau. Gastroenterology 119: 1087-1095.

812. Hammond EH, Yowell RL, Flinner RL (1998). Neuroendocrine carcinomas: role of immunocytochemistry and electron microscopy. Hum Pathol 29: 1367-1371.

813. Hamy A, Heymann MF, Bodic J, Visset J, Le Borgne J, Leneel JC, Le Bodic MF (2001). [Duodenal somatostatinoma. Anatomic/clinical study of 12 operated cases]. Ann Chir 126: 221-226.

814. Han SS, Cooper DN, Upadhyaya MN (2001). Evaluation of denaturing high performance liquid chromatography (DHPLC) for the mutational analysis of the neurofibromatosis type 1 (NF1) gene. Hum Genet 109: 487-497.

815. Hanahan D (1985). Heritable formation of pancreatic beta-cell tumours in transgenic mice expressing recombinant insulin/simian virus 40 oncogenes. Nature 315: 115-122.

816. Hansen WJ, Ohh M, Moslehi J, Kondo K, Kaelin WG, Welch WJ (2002). Diverse effects of mutations in exon II of the von Hippel-Lindau (VHL) tumor suppressor gene on the interaction of pVHL with the cytosolic chaperonin and pVHL-dependent ubiquitin ligase activity. Mol Cell Biol 22: 1947-1960.

817. Hansford JR, Mulligan LM (2000). Multiple endocrine neoplasia type 2 and RET: from neoplasia to neurogenesis. J Med Genet 37: 817-827.

818. Happle R (1986). The McCune-Albright syndrome: a lethal gene surviving by mosaicism. Clin Genet 29: 321-324.

819. Hara H, Fulton N, Yashiro T, Ito K, DeGroot LJ, Kaplan EL (1994). N-ras mutation: an independent prognostic factor for aggressiveness of papillary thyroid carcinoma. Surgery 116: 1010-1016.

820. Harach HR (1988). Solid cell nests of the thyroid. J Pathol 155: 191-200.

821. Harach HR (1991). Thyroglobulin in human thyroid follicles with acid mucin. J Pathol 164: 261-263.

822. Harach HR, Bergholm U (1988). Medullary (C cell) carcinoma of the thyroid with features of follicular oxyphilic cell tumours. Histopathology 13: 645-656.

823. Harach HR, Bergholm U (1992). Small cell variant of medullary carcinoma of the thyroid with neuroblastoma-like features. Histopathology 21: 378-380.

824. Harach HR, Bergholm U (1993). Medullary carcinoma of the thyroid with carcinoid-like features. J Clin Pathol 46: 113-117.

825. Harach HR, Escalante DA, Day ES (2002). Thyroid cancer and thyroiditis in salta, Argentina: a 40-yr study in relation to iodine prophylaxis. Endocr Pathol 13: 175-181.

826. Harach HR, Franssila KO, Wasenius VM (1985). Occult papillary carcinoma of the thyroid. A "normal" finding in Finland. A systematic autopsy study. Cancer 56: 531-538.

827. Harach HR, Lesueur F, Amati P, Brown A, Canzian F, Kraimps JL, Levillain P, Menet E, Romeo G, Bonneau D (1999). Histology of familial thyroid tumours linked to a gene mapping to chromosome 19p13.2. J Pathol 189: 387-393.

828. Harach HR, Saravia Day E, Franssila KO (1985). Thyroid spindle-cell tumor with mucous cysts. An intrathyroid thymoma? Am J Surg Pathol 9: 525-530.

829. Harach HR, Williams ED (1983). Glandular (tubular and follicular) variants of medullary carcinoma of the thyroid. Histopathology 7: 83-97.

830. Harach HR, Williams GT, Williams ED (1994). Familial adenomatous polyposis associated thyroid carcinoma: a distinct type of follicular cell neoplasm. Histopathology 25: 549-561.

831. Harada K, Arita K, Kurisu K, Tahara H (2000). Telomerase activity and the expression of telomerase components in pituitary adenoma with malignant transformation. Surg Neurol 53: 267-274.

832. Harada K, Nishizaki T, Ozaki S, Kubota H, Harada K, Okamura T, Ito H, Sasaki K (1999). Cytogenetic alterations in pituitary adenomas detected by comparative genomic hybridization. Cancer Genet Cytogenet 112: 38-41.

833. Hardy J, Vezina JL (1976). Transsphenoidal neurosurgery of intracranial neoplasm. Adv Neurol 15: 261-273.

834. Hargreaves HK, Wright TCJr (1981). A large functioning parathyroid lipoadenoma found in the posterior mediastinum. Am J Clin Pathol 76: 89-93.

835. Harrer P, Broecker M, Zint A, Schatz H, Zumtobel V, Derwahl M (1998). Thyroid nodules in recurrent multinodular goiters are predominantly polyclonal. J Endocrinol Invest 21: 380-385.

836. Harris S (1924). Hyperinsulinism and dysinsulinism. JAMA 83: 729-733.

837. Harris WH, Dudley HR, Barry RJ (1962). The natural history of fibrous dysplasia - an orthopaedic, pathological, and roentgenographic study. J Bone Joint Surg Am 44: 207-233.

838. Harrison LE, Gaudin PB, Brennan MF (1999). Pathologic features of prognostic significance for adrenocortical carcinoma after curative resection. Arch Surg 134: 181-185.

839. Harsh GR (2001). Chordomas and chondrosarcomas of the skull base. In: Brain Tumors: An Encyclopedic Approach , Kaye AH, Laws ERJr, eds., 2nd Edition ed. Churchill Livingstone: London , pp. 857-868.

840. Hartley L, Perry-Keene D (1985). Phaeochromocytoma in Queensland—1970-83. Aust N Z J Surg 55: 471-475.

841. Hartman WH (1978). Tumors of the Parathyroid Glands. 2nd ed. Armed Forces Institute of Pathology: Washington, DC.

842. Hashimoto K, Koga M, Motomura T, Kasayama S, Kouhara H, Ohnishi T, Arita N, Hayakawa T, Sato B, Kishimoto T (1995). Identification of alternatively spliced messenger ribonucleic acid encoding truncated growth hormone-releasing hormone receptor in human pituitary adenomas. J Clin Endocrinol Metab 80: 2933-2939.

843. Haslbeck KM, Eberhardt KE, Nissen U, Tomandl BF, Stefan H, Neundorfer B, Erbguth F (1999). Intracranial hypertension as a clinical manifestation of cauda equina paraganglioma. Neurology 52: 1297-1298.

844. Hatva E, Bohling T, Jaaskelainen J, Persico MG, Haltia M, Alitalo K (1996). Vascular growth factors and receptors in capillary hemangioblastomas and hemangiopericytomas. Am J Pathol 148: 763-775.

845. Haven CJ, Wong FK, van Dam EW, van der Juijt R, van Asperen C, Jansen J, Rosenberg C, de Wit M, Roijers J, Hoppener J, Lips CJ, Larsson C, Teh BT, Morreau H (2000). A genotypic and histopathological study of a large Dutch kindred with hyperparathyroidism-jaw tumor syndrome. J Clin Endocrinol Metab 85: 1449-1454.

846. Hayes WS, Davidson AJ, Grimley PM, Hartman DS (1990). Extraadrenal retroperitoneal paraganglioma: clinical, pathologic, and CT findings. AJR Am J Roentgenol 155: 1247-1250.

847. Hayward BE, Barlier A, Korbonits M, Grossman AB, Jacquet P, Enjalbert A, Bonthron DT (2001). Imprinting of the G(s)alpha gene GNAS1 in the pathogenesis of acromegaly. J Clin Invest 107: R31-R36.

848. Hayward BE, Kamiya M, Strain L, Moran V, Campbell R, Hayashizaki Y, Bonthron DT (1998). The human GNAS1 gene is imprinted and encodes distinct paternally and biallelically expressed G proteins. Proc Natl Acad Sci U S A 95: 10038-10043.

849. Hayward BE, Moran V, Strain L, Bonthron DT (1998). Bidirectional imprinting of a single gene: GNAS1 encodes maternally, paternally, and biallelically derived proteins. Proc Natl Acad Sci U S A 95: 15475-15480.

850. Hazard JB, Hawk WA, Crile GJr (1959). Medullary (solid) carcinoma of the thyroid; a clinicopathologic entity. J Clin Endocrinol Metab 19: 152-161.

851. Hazard JB, Kenyon R (1954). Atypical adenoma of the thyroid. Arch Pathol 58: 554-563.

852. Heaney AP, Fernando M, Yong WH, Melmed S (2002). Functional PPAR-gamma receptor is a novel therapeutic target for ACTH-secreting pituitary adenomas. Nat Med 8: 1281-1287.

853. Heaney AP, Melmed S (2000). New pituitary oncogenes. Endocr Relat Cancer 7: 3-15.

854. Heath HI, Hodgson SF, Kennedy MA (1980). Primary hyperparathyroidism. Incidence, morbidity, and potential economic impact in a community. N Engl J Med 302: 189-193.

855. Hedinger C (1981). Geographic pathology of thyroid diseases. Pathol Res

Pract 171: 285-292.
856. Hedinger CE, Williams ED, Sobin LH (1988). World Health Organization Histological Classification of Tumours. Histological Typing of Thyroid Tumours. 2nd ed. Springer Verlag: Berlin Heidelberg New York.
857. Heffess CS, Wenig BM, Thompson LD (2002). Metastatic renal cell carcinoma to the thyroid gland: a clinicopathologic study of 36 cases. Cancer 95: 1869-1878.
858. Heitz PU (1984). Pancreatic endocrine tumors. In: Pancreatic pathology, Kloppel G, Heitz PU, eds., Churchill Livingstone: Edinburgh/New York , pp. 206-232.
859. Heitz PU, Oberholzer M, Zenklusen HR, Kasper M, Reubi JC, Gudat F, Landolt AM, Staehli C (1988). Occurrence and pattern of cytokeratins in human pituitary adenomas. In: Advances in Pituitary Adenoma Research, Landolt AM, Girard J, Heitz PU, del Pozo E, Zapf J, eds., Pergamon Press: Oxford , pp. 27-37.
860. Held EL, Gal AA, DeRose PB, Cohen C (1997). Image cytometric nuclear DNA quantitation of paragangliomas in tissue sections. Prognostic significance. Anal Quant Cytol Histol 19: 501-506.
861. Hemmer S, Wasenius VM, Knuutila S, Franssila K, Joensuu H (1999). DNA copy number changes in thyroid carcinoma. Am J Pathol 154: 1539-1547.
862. Hemminki K, Dong C (2000). Familial relationships in thyroid cancer by histopathological type. Int J Cancer 85: 201-205.
863. Hemminki K, Li X (2003). Familial risk of cancer by site and histopathology. Int J Cancer 103: 105-109.
864. Hemminki K, Vaittinen P (1999). Familial cancers in a nationwide family cancer database: age distribution and prevalence. Eur J Cancer 35: 1109-1117.
865. Hendy GN, Arnold A (2002). Molecular basis of PTH overexpression. In: Principles of Bone Biology, Bilezikian JP, Raisz LG, Rodan GA, eds., 2nd ed. Academic Press: San Diego , pp. 1017-1030.
866. Henry I, Jeanpierre M, Couillin P, Barichard F, Serre JL, Journel H, Lamouroux A, Turleau C, de Grouchy J, Junien C (1989). Molecular definition of the 11p15.5 region involved in Beckwith-Wiedemann syndrome and probably in predisposition to adrenocortical carcinoma. Hum Genet 81: 273-277.
867. Henry JF, Sebag F, Iacobone M, Hubbard J, Maweja S (2002). [Lessons learned from 274 laparoscopic adrenalectomies]. Ann Chir 127: 512-519.
868. Heppner C, Bilimoria KY, Agarwal SK, Kester M, Whitty LJ, Guru SC, Chandrasekharappa SC, Collins FS, Spiegel AM, Marx SJ, Burns AL (2001). The tumor suppressor protein menin interacts with NF-kappaB proteins and inhibits NF-kappaB-mediated transactivation. Oncogene 20: 4917-4925.
869. Heppner C, Kester MB, Agarwal SK, Debelenko LV, Emmert-Buck MR, Guru SC, Manickam P, Olufemi SE, Skarulis MC, Doppman JL, Alexander RH, Kim YS, Saggar SK, Lubensky IA, Zhuang Z, Liotta LA, Chandrasekharappa SC, Collins FS, Spiegel AM, Burns AL, Marx SJ (1997). Somatic mutation of the MEN1 gene in parathyroid tumours. Nat Genet 16: 375-378.
870. Heppner C, Reincke M, Agarwal SK, Mora P, Allolio B, Burns AL, Spiegel AM, Marx SJ (1999). MEN1 gene analysis in sporadic adrenocortical neoplasms. J Clin Endocrinol Metab 84: 216-219.
871. Herfarth KK, Wick MR, Marshall HN, Gartner E, Lum S, Moley JF (1997). Absence of TP53 alterations in pheochromocytomas and medullary thyroid carcinomas. Genes Chromosomes Cancer 20: 24-29.
872. Hergovich A, Lisztwan J, Barry R, Ballschmieter P, Krek W (2003). Regulation of microtubule stability by the von Hippel-Lindau tumour suppressor protein pVHL. Nat Cell Biol 5: 64-70.
873. Herrera MF, Hay ID, Wu PS, Goellner JR, Ryan JJ, Ebersold JR, Bergstralh EJ, Grant CS (1992). Hurthle cell (oxyphilic) papillary thyroid carcinoma: a variant with more aggressive biologic behavior. World J Surg 16: 669-674.
874. Herrmann MA, Hay ID, Bartelt DHJr, Ritland SR, Dahl RJ, Grant CS, Jenkins RB (1991). Cytogenetic and molecular genetic studies of follicular and papillary thyroid cancers. J Clin Invest 88: 1596-1604.
875. Herrmann ME, Ciesla MC, Chejfec G, DeJong SA, Yong SL (2000). Primary nodal gastrinomas. Arch Pathol Lab Med 124: 832-835.
876. Herrmann ME, LiVolsi VA, Pasha TL, Roberts SA, Wojcik EM, Baloch ZW (2002). Immunohistochemical expression of galectin-3 in benign and malignant thyroid lesions. Arch Pathol Lab Med 126: 710-713.
877. Heshmati HM, Gharib H, van Heerden JA, Sizemore GW (1997). Advances and controversies in the diagnosis and management of medullary thyroid carcinoma. Am J Med 103: 60-69.
878. Heshmati HM, Scheithauer BW, Young WFJr (2002). Metastases to the pituitary gland. Endocrinologist 12: 45-49.
879. Hessman O, Lindberg D, Einarsson A, Lillhager P, Carling T, Grimelius L, Eriksson B, Akerstrom G, Westin G, Skogseid B (1999). Genetic alterations on 3p, 11q13, and 18q in nonfamilial and MEN 1-associated pancreatic endocrine tumors. Genes Chromosomes Cancer 26: 258-264.
880. Hessman O, Lindberg D, Skogseid B, Carling T, Hellman P, Rastad J, Akerstrom G, Westin G (1998). Mutation of the multiple endocrine neoplasia type 1 gene in nonfamilial, malignant tumors of the endocrine pancreas. Cancer Res 58: 377-379.
881. Heymann MF, Moreau A, Chetritt J, Murat A, Leborgne J, Le Neel JC, Visset J, Le Bodic MF (1996). [Pathologic study with immunohistochemistry of 61 pancreatic endocrine tumors in 16 patients suffering from multiple endocrine neoplasia type I (MEN I). Review of the literature]. Ann Pathol 16: 167-173.
882. Hibberts NA, Simpson DJ, Bicknell JE, Broome JC, Hoban PR, Clayton RN, Farrell WE (1999). Analysis of cyclin D1 (CCND1) allelic imbalance and overexpression in sporadic human pituitary tumors. Clin Cancer Res 5: 2133-2139.
883. Higgins GA, Recant L, Fischman AB (1979). The glucagonoma syndrome: surgically curable diabetes. Am J Surg 137: 142-148.
884. Higgins JP, Warnke RA (2000). Large B-cell lymphoma of thyroid. Two cases with a marginal zone distribution of the neoplastic cells. Am J Clin Pathol 114: 264-270.
885. Higuchi M, Tsuji M, Ikeda H (1997). Symptomatic hypophyseal granular cell tumour: endocrinological and clinicopathological analysis. Br J Neurosurg 11: 582-586.
886. Hill JH, Werkhaven JA, DeMay RM (1988). Hurthle cell variant of papillary carcinoma of the thyroid gland. Otolaryngol Head Neck Surg 98: 338-341.
887. Himelfarb MZ, Ostrzega NL, Samuel J, Shanon E (1983). Paraganglioma of the nasal cavity. Laryngoscope 93: 350-352.
888. Hinze R, Machens A, Schneider U, Holzhausen HJ, Dralle H, Rath FW (2000). Simultaneously occurring liver metastases of pheochromocytoma and medullary thyroid carcinoma—a diagnostic pitfall with clinical implications for patients with multiple endocrine neoplasia type 2a. Pathol Res Pract 196: 477-481.
889. Hirawake H, Taniwaki M, Tamura A, Amino H, Tomitsuka E, Kita K (1999). Characterization of the human SDHD gene encoding the small subunit of cytochrome b (cybS) in mitochondrial succinate-ubiquinone oxidoreductase. Biochim Biophys Acta 1412: 295-300.
890. Hirawake H, Taniwaki M, Tamura A, Kojima S, Kita K (1997). Cytochrome b in human complex II (succinate-ubiquinone oxidoreductase): cDNA cloning of the components in liver mitochondria and chromosome assignment of the genes for the large (SDHC) and small (SDHD) subunits to 1q21 and 11q23. Cytogenet Cell Genet 79: 132-138.
891. Hirokawa M, Carney JA (2000). Cell membrane and cytoplasmic staining for MIB-1 in hyalinizing trabecular adenoma of the thyroid gland. Am J Surg Pathol 24: 575-578.
892. Hirokawa M, Carney JA, Ohtsuki Y (2000). Hyalinizing trabecular adenoma and papillary carcinoma of the thyroid gland express different cytokeratin patterns. Am J Surg Pathol 24: 877-881.
893. Hirose T, Scheithauer BW, Sano T (1998). Perineurial malignant peripheral nerve sheath tumor (MPNST): a clinicopathologic, immunohistochemical, and ultrastructural study of seven cases. Am J Surg Pathol 22: 1368-1378.
894. Hirvonen O, Lakkakorpi J, Aaltonen V, Hirvonen H, Rossi M, Karvonen SL, Yla-Outinen H, Kalimo H, Peltonen J (1998). Developmental regulation of NF1 tumor suppressor gene in human peripheral nerve. J Neurocytol 27: 939-952.
895. Hjorth L, Thomsen LB, Nielsen VT (1986). Adenolipoma of the thyroid gland. Histopathology 10: 91-96.
896. Hoang MP, Hruban RH, Albores-Saavedra J (2001). Clear cell endocrine pancreatic tumor mimicking renal cell carcinoma: a distinctive neoplasm of von Hippel-Lindau disease. Am J Surg Pathol 25: 602-609.
897. Hobbs RD, Stewart AF, Ravin ND, Carter D (1984). Hypercalcemia in small cell carcinoma of the pancreas. Cancer 53: 1552-1554.
898. Hochstrasser H, Boltshauser E, Valavanis A (1988). Brain tumors in children with von Recklinghausen neurofibromatosis. Neurofibromatosis 1: 233-239.
899. Hochwald SN, Zee S, Conlon KC, Colleoni R, Louie O, Brennan MF, Klimstra DS (2002). Prognostic factors in pancreatic endocrine neoplasms: an analysis of 136 cases with a proposal for low-grade and intermediate-grade groups. J Clin Oncol 20: 2633-2642.
900. Hoegerle S, Nitzsche E, Altehoefer C, Ghanem N, Manz T, Brink I, Reincke M, Moser E, Neumann HP (2002). Pheochromocytomas: detection with 18F DOPA whole body PET—initial results. Radiology 222: 507-512.
901. Hoffman MA, Ohh M, Yang H, Klco JM, Ivan M, Kaelin WGJr (2001). von Hippel-Lindau protein mutants linked to type 2C VHL disease preserve the ability to downregulate HIF. Hum Mol Genet 10: 1019-1027.
902. Hoffman RW, Gardner DW, Mitchell FL (1982). Intrathoracic and multiple abdominal pheochromocytomas in von Hippel-Lindau disease. Arch Intern Med 142: 1962-1964.
903. Hofler H, Ruhri C, Putz B, Wirnsberger G, Hauser H (1988). Oncogene expression in endocrine pancreatic tumors. Virchows Arch B Cell Pathol Incl Mol Pathol 55: 355-361.
904. Hofman P, Mainguene C, Michiels JF, Pages A, Thyss A (1995). Thyroid spindle epithelial tumor with thymus-like differentiation (the "SETTLE" tumor). An immunohistochemical and electron microscopic study. Eur Arch Otorhinolaryngol 252: 316-320.
905. Hofstra RM, Fattoruso O, Quadro L, Wu Y, Libroia A, Verga U, Colantuoni V, Buys CH (1997). A novel point mutation in the intracellular domain of the ret protooncogene in a family with medullary thyroid carcinoma. J Clin Endocrinol Metab 82: 4176-4178.
906. Hofstra RM, Landsvater RM, Ceccherini I, Stulp RP, Stelwagen T, Luo Y, Pasini B, Hoppener JW, van Amstel HK, Romeo G, Lips CJM, Buys CH (1994). A mutation in the RET proto-oncogene associated with multiple endocrine neoplasia type 2B and sporadic medullary thyroid carcinoma. Nature 367: 375-376.
907. Hofstra RM, Stelwagen T, Stulp RP, de Jong D, Hulsbeek M, Kamsteeg EJ, van den Berg A, Landsvater RM, Vermey A, Molenaar WM, Lips CJ, Buys CH (1996). Extensive mutation scanning of RET in sporadic medullary thyroid carcinoma and of RET and VHL in sporadic pheochromocytoma reveals involvement of these genes in only a minority of cases. J Clin Endocrinol Metab 81: 2881-2884.
908. Holder CA, Elster AD (1997). Magnetization transfer imaging of the pituitary: further insights into the nature of the posterior "bright spot". J Comput Assist Tomogr 21: 171-174.
909. Holm R, Sobrinho-Simoes M, Nesland JM, Gould VE, Johannessen JV (1985). Medullary carcinoma of the thyroid gland: an immunocytochemical study. Ultrastruct Pathol 8: 25-41.
910. Holm R, Sobrinho-Simoes M, Nesland JM, Sambade C, Johannessen JV (1987). Medullary thyroid carcinoma with thyroglobulin immunoreactivity. A special entity? Lab Invest 57: 258-268.
911. Holmberg E, Wallgren A, Holm LE, Lundell M, Karlsson P (2002). Dose-response relationship for parathyroid adenoma after exposure to ionizing radiation in infancy. Radiat Res 158: 418-423.
912. Hoos A, Stojadinovic A, Singh B, Dudas ME, Leung DH, Shaha AR, Shah JP, Brennan MF, Cordon-Cardo C, Ghossein R (2002). Clinical significance of molecular expression profiles of Hurthle cell tumors of the thyroid gland analyzed via tissue microarrays. Am J Pathol 160: 175-183.
913. Horiguchi H, Sano T, Toi H, Kageji T, Hirokawa M, Nagahiro S (2001). Endolymphatic sac tumor associated with a von Hippel-Lindau disease patient: an immunohistochemical study. Mod Pathol 14: 727-732.
914. Horn RC (1951). Carcinoma of the

thyroid. Description of a distinctive morphological variant and report of 7 cases. Cancer 4: 697-707.
915. Horvath E, Kovacs K (1984). Gonadotroph adenomas of the human pituitary: sex-related fine-structural dichotomy. A histologic, immunocytochemical, and electron-microscopic study of 30 tumors. Am J Pathol 117: 429-440.
916. Horvath E, Kovacs K, Killinger DW, Smyth HS, Platts ME, Singer W (1980). Silent corticotropic adenomas of the human pituitary gland: a histologic, immunocytologic, and ultrastructural study. Am J Pathol 98: 617-638.
917. Horvath E, Kovacs K, Scheithauer BW, Lloyd RV, Smyth HS (1994). Pituitary adenoma with neuronal choristoma (PANCH): composite lesion or lineage infidelity? Ultrastruct Pathol 18: 565-574.
918. Horvath E, Kovacs K, Smyth HS, Killinger DW, Scheithauer BW, Randall R, Laws ERJr, Singer W (1988). A novel type of pituitary adenoma: morphological features and clinical correlations. J Clin Endocrinol Metab 66: 1111-1118.
919. Horvath E, Scheithauer BW, Kovacs K, Lloyd RV (2002). Hypothalamus and pituitary. In: Greenfield's Neuropathology, Graham DI, Lantos PL, eds., 7th ed. Edward Arnold: London , pp. 983-1062.
920. Horwitz CA, Myers WP, Foote FWJr (1972). Secondary malignant tumors of the parathyroid glands. Report of two cases with associated hypoparathyroidism. Am J Med 52: 797-808.
921. Hosaka N, Kitajiri S, Hiraumi H, Nogaki H, Toki J, Yang G, Hisha H, Ikehara S (2002). Ectopic pituitary adenoma with malignant transformation. Am J Surg Pathol 26: 1078-1082.
922. Hosokawa Y, Pollak MR, Brown EM, Arnold A (1995). Mutational analysis of the extracellular Ca(2+)-sensing receptor gene in human parathyroid tumors. J Clin Endocrinol Metab 80: 3107-3110.
923. Hough AJ, Hollifield JW, Page DL, Hartmann WH (1979). Prognostic factors in adrenal cortical tumors. A mathematical analysis of clinical and morphologic data. Am J Clin Pathol 72: 390-399.
924. Houlston RS, Stratton MR (1995). Genetics of non-medullary thyroid cancer. QJM 88: 685-693.
925. Howard TJ, Stabile BE, Zinner MJ, Chang S, Bhagavan BS, Passaro EJ (1990). Anatomic distribution of pancreatic endocrine tumors. Am J Surg 159: 258-264.
926. Howard TJ, Zinner MJ, Stabile BE, Passaro EJ (1990). Gastrinoma excision for cure. A prospective analysis. Ann Surg 211: 9-14.
927. Howell VM, Haven CJ, Kahnoski K, Khoo SK, Petillo D, Chen J, Fleuren GJ, Robinson BG, Delbridge LW, Philips J, Nelson AE, Krause U, Hammje K, Dralle H, Hoang-Vu C, Gimm O, Marsh DJ, Morreau H, Teh BT (2003). HRPT2 mutations are associated with malignancy in sporadic parathyroid tumours. J Med Genet 40: 657-663.
928. Howlett TA, Plowman PN, Wass JA, Rees LH, Jones AE, Besser GM (1989). Megavoltage pituitary irradiation in the management of Cushing's disease and Nelson's syndrome: long-term follow-up. Clin Endocrinol (Oxf) 31: 309-323.
929. Hoyt WF, Baghdassarian SA (1969). Optic glioma of childhood. Natural history and rationale for conservative management. Br J Ophthalmol 53: 793-798.
930. Hrafnkelsson J, Tulinius H, Jonasson JG, Olafsdottir G, Sigvaldason H (1989). Papillary thyroid carcinoma in Iceland. A study of the occurrence in families and the coexistence of other primary tumours. Acta Oncol 28: 785-788.
931. Hruban RH, Iacobuzio-Donahue C, Wilentz RE, Goggins M, Kern SE (2001). Molecular pathology of pancreatic cancer. Cancer J 7: 251-258.
932. Hsueh YP, Roberts AM, Volta M, Sheng M, Roberts RG (2001). Bipartite interaction between neurofibromatosis type I protein (neurofibromin) and syndecan transmembrane heparan sulfate proteoglycans. J Neurosci 21: 3764-3770.
933. Huang SC, Zhuang Z, Weil RJ, Pack S, Wang C, Krutzsch HC, Pham TA, Lubensky IA (1999). Nuclear/cytoplasmic localization of the multiple endocrine neoplasia type 1 gene product, menin. Lab Invest 79: 301-310.
934. Hug EB, Sweeney RA, Nurre PM, Holloway KC, Slater JD, Munzenrider JE (2002). Proton radiotherapy in management of pediatric base of skull tumors. Int J Radiat Oncol Biol Phys 52: 1017-1024.
935. Hui AB, Pang JC, Ko CW, Ng HK (1999). Detection of chromosomal imbalances in growth hormone-secreting pituitary tumors by comparative genomic hybridization. Hum Pathol 30: 1019-1023.
936. Huizenga NA, de Lange P, Koper JW, Clayton RN, Farrell WE, van der Lely AJ, Brinkmann AO, de Jong FH, Lamberts SW (1998). Human adrenocorticotropin-secreting pituitary adenomas show frequent loss of heterozygosity at the glucocorticoid receptor gene locus. J Clin Endocrinol Metab 83: 917-921.
937. Hull MT, Roth LM, Glover JL, Walker PD (1982). Metastatic carotid body paraganglioma in von Hippel-Lindau disease. An electron microscopic study. Arch Pathol Lab Med 106: 235-239.
938. Hull MT, Warfel KA, Muller J, Higgins JT (1979). Familial islet cell tumors in Von Hippel-Lindau's disease. Cancer 44: 1523-1526.
939. Hundahl SA, Cady B, Cunningham MP, Mazzaferri E, McKee RF, Rosai J, Shah JP, Fremgen AM, Stewart AK, Holzer S (2000). Initial results from a prospective cohort study of 5583 cases of thyroid carcinoma treated in the united states during 1996. U.S. and German Thyroid Cancer Study Group. An American College of Surgeons Commission on Cancer Patient Care Evaluation study. Cancer 89: 202-217.
940. Hundahl SA, Fleming ID, Fremgen AM, Menck HR (1998). A National Cancer Data Base report on 53,856 cases of thyroid carcinoma treated in the U.S., 1985-1995. Cancer 83: 2638-2648.
941. Hundahl SA, Fleming ID, Fremgen AM, Menck HR (1999). Two hundred eighty-six cases of parathyroid carcinoma treated in the U.S. between 1985-1995: a National Cancer Data Base Report. The American College of Surgeons Commission on Cancer and the American Cancer Society. Cancer 86: 538-544.
942. Hunt JL, LiVolsi VA, Baloch ZW, Swalsky PA, Bakker A, Sasatomi E, Finkelstein S, Barnes EL (2003). A novel microdissection and genotyping of follicular-derived thyroid tumors to predict aggressiveness. Hum Pathol 34: 375-380.
943. Hunt JL, Tometsko M, LiVolsi VA, Swalsky P, Finkelstein SD, Barnes EL (2003). Molecular evidence of anaplastic transformation in coexisting well-differentiated and anaplastic carcinomas of the thyroid. Am J Surg Pathol 27: 1559-1564.
944. Hurley TR, D'Angelo CM, Clasen RA, DiGianfilippo A, Ryan WG (1992). Adenocarcinoma metastatic to a growth-hormone-secreting pituitary adenoma: case report. Surg Neurol 37: 361-365.
945. Huson SM, Compston DA, Clark P, Harper PS (1989). A genetic study of von Recklinghausen neurofibromatosis in south east Wales. I. Prevalence, fitness, mutation rate, and effect of parental transmission on severity. J Med Genet 26: 704-711.
946. Huson SM, Compston DA, Harper PS (1989). A genetic study of von Recklinghausen neurofibromatosis in south east Wales. II. Guidelines for genetic counselling. J Med Genet 26: 712-721.
947. Huson SM, Harper PS, Compston DA (1988). Von Recklinghausen neurofibromatosis. A clinical and population study in south-east Wales. Brain 111 (Pt 6): 1355-1381.
948. Huss LJ, Mendelsohn G (1990). Medullary carcinoma of the thyroid gland: an encapsulated variant resembling the hyalinizing trabecular (paraganglioma-like) adenoma of thyroid. Mod Pathol 3: 581-585.
949. Hutcheon DF, Bayless TM, Cameron JL, Baylin SB (1979). Hormone-mediated watery diarrhea in a family with multiple endocrine neoplasms. Ann Intern Med 90: 932-934.
950. Icard P, Goudet P, Charpenay C, Andreassian B, Carnaille B, Chapuis Y, Cougard P, Henry JF, Proye C (2001). Adrenocortical carcinomas: surgical trends and results of a 253-patient series from the French Association of Endocrine Surgeons study group. World J Surg 25: 891-897.
951. Iglesias A, Arias M, Brasa J, Paramo C, Conde C, Fernandez R (2000). MR imaging findings in granular cell tumor of the neurohypophysis: a difficult preoperative diagnosis. Eur Radiol 10: 1871-1873.
952. Iino K, Sasano H, Yabuki N, Oki Y, Kikuchi A, Yoshimi T, Nagura H (1997). DNA topoisomerase II alpha and Ki-67 in human adrenocortical neoplasms: a possible marker of differentiation between adenomas and carcinomas. Mod Pathol 10: 901-907.
953. Ikeda T, Satoh M, Azuma K, Sawada N, Mori M (1998). Medullary thyroid carcinoma with a paraganglioma-like pattern and melanin production: a case report with ultrastructural and immunohistochemical studies. Arch Pathol Lab Med 122: 555-558.
954. Ilgren EB, Kinnier-Wilson LM, Stiller CA (1985). Gliomas in neurofibromatosis: a series of 89 cases with evidence for enhanced malignancy in associated cerebellar astrocytomas. Pathol Annu 20 Pt 1: 331-358.
955. Iliopoulos O, Levy AP, Jiang C, Kaelin WGJr, Goldberg MA (1996). Negative regulation of hypoxia-inducible genes by the von Hippel-Lindau protein. Proc Natl Acad Sci U S A 93: 10595-10599.
956. Ilizarov GA (1971). [Basic principles of transosseous compression and distraction osteosynthesis]. Ortop Travmatol Protez 32: 7-15.
957. Illyes G, Bucsek MJ, Kadar A, Horanyi J, Flautner L (1993). Ultrastructural study of a black insulinoma. Ultrastruct Pathol 17: 495-501.
958. Ilvesmaki V, Kahri AI, Miettinen PJ, Voutilainen R (1993). Insulin-like growth factors (IGFs) and their receptors in adrenal tumors: high IGF-II expression in functional adrenocortical carcinomas. J Clin Endocrinol Metab 77: 852-858.
959. Imam H, Eriksson B, Oberg K (2000). Expression of CD44 variant isoforms and association to the benign form of endocrine pancreatic tumours. Ann Oncol 11: 295-300.
960. Imamura M, Kanda M, Takahashi K, Shimada Y, Miyahara T, Wagata T, Hashimoto M, Tobe T, Soga J (1992). Clinicopathological characteristics of duodenal microgastrinomas. World J Surg 16: 703-709.
961. Imanishi Y, Hosokawa Y, Yoshimoto K, Schipani E, Mallya S, Papanikolaou A, Kifor O, Tokura T, Sablosky M, Ledgard F, Gronowicz G, Wang TC, Schmidt EV, Hall C, Brown EM, Bronson R, Arnold A (2001). Primary hyperparathyroidism caused by parathyroid-targeted overexpression of cyclin D1 in transgenic mice. J Clin Invest 107: 1093-1102.
962. Inabnet WB, Caragliano P, Pertsemlidis D (2000). Pheochromocytoma: inherited associations, bilaterality, and cortex preservation. Surgery 128: 1007-1011.
963. Inai K, Kobuke T, Yonehara S, Tokuoka S (1989). Duodenal gangliocytic paraganglioma with lymph node metastasis in a 17-year-old boy. Cancer 63: 2540-2545.
964. Inamo Y, Hanawa Y, Kin H, Okuni M (1993). Findings on magnetic resonance imaging of the spine and femur in a case of McCune-Albright syndrome. Pediatr Radiol 23: 15-18.
965. Inoue H, Miki H, Oshimo K, Tanaka K, Monden Y, Yamamoto A, Kagawa S, Sano N, Hayashi E, Nagayama M, Hayashi Y (1995). Familial hyperparathyroidism associated with jaw fibroma: case report and literature review. Clin Endocrinol (Oxf) 43: 225-229.
966. Isaacs RS, Donald PJ (1995). Sphenoid and sellar tumors. Otolaryngol Clin North Am 28: 1191-1229.
967. Isaia GC, Lala R, Defilippi C, Matarazzo P, Andreo M, Roggia C, Priolo G, de Sanctis C (2002). Bone turnover in children and adolescents with McCune-Albright syndrome treated with pamidronate for bone fibrous dysplasia. Calcif Tissue Int 71: 121-128.
968. Ishida T, Dorfman HD (1993). Massive chondroid differentiation in fibrous dysplasia of bone (fibrocartilaginous dysplasia). Am J Surg Pathol 17: 924-930.
969. Ishido H, Yamashita N, Kitaoka M, Tanaka Y, Ogata E (1994). A case of ectopic ACTH syndrome associated with Zollinger-Ellison syndrome: long-term survival with chemical adrenalectomy. Endocr J 41: 171-176.
970. Ishiguro A, Hirai Y, Hasegawa N, Nakamura J, Tamura M, Nishimura S, Kaimori M, Sasano H (2002). [WDHA syndrome by composite pheochromocytoma and ganglioneuroma]. Nippon Naika Gakkai Zasshi 91: 1585-1588.
971. Ishikawa Y, Sugano H, Matsumoto T, Furuichi Y, Miller RW, Goto M (1999). Unusual features of thyroid carcinomas in Japanese patients with Werner syndrome and possible genotype-phenotype relations to cell type and race. Cancer 85: 1345-1352.
972. Ishikawa Y, Sugano H, Miller RW, Goto M (1999). Author reply. Cancer 86: 729.
973. Ismail SM, Cole G (1984). Von Hippel-Lindau syndrome with microscopic hemangioblastomas of the spinal nerve roots. Case

report. J Neurosurg 60: 1279-1281.
974. Isotalo PA, Lloyd RV (2002). Presence of birefringent crystals is useful in distinguishing thyroid from parathyroid gland tissues. Am J Surg Pathol 26: 813-814.
975. Itakura Y, Sakurai A, Katai M, Ikeo Y, Hashizume K (2000). Enhanced sensitivity to alkylating agent in lymphocytes from patients with multiple endocrine neoplasia type 1. Biomed Pharmacother 54 Suppl 1: 187s-190s.
976. Ito T, Seyama T, Mizuno T, Tsuyama N, Hayashi T, Hayashi Y, Dohi K, Nakamura N, Akiyama M (1992). Unique association of p53 mutations with undifferentiated but not with differentiated carcinomas of the thyroid gland. Cancer Res 52: 1369-1371.
977. Ivan M, Kondo K, Yang H, Kim W, Valiando J, Ohh M, Salic A, Asara JM, Lane WS, Kaelin WGJr (2001). HIFalpha targeted for VHL-mediated destruction by proline hydroxylation: implications for O2 sensing. Science 292: 464-468.
978. Ivanova R, Soares P, Castro P, Sobrinho-Simoes M (2002). Diffuse (or multinodular) follicular variant of papillary thyroid carcinoma: a clinicopathologic and immunohistochemical analysis of ten cases of an aggressive form of differentiated thyroid carcinoma. Virchows Arch 440: 418-424.
979. Iwama T, Mishima Y, Utsunomiya J (1993). The impact of familial adenomatous polyposis on the tumorigenesis and mortality at the several organs. Its rational treatment. Ann Surg 217: 101-108.
980. Iwamura Y, Futagawa T, Kaneko M, Nakagawa K, Kawai K, Yamashita K, Nakamura T, Hayashi H (1992). Co-deletions of the retinoblastoma gene and Wilms' tumor gene and rearrangement of the Krev-1 gene in a human insulinoma. Jpn J Clin Oncol 22: 6-9.
981. Iwasa K, Imai MA, Noguchi M, Tanaka S, Sasaki T, Katsuda S, Kawahara E, Mizukami Y (2002). Spindle epithelial tumor with thymus-like differentiation (SETTLE) of the thyroid. Head Neck 24: 888-893.
982. Iwashita T, Kato M, Murakami H, Asai N, Ishiguro Y, Ito S, Iwata Y, Kawai K, Asai M, Kurokawa K, Kajita H, Takahashi M (1999). Biological and biochemical properties of Ret with kinase domain mutations identified in multiple endocrine neoplasia type 2B and familial medullary thyroid carcinoma. Oncogene 18: 3919-3922.
983. Jaakkola P, Mole DR, Tian YM, Wilson MI, Gielbert J, Gaskell SJ, von Kriegsheim A, Hebestreit HF, Mukherji M, Schofield CJ, Maxwell PH, Pugh CW, Ratcliffe PJ (2001). Targeting of HIF-alpha to the von Hippel-Lindau ubiquitylation complex by O2-regulated prolyl hydroxylation. Science 292: 468-472.
984. Jacks T, Shih TS, Schmitt EM, Bronson RT, Bernards A, Weinberg RA (1994). Tumour predisposition in mice heterozygous for a targeted mutation in Nf1. Nat Genet 7: 353-361.
985. Jackson CE, Norum RA, Boyd SB, Talpos GB, Wilson SD, Taggart RT, Mallette LE (1990). Hereditary hyperparathyroidism and multiple ossifying jaw fibromas: a clinically and genetically distinct syndrome. Surgery 108: 1006-1012.
986. Jacobi JM, Lloyd HM, Smith JF (1986). Nuclear diameter in parathyroid carcinomas. J Clin Pathol 39: 1353-1354.
987. Jacobsen O, Bardram L, Rehfeld JF (1986). The requirement for gastrin measurements. Scand J Clin Lab Invest 46: 423-426.
988. Jaffe CA, Barkan AL (1994). Acromegaly. Recognition and treatment. Drugs 47: 425-445.
989. Jaffe ES, Harris NL, Stein H, Vardiman JW (2001). World Health Organization Classification of Tumours. Pathology and Genetics of Tumours of Haematopoietic and Lymphoid Tissues. IARC Press: Lyon.
990. Jaffrain-Rea ML, Ferretti E, Toniato E, Cannita K, Santoro A, Di Stefano D, Ricevuto E, Maroder M, Tamburrano G, Cantore G, Gulino A, Martinotti S (1999). p16 (INK4a, MTS-1) gene polymorphism and methylation status in human pituitary tumours. Clin Endocrinol (Oxf) 51: 317-325.
991. James LA, Kelsey AM, Birch JM, Varley JM (1999). Highly consistent genetic alterations in childhood adrenocortical tumours detected by comparative genomic hybridization. Br J Cancer 81: 300-304.
992. James RLJr, Arsenis G, Stoler M, Nelson C, Baran D (1984). Hypophyseal metastatic renal cell carcinoma and pituitary adenoma. Case report and review of the literature. Am J Med 76: 337-340.
993. Jansen JC, van den Berg R, Kuiper A, van der Mey AG, Zwinderman AH, Cornelisse CJ (2000). Estimation of growth rate in patients with head and neck paragangliomas influences the treatment proposal. Cancer 88: 2811-2816.
994. Jansson S, Tisell LE, Hansson G (1988). Morphology of the adrenal medulla indicating multiple neuroectodermal abnormalities in pheochromocytoma patients. Acta Med Austriaca 15: 99-100.
995. Jaresch S, Kornely E, Kley HK, Schlaghecke R (1992). Adrenal incidentaloma and patients with homozygous or heterozygous congenital adrenal hyperplasia. J Clin Endocrinol Metab 74: 685-689.
996. Jayaram G (1999). Neurilemmoma (schwannoma) of the thyroid diagnosed by fine needle aspiration cytology. Acta Cytol 43: 743-744.
997. Jayawardene S, Owen WJ, Goldsmith DJ (2000). Parathyroid carcinoma in a dialysis patient. Am J Kidney Dis 36: E26.
998. Jee WH, Choi KH, Choe BY, Park JM, Shinn KS (1996). Fibrous dysplasia: MR imaging characteristics with radiopathologic correlation. AJR Am J Roentgenol 167: 1523-1527.
999. Jenkins RB, Hay ID, Herath JF, Schultz CG, Spurbeck JL, Grant CS, Goellner JR, Dewald GW (1990). Frequent occurrence of cytogenetic abnormalities in sporadic nonmedullary thyroid carcinoma. Cancer 66: 1213-1220.
1000. Jensen RT (1999). Pancreatic endocrine tumors: recent advances. Ann Oncol 10 Suppl 4: 170-176.
1001. Jensen RT, Gardner JD (1991). Zollinger-Ellison syndrome: clinical presentation, pathology, diagnosis and treatment. In: Peptic Ulcer Disease and Other Acid-Related Disorders, Zakim D, Dannenberg A, eds., Academic Research Associates: Armonk , pp. 117-211.
1002. Jensen RT, Gardner JD (1993). Gastrinoma. In: The Pancreas: Biology, Pathobiology and Disease, Go VLW, Dimagno EP, eds., 2nd ed. Raven Press: New York , pp. 512-530.
1003. Jensen RT, Gardner JD, Raufman JP, Pandol SJ, Doppman JL, Collen MJ (1983). Zollinger-Ellison syndrome: current concepts and management. Ann Intern Med 98: 59-75.
1004. Jhiang SM, Sagartz JE, Tong Q, Parker-Thornburg J, Capen CC, Cho JY, Xing S, Ledent C (1996). Targeted expression of the ret/PTC1 oncogene induces papillary thyroid carcinomas. Endocrinology 137: 375-378.
1005. Jimbow K, Szabo G, Fitzpatrick TB (1973). Ultrastructure of giant pigment granules (macromelanosomes) in the cutaneous pigmented macules of neurofibromatosis. J Invest Dermatol 61: 300-309.
1006. Jin L, Qian X, Kulig E, Sanno N, Scheithauer BW, Kovacs K, Young WFJr, Lloyd RV (1997). Transforming growth factor-beta, transforming growth factor-beta receptor II, and p27Kip1 expression in nontumorous and neoplastic human pituitaries. Am J Pathol 151: 509-519.
1007. Jin L, Qian X, Kulig E, Scheithauer BW, Calle-Rodrigue R, Abboud C, Davis DH, Kovacs K, Lloyd RV (1997). Prolactin receptor messenger ribonucleic acid in normal and neoplastic human pituitary tissues. J Clin Endocrinol Metab 82: 963-968.
1008. John H, Ziegler WH, Hauri D, Jaeger P (1999). Pheochromocytomas: can malignant potential be predicted? Urology 53: 679-683.
1009. Johnson MR, Look AT, DeClue JE, Valentine MB, Lowy DR (1993). Inactivation of the NF1 gene in human melanoma and neuroblastoma cell lines without impaired regulation of GTP.Ras. Proc Natl Acad Sci U S A 90: 5539-5543.
1010. Johnston LB, Carroll MJ, Britton KE, Lowe DG, Shand W, Besser GM, Grossman AB (1996). The accuracy of parathyroid gland localization in primary hyperparathyroidism using sestamibi radionuclide imaging. J Clin Endocrinol Metab 81: 346-352.
1011. Jonasson JG, Hrafnkelsson J, Bjornsson J (1989). Tumours in Iceland. 11. Malignant tumours of the thyroid gland. A histological classification and epidemiological considerations. APMIS 97: 625-630.
1012. Jordan RB, Gauderer MW (1988). Cervical teratomas: an analysis. Literature review and proposed classification. J Pediatr Surg 23: 583-591.
1013. Jordan S, Lidhar K, Korbonits M, Lowe DG, Grossman AB (2000). Cyclin D and cyclin E expression in normal and adenomatous pituitary. Eur J Endocrinol 143: R1-R6.
1014. Jouanneau E, Perrin G, Trouillas J (2002). [Corticotroph microadenomas of the pituitary stalk. Diagnostic and therapeutic difficulties]. Neurochirurgie 48: 215-222.
1015. Joubert D, Benlot C, Lagoguey A, Garnier P, Brandi AM, Gautron JP, Legrand JC, Peillon F (1989). Normal and growth hormone (GH)-secreting adenomatous human pituitaries release somatostatin and GH-releasing hormone. J Clin Endocrinol Metab 68: 572-577.
1016. Julian-Reynier C, Eisinger F, Vennin P, Chabal F, Aurran Y, Nogues C, Bignon YJ, Machelard-Roumagnac M, Maugard-Louboutin C, Serin D, Blanc B, Orsoni P, Sobol H (1996). Attitudes towards cancer predictive testing and transmission of information to the family. J Med Genet 33: 731-736.
1017. Juneau P, Schoene WC, Black P (1992). Malignant tumors in the pituitary gland. Arch Neurol 49: 555-558.
1018. Kadota M, Tamaki Y, Sekimoto M, Fujiwara Y, Aritake N, Hasegawa S, Kobayashi T, Ikeda T, Horii A, Monden M (2003). Loss of heterozygosity on chromosome 16p and 18q in anaplastic thyroid carcinoma. Oncol Rep 10: 35-38.
1019. Kainuma O, Ito Y, Taniguchi T, Shimizu T, Nakada H, Date Y, Hara T (1996). Ampullary somatostatinoma in a patient with von Recklinghausen's disease. J Gastroenterol 31: 460-464.
1020. Kaji H, Canaff L, Goltzman D, Hendy GN (1999). Cell cycle regulation of menin expression. Cancer Res 59: 5097-5101.
1021. Kaji H, Canaff L, Lebrun JJ, Goltzman D, Hendy GN (2001). Inactivation of menin, a Smad3-interacting protein, blocks transforming growth factor type beta signaling. Proc Natl Acad Sci U S A 98: 3837-3842.
1022. Kakinuma A, Morimoto I, Nakano Y, Fujimoto R, Ishida O, Okada Y, Inokuchi N, Fujihira T, Eto S (1994). Familial primary hyperparathyroidism complicated with Wilms' tumor. Intern Med 33: 123-126.
1023. Kakudo K, Miyauchi A, Takai S, Katayama S, Kuma K, Kitamura H (1979). C cell carcinoma of the thyroid—papillary type. Acta Pathol Jpn 29: 653-659.
1024. Kakudo K, Mori I, Tamaoki N, Watanabe K (1988). Carcinoma of possible thymic origin presenting as a thyroid mass: a new subgroup of squamous cell carcinoma of the thyroid. J Surg Oncol 38: 187-192.
1025. Kaleem Z, Davila RM (1997). Hyalinizing trabecular adenoma of the thyroid. A report of two cases with cytologic, histologic and immunohistochemical findings. Acta Cytol 41: 883-888.
1026. Kalff V, Shapiro B, Lloyd R, Nakajo M, Sisson JC, Beierwaltes WH (1984). Bilateral pheochromocytomas. J Endocrinol Invest 7: 387-392.
1027. Kaltsas GA, Mukherjee JJ, Plowman PN, Monson JP, Grossman AB, Besser GM (1998). The role of cytotoxic chemotherapy in the management of aggressive and malignant pituitary tumors. J Clin Endocrinol Metab 83: 4233-4238.
1028. Kameyama K, Takami H, Miyajima K, Mimura T, Hosoda Y, Ito K, Ito K (2001). Papillary carcinoma occurring within an adenomatous goiter of the thyroid gland in Cowden's disease. Endocr Pathol 12: 73-76.
1029. Kamio T, Shigematsu K, Sou H, Kawai K, Tsuchiyama H (1990). Immunohistochemical expression of epidermal growth factor receptors in human adrenocortical carcinoma. Hum Pathol 21: 277-282.
1030. Kamisawa T, Tu Y, Egawa N, Ishiwata J, Tsuruta K, Okamoto A, Hayashi Y, Koike M, Yamaguchi T (2002). Ductal and acinar differentiation in pancreatic endocrine tumors. Dig Dis Sci 47: 2254-2261.
1031. Kamura T, Koepp DM, Conrad MN, Skowyra D, Moreland RJ, Iliopoulos O, Lane WS, Kaelin WGJr, Elledge SJ, Conaway RC, Harper JW, Conaway JW (1999). Rbx1, a component of the VHL tumor suppressor complex and SCF ubiquitin ligase. Science 284: 657-661.
1032. Kane LA, Leinung MC, Scheithauer BW, Bergstralh EJ, Laws ERJr, Groover RV, Kovacs K, Horvath E, Zimmerman D (1994). Pituitary adenomas in childhood and adolescence. J Clin Endocrinol Metab 79: 1135-1140.
1033. Kannuki S, Matsumoto K, Sano T, Shintani Y, Bando H, Saito S (1996). Double pituitary adenoma—two case reports. Neurol Med Chir (Tokyo) 36: 818-821.
1034. Kanoh N, Nishimura Y, Nakamura M, Mori M, Uematsu K (1991). Primary nasopharyngeal paraganglioma: a case report. Auris Nasus Larynx 18: 307-314.
1035. Kao PC, van Heerden JA, Taylor RL

(1994). Intraoperative monitoring of parathyroid procedures by a 15-minute parathyroid hormone immunochemiluminometric assay. Mayo Clin Proc 69: 532-537.

1036. Kaplan SJ, Holbrook CT, McDaniel HG, Buntain WL, Crist WM (1980). Vasoactive intestinal peptide secreting tumors of childhood. Am J Dis Child 134: 21-24.

1037. Karasawa Y, Sakaguchi M, Minami S, Kitano K, Kawa S, Aoki Y, Itoh N, Sakurai A, Miyazaki M, Watanabe T, Akimoto M, Arakura N, Kiyosawa K (2001). Duodenal somatostatinoma and erythrocytosis in a patient with von Hippel-Lindau disease type 2A. Intern Med 40: 38-43.

1038. Karasov RS, Sheps SG, Carney JA, van Heerden JA, DeQuattro V (1982). Paragangliomatosis with numerous catecholamine-producing tumors. Mayo Clin Proc 57: 590-595.

1039. Karatzas G, Kouraklis G, Karayiannakis A, Patapis P, Givalos N, Kaperonis E (2000). Ampullary carcinoid and jejunal stromal tumour associated with von Recklinghausen's disease presenting as gastrointestinal bleeding and jaundice. Eur J Surg Oncol 26: 428-429.

1040. Karavitaki N, Vlassopoulou V, Tzanela M, Tzavara I, Thalassinos N (2002). Recurrent and/or metastatic thyroid cancer: therapeutic options. Expert Opin Pharmacother 3: 939-947.

1041. Karga HJ, Alexander JM, Hedley-Whyte ET, Klibanski A, Jameson JL (1992). Ras mutations in human pituitary tumors. J Clin Endocrinol Metab 74: 914-919.

1042. Karl M, Lamberts SW, Koper JW, Katz DA, Huizenga NE, Kino T, Haddad BR, Hughes MR, Chrousos GP (1996). Cushing's disease preceded by generalized glucocorticoid resistance: clinical consequences of a novel, dominant-negative glucocorticoid receptor mutation. Proc Assoc Am Physicians 108: 296-307.

1042A. Karl M, Von Wichert G, Kempter E, Katz DA, Reincke M, Monig H, Ali IU, Stratakis CA, Oldfield EH, Chrousos GP, Schulte HM (1996). Nelson's syndrome associated with a somatic frame shift mutation in the glucocorticoid receptor gene. J Clin Endocrinol Metab 81: 124-129.

1043. Kaserer K, Scheuba C, Neuhold N, Weinhausel A, Haas OA, Vierhapper H, Niederle B (2001). Sporadic versus familial medullary thyroid microcarcinoma: a histopathologic study of 50 consecutive patients. Am J Surg Pathol 25: 1245-1251.

1044. Kaserer K, Scheuba C, Neuhold N, Weinhausel A, Vierhapper H, Haas OA, Niederle B (1998). C-cell hyperplasia and medullary thyroid carcinoma in patients routinely screened for serum calcitonin. Am J Surg Pathol 22: 722-728.

1045. Kashima K, Yokoyama S, Inoue S, Daa T, Kodama M, Nakayama I, Noguchi S (1993). Mixed medullary and follicular carcinoma of the thyroid: report of two cases with an immunohistochemical study. Acta Pathol Jpn 43: 428-433.

1046. Kasprzak L, Nolet S, Gaboury L, Pavia C, Villabona C, Rivera-Fillat F, Oriola J, Foulkes WD (2001). Familial medullary thyroid carcinoma and prominent corneal nerves associated with the germline V804M and V778I mutations on the same allele of RET. J Med Genet 38: 784-787.

1047. Kassem M, Kruse TA, Wong FK, Larsson C, Teh BT (2000). Familial isolated hyperparathyroidism as a variant of multiple endocrine neoplasia type 1 in a large Danish pedigree. J Clin Endocrinol Metab 85: 165-167.

1048. Katai M, Sakurai A, Ichikawa K, Yamagata M, Ogiso Y, Kobayashi S, Hashizume K (1998). Pheochromocytoma arising from an accessory adrenal gland in a patient with multiple endocrine neoplasia type 2A: transient development of clinical manifestations after hemorrhagic necrosis. Endocr J 45: 329-334.

1049. Kato H, Uchimura I, Morohoshi M, Fujisawa K, Kobayashi Y, Numano F, Goseki N, Endo M, Tamura A, Nagashima C (1996). Multiple endocrine neoplasia type 1 associated with spinal ependymoma. Intern Med 35: 285-289.

1050. Kato N, Tsuchiya T, Tamura G, Motoyama T (2002). E-cadherin expression in follicular carcinoma of the thyroid. Pathol Int 52: 13-18.

1051. Katoh R, Harach HR, Williams ED (1998). Solitary, multiple, and familial oxyphil tumours of the thyroid gland. J Pathol 186: 292-299.

1052. Katoh R, Harach HR, Williams ED (1998). Solitary, multiple, and familial oxyphil tumours of the thyroid gland. J Pathol 186: 292-299.

1053. Katoh R, Sugai T, Ono S, Takayama K, Tomichi N, Kurihara H, Takamatsu M (1990). Mucoepidermoid carcinoma of the thyroid gland. Cancer 65: 2020-2027.

1054. Kattah JC, Silgals RM, Manz H, Toro JG, Dritschilo A, Smith FP (1985). Presentation and management of parasellar and suprasellar metastatic mass lesions. J Neurol Neurosurg Psychiatry 48: 44-49.

1055. Kaushik S, Smoker WR, Frable WJ (2002). Malignant transformation of fibrous dysplasia into chondroblastic osteosarcoma. Skeletal Radiol 31: 103-106.

1056. Kawahara E, Nakanishi I, Terahata S, Ikegaki S (1988). Leiomyosarcoma of the thyroid gland. A case report with a comparative study of five cases of anaplastic carcinoma. Cancer 62: 2558-2563.

1057. Kawashima A, Sandler CM, Fishman EK, Charnsangavej C, Yasumori K, Honda H, Ernst RD, Takahashi N, Raval BK, Masuda K, Goldman SM (1998). Spectrum of CT findings in nonmalignant disease of the adrenal gland. Radiographics 18: 393-412.

1058. Kayath MJ, Martin LC, Vieira JG, Roman LM, Nose-Alberti V (1998). A comparative study of p53 immunoexpression in parathyroid hyperplasias secondary to uremia, primary hyperplasias, adenomas and carcinomas. Eur J Endocrinol 139: 78-83.

1059. Kayes LM, Burke W, Riccardi VM, Bennett R, Ehrlich P, Rubenstein A, Stephens K (1994). Deletions spanning the neurofibromatosis 1 gene: identification and phenotype of five patients. Am J Hum Genet 54: 424-436.

1060. Kebebew E, Ituarte PH, Siperstein AE, Duh QY, Clark OH (2000). Medullary thyroid carcinoma: clinical characteristics, treatment, prognostic factors, and a comparison of staging systems. Cancer 88: 1139-1148.

1061. Keeler LLI, Klauber GT (1992). Von Hippel-Lindau disease and renal cell carcinoma in a 16-year-old boy. J Urol 147: 1588-1591.

1062. Keijser LC, Van Tienen TG, Schreuder HW, Lemmens JA, Pruszczynski M, Veth RP (2001). Fibrous dysplasia of bone: management and outcome of 20 cases. J Surg Oncol 76: 157-166.

1063. Kelijman M, Williams TC, Downs TR, Frohman LA (1988). Comparison of the sensitivity of growth hormone secretion to somatostatin in vivo and in vitro in acromegaly. J Clin Endocrinol Metab 67: 958-963.

1064. Kelly TR (1983). Pancreatic somatostatinoma. Am J Surg 146: 671-673.

1065. Kemink SA, Wesseling P, Pieters GF, Verhofstad AA, Hermus AR, Smals AG (1999). Progression of a Nelson's adenoma to pituitary carcinoma; a case report and review of the literature. J Endocrinol Invest 22: 70-75.

1066. Kendall CH, Roberts PA, Pringle JH, Lauder I (1991). The expression of parathyroid hormone messenger RNA in normal and abnormal parathyroid tissue. J Pathol 165: 111-118.

1067. Kendrick ML, Curlee K, Lloyd R, Farley DR, Grant CS, Thompson GB, Rowland C, Young WFJr, van Heerden JA (2002). Aldosterone-secreting adrenocortical carcinomas are associated with unique operative risks and outcomes. Surgery 132: 1008-1011.

1068. Kenny BD, Sloan JM, Hamilton PW, Watt PC, Johnston CF, Buchanan KD (1989). The role of morphometry in predicting prognosis in pancreatic islet cell tumors. Cancer 64: 460-465.

1069. Kent RBI, van Heerden JA, Weiland LH (1981). Nonfunctioning islet cell tumors. Ann Surg 193: 185-190.

1070. Kesmodel SB, Terhune KP, Canter RJ, Mandel SJ, LiVolsi VA, Baloch ZW, Fraker DL (2003). The diagnostic dilemma of follicular variant of papillary thyroid carcinoma. Surgery 134: 1005-1012.

1071. Khodaei-O'Brien S, Zablewska B, Fromaget M, Bylund L, Weber G, Gaudray P (2000). Heterogeneity at the 5'-end of MEN1 transcripts. Biochem Biophys Res Commun 276: 508-514.

1072. Khodaei S, O'Brien KP, Dumanski J, Wong FK, Weber G (1999). Characterization of the MEN1 ortholog in zebrafish. Biochem Biophys Res Commun 264: 404-408.

1073. Khoo ML, Beasley NJ, Ezzat S, Freeman JL, Asa SL (2002). Overexpression of cyclin D1 and underexpression of p27 predict lymph node metastases in papillary thyroid carcinoma. J Clin Endocrinol Metab 87: 1814-1818.

1074. Khoo ML, Freeman JL, Witterick IJ, Irish JC, Rotstein LE, Gullane PJ, Asa SL (2002). Underexpression of p27/Kip in thyroid papillary microcarcinomas with gross metastatic disease. Arch Otolaryngol Head Neck Surg 128: 253-257.

1075. Kiang DT, Bauer GE, Kennedy BJ (1973). Immunoassayable insulin in carcinoma of the cervix associated with hypoglycemia. Cancer 31: 801-805.

1076. Kie JH, Kim JY, Park YN, Lee MK, Yang WI, Park JS (1997). Solitary fibrous tumour of the thyroid. Histopathology 30: 365-368.

1077. Kim IS, Kim ER, Nam HJ, Chin MO, Moon YH, Oh MR, Yeo UC, Song SM, Kim JS, Uhm MR, Beck NS, Jin DK (1999). Activating mutation of GS alpha in McCune-Albright syndrome causes skin pigmentation by tyrosinase gene activation on affected melanocytes. Horm Res 52: 235-240.

1078. Kim YS, Burns AL, Goldsmith PK, Heppner C, Park SY, Chandrasekharappa SC, Collins FS, Spiegel AM, Marx SJ (1999). Stable overexpression of MEN1 suppresses tumorigenicity of RAS. Oncogene 18: 5936-5942.

1079. Kimura ET, Nikiforova MN, Zhu Z, Knauf JA, Nikiforov YE, Fagin JA (2003). High prevalence of BRAF mutations in thyroid cancer: genetic evidence for constitutive activation of the RET/PTC-RAS-BRAF signalling pathway in papillary thyroid carcinoma. Cancer Res 63: 1454-1457.

1080. Kimura N (2000). The adrenal medulla and extra-adrenal paraganglia. In: Molecular and Cellular Endocrine Pathology, Stefaneanu L, Sasano H, Kovacs K, eds., Edward Arnold: London .

1081. Kimura N, Miura W, Noshiro T, Miura Y, Ookura T, Nagura H (1994). Ki-67 is an indicator of progression in neuroendocrine tumours. Endocr Pathol 5: 223-228.

1082. Kimura N, Miura Y, Miura K, Takahashi N, Osamura RY, Nagatsu I, Nagura H (1991). Adrenal and retroperitoneal mixed neuroendocrine-neural tumors. Endocr Pathol 2: 139-147.

1083. Kimura N, Miura Y, Nagatsu I, Nagura H (1992). Catecholamine synthesizing enzymes in 70 cases of functioning and non-functioning phaeochromocytoma and extra-adrenal paraganglioma. Virchows Arch A Pathol Anat Histopathol 421: 25-32.

1084. Kimura N, Sasano N (1990). A comparative study between malignant and benign pheochromocytoma using morphometry, cytomorphometry, and immunohistochemistry. In: Endocrine Pathology Update, LeChago J, Kameya T, eds., Field and Wood: Blue Bell, PA , pp. 99-118.

1085. Kimura N, Watanabe T, Fukase M, Wakita A, Noshiro T, Kimura I (2002). Neurofibromin and NF1 gene analysis in composite pheochromocytoma and tumors associated with von Recklinghausen's disease. Mod Pathol 15: 183-188.

1086. Kimura W, Kuroda A, Morioka Y (1991). Clinical pathology of endocrine tumors of the pancreas. Analysis of autopsy cases. Dig Dis Sci 36: 933-942.

1087. Kindblom LG, Ahlden M, Meis-Kindblom JM, Stenman G (1995). Immunohistochemical and molecular analysis of p53, MDM2, proliferating cell nuclear antigen and Ki67 in benign and malignant peripheral nerve sheath tumours. Virchows Arch 427: 19-26.

1088. Kingsley DPE, Elton A, Bennett MH (1968). Malignant teratoma of the thyroid. Case report and a review of the literature. Br J Cancer 22: 7-11.

1089. Kinjo T, al Mefty O, Ciric I (1995). Diaphragma sellae meningiomas. Neurosurgery 36: 1082-1092.

1090. Kinney MA, Warner ME, vanHeerden JA, Horlocker TT, Young WFJr, Schroeder DR, Maxson PM, Warner MA (2000). Perianesthetic risks and outcomes of pheochromocytoma and paraganglioma resection. Anesth Analg 91: 1118-1123.

1091. Kirby PA, Ellison WA, Thomas PA (1999). Spindle epithelial tumor with thymus-like differentiation (SETTLE) of the thyroid with prominent mitotic activity and focal necrosis. Am J Surg Pathol 23: 712-716.

1092. Kirk JF, Flowers FP, Ramos-Caro FA, Browder JF (1991). Multiple endocrine neoplasia type III: case report and review. Pediatr Dermatol 8: 124-128.

1093. Kirk JM, Brain CE, Carson DJ, Hyde JC, Grant DB (1999). Cushing's syndrome caused by nodular adrenal hyperplasia in children with McCune-Albright syndrome. J Pediatr 134: 789-792.

1094. Kirschner LS, Carney JA, Pack SD, Taymans SE, Giatzakis C, Cho YS, Cho-Chung YS, Stratakis CA (2000). Mutations of the gene encoding the protein kinase A type I-alpha regulatory subunit in patients with

the Carney complex. Nat Genet 26: 89-92.
1095. Kirschner LS, Sandrini F, Monbo J, Lin JP, Carney JA, Stratakis CA (2000). Genetic heterogeneity and spectrum of mutations of the PRKAR1A gene in patients with the carney complex. Hum Mol Genet 9: 3037-3046.
1096. Kishi M, Tsukada T, Shimizu S, Futami H, Ito Y, Kanbe M, Obara T, Yamaguchi K (1998). A large germline deletion of the MEN1 gene in a family with multiple endocrine neoplasia type 1. Jpn J Cancer Res 89: 1-5.
1097. Kitahama S, Iitaka M, Shimizu T, Serizawa N, Fukasawa N, Miura S, Kawasaki S, Yamanaka K, Kawakami Y, Murakami S, Ishii J, Katayama S (1996). Thyroid involvement by malignant histiocytosis of Langerhans' cell type. Clin Endocrinol (Oxf) 45: 357-363.
1098. Kitamura Y, Shimizu K, Ito K, Tanaka S, Emi M (2001). Allelotyping of follicular thyroid carcinoma: frequent allelic losses in chromosome arms 7q, 11p, and 22q. J Clin Endocrinol Metab 86: 4268-4272.
1099. Kitamura Y, Shimizu K, Tanaka S, Ito K, Emi M (2000). Allelotyping of anaplastic thyroid carcinoma: frequent allelic losses on 1q, 9p, 11, 17, 19p, and 22q. Genes Chromosomes Cancer 27: 244-251.
1100. Kjellman M, Kallioniemi OP, Karhu R, Hoog A, Farnebo LO, Auer G, Larsson C, Backdahl M (1996). Genetic aberrations in adrenocortical tumors detected using comparative genomic hybridization correlate with tumor size and malignancy. Cancer Res 56: 4219-4223.
1101. Kjellman M, Roshani L, Teh BT, Kallioniemi OP, Hoog A, Gray S, Farnebo LO, Holst M, Backdahl M, Larsson C (1999). Genotyping of adrenocortical tumors: very frequent deletions of the MEN1 locus in 11q13 and of a 1-centimorgan region in 2p16. J Clin Endocrinol Metab 84: 730-735.
1102. Kleer CG, Bryant BR, Giordano TJ, Sobel M, Merino MJ (2000). Genetic Changes in Chromosomes 1p and 17p in Thyroid Cancer Progression. Endocr Pathol 11: 137-143.
1103. Kleer CG, Giordano TJ, Merino MJ (2000). Squamous cell carcinoma of the thyroid: an aggressive tumor associated with tall cell variant of papillary thyroid carcinoma. Mod Pathol 13: 742-746.
1104. Kleihues P, Cavenee WK (2000). World Health Organization Classification of Tumours. Pathology and Genetics of Tumours of the Nervous System. IARCPress: Lyon.
1105. Kleihues P, Schauble B, zur Hausen A, Esteve J, Ohgaki H (1997). Tumors associated with p53 germline mutations: a synopsis of 91 families. Am J Pathol 150: 1-13.
1106. Klimstra DS, Rosai J, Heffess CS (1994). Mixed acinar-endocrine carcinomas of the pancreas. Am J Surg Pathol 18: 765-778.
1107. Kloboves-Prevodnik V, Jazbec J, Us-Krasovec M, Lamovec J (2002). Thyroid spindle epithelial tumor with thymus-like differentiation (SETTLE): is cytopathological diagnosis possible? Diagn Cytopathol 26: 314-319.
1108. Klonoff DC, Greenspan FS (1982). The thyroid nodule. Adv Intern Med 27: 101-126.
1109. Kloos RT, Gross MD, Francis IR, Korobkin M, Shapiro B (1995). Incidentally discovered adrenal masses. Endocr Rev 16: 460-484.
1110. Kloppel G (2000). Mixed exocrine-endocrine tumors of the pancreas. Semin Diagn Pathol 17: 104-108.
1111. Kloppel G, Heitz PU (1988). Pancreatic endocrine tumors. Pathol Res Pract 183: 155-168.
1112. Kloppel G, Heitz PU (1990). Morphology and functional activity of gastroenteropancreatic neuroendocrine tumours. Recent Results Cancer Res 118: 27-36.
1113. Kloppel G, Hofler H, Heitz PU (1993). Pancreatic endocrine tumours in man. In: Diagnostic Histopathology of Neuroendocrine Tumours, Polak JM, ed., Churchill Livingstone: Edinburgh , pp. 91-121.
1114. Kloppel G, Willemer S, Stamm B, Hacki WH, Heitz PU (1986). Pancreatic lesions and hormonal profile of pancreatic tumors in multiple endocrine neoplasia type I. An immunocytochemical study of nine patients. Cancer 57: 1824-1832.
1115. Klugbauer S, Demidchik EP, Lengfelder E, Rabes HM (1998). Detection of a novel type of RET rearrangement (PTC5) in thyroid carcinomas after Chernobyl and analysis of the involved RET-fused gene RFG5. Cancer Res 58: 198-203.
1116. Klugbauer S, Jauch A, Lengfelder E, Demidchik E, Rabes HM (2000). A novel type of RET rearrangement (PTC8) in childhood papillary thyroid carcinomas and characterization of the involved gene (RFG8). Cancer Res 60: 7028-7032.
1117. Klugbauer S, Pfeiffer P, Gassenhuber H, Beimfohr C, Rabes HM (2001). RET rearrangements in radiation-induced papillary thyroid carcinomas: high prevalence of topoisomerase I sites at breakpoints and microhomology-mediated end joining in ELE1 and RET chimeric genes. Genomics 73: 149-160.
1118. Klugbauer S, Rabes HM (1999). The transcription coactivator HTIF1 and a related protein are fused to the RET receptor tyrosine kinase in childhood papillary thyroid carcinomas. Oncogene 18: 4388-4393.
1119. Kluwe L, Hagel C, Tatagiba M, Thomas S, Stavrou D, Ostertag H, von Deimling A, Mautner VF (2001). Loss of NF1 alleles distinguish sporadic from NF1-associated pilocytic astrocytomas. J Neuropathol Exp Neurol 60: 917-920.
1120. Kobayashi Y, Nakata M, Maekawa M, Takahashi M, Fujii H, Matsuno Y, Fujishiro M, Ono H, Saito D, Takenaka T, Hirase N, Nishimura J, Akioka T, Enomoto K, Mikuni C, Hishima T, Fukayama M, Sugano K, Hosoda F, Ohki M, Tobinai K (2001). Detection of t(l 1; 18) in MALT-type lymphoma with dual-color fluorescence in situ hybridization and reverse transcriptase-polymerase chain reaction analysis. Diagn Mol Pathol 10: 207-213.
1121. Koch CA, Mauro D, Walther MM, Linehan WM, Vortmeyer AO, Jaffe R, Pacak K, Chrousos GP, Zhuang Z, Lubensky IA (2002). Pheochromocytoma in von hippel-lindau disease: distinct histopathologic phenotype compared to pheochromocytoma in multiple endocrine neoplasia type 2. Endocr Pathol 13: 17-27.
1122. Koch CA, Pacak K, Chrousos GP (2002). The molecular pathogenesis of hereditary and sporadic adrenocortical and adrenomedullary tumors. J Clin Endocrinol Metab 87: 5367-5384.
1123. Koch CA, Vortmeyer AO, Huang SC, Alesci S, Zhuang Z, Pacak K (2001). Genetic aspects of pheochromocytoma. Endocr Regul 35: 43-52.
1124. Koga A, Tabata M, Kido H, Todo S, Nagamitsu S, Nakamura Y, Aono K (1979). [Successful treatment of ectopic insulinoma. Report of a case (author's transl)]. Nippon Shokakibyo Gakkai Zasshi 76: 279-284.
1125. Kogire M, Hosotani R, Kondo M, Itoh K, Doi R, Terachi T, Imamura M (2000). Pancreatic lesions in von Hippel-Lindau syndrome: the coexistence of metastatic tumors from renal cell carcinoma and multiple cysts. Surg Today 30: 380-382.
1126. Kogut MD, Kaplan SA (1962). Systemic manifestations of neurogenic tumors. J Pediatr 60: 694-704.
1127. Koivunen J, Yla-Outinen H, Korkiamaki T, Karvonen SL, Poyhonen M, Laato M, Karvonen J, Peltonen S, Peltonen J (2000). New function for NF1 tumor suppressor. J Invest Dermatol 114: 473-479.
1128. Komminoth P (1999). Review: multiple endocrine neoplasia type 1, sporadic neuroendocrine tumors, and MENIN. Diagn Mol Pathol 8: 107-112.
1129. Komminoth P, Heitz PU, Kloppel G (1998). Pathology of MEN-1: morphology, clinicopathologic correlations and tumour development. J Intern Med 243: 455-464.
1130. Komminoth P, Kunz E, Hiort O, Schroder S, Matias-Guiu X, Christiansen G, Roth J, Heitz PU (1994). Detection of RET proto-oncogene point mutations in paraffin-embedded pheochromocytoma specimens by nonradioactive single-strand conformation polymorphism analysis and direct sequencing. Am J Pathol 145: 922-929.
1131. Komminoth P, Roth J, Muletta-Feurer S, Saremaslani P, Seelentag WK, Heitz PU (1996). RET proto-oncogene point mutations in sporadic neuroendocrine tumors. J Clin Endocrinol Metab 81: 2041-2046.
1132. Komminoth P, Roth J, Schroder S, Saremaslani P, Heitz PU (1995). Overlapping expression of immunohistochemical markers and synaptophysin mRNA in pheochromocytomas and adrenocortical carcinomas. Implications for the differential diagnosis of adrenal gland tumors. Lab Invest 72: 424-431.
1133. Komminoth P, Seelentag WK, Saremaslani P, Heitz PU, Roth J (1996). CD44 isoform expression in the diffuse neuroendocrine system. II. Benign and malignant tumors. Histochem Cell Biol 106: 551-562.
1134. Kondo K, Klco J, Nakamura E, Lechpammer M, Kaelin WGJr (2002). Inhibition of HIF is necessary for tumor suppression by the von Hippel-Lindau protein. Cancer Cell 1: 237-246.
1135. Kontogeorgos G, Kapranos N (1996). Interphase Analysis of Chromosome 11 in Human Pituitary Somatotroph Adenomas by Direct Fluorescence In Situ Hybridization. Endocr Pathol 7: 203-206.
1136. Kontogeorgos G, Kapranos N, Orphanidis G, Rologis D, Kokka E (1999). Molecular cytogenetics of chromosome 11 in pituitary adenomas: a comparison of fluorescence in situ hybridization and DNA ploidy study. Hum Pathol 30: 1377-1382.
1137. Kontogeorgos G, Kapranos N, Rologis D, Vamvassakis E, Papadopoulos N (1996). DNA measurement in pituitary adenomas assessed on imprints by image analysis. Anal Quant Cytol Histol 18: 144-150.
1138. Kontogeorgos G, Kapranos N, Thoudou E (2001). Applications of FISH in pathology. In: Morphology Methods Cell and Molecular Biology Techniques, Lloyd RV, ed., Humana Press: Totowa , pp. 91-111.
1139. Kontogeorgos G, Kovacs K (1999). Surgical and non-surgical treatment of pituitary adenomas. In: Surgical Technology International, Szabo Z, Lewis JE, Fantini GA, Savalgi RS, eds., 8 ed. Universal Medical Press: San Francisco , pp. 295-304.
1140. Kontogeorgos G, Kovacs K, Horvath E, Scheithauer BW (1991). Multiple adenomas of the human pituitary. A retrospective autopsy study with clinical implications. J Neurosurg 74: 243-247.
1141. Kontogeorgos G, Kovacs K, Horvath E, Scheithauer BW (1993). Null cell adenomas, oncocytomas, and gonadotroph adenomas of the human pituitary: an immunocytochemical and ultrastructural analysis of 300 cases. Endocr Pathol 4: 20-27.
1142. Kontogeorgos G, Kovacs K, Scheithauer BW, Rologis D, Orphanidis G (1991). Alpha-subunit immunoreactivity in plurihormonal pituitary adenomas of patients with acromegaly. Mod Pathol 4: 191-195.
1143. Kontogeorgos G, Sambaziotis D, Piaditis G, Karameris A (1997). Apoptosis in human pituitary adenomas: a morphologic and in situ end-labeling study. Mod Pathol 10: 921-926.
1144. Kontogeorgos G, Scheithauer BW, Horvath E, Kovacs K, Lloyd RV, Smyth HS, Rologis D (1992). Double adenomas of the pituitary: a clinicopathological study of 11 tumors. Neurosurgery 31: 840-849.
1145. Kooijman CD (1988). Immature teratomas in children. Histopathology 12: 491-502.
1146. Korber C, Geling M, Werner E, Mortl M, Mader U, Reiners C, Farahati J (2000). [Incidence of familial non-medullary thyroid carcinoma in the patient register of the Clinic and Polyclinic of Nuclear Medicine, University of Wurzburg]. Nuklearmedizin 39: 27-32.
1147. Korbonits M, Chahal HS, Kaltsas G, Jordan S, Urmanova Y, Khalimova Z, Harris PE, Farrell WE, Claret FX, Grossman AB (2002). Expression of phosphorylated p27(Kip1) protein and Jun activation domain-binding protein 1 in human pituitary tumors. J Clin Endocrinol Metab 87: 2635-2643.
1148. Korbonits M, Jacobs RA, Aylwin SJ, Burrin JM, Dahia PL, Monson JP, Honegger J, Fahlbush R, Trainer PJ, Chew SL, Besser GM, Grossman AB (1998). Expression of the growth hormone secretagogue receptor in pituitary adenomas and other neuroendocrine tumors. J Clin Endocrinol Metab 83: 3624-3630.
1149. Korkiamaki T, Yla-Outinen H, Koivunen J, Karvonen SL, Peltonen J (2002). Altered calcium-mediated cell signaling in keratinocytes cultured from patients with neurofibromatosis type 1. Am J Pathol 160: 1981-1990.
1150. Kouhara H, Tatekawa T, Koga M, Hiraga S, Arita N, Mori H, Sato B (1992). Intracranial and intraspinal dissemination of an ACTH-secreting pituitary tumor. Endocrinol Jpn 39: 177-184.
1151. Kousseff BG, Espinoza C, Zamore GA (1991). Sipple syndrome with lichen amyloidosis as a paracrinopathy: pleiotropy, heterogeneity, or a contiguous gene? J Am Acad Dermatol 25: 651-657.
1152. Kovacs CS, Mase RM, Kovacs K, Nguyen GK, Chik CL (1994). Thyroid medullary carcinoma with thyroglobulin immunoreactivity in sporadic multiple endocrine neoplasia type 2-B. Cancer 74: 928-932.

1153. Kovacs K (1973). Metastatic cancer of the pituitary gland. Oncology 27: 533-542.
1154. Kovacs K, Asa SL (1998). Functional Endocrine Pathology. 2nd ed. Blackwell Science Inc.: Oxford, Boston.
1155. Kovacs K, Horvath E (2001). The differential diagnosis of lesions involving the sella turcica. Endocr Pathol 12: 389-395.
1156. Kovacs K, Horvath E, Bayley TA, Hassaram ST, Ezrin C (1978). Silent corticotroph cell adenoma with lysosomal accumulation and crinophagy. A distinct clinicopathologic entity. Am J Med 64: 492-499.
1157. Kovacs K, Horvath E, Ryan N, Ezrin C (1980). Null cell adenoma of the human pituitary. Virchows Arch A Pathol Anat Histol 387: 165-174.
1158. Kovacs K, Horvath E, Thorner MO, Rogol AD (1984). Mammosomatotroph hyperplasia associated with acromegaly and hyperprolactinemia in a patient with the McCune-Albright syndrome. A histologic, immunocytologic and ultrastructural study of the surgically-removed adenohypophysis. Virchows Arch A Pathol Anat Histopathol 403: 77-86.
1159. Kovacs K, Scheithauer BW, Horvath E, Lloyd RV (1996). The World Health Organization classification of adenohypophysial neoplasms. A proposed five-tier scheme. Cancer 78: 502-510.
1160. Kovacs K, Stefaneanu L, Ezzat S, Smyth HS (1994). Prolactin-producing pituitary adenoma in a male-to-female transsexual patient with protracted estrogen administration. A morphologic study. Arch Pathol Lab Med 118: 562-565.
1161. Kozasa T, Itoh H, Tsukamoto T, Kaziro Y (1988). Isolation and characterization of the human Gs alpha gene. Proc Natl Acad Sci U S A 85: 2081-2085.
1162. Krebs LJ, Arnold A (2002). Molecular basis of hyperparathyroidism and potential targets for drug development. Curr Drug Targets Immune Endocr Metabol Disord 2: 167-179.
1163. Krejs GJ (1987). VIPoma syndrome. Am J Med 82: 37-48.
1164. Krejs GJ, Orci L, Conlon JM, Ravazzola M, Davis GR, Raskin P, Collins SM, McCarthy DM, Baetens D, Rubenstein A, Aldor TA, Unger RH (1979). Somatostatinoma syndrome. Biochemical, morphologic and clinical features. N Engl J Med 301: 285-292.
1165. Krenning EP, Kwekkeboom DJ, Oei HY, de Jong RJ, Dop FJ, Reubi JC, Lamberts SW (1994). Somatostatin-receptor scintigraphy in gastroenteropancreatic tumors. An overview of European results. Ann N Y Acad Sci 733: 416-424.
1166. Krieg M, Haas R, Brauch H, Acker T, Flamme I, Plate KH (2000). Up-regulation of hypoxia-inducible factors HIF-1alpha and HIF-2alpha under normoxic conditions in renal carcinoma cells by von Hippel-Lindau tumor suppressor gene loss of function. Oncogene 19: 5435-5443.
1167. Krieg M, Marti HH, Plate KH (1998). Coexpression of erythropoietin and vascular endothelial growth factor in nervous system tumors associated with von Hippel-Lindau tumor suppressor gene loss of function. Blood 92: 3388-3393.
1168. Krohn K, Paschke R (2001). Clinical review 133: Progress in understanding the etiology of thyroid autonomy. J Clin Endocrinol Metab 86: 3336-3345.
1169. Krohn K, Paschke R (2002). Somatic mutations in thyroid nodular disease. Mol Genet Metab 75: 202-208.
1170. Krohn K, Reske A, Ackermann F, Muller A, Paschke R (2001). Ras mutations are rare in solitary cold and toxic thyroid nodules. Clin Endocrinol (Oxf) 55: 241-248.
1171. Kroll TG, Sarraf P, Pecciarini L, Chen CJ, Mueller E, Spiegelman BM, Fletcher JA (2000). PAX8-PPARgamma1 fusion oncogene in human thyroid carcinoma [corrected]. Science 289: 1357-1360.
1172. Kudva YC, Young WFJr, Thompson GB, Grant CS, van Heerden J (1999). Adrenal incidentaloma: an important component of the clinical presentation spectrum of benign sporadic adrenal pheochromocytoma. Endocrinologist 9: 77-80.
1173. Kuhel WI, Gonzales D, Hoda SA, Pan L, Chiu A, Giri D, DeLellis RA (2001). Synchronous water-clear cell double parathyroid adenomas a hitherto uncharacterized entity? Arch Pathol Lab Med 125: 256-259.
1174. Kuhn JA, Aronoff BL (1989). Nasal and nasopharyngeal paraganglioma. J Surg Oncol 40: 38-45.
1175. Kuhn JM, Lefebvre H, Duparc C, Pellerin A, Luton JP, Strauch G (2002). Cosecretion of estrogen and inhibin B by a feminizing adrenocortical adenoma: impact on gonadotropin secretion. J Clin Endocrinol Metab 87: 2367-2375.
1176. Kulig E, Jin L, Qian X, Horvath E, Kovacs K, Stefaneanu L, Scheithauer BW, Lloyd RV (1999). Apoptosis in nontumorous and neoplastic human pituitaries: expression of the Bcl-2 family of proteins. Am J Pathol 154: 767-774.
1177. Kumar K, Macaulay RJ, Kelly M, Pirlot T (2001). Absent p53 immunohistochemical staining in a pituitary carcinoma. Can J Neurol Sci 28: 174-178.
1178. Kumar PV, Malekhusseini SA, Talei AR (1999). Primary squamous cell carcinoma of the thyroid diagnosed by fine needle aspiration cytology. A report of two cases. Acta Cytol 43: 659-662.
1179. Kunwar S, Wilson CB (1999). Pediatric pituitary adenomas. J Clin Endocrinol Metab 84: 4385-4389.
1180. Kunz J, Amendt P, Hahn von Dorsche H, Gerl H, Knappe E, Lorenz D (1983). [The endocrine pancreas in pluriglandular neoplasia type I. A report of two cases and review of the literature]. Zentralbl Allg Pathol 127: 375-383.
1181. Kuratomi Y, Kumamoto Y, Sakai Y, Komiyama S (1994). Carotid body tumor associated with differentiated thyroid carcinoma. Eur Arch Otorhinolaryngol 251 Suppl 1: S91-S94.
1182. Kurihara N, Takahashi S, Higano S, Ikeda H, Mugikura S, Singh LN, Furuta S, Tamura H, Ishibashi T, Maruoka S, Yamada S (1998). Hemorrhage in pituitary adenoma: correlation of MR imaging with operative findings. Eur Radiol 8: 971-976.
1183. Kuroki M, Tanaka R, Yokoyama M, Shimbo Y, Ikuta F (1987). Subarachnoid dissemination of a pituitary adenoma. Surg Neurol 28: 71-76.
1184. Kurtkaya-Yapicier OWJr (2002). Pituitary adenoma in carney complex: an immunohistochemical, ultrastructural, and immunoelectron microscopic study. Ultrastruct Pathol 26: 345-353.
1185. Kwekkeboom DJ, Lamberts SW, Habbema JD, Krenning EP (1996). Cost-effectiveness analysis of somatostatin receptor scintigraphy. J Nucl Med 37: 886-892.
1186. Kwok CG, McDougall IR (1995). Familial differentiated carcinoma of the thyroid: report of five pairs of siblings. Thyroid 5: 395-397.
1187. Kwon Y, Koo H, Cho K, Kim Y, Ko Y, Ro J (2002). Clinicopathological and immunohistochemical studies in three ectopic cervical thymomas (ECT) and one carcinoma showing thymus-like differentiation (CASTLE). Korean J Pathol 36: S133.
1188. Kytola S, Farnebo F, Obara T, Isola J, Grimelius L, Farnebo LO, Sandelin K, Larsson C (2000). Patterns of chromosomal imbalances in parathyroid carcinomas. Am J Pathol 157: 579-586.
1189. Kytola S, Nord B, Elder EE, Carling T, Kjellman M, Cedermark B, Juhlin C, Hoog A, Isola J, Larsson C (2002). Alterations of the SDHD gene locus in midgut carcinoids, Merkel cell carcinomas, pheochromocytomas, and abdominal paragangliomas. Genes Chromosomes Cancer 34: 325-332.
1190. La Rosa S, Sessa F, Capella C, Riva C, Leone BE, Klersy C, Rindi G, Solcia E (1996). Prognostic criteria in nonfunctioning pancreatic endocrine tumours. Virchows Arch 429: 323-333.
1191. Labate AM, Klimstra DL, Zakowski MF (1997). Comparative cytologic features of pancreatic acinar cell carcinoma and islet cell tumor. Diagn Cytopathol 16: 112-116.
1192. Lack EE (1990). Pathology of the Adrenal Glands. Churchill Livingstone: New York.
1193. Lack EE (1994). Pathology of Adrenal and Extra-Adrenal Paraganglia. W. B. Saunders: Philadelphia.
1194. Lack EE (1995). Atlas of Tumor Pathology. 3rd series ed. Armed Forces Institute of Pathology: Washington, DC.
1195. Lack EE (1997). Tumors of the Adrenal Gland and Extra-Adrenal Paraganglia. 3rd ed. Armed Forces Institute of Pathology: Washington, DC.
1196. Lack EE, Cubilla AL, Woodruff JM, Farr HW (1977). Paragangliomas of the head and neck region: a clinical study of 69 patients. Cancer 39: 397-409.
1197. Ladisch S, Gadner H (1994). Treatment of Langerhans cell histiocytosis—evolution and current approaches. Br J Cancer Suppl 23: S41-S46.
1198. Ladurner D, Totsch M, Luze T, Bangerl I, Sandbichler P, Schmid KW (1990). [Malignant hemangioendothelioma of the thyroid gland. Pathology, clinical aspects and prognosis]. Wien Klin Wochenschr 102: 256-259.
1199. Lafferty AR, Torpy DJ, Stowasser M, Taymans SE, Lin JP, Huggard P, Gordon RD, Stratakis CA (2000). A novel genetic locus for low renin hypertension: familial hyperaldosteronism type II maps to chromosome 7 (7p22). J Med Genet 37: 831-835.
1200. Laforga JB, Vierna J (1996). Adenoma of thyroid gland containing fat (thyrolipoma). Report of a case. J Laryngol Otol 110: 1088-1089.
1201. Laguette J, Matias-Guiu X, Rosai J (1997). Thyroid paraganglioma: a clinicopathologic and immunohistochemical study of three cases. Am J Surg Pathol 21: 748-753.
1202. Lair-Milan F, Blevec GL, Carel JC, Chaussain JL, Adamsbaum C (1996). Thyroid sonographic abnormalities in McCune-Albright syndrome. Pediatr Radiol 26: 424-426.
1203. Lala R, Matarazzo P, Bertelloni S, Buzi F, Rigon F, de Sanctis C (2000). Pamidronate treatment of bone fibrous dysplasia in nine children with McCune-Albright syndrome. Acta Paediatr 89: 188-193.
1204. Lam KY, Chan AC, Chan KW, Leung ML, Srivastava G (1995). Expression of p53 and its relationship with human papillomavirus in penile carcinomas. Eur J Surg Oncol 21: 613-616.
1205. Lam KY, Chan AC, Ng IO (1997). Giant adrenal lipoma: a report of two cases and review of literature. Scand J Urol Nephrol 31: 89-90.
1206. Lam KY, Law S, Tin L, Tung PH, Wong J (1999). The clinicopathological significance of p21 and p53 expression in esophageal squamous cell carcinoma: an analysis of 153 patients. Am J Gastroenterol 94: 2060-2068.
1207. Lam KY, Lo CY (1997). Pancreatic endocrine tumour: a 22-year clinico-pathological experience with morphological, immunohistochemical observation and a review of the literature. Eur J Surg Oncol 23: 36-42.
1208. Lam KY, Lo CY (1998). Metastatic tumors of the thyroid gland: a study of 79 cases in Chinese patients. Arch Pathol Lab Med 122: 37-41.
1209. Lam KY, Lo CY (1999). Composite Pheochromocytoma-Ganglioneuroma of the Adrenal Gland: An Uncommon Entity with Distinctive Clinicopathologic Features. Endocr Pathol 10: 343-352.
1210. Lam KY, Lo CY (1999). Teratoma in the region of adrenal gland: a unique entity masquerading as lipomatous adrenal tumor. Surgery 126: 90-94.
1211. Lam KY, Lo CY (2001). Adrenal lipomatous tumours: a 30 year clinicopathological experience at a single institution. J Clin Pathol 54: 707-712.
1212. Lam KY, Lo CY (2002). Metastatic tumours of the adrenal glands: a 30-year experience in a teaching hospital. Clin Endocrinol (Oxf) 56: 95-101.
1213. Lam KY, Lo CY, Chan KW, Wan KY (2000). Insular and anaplastic carcinoma of the thyroid: a 45-year comparative study at a single institution and a review of the significance of p53 and p21. Ann Surg 231: 329-338.
1214. Lam KY, Lo CY, Fan ST, Luk JM (2000). Telomerase activity in pancreatic endocrine tumours: a potential marker for malignancy. Mol Pathol 53: 133-136.
1215. Lam KY, Lo CY, Liu MC (2001). Primary squamous cell carcinoma of the thyroid gland: an entity with aggressive clinical behaviour and distinctive cytokeratin expression profiles. Histopathology 39: 279-286.
1216. Lam KY, Lo CY, Wat NM, Luk JM, Lam KS (2001). The clinicopathological features and importance of p53, Rb, and mdm2 expression in phaeochromocytomas and paragangliomas. J Clin Pathol 54: 443-448.
1217. Lam KY, Loong F, Shek TW, Chu SM (1998). Composite Paraganglioma-Ganglioneuroma of the Urinary Bladder: A Clinicopathologic, Immunohistochemical, and Ultrastructural Study of a Case and Review of the Literature. Endocr Pathol 9: 353-361.
1218. Lam KY, Lui MC, Lo CY (2001). Cytokeratin expression profiles in thyroid carcinomas. Eur J Surg Oncol 27: 631-635.
1219. Lamberts SW, Tilanus HW, Klooswijk AI, Bruining HA, van der Lely AJ, de Jong FH (1988). Successful treatment with SMS 201-995 of Cushing's syndrome caused by ectopic adrenocorticotropin secretion from a metastatic gastrin-secreting pancreatic islet cell carcinoma. J Clin Endocrinol Metab 67: 1080-1083.
1220. Lamolet B, Pulichino AM,

Lamonerie T, Gauthier Y, Brue T, Enjalbert A, Drouin J (2001). A pituitary cell-restricted T box factor, Tpit, activates POMC transcription in cooperation with Pitx homeoproteins. Cell 104: 849-859.
1221. Lamovec J, Frkovic-Grazio S, Bracko M (1998). Nonsporadic cases and unusual morphological features in pheochromocytoma and paraganglioma. Arch Pathol Lab Med 122: 63-68.
1222. Lamovec J, Zidar A, Zidanik B (1994). Epithelioid angiosarcoma of the thyroid gland. Report of two cases. Arch Pathol Lab Med 118: 642-646.
1223. Landas SK, Leigh C, Bonsib SM, Layne K (1993). Occurrence of melanin in pheochromocytoma. Mod Pathol 6: 175-178.
1224. Landis CA, Masters SB, Spada A, Pace AM, Bourne HR, Vallar L (1989). GTPase inhibiting mutations activate the alpha chain of Gs and stimulate adenylyl cyclase in human pituitary tumours. Nature 340: 692-696.
1225. Landman RE, Horwith M, Peterson RE, Khandji AG, Wardlaw SL (2002). Long-term survival with ACTH-secreting carcinoma of the pituitary: a case report and review of the literature. J Clin Endocrinol Metab 87: 3084-3089.
1226. Landolt AM, Keller PJ, Froesch ER, Mueller J (1982). Bromocriptine: Does it jeopardise the result of later surgery for prolactinomas? Lancet 2: 657-658.
1227. Landolt AM, Shibata T, Kleihues P (1987). Growth rate of human pituitary adenomas. J Neurosurg 67: 803-806.
1228. Landon G, Ordonez NG (1985). Clear cell variant of medullary carcinoma of the thyroid. Hum Pathol 16: 844-847.
1229. Lang W, Choritz H, Hundeshagen H (1986). Risk factors in follicular thyroid carcinomas. A retrospective follow-up study covering a 14-year period with emphasis on morphological findings. Am J Surg Pathol 10: 246-255.
1230. Lang W, Georgii A, Stauch G, Kienzle E (1980). The differentiation of atypical adenomas and encapsulated follicular carcinomas in the thyroid gland. Virchows Arch A Pathol Anat Histol 385: 125-141.
1231. Langer P, Cupisti K, Bartsch DK, Nies C, Goretzki PE, Rothmund M, Roher HD (2002). Adrenal involvement in multiple endocrine neoplasia type 1. World J Surg 26: 891-896.
1232. Larkin DF, Dervan PA, Munnelly J, Finucane J (1986). Sinus histiocytosis with massive lymphadenopathy simulating subacute thyroiditis. Hum Pathol 17: 321-324.
1233. Larsen JB, Schroder HD, Sorensen AG, Bjerre P, Heim S (1999). Simple numerical chromosome aberrations characterize pituitary adenomas. Cancer Genet Cytogenet 114: 144-149.
1234. Larsson C, Skogseid B, Oberg K, Nakamura Y, Nordenskjold M (1988). Multiple endocrine neoplasia type 1 gene maps to chromosome 11 and is lost in insulinoma. Nature 332: 85-87.
1235. Larsson LI, Grimelius L, Hakanson R, Rehfeld JF, Stadil F, Holst J, Angervall L, Sundler F (1975). Mixed endocrine pancreatic tumors producing several peptide hormones. Am J Pathol 79: 271-284.
1236. Larsson LI, Hirsch MA, Holst JJ, Ingemansson S, Kuhl C, Jensen SL, Lundqvist G, Rehfeld JF, Schwartz TW (1977). Pancreatic somatostatinoma. Clinical features and physiological implications. Lancet 1: 666-668.
1237. Larsson LI, Ljungberg O, Sundler F, Hakanson R, Svensson SO, Rehfeld J, Stadil R, Holst J (1973). Antor-pyloric gastrinoma associated with pancreatic nesidioblastosis and proliferation of islets. Virchows Arch A Pathol Pathol Anat 360: 305-314.
1238. Larsson LI, Polak JM, Buffa R, Sundler F, Solcia E (1979). On the immunocytochemical localization of the vasoactive intestinal polypeptide. J Histochem Cytochem 27: 936-938.
1239. Larsson LI, Schwartz T, Lundqvist G, Chance RE, Sundler F, Rehfeld JF, Grimelius L, Fahrenkrug J, Schaffalitzky de Muckadell O, Moon N (1976). Occurrence of human pancreatic polypeptide in pancreatic endocrine tumors. Possible implication in the watery diarrhea syndrome. Am J Pathol 85: 675-684.
1240. Latham PD, Athanasou NA, Woods CG (1992). Fibrous dysplasia with locally aggressive malignant change. Arch Orthop Trauma Surg 111: 183-186.
1241. Latif F, Tory K, Gnarra J, Yao M, Duh FM, Orcutt ML, Stackhouse T, Kuzmin I, Modi W, Geil L, Schmidt L, Zhou FW, Li H, Wei MH, Chen F, Glenn G, Choyke P, Walther MM, Weng YK, Duan DSR, Dean M, Glavac D, Richards FM, Crossey PA, Ferguson-Smith MA, Lepaslier D, Chumakov I, Cohen D, Chinault AC, Maher ER, Linehan WM, Zbar B, Lerman MI (1993). Identification of the von Hippel-Lindau disease tumor suppressor gene. Science 260: 1317-1320.
1242. Latronico AC, Mendonca BB, Bianco AC, Villares SM, Lucon MA, Nicolau W, Wajchenberg BL (1994). Calcium-dependent protein kinase-C activity in human adrenocortical neoplasms, hyperplastic adrenals, and normal adrenocortical tissue. J Clin Endocrinol Metab 79: 736-739.
1243. Latronico AC, Pinto EM, Domenice S, Fragoso MC, Martin RM, Zerbini MC, Lucon AM, Mendonca BB (2001). An inherited mutation outside the highly conserved DNA-binding domain of the p53 tumor suppressor protein in children and adults with sporadic adrenocortical tumors. J Clin Endocrinol Metab 86: 4970-4973.
1244. Lau N, Feldkamp MM, Roncari L, Loehr AH, Shannon P, Gutmann DH, Guha A (2000). Loss of neurofibromin is associated with activation of RAS/MAPK and PI3-K/AKT signaling in a neurofibromatosis 1 astrocytoma. J Neuropathol Exp Neurol 59: 759-767.
1245. Lawrence DA (1978). A histological comparison of adenomatous and hyperplastic parathyroid glands. J Clin Pathol 31: 626-632.
1246. Laws ERJr, Vance ML (2000). Conventional radiotherapy for pituitary tumors. Neurosurg Clin N Am 11: 617-625.
1247. Lax SF, Beham A, Kronberger-Schonecker D, Langsteger W, Denk H (1994). Coexistence of papillary and medullary carcinoma of the thyroid gland-mixed or collision tumour? Clinicopathological analysis of three cases. Virchows Arch 424: 441-447.
1248. Layfield LJ, Glasgow BJ, Du Puis MH, Bhuta S (1987). Aspiration cytology and immunohistochemistry of a pheochromocytoma-ganglioneuroma of the adrenal gland. Acta Cytol 31: 33-39.
1249. Le Bodic MF, Fiche M, Aillet G, Sagan C, Bouc M, Liebault C, Legent F (1991). [Immunohistochemical study of 6 multiple familial cervical paragangliomas with lymph node metastasis in one case]. Ann Pathol 11: 176-180.
1250. Le Bodic MF, Heymann MF, Lecomte M, Berger N, Berger F, Louvel A, De Micco C, Patey M, de Mascarel A, Burtin F, Saint-Andre JP (1996). Immunohistochemical study of 100 pancreatic tumors in 28 patients with multiple endocrine neoplasia, type I. Am J Surg Pathol 20: 1378-1384.
1251. Le Dafniet M, Blumberg-Tick J, Gozlan H, Barret A, Joubert Bression D, Peillon F (1989). Altered balance between thyrotropin-releasing hormone and dopamine in prolactinomas and other pituitary tumors compared to normal pituitaries. J Clin Endocrinol Metab 69: 267-271.
1252. Le Dafniet M, Blumberg-Tick J, Yuan Li J, Brandi AM, Bression D, Barret A, Feinstein MC, Peillon F (1988). [Release of thyrotropin releasing hormone (TRH) from human prolactin-secreting pituitary adenoma cells. Modulation by dopamine]. C R Acad Sci III 306: 129-134.
1253. Le Douarin NM (1988). On the origin of pancreatic endocrine cells. Cell 53: 169-171.
1254. Le Hir H, Charlet-Berguerand N, de Franciscis V, Thermes C (2002). 5'-End RET splicing: absence of variants in normal tissues and intron retention in pheochromocytomas. Oncology 63: 84-91.
1255. Le Quesne LP, Nabarro JD, Kurtz A, Zweig S (1979). The management of insulin tumours of the pancreas. Br J Surg 66: 373-378.
1256. le Roux CW, Mulla A, Meeran K (2001). Pituitary carcinoma as a cause of acromegaly. N Engl J Med 345: 1645-1646.
1257. Leahy MA, Krejci SM, Friednash M, Stockert SS, Wilson H, Huff JC, Weston WL, Brice SL (1993). Human herpesvirus 6 is present in lesions of Langerhans cell histiocytosis. J Invest Dermatol 101: 642-645.
1258. Leath CAI, Huh WK, Straughn JMJr, Conner MG (2002). Uterine leiomyosarcoma metastatic to the thyroid. Obstet Gynecol 100: 1122-1124.
1259. Leboulleux S, Travagli JP, Caillou B, Laplanche A, Bidart JM, Schlumberger M, Baudin E (2002). Medullary thyroid carcinoma as part of a multiple endocrine neoplasia type 2B syndrome: influence of the stage on the clinical course. Cancer 94: 44-50.
1260. Leckschat S, Ream-Robinson D, Scheffler IE (1993). The gene for the iron sulfur protein of succinate dehydrogenase (SDH-IP) maps to human chromosome 1p35-36.1. Somat Cell Mol Genet 19: 505-511.
1261. Lecomte-Houcke M, Parent M, Carnaille B, Baranzelli MC, Chauvet-Hogedez G, Proye C, Dupont A (1992). [Primary malignant teratoma of the thyroid. Two cases involving immunohistochemical and ultrastructural studies]. Ann Pathol 12: 12-19.
1262. Lecomte P, Jan M, Combe H, Gervaise N, Trouillas J (2000). Les adénomes hypophysaires multiples. Rev Fr Endocrinol Clin 41-56.
1263. Lecube A, Hernandez C, Oriola J, Galard R, Gemar E, Mesa J, Simo R (2002). V804M RET mutation and familial medullary thyroid carcinoma: report of a large family with expression of the disease only in the homozygous gene carriers. Surgery 131: 509-514.
1264. Lee CH, Ching KN, Lui WY, P'eng FK, Franklin WA, Kaplan EL (1986). Carcinoid tumor of the pancreas causing the diarrheogenic syndrome: report of a case combined with multiple endocrine neoplasia, type I. Surgery 99: 123-129.
1265. Lee JH, Barich F, Karnell LH, Robinson RA, Zhen WK, Gantz BJ, Hoffman HT (2002). National Cancer Data Base report on malignant paragangliomas of the head and neck. Cancer 94: 730-737.
1266. Lee JS, FitzGibbon E, Butman JA, Dufresne CR, Kushner H, Wientroub S, Robey PG, Collins MT (2002). Normal vision despite narrowing of the optic canal in fibrous dysplasia. N Engl J Med 347: 1670-1676.
1267. Lee PA, Van Dop C, Migeon CJ (1986). McCune-Albright syndrome. Long-term follow-up. JAMA 256: 2980-2984.
1268. Leedham PW, Pollock DJ (1970). Intrafollicular amyloid in primary hyperparathyroidism. J Clin Pathol 23: 811-817.
1269. Leestma JE, Price EBJr (1971). Paraganglioma of the urinary bladder. Cancer 28: 1063-1073.
1270. Legius E, Marchuk DA, Collins FS, Glover TW (1993). Somatic deletion of the neurofibromatosis type 1 gene in a neurofibrosarcoma supports a tumour suppressor gene hypothesis. Nat Genet 3: 122-126.
1271. Leinung MC, Kane LA, Scheithauer BW, Carpenter PC, Laws ERJr, Zimmerman D (1995). Long term follow-up of transsphenoidal surgery for the treatment of Cushing's disease in childhood. J Clin Endocrinol Metab 80: 2475-2479.
1272. Lemmens I, Van de Ven WJ, Kas K, Zhang CX, Giraud S, Wautot V, Buisson N, De Witte K, Salandre J, Lenoir G, Pugeat M, Calender A, Parente F, Quincey D, Gaudray P, de Wit MJ, Lips CJ, Hoppener JW, Khodaei S, Grant AL, Weber G, Kytola S, Teh BT, Farnebo F, Phelan C, Hayward N, Larsson C, Pannett AA, Forbes SA, Bassett JH, Thakker RV (1997). Identification of the multiple endocrine neoplasia type 1 (MEN1) gene. The European Consortium on MEN1. Hum Mol Genet 6: 1177-1183.
1273. Lemmens IH, Forsberg L, Pannett AA, Meyen E, Piehl F, Turner JJ, Van de Ven WJ, Thakker RV, Larsson C, Kas K (2001). Menin interacts directly with the homeobox-containing protein Pem. Biochem Biophys Res Commun 286: 426-431.
1274. Lemoine NR, Mayall ES, Wyllie FS, Farr CJ, Hughes D, Padua RA, Thurston V, Williams ED, Wynford-Thomas D (1988). Activated ras oncogenes in human thyroid cancers. Cancer Res 48: 4459-4463.
1275. Lemoine NR, Mayall ES, Wyllie FS, Williams ED, Goyns M, Stringer B, Wynford-Thomas D (1989). High frequency of ras oncogene activation in all stages of human thyroid tumorigenesis. Oncogene 4: 159-164.
1276. Lenders JW, Keiser HR, Goldstein DS, Willemsen JJ, Friberg P, Jacobs MC, Kloppenborg PW, Thien T, Eisenhofer G (1995). Plasma metanephrines in the diagnosis of pheochromocytoma. Ann Intern Med 123: 101-109.
1277. Lenders JW, Pacak K, Walther MM, Linehan WM, Mannelli M, Friberg P, Keiser HR, Goldstein DS, Eisenhofer G (2002). Biochemical diagnosis of pheochromocytoma: which test is best? JAMA 287: 1427-1434.
1278. Leprat F, Bonichon F, Guyot M, Trouette H, Trojani M, Vergnot V, Longy M, Belleannee G, de Mascarel A, Roger P (1999). Familial non-medullary thyroid carcinoma: pathology review in 27 affected cases from 13 French families. Clin Endocrinol (Oxf) 50: 589-594.
1279. LeRiche VK, Asa SL, Ezzat S (1996).

Epidermal growth factor and its receptor (EGF-R) in human pituitary adenomas: EGF-R correlates with tumor aggressiveness. J Clin Endocrinol Metab 81: 656-662.
1280. Leteurtre E, Brami F, Kerr-Conte J, Quandalle P, Lecomte-Houcke M (2000). Mixed ductal-endocrine carcinoma of the pancreas: a possible pathogenic mechanism for arrhythmogenic right ventricular cardiomyopathy. Arch Pathol Lab Med 124: 284-286.
1281. Levey M (1976). An unusual thyroid tumor in a child. Laryngoscope 86: 1864-1868.
1282. Levin KE, Chew KL, Ljung BM, Mayall BH, Siperstein AE, Clark OH (1988). Deoxyribonucleic acid cytometry helps identify parathyroid carcinomas. J Clin Endocrinol Metab 67: 779-784.
1283. Levin KE, Galante M, Clark OH (1987). Parathyroid carcinoma versus parathyroid adenoma in patients with profound hypercalcemia. Surgery 101: 649-660.
1284. Levy A, Hall L, Yeudall WA, Lightman SL (1994). p53 gene mutations in pituitary adenomas: rare events. Clin Endocrinol (Oxf) 41: 809-814.
1285. Levy A, Lightman SL (1992). Growth hormone-releasing hormone transcripts in human pituitary adenomas. J Clin Endocrinol Metab 74: 1474-1476.
1286. Levy AP, Levy NS, Goldberg MA (1996). Hypoxia-inducible protein binding to vascular endothelial growth factor mRNA and its modulation by the von Hippel-Lindau protein. J Biol Chem 271: 25492-25497.
1287. Levy L, Bourdais J, Mouhieddine B, Benlot C, Villares S, Cohen P, Peillon F, Joubert D (1993). Presence and characterization of the somatostatin precursor in normal human pituitaries and in growth hormone secreting adenomas. J Clin Endocrinol Metab 76: 85-90.
1288. Lewis JE, Wick MR, Scheithauer BW, Bernatz PE, Taylor WF (1987). Thymoma. A clinicopathologic review. Cancer 60: 2727-2743.
1289. Li C, Cheng Y, Gutmann DA, Mangoura D (2001). Differential localization of the neurofibromatosis 1 (NF1) gene product, neurofibromin, with the F-actin or microtubule cytoskeleton during differentiation of telencephalic neurons. Brain Res Dev Brain Res 130: 231-248.
1290. Li M, Wenig BM (2000). Adrenal oncocytic pheochromocytoma. Am J Surg Pathol 24: 1552-1557.
1291. Li WP, Komminoth P, Zuber C, Kloppel G, Heitz PU, Roth J (1996). Can malignancy in insulinoma be predicted by the expression patterns of beta 1,6 branching of asparagine-linked oligosaccharides and polysialic acid of the neural cell adhesion molecule? Virchows Arch 429: 197-204.
1292. Li Y, Bollag G, Clark R, Stevens J, Conroy L, Fults D, Ward K, Friedman E, Samowitz W, Robertson M, Bradley P, McCormick F, White R, Cawthon RM (1992). Somatic mutations in the neurofibromatosis 1 gene in human tumors. Cell 69: 275-281.
1293. Li Y, Koga M, Kasayama S, Matsumoto K, Arita N, Hayakawa T, Sato B (1992). Identification and characterization of high molecular weight forms of basic fibroblast growth factor in human pituitary adenomas. J Clin Endocrinol Metab 75: 1436-1441.
1294. Li Z, Na X, Wang D, Schoen SR, Messing EM, Wu G (2002). Ubiquitination of a novel deubiquitinating enzyme requires direct binding to von Hippel-Lindau tumor suppressor protein. J Biol Chem 277: 4656-4662.
1295. Libutti SK, Choyke PL, Bartlett DL, Vargas H, Walther M, Lubensky I, Glenn G, Linehan WM, Alexander HR (1998). Pancreatic neuroendocrine tumors associated with von Hippel Lindau disease: diagnostic and management recommendations. Surgery 124: 1153-1159.
1296. Liccardo G, Pastore FS, Sherkat S, Signoretti S, Cavazzana A, Fraioli B (1999). Paraganglioma of the cauda equina. Case report with 33-month recurrence free follow-up and review of the literature. J Neurosurg Sci 43: 169-173.
1297. Lidhar K, Korbonits M, Jordan S, Khalimova Z, Kaltsas G, Lu X, Clayton RN, Jenkins PJ, Monson JP, Besser GM, Lowe DG, Grossman AB (1999). Low expression of the cell cycle inhibitor p27Kip1 in normal corticotroph cells, corticotroph tumors, and malignant pituitary tumors. J Clin Endocrinol Metab 84: 3823-3830.
1298. Liechty RD, Teter A, Suba EJ (1986). The tiny parathyroid adenoma. Surgery 100: 1048-1052.
1299. Liens D, Delmas PD, Meunier PJ (1994). Long-term effects of intravenous pamidronate in fibrous dysplasia of bone. Lancet 343: 953-954.
1300. Lifton RP, Dluhy RG, Powers M, Rich GM, Cook S, Ulick S, Lalouel JM (1992). A chimaeric 11 beta-hydroxylase/aldosterone synthase gene causes glucocorticoid-remediable aldosteronism and human hypertension. Nature 355: 262-265.
1301. Ligneau B, Lombard-Bohas C, Partensky C, Valette PJ, Calender A, Dumortier J, Gouysse G, Boulez J, Napoleon B, Berger F, Chayvialle JA, Scoazec JY (2001). Cystic endocrine tumors of the pancreas: clinical, radiologic, and histopathologic features in 13 cases. Am J Surg Pathol 25: 752-760.
1302. Lillehei KO, Kirschman DL, Kleinschmidt-DeMasters BK, Ridgway EC (1998). Reassessment of the role of radiation therapy in the treatment of endocrine-inactive pituitary macroadenomas. Neurosurgery 43: 432-438.
1303. Lin SR, Lee YJ, Tsai JH (1994). Mutations of the p53 gene in human functional adrenal neoplasms. J Clin Endocrinol Metab 78: 483-491.
1304. Lindholm J, Juul S, Jorgensen JO, Astrup J, Bjerre P, Feldt-Rasmussen U, Hagen C, Jorgensen J, Kosteljanetz M, Kristensen L, Laurberg P, Schmidt K, Weeke J (2001). Incidence and late prognosis of cushing's syndrome: a population-based study. J Clin Endocrinol Metab 86: 117-123.
1305. Lindley R, Hoile R, Schofield J, Ashton-Key M (1998). Langerhans cell histiocytosis associated with papillary carcinoma of the thyroid. Histopathology 32: 180.
1306. Linnoila RI, Keiser HR, Steinberg SM, Lack EE (1990). Histopathology of benign versus malignant sympathoadrenal paragangliomas: clinicopathologic study of 120 cases including unusual histologic features. Hum Pathol 21: 1168-1180.
1307. Linnoila RI, Lack EE, Steinberg SM, Keiser HR (1988). Decreased expression of neuropeptides in malignant paragangliomas: an immunohistochemical study. Hum Pathol 19: 41-50.
1308. Lips CJ (1998). Clinical management of the multiple endocrine neoplasia syndromes: results of a computerized opinion poll at the Sixth International Workshop on Multiple Endocrine Neoplasia and von Hippel-Lindau disease. J Intern Med 243: 589-594.
1309. Lips CJ, Landsvater RM, Hoppener JW, Geerdink RA, Blijham G, van Veen JM, van Gils AP, de Wit MJ, Zewald RA, Berends MJ, Beemer FA, Brouwers-Smalbraak J, Jansen RPM, van Amstel HK, van Vroonhoven TJM, Vroom TM (1994). Clinical screening as compared with DNA analysis in families with multiple endocrine neoplasia type 2A. N Engl J Med 331: 828-835.
1310. Listernick R, Charrow J, Greenwald MJ, Esterly NB (1989). Optic gliomas in children with neurofibromatosis type 1. J Pediatr 114: 788-792.
1311. Listernick R, Louis DN, Packer RJ, Gutmann DH (1997). Optic pathway gliomas in children with neurofibromatosis 1: consensus statement from the NF1 Optic Pathway Glioma Task Force. Ann Neurol 41: 143-149.
1312. Liu J, Kahri AI, Heikkila P, Voutilainen R (1997). Ribonucleic acid expression of the clustered imprinted genes, p57KIP2, insulin-like growth factor II, and H19, in adrenal tumors and cultured adrenal cells. J Clin Endocrinol Metab 82: 1766-1771.
1313. Liu J, Litman D, Rosenberg MJ, Yu S, Biesecker LG, Weinstein LS (2000). A GNAS1 imprinting defect in pseudohypoparathyroidism type IB. J Clin Invest 106: 1167-1174.
1314. Liu TH, Zhu Y, Cui QC, Cai LX, Ye SF, Zhong SX, Jia HP (1992). Nonfunctioning pancreatic endocrine tumors. An immunohistochemical and electron microscopic analysis of 26 cases. Pathol Res Pract 188: 191-198.
1315. LiVolsi VA (1990). Surgical Pathology of the Thyroid. Major Problems in Pathology. WB Saunders: Philadelphia.
1316. LiVolsi VA (1992). Papillary neoplasms of the thyroid. Pathologic and prognostic features. Am J Clin Pathol 97: 426-434.
1317. LiVolsi VA (1997). C cell hyperplasia/neoplasia. J Clin Endocrinol Metab 82: 39-41.
1318. LiVolsi VA (2003). Pure versus follicular variant of papillary thyroid carcinoma: clinical features, prognostic factors, treatment, and survival. Cancer 98: 1997-1998.
1319. LiVolsi VA, Asa SL (2002). Endocrine Pathology. Churchill Livingstone: New York.
1320. LiVolsi VA, Brooks JJ, Arendash-Durand B (1987). Anaplastic thyroid tumors. Immunohistology. Am J Clin Pathol 87: 434-442.
1321. LiVolsi VA, Feind CR (1979). Incidental medullary thyroid carcinoma in sporadic hyperparathyroidism. An expansion of the concept of C-cell hyperplasia. Am J Clin Pathol 71: 595-599.
1322. LiVolsi VA, Gupta PK (1992). Thyroid fine-needle aspiration: intranuclear inclusions, nuclear grooves and psammoma bodies—paraganglioma-like adenoma of the thyroid. Diagn Cytopathol 8: 82-83.
1323. Ljungberg O (1992). Biopsy Pathology of the Thyroid and Parathyroid. Chapman & Hall Medical: London.
1324. Ljungberg O, Bondeson L, Bondeson AG (1984). Differentiated thyroid carcinoma, intermediate type: a new tumor entity with features of follicular and parafollicular cell carcinoma. Hum Pathol 15: 218-228.
1325. Ljungberg O, Ericsson UB, Bondeson L, Thorell J (1983). A compound follicular-parafollicular cell carcinoma of the thyroid: a new tumor entity? Cancer 52: 1053-1061.
1326. Ljungberg O, Tibblin S (1979). Peroperative fat staining of frozen sections in primary hyperparathyroidism. Am J Pathol 95: 633-641.
1327. Lloyd HM, Jacobi JM, Cooke RA (1979). Nuclear diameter in parathyroid adenomas. J Clin Pathol 32: 1278-1281.
1328. Lloyd RV (2001). Molecular pathology of pituitary adenomas. J Neurooncol 54: 111-119.
1329. Lloyd RV, Blaivas M, Wilson BS (1985). Distribution of chromogranin and S100 protein in normal and abnormal adrenal medullary tissues. Arch Pathol Lab Med 109: 633-635.
1330. Lloyd RV, Carney JA, Ferreiro JA, Jin L, Thompson GB, van Heerden JA, Grant CS, Wollan PC (1995). Immunohistochemical Analysis of the Cell Cycle-Associated Antigens Ki-67 and Retinoblastoma Protein in Parathyroid Carcinomas and Adenomas. Endocr Pathol 6: 279-287.
1331. Lloyd RV, Chandler WF, Kovacs K, Ryan N (1986). Ectopic pituitary adenomas with normal anterior pituitary glands. Am J Surg Pathol 10: 546-552.
1332. Lloyd RV, Erickson LA, Jin L, Kulig E, Qian X, Cheville JC, Scheithauer BW (1999). p27kip1: a multifunctional cyclin-dependent kinase inhibitor with prognostic significance in human cancers. Am J Pathol 154: 313-323.
1333. Lloyd RV, Fields K, Jin L, Horvath E, Kovacs K (1990). Analysis of endocrine active and clinically silent corticotropic adenomas by in situ hybridization. Am J Pathol 137: 479-488.
1334. Lloyd RV, Jin L, Qian X, Kulig E (1997). Aberrant p27kip1 expression in endocrine and other tumors. Am J Pathol 150: 401-407.
1335. Lloyd RV, Johnson TL, Blaivas M, Sisson JC, Wilson BS (1985). Detection of HLA-DR antigens in paraffin-embedded thyroid epithelial cells with a monoclonal antibody. Am J Pathol 120: 106-111.
1336. Lloyd RV, Mervak T, Schmidt K, Warner TF, Wilson BS (1984). Immunohistochemical detection of chromogranin and neuron-specific enolase in pancreatic endocrine neoplasms. Am J Surg Pathol 8: 607-614.
1337. Lloyd RV, Scheithauer BW, Kovacs K, Roche PC (1996). The Immunophenotype of Pituitary Adenomas. Endocr Pathol 7: 145-150.
1338. Lloyd RV, Sisson JC, Marangos PJ (1983). Calcitonin, carcinoembryonic antigen and neuron-specific enolase in medullary thyroid carcinoma. Cancer 51: 2234-2239.
1339. Lloyd RV, Sisson JC, Shapiro B, Verhofstad AA (1986). Immunohistochemical localization of epinephrine, norepinephrine, catecholamine-synthesizing enzymes, and chromogranin in neuroendocrine cells and tumors. Am J Pathol 125: 45-54.
1340. Lloyd RV, Vidal S, Horvath E, Kovacs K, Scheithauer B (2003). Angiogenesis in normal and neoplastic pituitary tissues. Microsc Res Tech 60: 244-250.
1341. Lo CY, Lam KY, Wan KY (1999). Anaplastic carcinoma of the thyroid. Am J Surg 177: 337-339.
1342. Lo CY, van Heerden JA, Soreide JA,

Grant CS, Thompson GB, Lloyd RV, Harmsen WS (1996). Adrenalectomy for metastatic disease to the adrenal glands. Br J Surg 83: 528-531.
1343. Lockhart ME, Smith JK, Kenney PJ (2002). Imaging of adrenal masses. Eur J Radiol 41: 95-112.
1344. Loh KC (1997). Familial nonmedullary thyroid carcinoma: a meta-review of case series. Thyroid 7: 107-113.
1345. Loh KC, Greenspan FS, Gee L, Miller TR, Yeo PP (1997). Pathological tumor-node-metastasis (pTNM) staging for papillary and follicular thyroid carcinomas: a retrospective analysis of 700 patients. J Clin Endocrinol Metab 82: 3553-3562.
1346. Lohmann DR, Funk A, Niedermeyer HP, Haupel S, Hofler H (1993). Identification of p53 gene mutations in gastrointestinal and pancreatic carcinoids by nonradioisotopic SSCA. Virchows Arch B Cell Pathol Incl Mol Pathol 64: 293-296.
1347. Lombardo F, Baudin E, Chiefari E, Arturi F, Bardet S, Caillou B, Conte C, Dallapiccola B, Giuffrida D, Bidart JM, Schlumberger M, Filetti S (2002). Familial medullary thyroid carcinoma: clinical variability and low aggressiveness associated with RET mutation at codon 804. J Clin Endocrinol Metab 87: 1674-1680.
1348. Lonergan KM, Iliopoulos O, Ohh M, Kamura T, Conaway RC, Conaway JW, Kaelin WGJr (1998). Regulation of hypoxia-inducible mRNAs by the von Hippel-Lindau tumor suppressor protein requires binding to complexes containing elongins B/C and Cul2. Mol Cell Biol 18: 732-741.
1349. Long RG (1983). Vasoactive intestinal polypeptide-secreting tumours (vipomas) in childhood. J Pediatr Gastroenterol Nutr 2: 122-126.
1350. Lopes MB, Lanzino G, Cloft HJ, Winston DC, Vance ML, Laws ERJr (1998). Primary fibrosarcoma of the sella unrelated to previous radiation therapy. Mod Pathol 11: 579-584.
1351. Lopes MB, Salmon I, Nagy N, Decaestecker C, Pasteels JL, Laws ERJr, Kiss R (1997). Computer-Assisted Microscope Analysis of Feulgen-Stained Nuclei in Gonadotroph Adenomas and Null-Cell Adenomas of the Pituitary Gland. Endocr Pathol 8: 109-120.
1352. Lopez-Correa C, Brems H, Lazaro C, Estivill X, Clementi M, Mason S, Rutkowski JL, Marynen P, Legius E (1999). Molecular studies in 20 submicroscopic neurofibromatosis type 1 gene deletions. Hum Mutat 14: 387-393.
1353. Lopez-Egido J, Cunningham J, Berg M, Oberg K, Bongcam-Rudloff E, Gobl A (2002). Menin's interaction with glial fibrillary acidic protein and vimentin suggests a role for the intermediate filament network in regulating menin activity. Exp Cell Res 278: 175-183.
1354. Los M, Jansen GH, Kaelin WG, Lips CJ, Blijham GH, Voest EE (1996). Expression pattern of the von Hippel-Lindau protein in human tissues. Lab Invest 75: 231-238.
1355. Lote K, Andersen K, Nordal E, Brennhovd IO (1980). Familial occurrence of papillary thyroid carcinoma. Cancer 46: 1291-1297.
1356. Lubensky I (2002). Endocrine pancreas. In: Endocrine Pathology, LiVolsi VA, Asa SL, eds., Churchill Livingstone: Philadelphia , pp. 205-235.
1357. Lubensky IA, Pack S, Ault D, Vortmeyer AO, Libutti SK, Choyke PL, Walther MM, Linehan WM, Zhuang Z (1998). Multiple neuroendocrine tumors of the pancreas in von Hippel-Lindau disease patients: histopathological and molecular genetic analysis. Am J Pathol 153: 223-231.
1358. Lubke D, Saeger W (1995). Carcinomas of the pituitary: definition and review of the literature. Gen Diagn Pathol 141: 81-92.
1359. Lubke D, Saeger W, Ludecke DK (1995). Proliferation Markers and EGF in ACTH-Secreting Adenomas and Carcinomas of the Pituitary. Endocr Pathol 6: 45-55.
1360. Lubs ML, Bauer MS, Formas ME, Djokic B (1991). Lisch nodules in neurofibromatosis type 1. N Engl J Med 324: 1264-1266.
1361. Lucas E, Sundaram M, Boccini T (1995). Radiologic case study. Polyostotic fibrous dysplasia. Orthopedics 18: 311-313.
1362. Lucot H, David JF, Boneu A, Combes PF, Cabarrot E, Daly N (1979). [Thyroid trabecular carcinoma. A clinicopathological entity of poor prognosis? (author's transl)]. Bull Cancer 66: 279-286.
1363. Ludvikova M, Ryska A, Korabecna M, Rydlova M, Michal M (2001). Oncocytic papillary carcinoma with lymphoid stroma (Warthin-like tumour) of the thyroid: a distinct entity with favourable prognosis. Histopathology 39: 17-24.
1364. Lui W, Leibiger I, Leibiger B, Thoppe S, Enberg U, Liden J, Hoog A, Farnebo L, Fletcher J, Kroll T, Larsson C (2003). A novel gene, FTCF, is fused to PPARg in follicular thyroid carcinoma (SUBMITTED). Hum Mol Genet .
1365. Lui WO, Chen J, Glasker S, Bender BU, Madura C, Khoo SK, Kort E, Larsson C, Neumann HP, Teh BT (2002). Selective loss of chromosome 11 in pheochromocytomas associated with the VHL syndrome. Oncogene 21: 1117-1122.
1366. Lui WO, Kytola S, Anfalk L, Larsson C, Farnebo LO (2000). Balanced translocation (3;7)(p25;q34): another mechanism of tumorigenesis in follicular thyroid carcinoma? Cancer Genet Cytogenet 119: 109-112.
1367. Luketich JD, Burt ME (1996). Does resection of adrenal metastases from non-small cell lung cancer improve survival? Ann Thorac Surg 62: 1614-1616.
1368. Lupoli G, Vitale G, Caraglia M, Fittipaldi MR, Abbruzzese A, Tagliaferri P, Bianco AR (1999). Familial papillary thyroid microcarcinoma: a new clinical entity. Lancet 353: 637-639.
1369. Luton JP, Cerdas S, Billaud L, Thomas G, Guilhaume B, Bertagna X, Laudat MH, Louvel A, Chapuis Y, Blondeau P, Bonnin A, Bricaire H (1990). Clinical features of adrenocortical carcinoma, prognostic factors, and the effect of mitotane therapy. N Engl J Med 322: 1195-1201.
1370. Luton JP, Martinez M, Coste J, Bertherat J (2000). Outcome in patients with adrenal incidentaloma selected for surgery: an analysis of 88 cases investigated in a single clinical center. Eur J Endocrinol 143: 111-117.
1371. Luttges J, Pierre E, Zamboni G, Weh G, Lietz H, Kussmann J, Kloppel G (1997). [Malignant non-epithelial tumors of the pancreas]. Pathologe 18: 233-237.
1372. Luzi P, Miracco C, Lio R, Malandrini A, Piovani S, Giovanni Venezia S, Tosi P (1987). Endocrine inactive pituitary carcinoma metastasizing to cervical lymph nodes: a case report. Hum Pathol 18: 90-92.
1373. Lyons J, Landis CA, Harsh G, Vallar L, Grunewald K, Feichtinger H, Duh QY, Clark OH, Kawasaki E, Bourne HR, McCormick F (1990). Two G protein oncogenes in human endocrine tumors. Science 249: 655-659.
1374. Ma W, Ikeda H, Yoshimoto T (2002). Clinicopathologic study of 123 cases of prolactin-secreting pituitary adenomas with special reference to multihormone production and clonality of the adenomas. Cancer 95: 258-266.
1375. MacMahon HE (1971). Albirght's syndrome- thirty years later (polyostotic fibrous dysplasia). In: Pathology Annual, Sommers SC, ed., Appleton-Century-Crofts: New York , pp. 81-146.
1376. Macpherson P, Hadley DM, Teasdale E, Teasdale G (1989). Pituitary microadenomas. Does Gadolinium enhance their demonstration? Neuroradiology 31: 293-298.
1377. Magalhaes MC (1972). A new crystal-containing cell in human adrenal cortex. J Cell Biol 55: 126-133.
1378. Maher CO, Friedman JA, Meyer FB, Lynch JJ, Unni K, Raffel C (2002). Surgical treatment of fibrous dysplasia of the skull in children. Pediatr Neurosurg 37: 87-92.
1379. Maher ER, Eng C (2002). The pressure rises: update on the genetics of phaeochromocytoma. Hum Mol Genet 11: 2347-2354.
1380. Maher ER, Iselius L, Yates JR, Littler M, Benjamin C, Harris R, Sampson J, Williams A, Ferguson-Smith MA, Morton N (1991). Von Hippel-Lindau disease: a genetic study. J Med Genet 28: 443-447.
1381. Maher ER, Webster AR, Richards FM, Green JS, Crossey PA, Payne SJ, Moore AT (1996). Phenotypic expression in von Hippel-Lindau disease: correlations with germline VHL gene mutations. J Med Genet 33: 328-332.
1382. Maher ER, Yates JR, Ferguson-Smith MA (1990). Statistical analysis of the two stage mutation model in von Hippel-Lindau disease, and in sporadic cerebellar haemangioblastoma and renal cell carcinoma. J Med Genet 27: 311-314.
1383. Maher ER, Yates JR, Harries R, Benjamin C, Harris R, Moore AT, Ferguson-Smith MA (1990). Clinical features and natural history of von Hippel-Lindau disease. Q J Med 77: 1151-1163.
1384. Mahler C, Verhelst J, Klaes R, Trouillas J (1991). Cushing's disease and hyperprolactinemia due to a mixed. Pathol Res Pract 187: 598-602.
1385. Mahzoon S, Wood MG (1980). Multifocal eosinophilic granuloma with skin ulceration. Histiocytosis X of the Hand-Schuller-Christian type. Arch Dermatol 116: 218-220.
1386. Mai KT, Landry DC, Thomas J, Burns BF, Commons AS, Yazdi HM, Odell PF (2001). Follicular adenoma with papillary architecture: a lesion mimicking papillary thyroid carcinoma. Histopathology 39: 25-32.
1387. Maiorana A, Collina G, Cesinaro AM, Fano RA, Eusebi V (1996). Epithelioid angiosarcoma of the thyroid. Clinicopathological analysis of seven cases from non-Alpine areas. Virchows Arch 429: 131-137.
1388. Majewski JT, Wilson SD (1979). The MEA-I syndrome: an all or none phenomenon? Surgery 86: 475-484.
1389. Maki M, Kaneko Y, Ohta Y, Nakamura T, Machinami R, Kurokawa K (1995). Somatostatinoma of the pancreas associated with von Hippel-Lindau disease. Intern Med 34: 661-665.
1390. Maki M, Saitoh K, Horiuchi H, Morohoshi T, Fukayama M, Machinami R (2001). Comparative study of fibrous dysplasia and osteofibrous dysplasia: histopathological, immunohistochemical, argyrophilic nucleolar organizer region and DNA ploidy analysis. Pathol Int 51: 603-611.
1391. Malchoff CD, Malchoff DM (1999). Familial nonmedullary thyroid carcinoma. Semin Surg Oncol 16: 16-18.
1392. Malchoff CD, Malchoff DM (2002). The genetics of hereditary nonmedullary thyroid carcinoma. J Clin Endocrinol Metab 87: 2455-2459.
1393. Malchoff CD, Sarfarazi M, Tendler B, Forouhar F, Whalen G, Joshi V, Arnold A, Malchoff DM (2000). Papillary thyroid carcinoma associated with papillary renal neoplasia: genetic linkage analysis of a distinct heritable tumor syndrome. J Clin Endocrinol Metab 85: 1758-1764.
1394. Malchoff CD, Sarfarazi M, Tendler B, Forouhar F, Whalen G, Malchoff DM (1999). Familial papillary thyroid carcinoma is genetically distinct from familial adenomatous polyposis coli. Thyroid 9: 247-252.
1395. Mallette LE (1992). DNA quantitation in the study of parathyroid lesions. A review. Am J Clin Pathol 98: 305-311.
1396. Mallette LE, Malini S, Rappaport MP, Kirkland JL (1987). Familial cystic parathyroid adenomatosis. Ann Intern Med 107: 54-60.
1397. Mallinson CN, Bloom SR, Warin AP, Salmon PR, Cox B (1974). A glucagonoma syndrome. Lancet 2: 1-5.
1398. Manenti G, Pilotti S, Re FC, Della Porta G, Pierotti MA (1994). Selective activation of ras oncogenes in follicular and undifferentiated thyroid carcinomas. Eur J Cancer 30A: 987-993.
1399. Manetto V, Lorenzini R, Cordon-Cardo C, Krajewski S, Rosai J, Reed JC, Eusebi V (1997). Bcl-2 and Bax expression in thyroid tumours. An immunohistochemical and western blot analysis. Virchows Arch 430: 125-130.
1400. Manger WM, Gifford RW (2002). Pheochromocytoma. J Clin Hypertens (Greenwich) 4: 62-72.
1401. Mannelli M, Ianni L, Cilotti A, Conti A (1999). Pheochromocytoma in Italy: a multicentric retrospective study. Eur J Endocrinol 141: 619-624.
1402. Manski TJ, Heffner DK, Glenn GM, Patronas NJ, Pikus AT, Katz D, Lebovics R, Sledjeski K, Choyke PL, Zbar B, Linehan WM, Oldfield EH (1997). Endolymphatic sac tumors. A source of morbid hearing loss in von Hippel-Lindau disease. JAMA 277: 1461-1466.
1403. Mantovani G, Ballare E, Giammona E, Beck-Peccoz P, Spada A (2002). The gsalpha gene: predominant maternal origin of transcription in human thyroid gland and gonads. J Clin Endocrinol Metab 87: 4736-4740.
1404. Maranchie JK, Vasselli JR, Riss J, Bonifacino JS, Linehan WM, Klausner RD (2002). The contribution of VHL substrate binding and HIF1-alpha to the phenotype of VHL loss in renal cell carcinoma. Cancer Cell 1: 247-255.
1405. Marcus JN, Dise CA, LiVolsi VA (1982). Melanin production in a medullary thyroid carcinoma. Cancer 49: 2518-2526.
1406. Margolis RM, Jang N (1984). Zollinger-Ellison syndrome associated with pancreatic cystadenocarcinoma. N Engl J Med 311: 1380-1381.
1407. Marie P (1886). Sur deux cas d'acromégalie ; hypertrophie singulière non congénitale des extrémites supérieures, inférieures et céphalique. Rev

Med 6: 297-333.
1408. Mariman EC, van Beersum SE, Cremers CW, Struycken PM, Ropers HH (1995). Fine mapping of a putatively imprinted gene for familial non-chromaffin paragangliomas to chromosome 11q13.1: evidence for genetic heterogeneity. Hum Genet 95: 56-62.
1409. Mark L, Pech P, Daniels D, Charles C, Williams A, Haughton V (1984). The pituitary fossa: a correlative anatomic and MR study. Radiology 153: 453-457.
1410. Marks IN, Bank S, Louw JH (1967). Islet cell tumor of the pancreas with reversible watery diarrhea and achylorhydraia. Gastroenterology 52: 695-708.
1411. Marques AR, Espadinha C, Catarino AL, Moniz S, Pereira T, Sobrinho LG, Leite V (2002). Expression of PAX8-PPAR gamma 1 rearrangements in both follicular thyroid carcinomas and adenomas. J Clin Endocrinol Metab 87: 3947-3952.
1412. Marsh DJ, Coulon V, Lunetta KL, Rocca-Serra P, Dahia PL, Zheng Z, Liaw D, Caron S, Duboue B, Lin AY, Richardson AL, Bonnetblanc JM, Bressieux JM, Cabarrot-Moreau A, Chompret A, Demange L, Eeles RA, Yahanda AM, Fearon ER, Fricker JP, Gorlin RJ, Hodgson SV, Huson S, Lacombe D, Leprat F, Odent S, Toulouse C, Olopade OI, Sobol H, Tishler S, Woods CG, Robinson BG, Weber HC, Parsons R, Peacocke M, Longy M, Eng C (1998). Mutation spectrum and genotype-phenotype analyses in Cowden disease and Bannayan-Zonana syndrome, two hamartoma syndromes with germline PTEN mutation. Hum Mol Genet 7: 507-515.
1413. Marsh DJ, Theodosopoulos G, Martin-Schulte K, Richardson AL, Philips J, Roher HD, Delbridge L, Robinson BG (2003). Genome-wide copy number imbalances identified in familial and sporadic medullary thyroid carcinoma. J Clin Endocrinol Metab 88: 1866-1872.
1414. Martella EM, Ferraro G, Azzoni C, Marignani M, Bordi C (1997). Pancreatic-polypeptide cell hyperplasia associated with pancreatic or duodenal gastrinomas. Hum Pathol 28: 149-153.
1415. Martelli ML, Iuliano R, Le Pera I, Sama' I, Monaco C, Cammarota S, Kroll T, Chiariotti L, Santoro M, Fusco A (2002). Inhibitory effects of peroxisome poliferator-activated receptor gamma on thyroid carcinoma cell growth. J Clin Endocrinol Metab 87: 4728-4735.
1416. Martignoni ME, Friess H, Lubke D, Uhl W, Maurer C, Muller M, Richard H, Reubi JC, Buchler MW (1999). Study of a primary gastrinoma in the common hepatic duct - a case report. Digestion 60: 187-190.
1417. Martin-Lacave I, Gonzalez-Campora R, Moreno-Fernandez A, Sachez-Gallego F, Montero C, Galera-Davidson H (1988). Mucosubstances in medullary carcinoma of the thyroid. Histopathology 13: 55-66.
1418. Martin-Zanca D, Hughes SH, Barbacid M (1986). A human oncogene formed by the fusion of truncated tropomyosin and protein tyrosine kinase sequences. Nature 319: 743-748.
1419. Martin JM, Randhawa G, Temple WJ (1986). Cervical thymoma. Arch Pathol Lab Med 110: 354-357.
1420. Martinez AJ (1986). The pathology of nonfunctional pituitary adenomas. Semin Diagn Pathol 3: 83-94.
1421. Marx S (2001). Multiple endocrine neoplasia type 1. In: The Metabolic and Molecular Bases of Inherited Disease, Scriver CR, Sly WS, Childs B, eds., 8th ed. McGraw-Hill Professional: New York , pp. 943-966.
1422. Marx SJ, Nieman LK (2002). Aggressive pituitary tumors in MEN1: do they refute the two-hit model of tumorigenesis? J Clin Endocrinol Metab 87: 453-456.
1423. Marx SJ, Simonds WF, Agarwal SK, Burns AL, Weinstein LS, Cochran C, Skarulis MC, Spiegel AM, Libutti SK, Alexander HRJr, Chen CC, Chang R, Chandrasekharappa SC, Collins FS (2002). Hyperparathyroidism in hereditary syndromes: special expressions and special managements. J Bone Miner Res 17 Suppl 2: N37-N43.
1424. Marzano AV, Gasparini G, Grammatica A, de Juli E, Caputo R (1998). Langerhans cell histiocytosis and thyroid carcinoma. Br J Dermatol 138: 909-910.
1425. Masse SR, Wolk RW, Conklin RH (1973). Peripituitary gland involvement in acute leukemia in adults. Arch Pathol 96: 141-142.
1426. Mastorakos G, Mitsiades NS, Doufas AG, Koutras DA (1997). Hyperthyroidism in McCune-Albright syndrome with a review of thyroid abnormalities sixty years after the first report. Thyroid 7: 433-439.
1427. Masuoka J, Brandner S, Paulus W, Soffer D, Vital A, Chimelli L, Jouvet A, Yonekawa Y, Kleihues P, Ohgaki H (2001). Germline SDHD mutation in paraganglioma of the spinal cord. Oncogene 20: 5084-5086.
1428. Matias-Guiu X (1999). Mixed medullary and follicular carcinoma of the thyroid. On the search for its histogenesis. Am J Pathol 155: 1413-1418.
1429. Matias-Guiu X, Caixas A, Costa I, Cabezas R, Prat J (1994). Compound medullary-papillary carcinoma of the thyroid: true mixed versus collision tumour [corrected]. Histopathology 25: 183-185.
1430. Matias-Guiu X, Colomer A, Mato E, Cuatrecasas M, Komminoth P, Prat J, Wolfe H (1995). Expression of the ret protooncogene in phaeochromocytoma. An in situ hybridization and northern blot study. J Pathol 176: 63-68.
1431. Matias-Guiu X, Garrastazu MT (1998). Composite phaeochromocytoma-ganglioneuroblastoma in a patient with multiple endocrine neoplasia type IIA. Histopathology 32: 281-282.
1432. Matias-Guiu X, Laguette J, Puras-Gil AM, Rosai J (1997). Metastatic neuroendocrine tumors to the thyroid gland mimicking medullary carcinoma: a pathologic and immunohistochemical study of six cases. Am J Surg Pathol 21: 754-762.
1433. Matias-Guiu X, Machin P, Pons C, Lagarda E, De Leiva A, Prat J (1998). Sustentacular cells occur frequently in the familial form of medullary thyroid carcinoma. J Pathol 184: 420-423.
1434. Matias-Guiu X, Peiro G, Esquius J, Oliva E, Cabezas R, Colomer A, Prat J (1995). Proliferative activity in C-cell hyperplasia and medullary thyroid carcinoma. Evaluation by PCNA immunohistochemistry and AgNORs staining. Pathol Res Pract 191: 42-47.
1435. Matias-Guiu X, Villanueva A, Cuatrecasas M, Capella G, De Leiva A, Prat J (1996). p53 in a thyroid follicular carcinoma with foci of poorly differentiated and anaplastic carcinoma. Pathol Res Pract 192: 1242-1249.
1436. Maton PN, Gardner JD, Jensen RT (1986). Cushing's syndrome in patients with the Zollinger-Ellison syndrome. N Engl J Med 315: 1-5.
1437. Matsumoto KK, Peter JB, Schultze RG, Hakim AA, Franck PT (1966). Watery diarrhea and hypokalemia associated with pancreatic islet cell adenoma. Gastroenterology 50: 231-242.
1438. Matsumoto T, Imamura O, Yamabe Y, Kuromitsu J, Tokutake Y, Shimamoto A, Suzuki N, Satoh M, Kitao S, Ichikawa K, Kataoka H, Sugawara K, Thomas W, Mason B, Tsuchihashi Z, Drayna D, Sugawara M, Sugimoto M, Furuichi Y, Goto M (1997). Mutation and haplotype analyses of the Werner's syndrome gene based on its genomic structure: genetic epidemiology in the Japanese population. Hum Genet 100: 123-130.
1439. Matsumura A, Meguro K, Doi M, Tsurushima H, Tomono Y (1990). Suprasellar ectopic pituitary adenoma: case report and review of the literature. Neurosurgery 26: 681-685.
1440. Matsuo K, Tang SH, Fagin JA (1991). Allelotype of human thyroid tumors: loss of chromosome 11q13 sequences in follicular neoplasms. Mol Endocrinol 5: 1873-1879.
1441. Matthews P, Jones CJ, Skinner J, Haughton M, De Micco C, Wynford-Thomas D (2001). Telomerase activity and telomere length in thyroid neoplasia: biological and clinical implications. J Pathol 194: 183-193.
1442. Mauras N, Blizzard RM (1986). The McCune-Albright syndrome. Acta Endocrinol Suppl (Copenh) 279: 207-217.
1443. Maurea S, Cuocolo A, Reynolds JC, Neumann RD, Salvatore M (1996). Diagnostic imaging in patients with paragangliomas. Computed tomography, magnetic resonance and MIBG scintigraphy comparison. Q J Nucl Med 40: 365-371.
1444. Maurea S, Lastoria S, Klain M, Brunetti A, Boscaino A, Lupoli G, Salvatore M (1994). Diagnostic evaluation of thyroid involvement by histiocytosis X. J Nucl Med 35: 263-265.
1445. Maury CP (1990). beta 2-Microglobulin amyloidosis. A systemic amyloid disease affecting primarily synovium and bone in long-term dialysis patients. Rheumatol Int 10: 1-8.
1446. Max MB, Deck MD, Rottenberg DA (1981). Pituitary metastasis: incidence in cancer patients and clinical differentiation from pituitary adenoma. Neurology 31: 998-1002.
1447. Maximo V, Soares P, Lima J, Cameselle-Teijeiro J, Sobrinho-Simoes M (2002). Mitochondrial DNA somatic mutations (point mutations and large deletions) and mitochondrial DNA variants in human thyroid pathology: a study with emphasis on Hurthle cell tumors. Am J Pathol 160: 1857-1865.
1448. Maxwell PH, Wiesener MS, Chang GW, Clifford SC, Vaux EC, Cockman ME, Wykoff CC, Pugh CW, Maher ER, Ratcliffe PJ (1999). The tumour suppressor protein VHL targets hypoxia-inducible factors for oxygen-dependent proteolysis. Nature 399: 271-275.
1449. Mayo-Smith WW, Boland GW, Noto RB, Lee MJ (2001). State-of-the-art adrenal imaging. Radiographics 21: 995-1012.
1450. Mayr NA, Yuh WT, Muhonen MG, Koci TM, Tali ET, Nguyen HD, Bergman RA, Jinkins JR (1993). Pituitary metastases: MR findings. J Comput Assist Tomogr 17: 432-437.
1451. Mazzaferri EL, Jhiang SM (1994). Long-term impact of initial surgical and medical therapy on papillary and follicular thyroid cancer. Am J Med 97: 418-428.
1452. Mazzaferri EL, Robbins RJ, Spencer CA, Braverman LE, Pacini F, Wartofsky L, Haugen BR, Sherman SI, Cooper DS, Braunstein GD, Lee S, Davies TF, Arafah BM, Ladenson PW, Pinchera A (2003). A consensus report of the role of serum thyroglobulin as a monitoring method for low-risk patients with papillary thyroid carcinoma. J Clin Endocrinol Metab 88: 1433-1441.
1453. McCaffrey TV, Meyer FB, Michels VV, Piepgras DG, Marion MS (1994). Familial paragangliomas of the head and neck. Arch Otolaryngol Head Neck Surg 120: 1211-1216.
1454. McCall A, Jarosz H, Lawrence AM, Paloyan E (1986). The incidence of thyroid carcinoma in solitary cold nodules and in multinodular goiters. Surgery 100: 1128-1132.
1455. McClain K, Weiss RA (1994). Viruses and Langerhans cell histiocytosis: is there a link? Br J Cancer Suppl 23: S34-S36.
1456. McCluggage WG, Sloan JM (1996). Hyalinizing trabecular carcinoma of thyroid gland. Histopathology 28: 357-362.
1457. McComb DJ, Ryan N, Horvath E, Kovacs K (1983). Subclinical adenomas of the human pituitary. New light on old problems. Arch Pathol Lab Med 107: 488-491.
1458. McCormick PC, Post KD, Kandji AD, Hays AP (1989). Metastatic carcinoma to the pituitary gland. Br J Neurosurg 3: 71-79.
1459. McCune DJ, Bruch H (1937). Osteodystrophia fibrosa. Report of a case in which the condition was combined with precocious puberty, pathologic pigmentation of the skin and hyperthyroidism, a review of the literature. Am J Dis Child 54: 806-848.
1460. McCutcheon IE, Pieper DR, Fuller GN, Benjamin RS, Friend KE, Gagel RF (2000). Pituitary carcinoma containing gonadotropins: treatment by radical excision and cytotoxic chemotherapy: case report. Neurosurgery 46: 1233-1239.
1461. McDermott MB, Swanson PE, Wick MR (1995). Immunostains for collagen type IV discriminate between C-cell hyperplasia and microscopic medullary carcinoma in multiple endocrine neoplasia, type 2a. Hum Pathol 26: 1308-1312.
1462. McGaughran JM, Harris DI, Donnai D, Teare D, MacLeod R, Westerbeek R, Kingston H, Super M, Harris R, Evans DG (1999). A clinical study of type 1 neurofibromatosis in north west England. J Med Genet 36: 197-203.
1463. McGregor DH, Lotuaco LG, Rao MS, Chu LL (1978). Functioning oxyphil adenoma of parathyroid gland. An ultrastructural and biochemical study. Am J Pathol 92: 691-711.
1464. McIver B, Hay ID, Giuffrida DF, Dvorak CE, Grant CS, Thompson GB, van Heerden JA, Goellner JR (2001). Anaplastic thyroid carcinoma: a 50-year experience at a single institution. Surgery 130: 1028-1034.
1465. McKay JD, Lesueur F, Jonard L, Pastore A, Williamson J, Hoffman L, Burgess J, Duffield A, Papotti M, Stark M, Sobol H, Maes B, Murat A, Kaariainen H, Bertholon-Gregoire M, Zini M, Rossing MA, Toubert ME, Bonichon F, Cavarec M, Bernard AM, Boneu A, Leprat F, Haas O, Lasset C, Schlumberger M, Canzian F, Goldgar DE, Romeo G (2001). Localization of a susceptibility gene for familial non-medullary thyroid carcinoma to chromosome 2q21. Am J Hum Genet 69: 440-446.
1466. McKeeby JL, Li X, Zhuang Z, Vortmeyer AO, Huang S, Pirner M, Skarulis MC, James-Newton L, Marx SJ, Lubensky

IA (2001). Multiple leiomyomas of the esophagus, lung, and uterus in multiple endocrine neoplasia type 1. Am J Pathol 159: 1121-1127.

1467. McKeever PE, Blaivas M, Sima AAF (1993). Neoplasms of the sellar region. In: Surgical Pathology of the Pituitary Gland, Lloyd RV, ed., WB Saunders: Philadelphia , pp. 141-210.

1468. McKusick VA (2000). Online Mendelian Inheritance in Man, OMIM (TM). McKusick-Nathans Institute for Genetic Medicine, Johns Hopkins University (Baltimore, MD) and National Center for Biotechnology Information, National Library of Medicine (Bethesda, MD), 2000 http://www.ncbi.nlm.nih.gov/omim/ .

1469. McLeod MK, Thompson NW, Hudson JL, Gaglio JA, Lloyd RV, Harness JK, Nishiyama R, Cheung PS (1988). Flow cytometric measurements of nuclear DNA and ploidy analysis in Hurthle cell neoplasms of the thyroid. Arch Surg 123: 849-854.

1470. McMillan PJ, Hooker WM, Deptos LJ (1974). Distribution of calcitonin-containing cells in the human thyroid. Am J Anat 140: 73-79.

1471. McNicol AM (2001). Differential diagnosis of pheochromocytomas and paragangliomas. Endocr Pathol 12: 407-415.

1472. McNicol AM, Struthers AL, Nolan CE, Hermans J, Haak HR (1997). Proliferation in Adrenocortical Tumors: Correlation with Clinical Outcome and p53 Status. Endocr Pathol 8: 29-36.

1473. McNicol AM, Teasdale GM, Beastall GH (1986). A study of corticotroph adenomas in Cushing's disease: no evidence of intermediate lobe origin. Clin Endocrinol (Oxf) 24: 715-722.

1474. Medeiros-Neto G, Gil-Da-Costa MJ, Santos CL, Medina AM, Silva JC, Tsou RM, Sobrinho-Simoes M (1998). Metastatic thyroid carcinoma arising from congenital goiter due to mutation in the thyroperoxidase gene. J Clin Endocrinol Metab 83: 4162-4166.

1475. Medeiros LJ, Weiss LM, Vickery ALJr (1989). Epithelial-lined (true) cyst of the adrenal gland: a case report. Hum Pathol 20: 491-492.

1476. Medeiros LJ, Wolf BC, Balogh K, Federman M (1985). Adrenal pheochromocytoma: a clinicopathologic review of 60 cases. Hum Pathol 16: 580-589.

1477. Meier CA, Biller BM (1997). Clinical and biochemical evaluation of Cushing's syndrome. Endocrinol Metab Clin North Am 26: 741-762.

1477A. Meij BP, Lopes MB, Ellegala DB, Alden TD, Laws ERJr (2002). The long-term significance of microscopic dural invasion in 354 patients with pituitary adenomas treated with transsphenoidal surgery. J Neurosurg 96: 195-208.

1478. Melicow MM (1977). One hundred cases of pheochromocytoma (107 tumors) at the Columbia-Presbyterian Medical Center, 1926-1976: a clinicopathological analysis. Cancer 40: 1987-2004.

1479. Melmed S (1990). Acromegaly. N Engl J Med 322: 966-977.

1480. Melmed S, Kleinberg D (2002). Anterior pituitary. In: Williams Textbook of Endocrinology, Larsen PR, Kronenberg HM, Melmed S, Williams RH, Wilson JD, Foster DW, eds., Saunders: Philadelphia , pp. 177-279.

1481. Memoli VA, Brown EF, Gould VE (1984). Glial fibrillary acidic protein (GFAP) immunoreactivity in peripheral nerve sheath tumors. Ultrastruct Pathol 7: 269-275.

1482. Mendelsohn G (1984). Signet-cell-simulating microfollicular adenoma of the thyroid. Am J Surg Pathol 8: 705-708.

1483. Mendelsohn G, Baylin SB, Bigner SH, Wells SAJr, Eggleston JC (1980). Anaplastic variants of medullary thyroid carcinoma: a light-microscopic and immunohistochemical study. Am J Surg Pathol 4: 333-341.

1484. Mendelsohn G, Wells SAJr, Baylin SB (1984). Relationship of tissue carcinoembryonic antigen and calcitonin to tumor virulence in medullary thyroid carcinoma. An immunohistochemical study in early, localized, and virulent disseminated stages of disease. Cancer 54: 657-662.

1485. Meng X, Lindahl M, Hyvonen ME, Parvinen M, de Rooij DG, Hess MW, Raatikainen-Ahokas A, Sainio K, Rauvala H, Lakso M, Pichel JG, Westphal H, Saarma M, Sariola H (2000). Regulation of cell fate decision of undifferentiated spermatogonia by GDNF. Science 287: 1489-1493.

1486. Menko FH, van der Luijt RB, de Valk IA, Toorians AW, Sepers JM, van Diest PJ, Lips CJ (2002). Atypical MEN type 2B associated with two germline RET mutations on the same allele not involving codon 918. J Clin Endocrinol Metab 87: 393-397.

1487. Messiaen LM, Callens T, Mortier G, Beysen D, Vandenbroucke I, Van Roy N, Speleman F, Paepe AD (2000). Exhaustive mutation analysis of the NF1 gene allows identification of 95% of mutations and reveals a high frequency of unusual splicing defects. Hum Mutat 15: 541-555.

1488. Metzger AK, Mohapatra G, Minn YA, Bollen AW, Lamborn K, Waldman FM, Wilson CB, Feuerstein BG (1999). Multiple genetic aberrations including evidence of chromosome 11q13 rearrangement detected in pituitary adenomas by comparative genomic hybridization. J Neurosurg 90: 306-314.

1489. Meyer JS, Abdel-Bari W (1968). Granules and thyrocalcitonin-like activity in medullary carcinoma of the thyroid gland. N Engl J Med 278: 523-529.

1490. Mickley V, Mattfeld T, Orend KH (1996). [Cervical sympathetic paraganglioma]. Chirurg 67: 199-201.

1491. Miedlich S, Krohn K, Lamesch P, Muller A, Paschke R (2000). Frequency of somatic MEN1 gene mutations in monoclonal parathyroid tumours of patients with primary hyperparathyroidism. Eur J Endocrinol 143: 47-54.

1492. Miettinen M, Clark R, Lehto VP, Virtanen I, Damjanov I (1985). Intermediate-filament proteins in parathyroid glands and parathyroid adenomas. Arch Pathol Lab Med 109: 986-989.

1493. Miettinen M, Franssila K, Lehto VP, Paasivuo R, Virtanen I (1984). Expression of intermediate filament proteins in thyroid gland and thyroid tumors. Lab Invest 50: 262-270.

1494. Miettinen M, Franssila KO (2000). Variable expression of keratins and nearly uniform lack of thyroid transcription factor 1 in thyroid anaplastic carcinoma. Hum Pathol 31: 1139-1145.

1495. Miettinen M, Karkkainen P (1996). Differential reactivity of HBME-1 and CD15 antibodies in benign and malignant thyroid tumours. Preferential reactivity with malignant tumours. Virchows Arch 429: 213-219.

1496. Miettinen M, Lehto VP, Virtanen I (1985). Immunofluorescence microscopic evaluation of the intermediate filament expression of the adrenal cortex and medulla and their tumors. Am J Pathol 118: 360-366.

1497. Miettinen M, Saari A (1988). Pheochromocytoma combined with malignant schwannoma: unusual neoplasm of the adrenal medulla. Ultrastruct Pathol 12: 513-527.

1498. Migliori M, Tomassetti P, Lalli S, Casadei R, Santini D, Corinaldesi R, Gullo L (2002). Carcinoid of the pancreas. Pancreatology 2: 163-166.

1499. Mikhail RA, Moore JB, Reed DNJr, Abbott RR (1986). Malignant retroperitoneal paragangliomas. J Surg Oncol 32: 32-36.

1500. Miki Y, Matsuo M, Nishizawa S, Kuroda Y, Keyaki A, Makita Y, Kawamura J (1990). Pituitary adenomas and normal pituitary tissue: enhancement patterns on gadopentetate-enhanced MR imaging. Radiology 177: 35-38.

1501. Miller GM, Alexander JM, Bikkal HA, Katznelson L, Zervas NT, Klibanski A (1995). Somatostatin receptor subtype gene expression in pituitary adenomas. J Clin Endocrinol Metab 80: 1386-1392.

1502. Mills SE, Gaffey MJ, Watts JC, Swanson PE, Wick MR, LiVolsi VA, Nappi O, Weiss LM (1994). Angiomatoid carcinoma and 'angiosarcoma' of the thyroid gland. A spectrum of endothelial differentiation. Am J Clin Pathol 102: 322-330.

1503. Mills SE, Stallings RG, Austin MB (1986). Angiomatoid carcinoma of the thyroid gland. Anaplastic carcinoma with follicular and medullary features mimicking angiosarcoma. Am J Clin Pathol 86: 674-678.

1504. Milunsky JM, Maher TA, Michels VV, Milunsky A (2001). Novel mutations and the emergence of a common mutation in the SDHD gene causing familial paraganglioma. Am J Med Genet 100: 311-314.

1505. Min KW, Clemens A, Bell J, Dick H (1988). Malignant peripheral nerve sheath tumor and pheochromocytoma. A composite tumor of the adrenal. Arch Pathol Lab Med 112: 266-270.

1506. Minagawa A, Iitaka M, Suzuki M, Yasuda S, Kameyama K, Shimada S, Kitahama S, Wada S, Katayama S (2002). A case of primary mucoepidermoid carcinoma of the thyroid: molecular evidence of its origin. Clin Endocrinol (Oxf) 57: 551-556.

1507. Mindermann T, Wilson CB (1994). Age-related and gender-related occurrence of pituitary adenomas. Clin Endocrinol (Oxf) 41: 359-364.

1508. Minkowski O (1887). Ueber einen all Fall von Akromegalie. Berl Klin Wochenschr 21: 371-374.

1509. Minutoli F, Pecorella GR, Cosentino S, Lipari R, Baldari S (2002). Scintigraphic features of a pure estrogen-secreting adrenocortical adenoma in a patient with gynecomastia. Clin Nucl Med 27: 741-742.

1510. Misago N, Ishii Y, Kohda H (1996). Malignant peripheral nerve sheath tumor of the skin: a superficial form of this tumor. J Cutan Pathol 23: 182-188.

1511. Missale C, Boroni F, Sigala S, Buriani A, Fabris M, Leon A, Dal Toso R, Spano P (1996). Nerve growth factor in the anterior pituitary: localization in mammotroph cells and cosecretion with prolactin by a dopamine-regulated mechanism. Proc Natl Acad Sci U S A 93: 4240-4245.

1512. Missiaglia E, Moore PS, Williamson J, Lemoine NR, Falconi M, Zamboni G, Scarpa A (2002). Sex chromosome anomalies in pancreatic endocrine tumors. Int J Cancer 98: 532-538.

1513. Mitrovic D, Mazabraud A, Ryckewaert A, Hioco D, de Seze S (1967). [Parathyroid adenoma with dark and clear cells. 2 ultrastructural aspects of the clear cells. Cytochemical study and electron microscopy]. Arch Anat Pathol (Paris) 15: 225-230.

1514. Miwa H, Takakuwa T, Nakatsuka S, Tomita Y, Matsuzuka F, Aozasa K (2001). DNA sequence of immunoglobulin heavy chain variable region gene in thyroid lymphoma. Jpn J Cancer Res 92: 1041-1047.

1515. Mixson AJ, Friedman TC, Katz DA, Feuerstein IM, Taubenberger JK, Colandrea JM, Doppman JL, Oldfield EH, Weintraub BD (1993). Thyrotropin-secreting pituitary carcinoma. J Clin Endocrinol Metab 76: 529-533.

1516. Miyauchi A, Futami H, Hai N, Yokozawa T, Kuma K, Aoki N, Kosugi S, Sugano K, Yamaguchi K (1999). Two germline missense mutations at codons 804 and 806 of the RET proto-oncogene in the same allele in a patient with multiple endocrine neoplasia type 2B without codon 918 mutation. Jpn J Cancer Res 90: 1-5.

1517. Miyauchi A, Kuma K, Matsuzuka F, Matsubayashi S, Kobayashi A, Tamai H, Katayama S (1985). Intrathyroidal epithelial thymoma: an entity distinct from squamous cell carcinoma of the thyroid. World J Surg 9: 128-135.

1518. Mizukami Y, Kurumaya H, Yamada T, Minato H, Nonomura A, Noguchi M, Matsubara F (1995). Thymic carcinoma involving the thyroid gland: report of two cases. Hum Pathol 26: 576-579.

1519. Mizukami Y, Michigishi T, Nonomura A, Nakamura S, Noguchi M, Hashimoto T, Itoh N (1993). Mixed medullary-follicular carcinoma of the thyroid occurring in familial form. Histopathology 22: 284-287.

1520. Mockridge KA, Levine MA, Reed LA, Post E, Kaplan FS, de Beur SMJ, Deng Z, Ding C, Howard C, Schnur RE (1999). Polyendocrinopathy, skeletal dysplasia, organomegaly, and distinctive facies associated with a novel, widely-expressed Gs alpha mutation. Am J Hum Genet 65: 2416.

1521. Modigliani E, Vasen HM, Raue K, Dralle H, Frilling A, Gheri RG, Brandi ML, Limbert E, Niederle B, Forgas L, Rosenberg-Bourgin M, Calmettes C (1995). Pheochromocytoma in multiple endocrine neoplasia type 2: European study. The Euromen Study Group. J Intern Med 238: 363-367.

1522. Modlin IM, Farndon JR, Shepherd A, Johnston ID, Kennedy TL, Montgomery DA, Welbourn RB (1979). Phaeochromocytomas in 72 patients: clinical and diagnostic features, treatment and long term results. Br J Surg 66: 456-465.

1523. Mohr VH, Vortmeyer AO, Zhuang Z, Libutti SK, Walther MM, Choyke PL, Zbar B, Linehan WM, Lubensky IA (2000). Histopathology and molecular genetics of multiple cysts and microcystic (serous) adenomas of the pancreas in von Hippel-Lindau patients. Am J Pathol 157: 1615-1621.

1524. Molberg K, Albores-Saavedra J (1994). Hyalinizing trabecular carcinoma of the thyroid gland. Hum Pathol 25: 192-197.

1525. Moley JF, Brother MB, Fong CT, White PS, Baylin SB, Nelkin B, Wells SA, Brodeur GM (1992). Consistent association of 1p loss of heterozygosity with pheochromocytomas from patients with multiple endocrine neoplasia type 2 syndromes. Cancer Res 52: 770-774.

1526. Molitch ME (2001). Medical therapy of pituitary tumors. In: Diagnosis and Management of Pituitary Tumors, Thapar K, Kovacs K, Scheithauer BW, Lloyd RV, eds., Humana Press: Totowa, NJ , pp. 247-267.

1527. Molloy PT, Bilaniuk LT, Vaughan SN, Needle MN, Liu GT, Zackai EH, Phillips PC (1995). Brainstem tumors in patients with neurofibromatosis type 1: a distinct clinical entity. Neurology 45: 1897-1902.

1528. Monnat RJJr (1999). Unusual features of thyroid carcinomas in Japanese patients with Werner syndrome and possible genotype-phenotype relations to cell type and race. Cancer 86: 728-729.

1529. Montori VM, Young WFJr (2002). Use of plasma aldosterone concentration-to-plasma renin activity ratio as a screening test for primary aldosteronism. A systematic review of the literature. Endocrinol Metab Clin North Am 31: 619-32, xi.

1530. Moore PS, Missiaglia E, Antonello D, Zamo A, Zamboni G, Corleto V, Falconi M, Scarpa A (2001). Role of disease-causing genes in sporadic pancreatic endocrine tumors: MEN1 and VHL. Genes Chromosomes Cancer 32: 177-181.

1531. Moore PS, Orlandini S, Zamboni G, Capelli P, Rigaud G, Falconi M, Bassi C, Lemoine NR, Scarpa A (2001). Pancreatic tumours: molecular pathways implicated in ductal cancer are involved in ampullary but not in exocrine nonductal or endocrine tumorigenesis. Br J Cancer 84: 253-262.

1532. Moran CA, Rush W, Mena H (1997). Primary spinal paragangliomas: a clinicopathological and immunohistochemical study of 30 cases. Histopathology 31: 167-173.

1533. Morant R, Bruckner HW (1989). Complete remission of refractory small cell carcinoma of the pancreas with cisplatin and etoposide. Cancer 64: 2007-2009.

1534. Moreno AM, Castilla-Guerra L, Martinez-Torres MC, Torres-Olivera F, Fernandez E, Galera-Davidson H (1999). Expression of neuropeptides and other neuroendocrine markers in human phaeochromocytomas. Neuropeptides 33: 159-163.

1535. Mornex R, Badet C, Peyrin L (1992). Malignant pheochromocytoma: a series of 14 cases observed between 1966 and 1990. J Endocrinol Invest 15: 643-649.

1536. Morohoshi T, Held G, Kloppel G (1983). Exocrine pancreatic tumours and their histological classification. A study based on 167 autopsy and 97 surgical cases. Histopathology 7: 645-661.

1537. Morohoshi T, Kanda M, Horie A, Chott A, Dreyer T, Kloppel G, Heitz PU (1987). Immunocytochemical markers of uncommon pancreatic tumors. Acinar cell carcinoma, pancreatoblastoma, and solid cystic (papillary-cystic) tumor. Cancer 59: 739-747.

1538. Morrison AB (1980). Islet cell tumors and the diarrheogenic syndrome. Monogr Pathol 21: 185-207.

1539. Morrison AB, Fitts WT, Rawson AJ (1962). Syndrome of refractory watery diarrhea and hypokalemia in patients with a non-insulin-secreting islet cell tumor. Am J Med 32: 119-127.

1540. Morrison PJ, Nevin NC (1996). Multiple endocrine neoplasia type 2B (mucosal neuroma syndrome, Wagenmann-Froboese syndrome). J Med Genet 33: 779-782.

1541. Morrissy RT (1982). Congenital pseudarthrosis of the tibia. Factors that affect results. Clin Orthop 21-27.

1542. Moss NH, Rhoades JE (1960). Hyperinsulinism and islet cell tumors of the pancreas. In: Surgical Diseases of the Pancreas, Howard JM, Jordan GL, eds., Lippincott: Philadelphia , pp. 321-441.

1543. Mossner R, Keidel M (2000). Malignant pheochromocytoma with progressive paraparesis in von Hippel-Lindau disease. Eur J Neurol 7: 439-442.

1544. Motoi N, Sakamoto A, Yamochi T, Horiuchi H, Motoi T, Machinami R (2000). Role of ras mutation in the progression of thyroid carcinoma of follicular epithelial origin. Pathol Res Pract 196: 1-7.

1545. Motokura T, Bloom T, Kim HG, Juppner H, Ruderman JV, Kronenberg HM, Arnold A (1991). A novel cyclin encoded by a bcl1-linked candidate oncogene. Nature 350: 512-515.

1546. Moul JW, Bishoff JT, Theune SM, Chang EH (1993). Absent ras gene mutations in human adrenal cortical neoplasms and pheochromocytomas. J Urol 149: 1389-1394.

1547. Mounier C, Trouillas J, Claustrat B, Duthel R, Estour B (2003). Macroprolactinaemia associated with prolactin adenoma. Hum Reprod 18: 853-857.

1548. Mouse BD, Shaw EG (2001). Radiation therapy of pituitary tumors. Including stereotactic radiosurgery. In: Diagnosis and Management of Pituitary Tumors, Thapar K, Kovacs K, Scheithauer BW, Lloyd RV, eds., Humana Press: Totowa, NJ , pp. 269-277.

1549. Movahedi-Lankarani S, Hruban RH, Westra WH, Klimstra DS (2002). Primitive neuroectodermal tumors of the pancreas: a report of seven cases of a rare neoplasm. Am J Surg Pathol 26: 1040-1047.

1550. Moyana TN, Kontozoglou T (1988). Urinary bladder paragangliomas. An immunohistochemical study. Arch Pathol Lab Med 112: 70-72.

1551. Mukai K, Grotting JC, Greider MH, Rosai J (1982). Retrospective study of 77 pancreatic endocrine tumors using the immunoperoxidase method. Am J Surg Pathol 6: 387-399.

1552. Muller-Leisse CR, Klose KC (1990). [Calcified liver metastases from a calcified pancreatic vipoma. Computed tomographic visualization]. Radiologe 30: 487-488.

1553. Mulligan LM, Eng C, Attie T, Lyonnet S, Marsh DJ, Hyland VJ, Robinson BG, Frilling A, Verellen-Dumoulin C, Safar A, Venter DJ, Munnich A, Ponder BA (1994). Diverse phenotypes associated with exon 10 mutations of the RET proto-oncogene. Hum Mol Genet 3: 2163-2167.

1554. Mulligan LM, Eng C, Healey CS, Clayton D, Kwok JB, Gardner E, Ponder MA, Frilling A, Jackson CE, Lehnert H, Neumann HP, Thibodeau SN, Ponder BA (1994). Specific mutations of the RET proto-oncogene are related to disease phenotype in MEN 2A and FMTC. Nat Genet 6: 70-74.

1555. Mulligan LM, Gardner E, Smith BA, Mathew CG, Ponder BA (1993). Genetic events in tumour initiation and progression in multiple endocrine neoplasia type 2. Genes Chromosomes Cancer 6: 166-177.

1556. Mulligan LM, Kwok JB, Healey CS, Elsdon MJ, Eng C, Gardner E, Love DR, Mole SE, Moore JK, Papi L (1993). Germ-line mutations of the RET proto-oncogene in multiple endocrine neoplasia type 2A. Nature 363: 458-460.

1557. Mundy GR, Cove DH, Fisken R (1980). Primary hyperparathyroidism: changes in the pattern of clinical presentation. Lancet 1: 1317-1320.

1558. Munro LM, Kennedy A, McNicol AM (1999). The expression of inhibin/activin subunits in the human adrenal cortex and its tumours. J Endocrinol 161: 341-347.

1559. Murao T, Nakanishi M, Toda K, Konishi H (1979). Malignant teratoma of the thyroid gland in an adolescent female. Acta Pathol Jpn 29: 109-117.

1560. Murat A, Heymann MF, Bernat S, Dupas B, Delajartre AY, Calender A, Despins P, Michaud JL, Giraud S, Le Bodic MF, Charbonnel B (1997). [Thymic and bronchial neuroendocrine tumors in multiple endocrine neoplasia type 1. GENEM1]. Presse Med 26: 1616-1621.

1561. Murray HH, Lovell WW (1982). Congenital pseudarthrosis of the tibia. A long-term follow-up study. Clin Orthop 14-20.

1562. Murray IP, Thomson JA, McGirr EM, Macdonald EM, Kennedy JS, McLennan I (1966). Unusual familial goiter associated with intrathyroidal calcification. J Clin Endocrinol Metab 26: 1039-1049.

1563. Musholt TJ, Musholt PB, Khaladj N, Schulz D, Scheumann GF, Klempnauer J (2000). Prognostic significance of RET and NTRK1 rearrangements in sporadic papillary thyroid carcinoma. Surgery 128: 984-993.

1564. Musso C, Paraf F, Petit B, Archambeaud-Mouveroux F, Valleix D, Labrousse F (2000). [Pancreatic neuroendocrine tumors and von Hippel-Lindau disease]. Ann Pathol 20: 130-133.

1565. Myers EN, Suen JY (1996). Cancer of the Head and Neck. 3rd ed. WB Saunders: Philadelphia.

1566. Myers SM, Eng C, Ponder BA, Mulligan LM (1995). Characterization of RET proto-oncogene 3' splicing variants and polyadenylation sites: a novel C-terminus for RET. Oncogene 11: 2039-2045.

1567. Naccarato AG, Marcocci C, Miccoli P, Bonadio AG, Cianferotti L, Vignali E, Cipollini G, Viacava P (1998). Bcl-2, p53 and MIB-1 expression in normal and neoplastic parathyroid tissues. J Endocrinol Invest 21: 136-141.

1568. Naganuma H, Iwama N, Nakamura Y, Ohtani N, Ohtani H, Takaya K, Sakai N (2002). Papillary carcinoma of the thyroid gland forming a myofibroblastic nodular tumor: report of two cases and review of the literature. Pathol Int 52: 54-58.

1569. Nagaya T, Kuwayama A, Seo H, Tsukamoto N, Matsui N, Sugita K (1992). Endocrinological evaluation of ACTH-secreting pituitary microadenomas: their location and alpha-melanocyte stimulating hormone immunoreactivity. J Neurosurg 76: 944-947.

1570. Nager GT, Kennedy DW, Kopstein E (1982). Fibrous dysplasia: a review of the disease and its manifestations in the temporal bone. Ann Otol Rhinol Laryngol Suppl 92: 1-52.

1571. Nagura S, Katoh R, Kawaoi A, Kobayashi M, Obara T, Omata K (1999). Immunohistochemical estimations of growth activity to predict biological behavior of pheochromocytomas. Mod Pathol 12: 1107-1111.

1572. Nakabayashi H, Sunada I, Hara M (2001). Immunohistochemical analyses of cell cycle-related proteins, apoptosis, and proliferation in pituitary adenomas. J

Histochem Cytochem 49: 1193-1194.

1573. Nakagawara A, Ikeda K, Tsuneyoshi M, Daimaru Y, Enjoji M (1985). Malignant pheochromocytoma with ganglioneuroblastoma elements in a patient with von Recklinghausen's disease. Cancer 55: 2794-2798.

1574. Nakata T, Kitamura Y, Shimizu K, Tanaka S, Fujimori M, Yokoyama S, Ito K, Emi M (1999). Fusion of a novel gene, ELKS, to RET due to translocation t(10;12)(q11;p13) in a papillary thyroid carcinoma. Genes Chromosomes Cancer 25: 97-103.

1575. Nakayama H (2002). RecQ family helicases: roles as tumor suppressor proteins. Oncogene 21: 9008-9021.

1576. Nakazumi H, Sasano H, Iino K, Ohashi Y, Orikasa S (1998). Expression of cell cycle inhibitor p27 and Ki-67 in human adrenocortical neoplasms. Mod Pathol 11: 1165-1170.

1577. Nakhjavani MK, Gharib H, Goellner JR, van Heerden JA (1997). Metastasis to the thyroid gland. A report of 43 cases. Cancer 79: 574-578.

1578. Namba H, Gutman RA, Matsuo K, Alvarez A, Fagin JA (1990). H-ras protooncogene mutations in human thyroid neoplasms. J Clin Endocrinol Metab 71: 223-229.

1579. Namba H, Rubin SA, Fagin JA (1990). Point mutations of ras oncogenes are an early event in thyroid tumorigenesis. Mol Endocrinol 4: 1474-1479.

1580. Nativ O, Grant CS, Sheps SG, O'Fallon JR, Farrow GM, van Heerden JA, Lieber MM (1992). The clinical significance of nuclear DNA ploidy pattern in 184 patients with pheochromocytoma. Cancer 69: 2683-2687.

1581. Neblett WW, Frexes-Steed M, Scott HWJr (1987). Experience with adrenocortical neoplasms in childhood. Am Surg 53: 117-125.

1582. Negri E, Dal Maso L, Ron E, La Vecchia C, Mark SD, Preston-Martin S, McTiernan A, Kolonel L, Yoshimoto Y, Jin F, Wingren G, Rosaria Galanti M, Hardell L, Glattre E, Lund E, Levi F, Linos D, Braga C, Franceschi S (1999). A pooled analysis of case-control studies of thyroid cancer. II. Menstrual and reproductive factors. Cancer Causes Control 10: 143-155.

1583. Netterville JL, Jackson CG, Miller FR, Wanamaker JR, Glasscock ME (1998). Vagal paraganglioma: a review of 46 patients treated during a 20-year period. Arch Otolaryngol Head Neck Surg 124: 1133-1140.

1584. Netterville JL, Reilly KM, Robertson D, Reiber ME, Armstrong WB, Childs P (1995). Carotid body tumors: a review of 30 patients with 46 tumors. Laryngoscope 105: 115-126.

1585. Neumann HP, Bausch B, McWhinney SR, Bender BU, Gimm O, Franke G, Schipper J, Klisch J, Altehoefer C, Zerres K, Januszewicz A, Eng C, Smith WM, Munk R, Manz T, Glaesker S, Apel TW, Treier M, Reineke M, Walz MK, Hoang-Vu C, Brauckhoff M, Klein-Franke A, Klose P, Schmidt H, Maier-Woelfle M, Peczkowska M, Szmigielski C, Eng C (2002). Germ-line mutations in nonsyndromic pheochromocytoma. N Engl J Med 346: 1459-1466.

1586. Neumann HP, Bender BU, Berger DP, Laubenberger J, Schultze-Seemann W, Wetterauer U, Ferstl FJ, Herbst EW, Schwarzkopf G, Hes FJ, Lips CJ, Lamiell JM, Masek O, Riegler P, Mueller B, Glavac

D, Brauch H (1998). Prevalence, morphology and biology of renal cell carcinoma in von Hippel-Lindau disease compared to sporadic renal cell carcinoma. J Urol 160: 1248-1254.

1587. Neumann HP, Berger DP, Sigmund G, Blum U, Schmidt D, Parmer RJ, Volk B, Kirste G (1993). Pheochromocytomas, multiple endocrine neoplasia type 2, and von Hippel-Lindau disease. N Engl J Med 329: 1531-1538.

1588. Neumann HP, Eggert HR, Scheremet R, Schumacher M, Mohadjer M, Wakhloo AK, Volk B, Hettmannsperger U, Riegler P, Schollmeyer P, Wiestler OD (1992). Central nervous system lesions in von Hippel-Lindau syndrome. J Neurol Neurosurg Psychiatry 55: 898-901.

1589. Neumann HP, Eng C, Mulligan LM, Glavac D, Zauner I, Ponder BA, Crossey PA, Maher ER, Brauch H (1995). Consequences of direct genetic testing for germline mutations in the clinical management of families with multiple endocrine neoplasia, type II. JAMA 274: 1149-1151.

1590. Neumann HP, Wiestler OD (1991). Clustering of features of von Hippel-Lindau syndrome: evidence for a complex genetic locus. Lancet 337: 1052-1054.

1591. Neumann S, Willgerodt H, Ackermann F, Reske A, Jung M, Reis A, Paschke R (1999). Linkage of familial euthyroid goiter to the multinodular goiter-1 locus and exclusion of the candidate genes thyroglobulin, thyroperoxidase, and Na+/I-symporter. J Clin Endocrinol Metab 84: 3750-3756.

1592. Nezelof C, Basset F, Rousseau MF (1973). Histiocytosis X histogenetic arguments for a Langerhans cell origin. Biomedicine 18: 365-371.

1593. Nguyen DT, Diamond LW, Hansmann ML, Hill K, Fisher R (1994). Follicular dendritic cell sarcoma, identification by monoclonal antibodies in paraffin sections. Appl Immunohistochem 2: 60-64.

1594. Nguyen GK, Akin MR (2001). Cytopathology of insular carcinoma of the thyroid. Diagn Cytopathol 25: 325-330.

1595. Niccoli-Sire P, Murat A, Baudin E, Henry JF, Proye C, Bigorgne JC, Bstandig B, Modigliani E, Morange S, Schlumberger M, Conte-Devolx B (1999). Early or prophylactic thyroidectomy in MEN 2/FMTC gene carriers: results in 71 thyroidectomized patients. The French Calcitonin Tumours Study Group (GETC). Eur J Endocrinol 141: 468-474.

1596. Nicolis G, Shimshi M, Allen C, Halmi NS, Kourides IA (1988). Gonadotropin-producing pituitary adenoma in a man with long-standing primary hypogonadism. J Clin Endocrinol Metab 66: 237-241.

1597. Nieman LK (2002). Diagnostic tests for Cushing's syndrome. Ann N Y Acad Sci 970: 112-118.

1598. Niemann S, Becker-Follmann J, Nurnberg G, Ruschendorf F, Sieweke N, Hugens-Penzel M, Traupe H, Wienker TF, Reis A, Muller U (2001). Assignment of PGL3 to chromosome 1 (q21-q23) in a family with autosomal dominant non-chromaffin paraganglioma. Am J Med Genet 98: 32-36.

1599. Niemann S, Muller U (2000). Mutations in SDHC cause autosomal dominant paraganglioma, type 3. Nat Genet 26: 268-270.

1600. Niemann S, Steinberger D, Muller U (1999). PGL3, a third, not maternally imprinted locus in autosomal dominant paraganglioma. Neurogenetics 2: 167-170.

1601. Nigawara K, Suzuki T, Tazawa H, Funyu T, Yagihashi S, Yamaya K, Terayama Y, Yamaguchi K (1987). A case of recurrent malignant pheochromocytoma complicated by watery diarrhea, hypokalemia, achlorhydria syndrome. J Clin Endocrinol Metab 65: 1053-1056.

1602. Nikiforov YE, Koshoffer A, Nikiforova M, Stringer J, Fagin JA (1999). Chromosomal breakpoint positions suggest a direct role for radiation in inducing illegitimate recombination between the ELE1 and RET genes in radiation-induced thyroid carcinomas. Oncogene 18: 6330-6334.

1603. Nikiforov YE, Rowland JM, Bove KE, Monforte-Munoz H, Fagin JA (1997). Distinct pattern of ret oncogene rearrangements in morphological variants of radiation-induced and sporadic thyroid papillary carcinomas in children. Cancer Res 57: 1690-1694.

1604. Nikiforova MN, Biddinger PW, Caudill CM, Kroll TG, Nikiforov YE (2002). PAX8-PPARgamma rearrangement in thyroid tumors: RT-PCR and immunohistochemical analyses. Am J Surg Pathol 26: 1016-1023.

1605. Nikiforova MN, Kimura ET, Gandhi M, Biddinger PW, Knauf JA, Basolo F, Zhu Z, Giannini R, Salvatore G, Fusco A, Santoro M, Fagin JA, Nikiforov YE (2003). BRAF mutations in thyroid tumors are restricted to papillary carcinomas and anaplastic or poorly differentiated carcinomas arising from papillary carcinomas. J Clin Endocrinol Metab 88: 5399-5404.

1606. Nikiforova MN, Lynch RA, Biddinger PW, Alexander EK, Dorn GW, Tallini G, Kroll TG, Nikiforov YE (2003). Ras point mutations and PAX8-PPAR gamma rearrangement in thyroid tumors: evidence for distinct molecular pathways in thyroid follicular carcinoma. J Clin Endocrinol Metab 88: 2318-2326.

1607. Nikiforova MN, Stringer JR, Blough R, Medvedovic M, Fagin JA, Nikiforov YE (2000). Proximity of chromosomal loci that participate in radiation-induced rearrangements in human cells. Science 290: 138-141.

1608. Nilsson O (1977). Studies on the ultrastructure of the human parathyroid glands in various pathological conditions. Acta Pathol Microbiol Scand Suppl 1-88.

1609. Nilsson O, Lindeberg J, Zedenius J, Ekman E, Tennvall J, Blomgren H, Grimelius L, Lundell G, Wallin G (1998). Anaplastic giant cell carcinoma of the thyroid gland: treatment and survival over a 25-year period. World J Surg 22: 725-730.

1610. Nilsson O, Tisell LE, Jansson S, Ahlman H, Gimm O, Eng C (1999). Adrenal and extra-adrenal pheochromocytomas in a family with germline RET V804L mutation. JAMA 281: 1587-1588.

1611. Nishida S, Tanimura A, Takasaki S, Nagaoka S, Fukueda M, Ikeda S, Matsuo K, Akao M, Tokunaga M (1995). Surgically resected adrenal leiomyoma: report of a case. Surg Today 25: 455-457.

1612. Nishida T, Katayama S, Tsujimoto M, Nakamura J, Matsuda H (1999). Clinicopathological significance of poorly differentiated thyroid carcinoma. Am J Surg Pathol 23: 205-211.

1613. Nishioka H, Haraoka J, Akada K, Azuma S (2002). Gender-related differences in prolactin secretion in pituitary prolactinomas. Neuroradiology 44: 407-410.

1614. Noel M, Delehaye MC, Segond N, Lasmoles F, Caillou B, Gardet P, Fragu P, Moukhtar MS (1991). Study of calcitonin and thyroglobulin gene expression in human mixed follicular and medullary thyroid carcinoma. Thyroid 1: 249-256.

1615. Nord B, Platz A, Smoczynski K, Kytola S, Robertson G, Calender A, Murat A, Weintraub D, Burgess J, Edwards M, Skogseid B, Owen D, Lassam N, Hogg D, Larsson C, Teh BT (2000). Malignant melanoma in patients with multiple endocrine neoplasia type 1 and involvement of the MEN1 gene in sporadic melanoma. Int J Cancer 87: 463-467.

1616. Nord KS, Joshi V, Hanna M, Khademi M, Saad S, Marquis J, Pelzman H, Verner E (1986). Zollinger-Ellison syndrome associated with a renal gastrinoma in a child. J Pediatr Gastroenterol Nutr 5: 980-986.

1617. Norton JA, Doppman JL, Collen MJ, Harmon JW, Maton PN, Gardner JD, Jensen RT (1986). Prospective study of gastrinoma localization and resection in patients with Zollinger-Ellison syndrome. Ann Surg 204: 468-479.

1618. Norton JA, Doppman JL, Jensen RT (1992). Curative resection in Zollinger-Ellison syndrome. Results of a 10-year prospective study. Ann Surg 215: 8-18.

1619. Norton JA, Fraker DL, Alexander HR, Venzon DJ, Doppman JL, Serrano J, Goebel SU, Peghini PL, Roy PK, Gibril F, Jensen RT (1999). Surgery to cure the Zollinger-Ellison syndrome. N Engl J Med 341: 635-644.

1620. Norton JA, Shawker TH, Doppman JL, Miller DL, Fraker DL, Cromack DT, Gorden P, Jensen RT (1990). Localization and surgical treatment of occult insulinomas. Ann Surg 212: 615-620.

1621. Norum RA, Lafreniere RG, O'Neal LW, Nikolai TF, Delaney JP, Sisson JC, Sobol H, Lenoir GM, Ponder BA, Willard HF, Jackson CE (1990). Linkage of the multiple endocrine neoplasia type 2B gene (MEN2B) to chromosome 10 markers linked to MEN2A. Genomics 8: 313-317.

1622. Nose-Alberti V, Mesquita MI, Martin LC, Kayath MJ (1998). Adrenocorticotropin-Producing Pituitary Carcinoma with Expression of c-erbB-2 and High PCNA Index: A Comparative Study with Pituitary Adenomas and Normal Pituitary Tissues. Endocr Pathol 9: 53-62.

1623. Nunziata V, di Giovanni G, Lettera AM, D'Armiento M, Mancini M (1989). Cutaneous lichen amyloidosis associated with multiple endocrine neoplasia type 2A. Henry Ford Hosp Med J 37: 144-146.

1624. Nussbaum SR, Thompson AR, Hutcheson KA, Gaz RD, Wang CA (1988). Intraoperative measurement of parathyroid hormone in the surgical management of hyperparathyroidism. Surgery 104: 1121-1127.

1625. Nwokoro NA, Korytkowski MT, Rose S, Gorin MB, Penles Stadler M, Witchel SF, Mulvihill JJ (1997). Spectrum of malignancy and premalignancy in Carney syndrome. Am J Med Genet 73: 369-377.

1626. O'Brien T, O'Riordan DS, Gharib H, Scheithauer BW, Ebersold MJ, van Heerden JA (1996). Results of treatment of pituitary disease in multiple endocrine neoplasia, type I. Neurosurgery 39: 273-278.

1627. O'Brien WM, Lynch JH (1987). Adrenal metastases by renal cell carcinoma. Incidence at nephrectomy. Urology 29: 605-607.

1628. O'Byrne KJ, Goggins MG, McDonald GS, Daly PA, Kelleher DP, Weir DG (1994). A metastatic neuroendocrine anaplastic small cell tumor in a patient with multiple endocrine neoplasia type 1 syndrome. Assessment of disease status and response to doxorubicin, cyclophosphamide, etoposide chemotherapy through scintigraphic imaging with 111In-pentetreotide. Cancer 74: 2374-2378.

1629. O'Connor TP, Wade TP, Sunwoo YC, Reimers HJ, Palmer DC, Silverberg AB, Johnson FE (1992). Small cell undifferentiated carcinoma of the pancreas. Report of a patient with tumor marker studies. Cancer 70: 1514-1519.

1630. Obara T, Fujimoto Y, Tanaka R, Ito Y, Kodama T, Yashiro T, Kanaji Y, Yamashita T, Fukuuchi A (1990). Mid-mediastinal parathyroid lesions: preoperative localization and surgical approach in two cases. Jpn J Surg 20: 481-486.

1631. Obara T, Okamoto T, Kanbe M, Iihara M (1997). Functioning parathyroid carcinoma: clinicopathologic features and rational treatment. Semin Surg Oncol 13: 134-141.

1632. Ober WB, Kaiser GA (1958). Hamartoma of the parathyroid. Cancer 601-606.

1633. Odze R, Begin LR (1990). Malignant paraganglioma of the posterior mediastinum. A case report and review of the literature. Cancer 65: 564-569.

1634. Ogawa T, Mitsukawa T, Ishikawa T, Tamura K (1994). Familial pheochromocytoma associated with von Recklinghausen's disease. Intern Med 33: 110-114.

1635. Oh YL, Ko YH, Ree HJ (1998). Aspiration cytology of ectopic cervical thymoma mimicking a thyroid mass. A case report. Acta Cytol 42: 1167-1171.

1636. Ohgaki H, Kleihues P, Heitz PU (1993). p53 mutations in sporadic adrenocortical tumors. Int J Cancer 54: 408-410.

1637. Ohh M, Yauch RL, Lonergan KM, Whaley JM, Stemmer-Rachamimov AO, Louis DN, Gavin BJ, Kley N, Kaelin WGJr, Iliopoulos O (1998). The von Hippel-Lindau tumor suppressor protein is required for proper assembly of an extracellular fibronectin matrix. Mol Cell 1: 959-968.

1638. Ohike N, Jurgensen A, Pipeleers-Marichal M, Kloppel G (2003). Mixed ductal-endocrine carcinomas of the pancreas and ductal adenocarcinomas with scattered endocrine cells: characterization of the endocrine cells. Virchows Arch 442: 258-265.

1639. Ohkura N, Kishi M, Tsukada T, Yamaguchi K (2001). Menin, a gene product responsible for multiple endocrine neoplasia type 1, interacts with the putative tumor metastasis suppressor nm23. Biochem Biophys Res Commun 282: 1206-1210.

1640. Ohneda A, Otsuki M, Fujiya H, Yaginuma N, Kokubo T, Ohtani H (1979). A malignant insulinoma transformed into a glucagonoma syndrome. Diabetes 28: 962-969.

1641. Ohta K, Yasuo K, Morikawa M, Nagashima T, Tamaki N (2001). Treatment of tuberculum sellae meningiomas: a long-term follow-up study. J Clin Neurosci 8 Suppl 1: 26-31.

1642. Ohta S, Ryu H, Miura K (1999). Eighteen-year survival of a patient with malignant pleomorphic xanthoastrocytoma associated with von Recklinghausen neurofibromatosis. Br J Neurosurg 13: 420-422.

1643. Okamoto S, Hisaoka M, Meis-Kindblom JM, Kindblom LG, Hashimoto H (2002). Juxta-articular myxoma and intramuscular myxoma are two distinct entities. Activating Gs alpha mutation at Arg 201

codon does not occur in juxta-articular myxoma. Virchows Arch 440: 12-15.
1644. Okamoto S, Hisaoka M, Ushijima M, Nakahara S, Toyoshima S, Hashimoto H (2000). Activating Gs(alpha) mutation in intramuscular myxomas with and without fibrous dysplasia of bone. Virchows Arch 437: 133-137.
1645. Okuda H, Saitoh K, Hirai S, Iwai K, Takaki Y, Baba M, Minato N, Ohno S, Shuin T (2001). The von Hippel-Lindau tumor suppressor protein mediates ubiquitination of activated atypical protein kinase C. J Biol Chem 276: 43611-43617.
1646. Oliveira AM, Tazelaar HD, Myers JL, Erickson LA, Lloyd RV (2001). Thyroid transcription factor-1 distinguishes metastatic pulmonary from well-differentiated neuroendocrine tumors of other sites. Am J Surg Pathol 25: 815-819.
1647. Olufemi SE, Green JS, Manickam P, Guru SC, Agarwal SK, Kester MB, Dong Q, Burns AL, Spiegel AM, Marx SJ, Collins FS, Chandrasekharappa SC (1998). Common ancestral mutation in the MEN1 gene is likely responsible for the prolactinoma variant of MEN1 (MEN1Burin) in four kindreds from Newfoundland. Hum Mutat 11: 264-269.
1648. Onal C, Bayindir C (1999). Gliomatosis cerebri with neurofibromatosis: an autopsy-proven case. Childs Nerv Syst 15: 219-221.
1649. Ooi A, Kameya T, Tsumuraya M, Yamaguchi K, Abe K, Shimosato Y, Yanaihara N (1985). Pancreatic endocrine tumours associated with WDHA syndrome. An immunohistochemical and electron microscopic study. Virchows Arch A Pathol Anat Histopathol 405: 311-323.
1650. Orchard T, Grant CS, van Heerden JA, Weaver A (1993). Pheochromocytoma—continuing evolution of surgical therapy. Surgery 114: 1153-1158.
1651. Ordonez NG (2000). Thyroid transcription factor-1 is a marker of lung and thyroid carcinomas. Adv Anat Pathol 7: 123-127.
1652. Ordonez NG (2000). Value of thyroid transcription factor-1, E-cadherin, BG8, WT1, and CD44S immunostaining in distinguishing epithelial pleural mesothelioma from pulmonary and nonpulmonary adenocarcinoma. Am J Surg Pathol 24: 598-606.
1653. Ordonez NG, el Naggar AK, Hickey RC, Samaan NA (1991). Anaplastic thyroid carcinoma. Immunocytochemical study of 32 cases. Am J Clin Pathol 96: 15-24.
1654. Ordonez NG, Ibanez ML, Mackay B, Samaan NA, Hickey RC (1982). Functioning oxyphil cell adenomas of parathyroid gland: immunoperoxidase evidence of hormonal activity in oxyphil cells. Am J Clin Pathol 78: 681-689.
1655. Ordonez NG, Ibanez ML, Samaan NA, Hickey RC (1983). Immunoperoxidase study of uncommon parathyroid tumors. Report of two cases of nonfunctioning parathyroid carcinoma and one intrathyroid parathyroid tumor-producing amyloid. Am J Surg Pathol 7: 535-542.
1656. Ordonez NG, Manning JTJr, Raymond AK (1985). Argentaffin endocrine carcinoma (carcinoid) of the pancreas with concomitant breast metastasis: an immunohistochemical and electron microscopic study. Hum Pathol 16: 746-751.
1657. Orlandi F, Chiefari E, Caraci P, Mussa A, Gonzatto I, De Giuli P, Giuffrida D, Angeli A, Filetti S (2001). RET proto-oncogene mutation in a mixed medullary-follicular thyroid carcinoma. J Endocrinol Invest 24: 51-55.
1658. Ornvold K, Ralfkiaer E, Carstensen H (1990). Immunohistochemical study of the abnormal cells in Langerhans cell histiocytosis (histiocytosis x). Virchows Arch A Pathol Anat Histopathol 416: 403-410.
1659. Orringer RD, Lynch JA, McDermott WV (1983). Cavernous hemangioma of the adrenal gland. J Surg Oncol 22: 106-108.
1660. Orselli RC, Bassler TJ (1973). Theca granuloma cell tumor arising in adrenal. Cancer 31: 474-477.
1661. Osamura RY, Yasuda O, Kawai K, Hori S, Suemizu S, Joh TH (1990). Immunohistochemical localization of catecholamine-synthesizing enzymes in human pheochromocytomas. Endocr Pathol 1: 102-108.
1662. Osborn AG (1994). Sellar/ suprasellar masses. In: Diagnostic Neuroradiology, Osborn AG, ed., Mosby: St Louis pp. 461-483.
1663. Ostrowski ML, Merino MJ (1996). Tall cell variant of papillary thyroid carcinoma: a reassessment and immunohistochemical study with comparison to the usual type of papillary carcinoma of the thyroid. Am J Surg Pathol 20: 964-974.
1664. Otal P, Escourrou G, Mazerolles C, Janne d'Othee B, Mezghani S, Musso S, Colombier D, Rousseau H, Joffre F (1999). Imaging features of uncommon adrenal masses with histopathologic correlation. Radiographics 19: 569-581.
1665. Oyama K, Sanno N, Teramoto A, Osamura RY (2001). Expression of neuro D1 in human normal pituitaries and pituitary adenomas. Mod Pathol 14: 892-899.
1666. Ozaki O, Ito K, Kobayashi K, Suzuki A, Manabe Y, Hosoda Y (1988). Familial occurrence of differentiated, nonmedullary thyroid carcinoma. World J Surg 12: 565-571.
1667. Ozaki O, Ito K, Sugino K, Yasuda K, Yamashita T, Toshima K (1992). Solid cell nests of the thyroid gland: precursor of mucoepidermoid carcinoma? World J Surg 16: 685-688.
1668. Pacak K, Eisenhofer G, Carrasquillo JA, Chen CC, Li ST, Goldstein DS (2001). 6-[18F]fluorodopamine positron emission tomographic (PET) scanning for diagnostic localization of pheochromocytoma. Hypertension 38: 6-8.
1669. Pachnis V, Mankoo B, Costantini F (1993). Expression of the c-ret proto-oncogene during mouse embryogenesis. Development 119: 1005-1017.
1670. Pacini F, Fontanelli M, Fugazzola L, Elisei R, Romei C, Di Coscio G, Miccoli P, Pinchera A (1994). Routine measurement of serum calcitonin in nodular thyroid diseases allows the preoperative diagnosis of unsuspected sporadic medullary thyroid carcinoma. J Clin Endocrinol Metab 78: 826-829.
1671. Pack SD, Kirschner LS, Pak E, Zhuang Z, Carney JA, Stratakis CA (2000). Genetic and histologic studies of somatomammotropic pituitary tumors in patients with the "complex of spotty skin pigmentation, myxomas, endocrine overactivity and schwannomas" (Carney complex). J Clin Endocrinol Metab 85: 3860-3865.
1672. Pack SD, Zbar B, Pak E, Ault DO, Humphrey JS, Pham T, Hurley K, Weil RJ, Park WS, Kuzmin I, Stolle C, Glenn G, Liotta LA, Lerman MI, Klausner RD, Linehan WM, Zhuang Z (1999). Constitutional von Hippel-Lindau (VHL) gene deletions detected in VHL families by fluorescence in situ hybridization. Cancer Res 59: 5560-5564.
1673. Page DL, DeLellis RA, Hough AJJ (1986). Tumors of the Adrenal. 2nd ed. Armed Forces Institute of Pathology: Washington, DC.
1674. Pagotto U, Arzberger T, Theodoropoulou M, Grubler Y, Pantaloni C, Saeger W, Losa M, Journot L, Stalla GK, Spengler D (2000). The expression of the antiproliferative gene ZAC is lost or highly reduced in nonfunctioning pituitary adenomas. Cancer Res 60: 6794-6799.
1675. Paivansalo M, Siniluoto T, Seppanen U (1986). Cavernous hemangioma of the adrenal gland. Diagn Imaging Clin Med 55: 168-171.
1676. Pal T, Vogl FD, Chappuis PO, Tsang R, Brierley J, Renard H, Sanders K, Kantemiroff T, Bagha S, Goldgar DE, Narod SA, Foulkes WD (2001). Increased risk for nonmedullary thyroid cancer in the first degree relatives of prevalent cases of nonmedullary thyroid cancer: a hospital-based study. J Clin Endocrinol Metab 86: 5307-5312.
1677. Paleologos TS, Gouliamos AD, Kourousis DD, Papanicolaou P, Vlahos C, Kyriakou T (1998). Paraganglioma of the cauda equina: a case presenting features of increased intracranial pressure. J Spinal Disord 11: 362-365.
1678. Palmer M, Adami HO, Bergstrom R, Akerstrom G, Ljunghall S (1987). Mortality after surgery for primary hyperparathyroidism: a follow-up of 441 patients operated on from 1956 to 1979. Surgery 102: 1-7.
1679. Pang LC, Tsao KC (1993). Flow cytometric DNA analysis for the determination of malignant potential in adrenal and extra-adrenal pheochromocytomas or paragangliomas. Arch Pathol Lab Med 117: 1142-1147.
1680. Papillon E, Rolachon A, Calender A, Chabre O, Barnoud R, Fournet J (2001). A malignant gastrointestinal stromal tumour in a patient with multiple endocrine neoplasia type 1. Eur J Gastroenterol Hepatol 13: 207-211.
1681. Papotti M, Bongiovanni M, Volante M, Allia E, Landolfi S, Helboe L, Schindler M, Cole SL, Bussolati G (2002). Expression of somatostatin receptor types 1-5 in 81 cases of gastrointestinal and pancreatic endocrine tumors. A correlative immunohistochemical and reverse-transcriptase polymerase chain reaction analysis. Virchows Arch 440: 461-475.
1682. Papotti M, Botto Micca F, Favero A, Palestini N, Bussolati G (1993). Poorly differentiated thyroid carcinomas with primordial cell component. A group of aggressive lesions sharing insular, trabecular, and solid patterns. Am J Surg Pathol 17: 291-301.
1683. Papotti M, Negro F, Carney JA, Bussolati G, Lloyd RV (1997). Mixed medullary-follicular carcinoma of the thyroid. A morphological, immunohistochemical and in situ hybridization analysis of 11 cases. Virchows Arch 430: 397-405.
1684. Papotti M, Sambataro D, Pecchioni C, Bussolati G (1996). The Pathology of Medullary Carcinoma of the Thyroid: Review of the Literature and Personal Experience on 62 Cases. Endocr Pathol 7: 1-20.
1685. Papotti M, Sapino A, Abbona GC, Palestini N, Bussolati G (1995). Pseudosarcomatous features in medullary carcinomas of the thyroid. Report of two cases. Int J Surg Pathol 3: 29-34.
1686. Papotti M, Torchio B, Grassi L, Favero A, Bussolati G (1996). Poorly differentiated oxyphilic (Hurthle cell) carcinomas of the thyroid. Am J Surg Pathol 20: 686-694.
1687. Papotti M, Volante M, Giuliano A, Fassina A, Fusco A, Bussolati G, Santoro M, Chiappetta G (2000). RET/PTC activation in hyalinizing trabecular tumors of the thyroid. Am J Surg Pathol 24: 1615-1621.
1688. Papotti M, Volante M, Komminoth P, Sobrinho-Simoes M, Bussolati G (2000). Thyroid carcinomas with mixed follicular and C-cell differentiation patterns. Semin Diagn Pathol 17: 109-119.
1689. Papotti M, Volante M, Negro F, Eusebi V, Bussolati G (2000). Thyroglobulin mRNA expression helps to distinguish anaplastic carcinoma from angiosarcoma of the thyroid. Virchows Arch 437: 635-642.
1690. Park DH, Park YK, Oh JI, Kwon TH, Chung HS, Cho HD, Suh YL (2002). Oncocytic paraganglioma of the cauda equina in a child. Case report and review of the literature. Pediatr Neurosurg 36: 260-265.
1691. Park SK, O'Dorisio MS, O'Dorisio TM (1996). Vasoactive intestinal polypeptide-secreting tumours: biology and therapy. Baillieres Clin Gastroenterol 10: 673-696.
1692. Parker LN, Kollin J, Wu SY, Rypins EB, Juler GL (1985). Carcinoma of the thyroid with a mixed medullary, papillary, follicular, and undifferentiated pattern. Arch Intern Med 145: 1507-1509.
1693. Parl FF, Cruz VE, Cobb CA, Bradley CA, Aleshire SL (1986). Late recurrence of surgically removed prolactinomas. Cancer 57: 2422-2426.
1694. Parsa CF, Hoyt CT, Lesser RL, Weinstein JM, Strother CM, Muci-Mendoza R, Ramella M, Manor RS, Fletcher WA, Repka MX, Garrity JA, Ebner RN, Monteiro ML, McFadzean RM, Rubtsova IV, Hoyt WF (2001). Spontaneous regression of optic gliomas: thirteen cases documented by serial neuroimaging. Arch Ophthalmol 119: 516-529.
1695. Partington MD, Davis DH, Laws ERJr, Scheithauer BW (1994). Pituitary adenomas in childhood and adolescence. Results of transsphenoidal surgery. J Neurosurg 80: 209-216.
1696. Pasini A, Geneste O, Legrand P, Schlumberger M, Rossel M, Fournier L, Rudkin BB, Schuffenecker I, Lenoir GM, Billaud M (1997). Oncogenic activation of RET by two distinct FMTC mutations affecting the tyrosine kinase domain. Oncogene 15: 393-402.
1697. Pasini B, Hofstra RM, Yin L, Bocciardi R, Santamaria G, Grootscholten PM, Ceccherini I, Patrone G, Priolo M, Buys CH, Romeo G (1995). The physical map of the human RET proto-oncogene. Oncogene 11: 1737-1743.
1698. Passarge E (1967). The genetics of Hirschsprung's disease. Evidence for heterogeneous etiology and a study of sixty-three families. N Engl J Med 276: 138-143.
1699. Pastolero GC, Coire CI, Asa SL (1996). Concurrent medullary and papillary carcinomas of thyroid with lymph node metastases. A collision phenomenon. Am J Surg Pathol 20: 245-250.
1700. Pastore YD, Jelinek J, Ang S, Guan Y, Liu E, Jedlickova K, Krishnamurti L, Prchal JT (2003). Mutations in the VHL gene in sporadic apparently congenital polycythemia. Blood 101: 1591-1595.
1701. Patchefsky AS, Solit R, Phillips LD, Craddock M, Harrer MV, Cohn HE, Kowlessar OD (1972). Hydroxyindole-producing tumors of the pancreas. Carcinoid-islet cell tumor and oat cell carcinoma. Ann Intern Med 77: 53-61.

1702. Patetsios P, Gable DR, Garrett WV, Lamont JP, Kuhn JA, Shutze WP, Kourlis H, Grimsley B, Pearl GJ, Smith BL, Talkington CM, Thompson JE (2002). Management of carotid body paragangliomas and review of a 30-year experience. Ann Vasc Surg 16: 331-338.
1703. Pause A, Lee S, Lonergan KM, Klausner RD (1998). The von Hippel-Lindau tumor suppressor gene is required for cell cycle exit upon serum withdrawal. Proc Natl Acad Sci U S A 95: 993-998.
1704. Pause A, Lee S, Worrell RA, Chen DY, Burgess WH, Linehan WM, Klausner RD (1997). The von Hippel-Lindau tumor-suppressor gene product forms a stable complex with human CUL-2, a member of the Cdc53 family of proteins. Proc Natl Acad Sci U S A 94: 2156-2161.
1705. Peczkowska M, Gessek J, Januszewicz A, Neumann HP, Januszewicz M, Janaszek-Sitkowska H, Prejbisz A, Kabat M, Skierski J, Ciesla W, Szostek M (2002). Pheochromocytoma of the urinary bladder coexisting with another extra-adrenal tumour—case report of a 19-year-old male patient. Blood Press 11: 101-105.
1706. Pedersen RK, Pedersen NT (1996). Primary non-Hodgkin's lymphoma of the thyroid gland: a population based study. Histopathology 28: 25-32.
1707. Peghini PL, Iwamoto M, Raffeld M, Chen YJ, Goebel SU, Serrano J, Jensen RT (2002). Overexpression of epidermal growth factor and hepatocyte growth factor receptors in a proportion of gastrinomas correlates with aggressive growth and lower curability. Clin Cancer Res 8: 2273-2285.
1708. Pei L, Melmed S (1997). Isolation and characterization of a pituitary tumor-transforming gene (PTTG). Mol Endocrinol 11: 433-441.
1709. Pei L, Melmed S, Scheithauer B, Kovacs K, Benedict WF, Prager D (1995). Frequent loss of heterozygosity at the retinoblastoma susceptibility gene (RB) locus in aggressive pituitary tumors: evidence for a chromosome 13 tumor suppressor gene other than RB. Cancer Res 55: 1613-1616.
1710. Pei L, Melmed S, Scheithauer B, Kovacs K, Prager D (1994). H-ras mutations in human pituitary carcinoma metastases. J Clin Endocrinol Metab 78: 842-846.
1711. Peillon F, Le Dafniet M, Garnier P, Feinstein MC, Donnadieu M, Barret A, Gautron JP, Brandi AM, Benlot C, Lagoguey A, Lefebvre P, Blumberg-Tick J, Joubert D (1989). [Neurohormones coming from the normal and tumoral human anterior pituitary. Secretion and regulation in vitro]. Pathol Biol (Paris) 37: 840-845.
1712. Peillon F, Liappi G, Garnier P, Brandi AM, Evain-Brion D, Dodeur M, Gautron JP, Donnadieu M, Michard M, Racadot J, Joubert D (1988). [In vitro secretion of somatostatin (SRIH) by human adenomatous somatotropic cells. Relation with somatotropic hormone (GH) release and modulation by thyroliberin (TRH)]. C R Acad Sci III 306: 161-166.
1713. Pelkey TJ, Frierson HFJr, Mills SE, Stoler MH (1998). The alpha subunit of inhibin in adrenal cortical neoplasia. Mod Pathol 11: 516-524.
1714. Pelletier G, Cortot A, Launay JM, Debons-Guillemain MC, Nemeth J, Le Charpentier Y, Celerier M, Modigliani R (1984). Serotonin-secreting and insulin-secreting ileal carcinoid tumor and the use of in vitro culture of tumoral cells. Cancer 54: 319-322.
1715. Pelosi G, Bresaola E, Bogina G, Pasini F, Rodella S, Castelli P, Iacono C, Serio G, Zamboni G (1996). Endocrine tumors of the pancreas: Ki-67 immunoreactivity on paraffin sections is an independent predictor for malignancy: a comparative study with proliferating-cell nuclear antigen and progesterone receptor protein immunostaining, mitotic index, and other clinicopathologic variables. Hum Pathol 27: 1124-1134.
1716. Penabad JL, Bashey HM, Asa SL, Haddad G, Davis KD, Herbst AB, Gennarelli TA, Kaiser UB, Chin WW, Snyder PJ (1996). Decreased follistatin gene expression in gonadotroph adenomas. J Clin Endocrinol Metab 81: 3397-3403.
1717. Perez-Montiel MD, Frankel WL, Suster S (2003). Neuroendocrine carcinomas of the pancreas with 'Rhabdoid' features. Am J Surg Pathol 27: 642-649.
1718. Perez-Ordonez B, Erlandson RA, Rosai J (1996). Follicular dendritic cell tumor: report of 13 additional cases of a distinctive entity. Am J Surg Pathol 20: 944-955.
1719. Perkel VS, Gail MH, Lubin J, Pee DY, Weinstein R, Shore-Freedman E, Schneider AB (1988). Radiation-induced thyroid neoplasms: evidence for familial susceptibility factors. J Clin Endocrinol Metab 66: 1316-1322.
1720. Pernicone PJ, Scheithauer BW, Sebo TJ, Kovacs KT, Horvath E, Young WFJr, Lloyd RV, Davis DH, Guthrie BL, Schoene WC (1997). Pituitary carcinoma: a clinicopathologic study of 15 cases. Cancer 79: 804-812.
1721. Perren A, Barghorn A, Schmid S, Saremaslani P, Roth J, Heitz PU, Komminoth P (2002). Absence of somatic SDHD mutations in sporadic neuroendocrine tumors and detection of two germline variants in paraganglioma patients. Oncogene 21: 7605-7608.
1722. Perren A, Hurlimann S, Saremaslani P, Schmid S, Bonvin C, Roth J, Heitz PU, Komminoth P (2002). DPC4/Smad4 expression is lost in a subset of ductal adenocarcinomas of the pancreas but not in endocrine pancreatic tumors and chronic pancreatitis. Mod Pathol 15: 119A.
1723. Perren A, Komminoth P, Saremaslani P, Matter C, Feurer S, Lees JA, Heitz PU, Eng C (2000). Mutation and expression analyses reveal differential subcellular compartmentalization of PTEN in endocrine pancreatic tumors compared to normal islet cells. Am J Pathol 157: 1097-1103.
1724. Perren A, Roth J, Muletta-Feurer S, Saremaslani P, Speel EJ, Heitz PU, Komminoth P (1998). Clonal analysis of sporadic pancreatic endocrine tumours. J Pathol 186: 363-371.
1725. Perren A, Saremaslani P, Bonvin C, Schmid S, Locher T, Heitz PU, Komminoth P (2003). Absence of BRAF Exon 11 and 15 mutations in neuroendocrine tumors. Mod Pathol 16: 108A.
1726. Perrier ND, Batts KP, Thompson GB, Grant CS, Plummer TB (1995). An immunohistochemical survey for neuroendocrine cells in regional pancreatic lymph nodes: a plausible explanation for primary nodal gastrinomas? Mayo Clinic Pancreatic Surgery Group. Surgery 118: 957-965.
1727. Perrier ND, van Heerden JA, Goellner JR, Williams ED, Gharib H, Marchesa P, Church JM, Fazio VW, Larson DR (1998). Thyroid cancer in patients with familial adenomatous polyposis. World J Surg 22: 738-742.
1728. Perry A, Molberg K, Albores-Saavedra J (1996). Physiologic versus neoplastic C-cell hyperplasia of the thyroid: separation of distinct histologic and biologic entities. Cancer 77: 750-756.
1729. Perry A, Stafford SL, Scheithauer BW, Suman VJ, Lohse CM (1998). The prognostic significance of MIB-1, p53, and DNA flow cytometry in completely resected primary meningiomas. Cancer 82: 2262-2269.
1730. Persaud V, Walrond ER (1971). Carcinoid tumor and cystadenoma of the pancreas. Arch Pathol 92: 28-30.
1731. Pesce C, Tobia F, Carli F, Antoniotti GV (1989). The sites of hormone storage in normal and diseased parathyroid glands: a silver impregnation and immunohistochemical study. Histopathology 15: 157-166.
1732. Peters J (1999). Components of a genetic cancer risk clinic. In: Cancer Genetics for the Clinician, Shaw GL, ed., Kluwer Academic/Plenum Publishers: New York , pp. 1-26.
1733. Pfaltz M, Hedinger C, Saremaslani P, Egloff B (1983). Malignant hemangioendothelioma of the thyroid and factor VIII-related antigen. Virchows Arch A Pathol Anat Histopathol 401: 177-184.
1734. Phay JE, Moley JF, Lairmore TC (2000). Multiple endocrine neoplasias. Semin Surg Oncol 18: 324-332.
1735. Pichard C, Gerber S, Laloi M, Kujas M, Clemenceau S, Ponvert D, Bruckert E, Turpin G (2002). Pituitary carcinoma: report of an exceptional case and review of the literature. J Endocrinol Invest 25: 65-72.
1736. Pierce SM, Barnes PD, Loeffler JS, McGinn C, Tarbell NJ (1990). Definitive radiation therapy in the management of symptomatic patients with optic glioma. Survival and long-term effects. Cancer 65: 45-52.
1737. Pierie JP, Muzikansky A, Gaz RD, Faquin WC, Ott MJ (2002). The effect of surgery and radiotherapy on outcome of anaplastic thyroid carcinoma. Ann Surg Oncol 9: 57-64.
1738. Piersanti M, Ezzat S, Asa SL (2003). Controversies in papillary microcarcinoma of the thyroid. Endocr Pathol 14: 183-191.
1739. Pietribiasi F, Sapino A, Papotti M, Bussolati G (1990). Cytologic features of poorly differentiated 'insular' carcinoma of the thyroid, as revealed by fine-needle aspiration biopsy. Am J Clin Pathol 94: 687-692.
1740. Pikkarainen L, Sane T, Reunanen A (1999). The survival and well-being of patients treated for Cushing's syndrome. J Intern Med 245: 463-468.
1741. Pilato FP, D'Adda T, Banchini E, Bordi C (1988). Nonrandom expression of polypeptide hormones in pancreatic endocrine tumors. An immunohistochemical study in a case of multiple islet cell neoplasia. Cancer 61: 1815-1820.
1742. Pilon C, Pistorello M, Moscon A, Altavilla G, Pagotto U, Boscaro M, Fallo F (1999). Inactivation of the p16 tumor suppressor gene in adrenocortical tumors. J Clin Endocrinol Metab 84: 2776-2779.
1743. Pilotti S, Collini P, Del Bo R, Cattoretti G, Pierotti MA, Rilke F (1994). A novel panel of antibodies that segregates immunocytochemically poorly differentiated carcinoma from undifferentiated carcinoma of the thyroid gland. Am J Surg Pathol 18: 1054-1064.
1744. Pilotti S, Collini P, Mariani L, Placucci M, Bongarzone I, Vigneri P, Cipriani S, Falcetta F, Miceli R, Pierotti MA, Rilke F (1997). Insular carcinoma: a distinct de novo entity among follicular carcinomas of the thyroid gland. Am J Surg Pathol 21: 1466-1473.
1745. Pinkus GS, Lones MA, Matsumura F, Yamashiro S, Said JW, Pinkus JL (2002). Langerhans cell histiocytosis immunohistochemical expression of fascin, a dendritic cell marker. Am J Clin Pathol 118: 335-343.
1746. Pinzone JJ, Katznelson L, Danila DC, Pauler DK, Miller CS, Klibanski A (2000). Primary medical therapy of micro- and macroprolactinomas in men. J Clin Endocrinol Metab 85: 3053-3057.
1747. Pioli PA, Rigby WF (2001). The von Hippel-Lindau protein interacts with heteronuclear ribonucleoprotein a2 and regulates its expression. J Biol Chem 276: 40346-40352.
1748. Pipeleers-Marichal M, Somers G, Willems G, Foulis A, Imrie C, Bishop AE, Polak JM, Hacki WH, Stamm B, Heitz PU, Kloppel G (1990). Gastrinomas in the duodenums of patients with multiple endocrine neoplasia type 1 and the Zollinger-Ellison syndrome. N Engl J Med 322: 723-727.
1749. Pizzi S, D'Adda T, Azzoni C, Rindi G, Grigolato P, Pasquali C, Corleto VD, Delle Fave G, Bordi C (2002). Malignancy-associated allelic losses on the X-chromosome in foregut but not in midgut endocrine tumours. J Pathol 196: 401-407.
1750. Plaut A (1962). Locally invasive lymphangioma of adrenal gland. Cancer 15: 1165-1169.
1751. Plawner J (1991). Results of surgical treatment of kidney cancer with solitary metastasis to contralateral adrenal. Urology 37: 233-236.
1752. Pledge S, Bessell EM, Leach IH, Pegg CA, Jenkins D, Dowling F, Moloney A (1996). Non-Hodgkin's lymphoma of the thyroid: a retrospective review of all patients diagnosed in Nottinghamshire from 1973 to 1992. Clin Oncol (R Coll Radiol) 8: 371-375.
1753. Plockinger U, Wiedenmann B (2002). Neuroendocrine tumors of the gastro-entero-pancreatic system: the role of early diagnosis, genetic testing and preventive surgery. Dig Dis 20: 49-60.
1754. Plukker JT, Brongers EP, Vermey A, Krikke A, van den Dungen JJ (2001). Outcome of surgical treatment for carotid body paraganglioma. Br J Surg 88: 1382-1386.
1755. Pojunas KW, Daniels DL, Williams AL, Haughton VM (1986). MR imaging of prolactin-secreting microadenomas. AJNR Am J Neuroradiol 7: 209-213.
1756. Polga JP, Balikian JP (1971). Partially calcified functioning parathyroid adenoma. Casedemonstrated roentgenographically. Radiology 99: 55-56.
1757. Pollack IF, Shultz B, Mulvihill JJ (1996). The management of brainstem gliomas in patients with neurofibromatosis 1. Neurology 46: 1652-1660.
1758. Pollock BE, Kondziolka D, Lunsford LD, Flickinger JC (1994). Stereotactic radiosurgery for pituitary adenomas: imaging, visual and endocrine results. Acta Neurochir Suppl (Wien) 62: 33-38.
1759. Pollock WJ, McConnell CF, Hilton C, Lavine RL (1986). Virilizing Leydig cell adenoma of adrenal gland. Am J Surg Pathol 10: 816-822.
1760. Pommier RF, Vetto JT, Billingsly K, Woltering EA, Brennan MF (1993).

Comparison of adrenal and extraadrenal pheochromocytomas. Surgery 114: 1160-1165.
1761. Ponder BA (1997). Multiple endocrine neoplasia type 2. In: The Genetic Basis of Human Cancer, Vogelstein B., Kinzler KW, eds., 1st ed. McGraw-Hill: New York , pp. 475-487.
1762. Ponder BA, Ponder MA, Coffey R, Pembrey ME, Gagel RF, Telenius-Berg M, Semple P, Easton DF (1988). Risk estimation and screening in families of patients with medullary thyroid carcinoma. Lancet 1: 397-401.
1763. Poole GVJr, Albertson DA, Marshall RB, Myers RT (1982). Oxyphil cell adenoma and hyperparathyroidism. Surgery 92: 799-805.
1764. Post KD, McCormick PC, Hays AP, Kandji AG (1988). Metastatic carcinoma to pituitary adenoma. Report of two cases. Surg Neurol 30: 286-292.
1765. Poston CD, Jaffe GS, Lubensky IA, Solomon D, Zbar B, Linehan WM, Walther MM (1995). Characterization of the renal pathology of a familial form of renal cell carcinoma associated with von Hippel-Lindau disease: clinical and molecular genetic implications. J Urol 153: 22-26.
1766. Powell DJJr, Russell J, Nibu K, Li G, Rhee E, Liao M, Goldstein M, Keane WM, Santoro M, Fusco A, Rothstein JL (1998). The RET/PTC3 oncogene: metastatic solid-type papillary carcinomas in murine thyroids. Cancer Res 58: 5523-5528.
1767. Powell J, Sahin M, Wang X, Hay I, Zhao Y, Hiddinga H, Goellner J, Kroll T, Grebe S, Eberhardt N, McIver B (2003). The PAX8-PPARg fusion gene transforms human thyrocytes and functions as a morphotype specific oncogene in follicular thyroid carcinoma. Cancer Res .
1768. Powell JG, Goellner JR, Nowak LE, McIver B (2003). Rosai-dorfman disease of the thyroid masquerading as anaplastic carcinoma. Thyroid 13: 217-221.
1769. Premkumar A, Stratakis CA, Shawker TH, Papanicolaou DA, Chrousos GP (1997). Testicular ultrasound in Carney complex: report of three cases. J Clin Ultrasound 25: 211-214.
1770. Preto A, Cameselle-Teijeiro J, Moldes-Boullosa J, Soares P, Cameselle-Teijeiro JF, Silva P, Reis-Filho JS, Reyes-Santias RM, Alfonsin-Barreiro N, Forteza J, Sobrinho-Simoes M (2004). Telomerase expression and proliferative activity suggest a stem cell role for thyroid solid cell nests. Mod Pathol 17: 819-826.
1771. Prinz RA, Dorsch TR, Lawrence AM (1981). Clinical aspects of glucagon-producing islet cell tumors. Am J Gastroenterol 76: 125-131.
1772. Proppe KH, Scully RE (1980). Large-cell calcifying Sertoli cell tumor of the testis. Am J Clin Pathol 74: 607-619.
1773. Prowse AH, Webster AR, Richards FM, Richard S, Olschwang S, Resche F, Affara NA, Maher ER (1997). Somatic inactivation of the VHL gene in Von Hippel-Lindau disease tumors. Am J Hum Genet 60: 765-771.
1774. Proye C, Racadot-Leroy N, Vix M, Vermesse B, Carnaille B (1994). [Comparative secretory profiles of benign and malignant pheochromocytomas]. Ann Chir 48: 430-434.
1775. Puchner MJ, Ludecke DK, Saeger W, Riedel M, Asa SL (1995). Gangliocytomas of the sellar region—a review. Exp Clin Endocrinol Diabetes 103: 129-149.
1776. Puchner MJ, Ludecke DK, Valdueza JM, Saeger W, Willig RP, Stalla GK, Odink RJ (1993). Cushing's disease in a child caused by a corticotropin-releasing hormone-secreting intrasellar gangliocytoma associated with an adrenocorticotropic hormone-secreting pituitary adenoma. Neurosurgery 33: 920-924.
1777. Pujol P, Bringer J, Faurous P, Jaffiol C (1995). Metastatic phaeochromocytoma with a long-term response after iodine-131 metaiodobenzylguanidine therapy. Eur J Nucl Med 22: 382-384.
1778. Pujol RM, Matias-Guiu X, Miralles J, Colomer A, de Moragas JM (1997). Multiple idiopathic mucosal neuromas: a minor form of multiple endocrine neoplasia type 2B or a new entity? J Am Acad Dermatol 37: 349-352.
1779. Puri P, Motwani N, Pande M (2001). Squamous carcinoma of the thyroid metastatic to the choroid: a report. Eur J Cancer Care (Engl) 10: 63-64.
1780. Pusel J, Rodier JF, Auge B, Janser JC (1993). [Malignant hemangioendothelioma of the thyroid. Pathologic study of a case]. Ann Pathol 13: 253-255.
1781. Qian X, Jin L, Grande JP, Lloyd RV (1996). Transforming growth factor-beta and p27 expression in pituitary cells. Endocrinology 137: 3051-3060.
1782. Quissel B, Mohammad A, Bauer JH, Hakami N (1979). Malignant pheochromocytoma in childhood: report of a case with familial neurofibromatosis. Med Pediatr Oncol 7: 327-333.
1783. Raaf HN, Grant LD, Santoscoy C, Levin HS, Abdul-Karim FW (1996). Adenomatoid tumor of the adrenal gland: a report of four new cases and a review of the literature. Mod Pathol 9: 1046-1051.
1784. Rabes HM, Demidchik EP, Sidorow JD, Lengfelder E, Beimfohr C, Hoelzel D, Klugbauer S (2000). Pattern of radiation-induced RET and NTRK1 rearrangements in 191 post-chernobyl papillary thyroid carcinomas: biological, phenotypic, and clinical implications. Clin Cancer Res 6: 1093-1103.
1785. Raco A, Bristot R, Domenicucci M, Cantore G (1999). Meningiomas of the tuberculum sellae. Our experience in 69 cases surgically treated between 1973 and 1993. J Neurosurg Sci 43: 253-260.
1786. Radi MJ, Fenoglio-Preiser CM, Chiffelle T (1985). Functioning oncocytic islet-cell carcinoma. Report of a case with electron-microscopic and immunohistochemical confirmation. Am J Surg Pathol 9: 517-524.
1787. Radice P, Sozzi G, Miozzo M, De Benedetti V, Cariani T, Bongarzone I, Spurr NK, Pierotti MA, Della Porta G (1991). The human tropomyosin gene involved in the generation of the TRK oncogene maps to chromosome 1q31. Oncogene 6: 2145-2148.
1788. Raff SB, Carney JA, Krugman D, Doppman JL, Stratakis CA (2000). Prolactin secretion abnormalities in patients with the "syndrome of spotty skin pigmentation, myxomas, endocrine overactivity and schwannomas" (Carney complex). J Pediatr Endocrinol Metab 13: 373-379.
1789. Rahmani M, Peron P, Weitzman J, Bakiri L, Lardeux B, Bernuau D (2001). Functional cooperation between JunD and NF-kappaB in rat hepatocytes. Oncogene 20: 5132-5142.
1790. Rajasoorya C, Scheithauer BW, Tan L, Young WFJr (1999). Pituitary gigantism with intracerebral metastases. Endocrinologist 9: 497-501.
1791. Ramsay JA, Asa SL, van Nostrand AW, Hassaram ST, de Harven EP (1987). Lipid degeneration in pheochromocytomas mimicking adrenal cortical tumors. Am J Surg Pathol 11: 480-486.
1792. Ramsay JA, Kovacs K, Scheithauer BW, Ezrin C, Weiss MH (1988). Metastatic carcinoma to pituitary adenomas: a report of two cases. Exp Clin Endocrinol 92: 69-76.
1793. Randolph GW (2003). Follicular carcinoma of the thyroid. Saunders: Philadelphia.
1794. Raphael SJ, Apel RL, Asa SL (1995). Brief report: detection of high-molecular-weight cytokeratins in neoplastic and non-neoplastic thyroid tumors using microwave antigen retrieval. Mod Pathol 8: 870-872.
1795. Raphael SJ, McKeown-Eyssen G, Asa SL (1994). High-molecular-weight cytokeratin and cytokeratin-19 in the diagnosis of thyroid tumors. Mod Pathol 7: 295-300.
1796. Rasbach DA, Monchik JM, Geelhoed GW, Harrison TS (1984). Solitary parathyroid microadenoma. Surgery 96: 1092-1098.
1797. Rasmuson T, Damber L, Johansson L, Johansson R, Larsson LG (2002). Increased incidence of parathyroid adenomas following X-ray treatment of benign diseases in the cervical spine in adult patients. Clin Endocrinol (Oxf) 57: 731-734.
1798. Rasmussen SA, Yang Q, Friedman JM (2001). Mortality in neurofibromatosis 1: an analysis using U.S. death certificates. Am J Hum Genet 68: 1110-1118.
1799. Rechitsky S, Verlinsky O, Chistokhina A, Sharapova T, Ozen S, Masciangelo C, Kuliev A, Verlinsky Y (2002). Preimplantation genetic diagnosis for cancer predisposition. Reprod Biomed Online 5: 148-155.
1800. Redman BG, Pazdur R, Zingas AP, Loredo R (1987). Prospective evaluation of adrenal insufficiency in patients with adrenal metastasis. Cancer 60: 103-107.
1801. Reed RJ, Caroca PJJr, Harkin JC (1977). Gangliocytic paraganglioma. Am J Surg Pathol 1: 207-216.
1802. Regan PT, Malagelada JR (1978). A reappraisal of clinical, roentgenographic, and endoscopic features of the Zollinger-Ellison syndrome. Mayo Clin Proc 53: 19-23.
1803. Reichardt P, Apel TW, Domula M, Trobs RB, Krause I, Bierbach U, Neumann HP, Kiess W (2002). Recurrent polytopic chromaffin paragangliomas in a 9-year-old boy resulting from a novel germline mutation in the von Hippel-Lindau gene. J Pediatr Hematol Oncol 24: 145-148.
1804. Reincke M (1998). Mutations in adrenocortical tumors. Horm Metab Res 30: 447-455.
1805. Reincke M, Allolio B, Saeger W, Kaulen D, Winkelmann W (1987). A pituitary adenoma secreting high molecular weight adrenocorticotropin without evidence of Cushing's disease. J Clin Endocrinol Metab 65: 1296-1300.
1806. Reincke M, Beuschlein F, Slawik M, Borm K (2000). Molecular adrenocortical tumourigenesis. Eur J Clin Invest 30 Suppl 3: 63-68.
1807. Reincke M, Karl M, Travis WH, Mastorakos G, Allolio B, Linehan HM, Chrousos GP (1994). p53 mutations in human adrenocortical neoplasms: immunohistochemical and molecular studies. J Clin Endocrinol Metab 78: 790-794.
1808. Reincke M, Mora P, Beuschlein F, Arlt W, Chrousos GP, Allolio B (1997). Deletion of the adrenocorticotropin receptor gene in human adrenocortical tumors: implications for tumorigenesis. J Clin Endocrinol Metab 82: 3054-3058.
1809. Reis-Filho JS, Preto A, Soares P, Ricardo S, Cameselle-Teijeiro J, Sobrinho-Simoes M (2003). p63 Expression in Solid Cell Nests of the Thyroid: Further Evidence for a Stem Cell Origin. Mod Pathol 16: 43-48.
1810. ReMine WH, Chong GC, van Heerden JA, Sheps SG, Harrison EGJr (1974). Current management of pheochromocytoma. Ann Surg 179: 740-748.
1811. Renard L, Godfraind C, Boon LM, Vikkula M (2003). A novel mutation in the SDHD gene in a family with inherited paragangliomas-implications of genetic diagnosis for follow up and treatment. Head Neck 25: 146-151.
1812. Renshaw AA (2002). Hurthle cell carcinoma is a better gold standard than Hurthle cell neoplasm for fine-needle aspiration of the thyroid: defining more consistent and specific cytologic criteria. Cancer 96: 261-266.
1813. Renshaw AA (2003). Fine-needle aspiration of Hurthle cell lesions: making the best of what consumers want. Diagn Cytopathol 29: 183-184.
1814. Renshaw AA, Granter SR (1998). A comparison of A103 and inhibin reactivity in adrenal cortical tumors: distinction from hepatocellular carcinoma and renal tumors. Mod Pathol 11: 1160-1164.
1815. Reubi JC, Heitz PU, Gyr K (1987). Vasoactive intestinal peptide producing tumour contains high density of somatostatin receptors. Lancet 1: 741-742.
1816. Reubi JC, Landolt AM (1989). The growth hormone responses to octreotide in acromegaly correlate with adenoma somatostatin receptor status. J Clin Endocrinol Metab 68: 844-850.
1817. Reyes CV, Wang T (1981). Undifferentiated small cell carcinoma of the pancreas: a report of five cases. Cancer 47: 2500-2502.
1818. Ribeiro RC, Sandrini Neto RS, Schell MJ, Lacerda L, Sambaio GA, Cat I (1990). Adrenocortical carcinoma in children: a study of 40 cases. J Clin Oncol 8: 67-74.
1819. Riccardi VM, Eichner JE (1981). Psychosocial aspects. In: Neurofibromatosis: Phenotype, Natural History, and Pathogenesis, Riccardi VM, Eichner JE, eds., John Hopkins University Press: Baltimore , pp. 150-161.
1820. Richards FM, Crossey PA, Phipps ME, Foster K, Latif F, Evans G, Sampson J, Lerman MI, Zbar B, Affara NA, Ferguson-Smith MA, Maher ER (1994). Detailed mapping of germline deletions of the von Hippel-Lindau disease tumour suppressor gene. Hum Mol Genet 3: 595-598.
1821. Richards FM, Payne SJ, Zbar B, Affara NA, Ferguson-Smith MA, Maher ER (1995). Molecular analysis of de novo germline mutations in the von Hippel-Lindau disease gene. Hum Mol Genet 4: 2139-2143.
1822. Richards FM, Schofield PN, Fleming S, Maher ER (1996). Expression of the von Hippel-Lindau disease tumour suppressor gene during human embryogenesis. Hum Mol Genet 5: 639-644.
1823. Richmond J, Sherman RS, Diamond H, Craver LF (1962). Renal lesions associated with malignant lymphomas. Am J Med 32: 184-207.
1824. Rickert CH, Dockhorn-Dworniczak B, Busch G, Moskopp D, Albert FK, Rama B, Paulus W (2001). Increased chromosomal imbalances in recurrent pituitary adenomas. Acta Neuropathol (Berl) 102: 615-620.
1825. Rickert CH, Scheithauer BW, Paulus W (2001). Chromosomal aberrations in pitu-

itary carcinoma metastases. Acta Neuropathol (Berl) 102: 117-120.
1826. Riddle PE, Dincsoy HP (1987). Primary squamous cell carcinoma of the thyroid associated with leukocytosis and hypercalcemia. Arch Pathol Lab Med 111: 373-374.
1827. Rieth KG, Comite F, Shawker TH, Cutler GBJr (1984). Pituitary and ovarian abnormalities demonstrated by CT and ultrasound in children with features of the McCune-Albright syndrome. Radiology 153: 389-393.
1828. Rieu M, Lame MC, Richard A, Lissak B, Sambort B, Vuong-Ngoc P, Berrod JL, Fombeur JP (1995). Prevalence of sporadic medullary thyroid carcinoma: the importance of routine measurement of serum calcitonin in the diagnostic evaluation of thyroid nodules. Clin Endocrinol (Oxf) 42: 453-460.
1829. Rigaud C, Peltier F, Bogomoletz WV (1985). Mucin producing microfollicular adenoma of the thyroid. J Clin Pathol 38: 277-280.
1830. Rigaud G, Missiaglia E, Moore PS, Zamboni G, Falconi M, Talamini G, Pesci A, Baron A, Lissandrini D, Rindi G, Grigolato P, Pederzoli P, Scarpa A (2001). High resolution allelotype of nonfunctional pancreatic endocrine tumors: identification of two molecular subgroups with clinical implications. Cancer Res 61: 285-292.
1831. Riminucci M, Fisher LW, Majolagbe A, Corsi A, Lala R, de Sanctis C, Robey PG, Bianco P (1999). A novel GNAS1 mutation, R201G, in McCune-albright syndrome. J Bone Miner Res 14: 1987-1989.
1832. Riminucci M, Fisher LW, Shenker A, Spiegel AM, Bianco P, Gehron Robev P (1997). Fibrous dysplasia of bone in the McCune-Albright syndrome: abnormalities in bone formation. Am J Pathol 151: 1587-1600.
1833. Riminucci M, Liu B, Corsi A, Shenker A, Spiegel AM, Robey PG, Bianco P (1999). The histopathology of fibrous dysplasia of bone in patients with activating mutations of the Gs alpha gene: site-specific patterns and recurrent histological hallmarks. J Pathol 187: 249-258.
1834. Rindi G, Bishop AE, Murphy D, Solcia E, Hogan B, Polak JM (1988). A morphological analysis endocrine tumour genesis in pancreas and anterior pituitary of AVP/SV40 transgenic mice. Virchows Arch A Pathol Anat Histopathol 412: 255-266.
1835. Rindi G, Candusso ME, Marchetti AL (1999). Origin and Genetic Background of Insulinomas. Endocr Pathol 10: 283-290.
1836. Rindi G, Candusso ME, Solcia E (1999). Molecular aspects of the endocrine tumours of the pancreas and the gastrointestinal tract. Ital J Gastroenterol Hepatol 31 Suppl 2: S135-S138.
1837. Rindi G, Grant SG, Yiangou Y, Ghatei MA, Bloom SR, Bautch VL, Solcia E, Polak JM (1990). Development of neuroendocrine tumors in the gastrointestinal tract of transgenic mice. Heterogeneity of hormone expression. Am J Pathol 136: 1349-1363.
1838. Rindi G, Villanacci V, Ubiali A, Scarpa A (2001). Endocrine tumors of the digestive tract and pancreas: histogenesis, diagnosis and molecular basis. Expert Rev Mol Diagn 1: 323-333.
1839. Rippe V, Belge G, Meiboom M, Kazmierczak B, Fusco A, Bullerdiek J (1999). A KRAB zinc finger protein gene is the potential target of 19q13 translocation in benign thyroid tumors. Genes Chromosomes Cancer 26: 229-236.
1840. Rippe V, Drieschner N, Meiboom M, Murua-Escobar H, Bonk U, Belge G, Bullerdiek J (2003). Identification of a gene rearranged by 2p21 aberrations in thyroid adenomas. Oncogene 22: 6111-6114.
1841. Robbins AW, Peacock JA (1985). Case report: cervical thymoma. J Med Soc N J 82: 221-224.
1842. Robert F, Hardy J (1986). Human corticotroph cell adenomas. Semin Diagn Pathol 3: 34-41.
1843. Robert F, Hardy J (1991). Cushing's disease: a correlation of radiological, surgical and pathological findings with therapeutic results. Pathol Res Pract 187: 617-621.
1844. Robert F, Pelletier G, Hardy J (1978). Pituitary adenomas in Cushing's disease. A histologic, ultrastructural, and immunocytochemical study. Arch Pathol Lab Med 102: 448-455.
1845. Robinson DW, Orr TG (1955). Carcinoma of the thyroid and other diseases of the thyroid in identical twins. Arch Surg 70: 923-928.
1846. Rocha AS, Soares P, Fonseca E, Cameselle-Teijeiro J, Oliveira MC, Sobrinho-Simoes M (2003). E-cadherin loss rather than beta-catenin alterations is a common feature of poorly differentiated thyroid carcinomas. Histopathology 42: 580-587.
1847. Rocha AS, Soares P, Machado JC, Maximo V, Fonseca E, Franssila K, Sobrinho-Simoes M (2002). Mucoepidermoid carcinoma of the thyroid: a tumour histotype characterised by P-cadherin neoexpression and marked abnormalities of E-cadherin/catenins complex. Virchows Arch 440: 498-504.
1848. Rocha AS, Soares P, Seruca R, Maximo V, Matias-Guiu X, Cameselle-Teijeiro J, Sobrinho-Simoes M (2001). Abnormalities of the E-cadherin/catenin adhesion complex in classical papillary thyroid carcinoma and in its diffuse sclerosing variant. J Pathol 194: 358-366.
1849. Rodriguez-Cuevas S, Lopez-Garza J, Labastida-Almendaro S (1998). Carotid body tumors in inhabitants of altitudes higher than 2000 meters above sea level. Head Neck 20: 374-378.
1850. Rodriguez I, Ayala E, Caballero C, De Miguel C, Matias-Guiu X, Cubilla AL, Rosai J (2001). Solitary fibrous tumor of the thyroid gland: report of seven cases. Am J Surg Pathol 25: 1424-1428.
1851. Roessmann U, Kaufman B, Friede RL (1970). Metastatic lesions in the sella turcica and pituitary gland. Cancer 25: 478-480.
1852. Roggli VL, Judge DM, McGavran MH (1979). Duodenal glucagonoma: a case report. Hum Pathol 10: 350-353.
1853. Rojiani AM, Owen DA, Berry K, Woodhurst B, Anderson FH, Scudamore CH, Erb S (1991). Hepatic hemangioblastoma. An unusual presentation in a patient with von Hippel-Lindau disease. Am J Surg Pathol 15: 81-86.
1854. Ron E, Kleinerman RA, Boice JDJr, LiVolsi VA, Flannery JT, Fraumeni JFJr (1987). A population-based case-control study of thyroid cancer. J Natl Cancer Inst 79: 1-12.
1855. Ron E, Lubin JH, Shore RE, Mabuchi K, Modan B, Pottern LM, Schneider AB, Tucker MA, Boice JDJr (1995). Thyroid cancer after exposure to external radiation: a pooled analysis of seven studies. Radiat Res 141: 259-277.
1856. Roncaroli F, Nose V, Scheithauer BW, Kovacs K, Horvath E, Young WFJr, Lloyd RV, Bishop MC, Hsi B, Fletcher JA (2003). Gonadotrophic pituitary carcinoma: HER-2/neu expression and gene amplification. Report of two cases. J Neurosurg 99: 402-408.
1857. Roncaroli F, Scheithauer BW, Young WFJr, Horvath E, Kovacs KT, Kros JM, Al-Sarraj S, Lloyd RV, Faustini-Fustini M (2003). Silent corticotroph carcinoma of the adenohypophysis: a report of five cases. Am J Surg Pathol 27: 477-486.
1858. Rood RP, DeLellis RA, Dayal Y, Donowitz M (1988). Pancreatic cholera syndrome due to a vasoactive intestinal polypeptide-producing tumor: further insights into the pathophysiology. Gastroenterology 94: 813-818.
1859. Roque L, Castedo S, Clode A, Soares J (1993). Deletion of 3p25—>pter in a primary follicular thyroid carcinoma and its metastasis. Genes Chromosomes Cancer 8: 199-203.
1860. Roque L, Clode A, Belge G, Pinto A, Bartnitzke S, Santos JR, Thode B, Bullerdiek J, Castedo S, Soares J (1998). Follicular thyroid carcinoma: chromosome analysis of 19 cases. Genes Chromosomes Cancer 21: 250-255.
1861. Roque L, Serpa A, Clode A, Castedo S, Soares J (1999). Significance of trisomy 7 and 12 in thyroid lesions with follicular differentiation: a cytogenetic and in situ hybridization study. Lab Invest 79: 369-378.
1862. Rosai J, Carcangiu ML, DeLellis RA (1992). Tumors of the Thyroid Gland. 3rd ed. Armed Forces Institute of Pathology: Washington, DC.
1863. Rosai J, LiVolsi VA, Sobrinho-Simoes M, Williams ED (2003). Renaming papillary microcarcinoma of the thyroid gland: the porto proposal. Int J Surg Pathol 11: 249-251.
1864. Rosen IB, Palmer JA (1981). Fibroosseous tumors of the facial skeleton in association with primary hyperparathyroidism: an endocrine syndrome or coincidence? Am J Surg 142: 494-498.
1865. Rosenberg D, Groussin L, Jullian E, Perlemoine K, Bertagna X, Bertherat J (2002). Role of the PKA-regulated transcription factor CREB in development and tumorigenesis of endocrine tissues. Ann N Y Acad Sci 968: 65-74.
1866. Rosenberg SA, Diamond HD, Jaslowitz B, Craver LF (1961). Lymphosarcoma. A review of 1269 cases. Medicine 40: 31-84.
1867. Rosenfeld MG (1991). POU-domain transcription factors: pou-er-ful developmental regulators. Genes Dev 5: 897-907.
1868. Ross EJ, Griffith DN (1989). The clinical presentation of phaeochromocytoma. Q J Med 71: 485-496.
1869. Rossi E, Regolisti G, Negro A, Sani C, Davoli S, Perazzoli F (2002). High prevalence of primary aldosteronism using post-captopril plasma aldosterone to renin ratio as a screening test among Italian hypertensives. Am J Hypertens 15: 896-902.
1870. Rossi R, Tauchmanova L, Luciano A, Di Martino M, Battista C, Del Viscovo L, Nuzzo V, Lombardi G (2000). Subclinical Cushing's syndrome in patients with adrenal incidentaloma: clinical and biochemical features. J Clin Endocrinol Metab 85: 1440-1448.
1871. Roth J, Kasper M, Stamm B, Hacki WH, Storch MJ, Madsen OD, Kloppel G, Heitz PU (1989). Localization of proinsulin and insulin in human insulinoma: preliminary immunohistochemical results. Virchows Arch B Cell Pathol Incl Mol Pathol 56: 287-292.
1872. Roth J, Kloppel G, Madsen OD, Storch MJ, Heitz PU (1992). Distribution patterns of proinsulin and insulin in human insulinomas: an immunohistochemical analysis in 76 tumors. Virchows Arch B Cell Pathol Incl Mol Pathol 63: 51-61.
1873. Roth J, Komminoth P, Heitz PU (1995). Topographic abnormalities of proinsulin to insulin conversion in functioning human insulinomas. Comparison of immunoelectron microscopic and clinical data. Am J Pathol 147: 489-502.
1874. Roth J, Komminoth P, Kloppel G, Heitz PU (1996). Diabetes and the endocrine pancreas. In: Anderson's Pathology, Damjanov I, Linder J, eds., 10th ed. Mosby-Year Book Inc: St. Louis , pp. 2042-2070.
1875. Roth SI, Gallagher MJ (1976). The rapid identification of "normal" parathyroid glands by the presence of intracellular fat. Am J Pathol 84: 521-528.
1876. Roth SI, Munger BL (1962). The cytology of the adenomatous atrophic and hyperplastic parathyroid glands of man. A light and electron microscopic study. Virchows Arch A 335: 389-410.
1877. Rothenberg HJ, Goellner JR, Carney JA (1999). Hyalinizing trabecular adenoma of the thyroid gland: recognition and characterization of its cytoplasmic yellow body. Am J Surg Pathol 23: 118-125.
1878. Roy J, Pompilio M, Samama G (1996). [Pancreatic somatostatinoma and MEN 1. Apropos of a case. Review of the literature]. Ann Endocrinol (Paris) 57: 71-76.
1879. Ruben Harach H (2001). Familial nonmedullary thyroid neoplasia. Endocr Pathol 12: 97-112.
1880. Ruco LP, Pulford KA, Mason DY, Ceccamea A, Uccini S, Pileri S, Baglioni P, Baroni CD (1989). Expression of macrophage-associated antigens in tissues involved by Langerhans' cell histiocytosis (histiocytosis X). Am J Clin Pathol 92: 273-279.
1881. Rudy FR, Bates RD, Cimorelli AJ, Hill GS, Engelman K (1980). Adrenal medullary hyperplasia: a clinicopathologic study of four cases. Hum Pathol 11: 650-657.
1882. Ruebel KH, Jin L, Zhang S, Scheithauer BW, Lloyd RV (2001). Inactivation of the p16 gene in human pituitary nonfunctioning tumors by hypermethylation is more common in null cell adenomas. Endocr Pathol 12: 281-289.
1883. Ruggieri P, Sim FH, Bond JR, Unni KK (1994). Malignancies in fibrous dysplasia. Cancer 73: 1411-1424.
1884. Russell DS, Rubinstein LJ (1989). Tumors of the neurohypophysis. In: Pathology of the Tumors of the Nervous System, Russell DS, Rubinstein LJ, eds., Williams & Wilkins: Baltimore , pp. 376-380.
1885. Ruttman E, Kloppel G, Bommer G, Kiehn M, Heitz PU (1980). Pancreatic glucagonoma with and without syndrome. Immunocytochemical study of 5 tumour cases and review of the literature. Virchows Arch A Pathol Anat Histol 388: 51-67.
1886. Saarma M (2000). GDNF - a stranger in the TGF-beta superfamily? Eur J Biochem 267: 6968-6971.
1887. Sachse R, Shao XJ, Rico A, Finckh U, Rolfs A, Reincke M, Hensen J (1997). Absence of angiotensin II type 1 receptor gene mutations in human adrenal tumors. Eur J Endocrinol 137: 262-266.
1888. Saeger W (1995). Latent hyper-

plasias and adenomas in post-mortem pituitaries. Endocr Pathol 6: 379-380.
1889. Saeger W (2003). Hypophysentumoren. Pathologe .
1890. Saeger W, Schreiber S, Ludecke DK (2001). Cyclins D1 and D3 and topoisomerase II alpha in inactive pituitary adenomas. Endocr Pathol 12: 39-47.
1891. Safer JD, Colan SD, Fraser LM, Wondisford FE (2001). A pituitary tumor in a patient with thyroid hormone resistance: a diagnostic dilemma. Thyroid 11: 281-291.
1892. Saffos RO, Rhatigan RM, Urgulu S (1984). The normal parathyroid and the borderline with early hyperplasia: a light microscopic study. Histopathology 8: 407-422.
1893. Sagalowsky AI, Molberg K (1999). Solitary metastasis of renal cell carcinoma to the contralateral adrenal gland 22 years after nephrectomy. Urology 54: 162.
1894. Sahagian-Edwards A, Holland JF (1954). Metastatic carcinoma to the adrenal glands with cortical hypofunction. Cancer 7: 1242-1245.
1895. Sahin A, Robinson RA (1988). Papillae formation in parathyroid adenoma. A source of possible diagnostic error. Arch Pathol Lab Med 112: 99-100.
1896. Sahoo M, Karak AK, Bhatnagar D, Bal CS (1998). Fine-needle aspiration cytology in a case of isolated involvement of thyroid with Langerhans cell histiocytosis. Diagn Cytopathol 19: 33-37.
1897. Saito K, Kuratomi Y, Yamamoto K, Saito T, Kuzuya T, Yoshida S, Moriyama SI, Takahashi A (1981). Primary squamous cell carcinoma of the thyroid associated with marked leukocytosis and hypercalcemia. Cancer 48: 2080-2083.
1898. Saito K, Sato O, Tsuruta J, Suematsu K (1982). [A case of pheochromocytoma originating from the superior cervical sympathetic ganglion (author's transl)]. Neurol Med Chir (Tokyo) 22: 154-158.
1899. Saiz E, Bakotic BW (2000). Isolated Langerhans cell histiocytosis of the thyroid: a report of two cases with nuclear imaging-pathologic correlation. Ann Diagn Pathol 4: 23-28.
1900. Sakaguchi N, Sano K, Ito M, Baba T, Fukuzawa M, Hotchi M (1996). A case of von Recklinghausen's disease with bilateral pheochromocytoma-malignant peripheral nerve sheath tumors of the adrenal and gastrointestinal autonomic nerve tumors. Am J Surg Pathol 20: 889-897.
1901. Sakamoto A, Kasai N, Sugano H (1983). Poorly differentiated carcinoma of the thyroid. A clinicopathologic entity for a high-risk group of papillary and follicular carcinomas. Cancer 52: 1849-1855.
1902. Sakamoto A, Oda Y, Iwamoto Y, Tsuneyoshi M (2000). A comparative study of fibrous dysplasia and osteofibrous dysplasia with regard to Gsalpha mutation at the Arg201 codon: polymerase chain reaction-restriction fragment length polymorphism analysis of paraffin-embedded tissues. J Mol Diagn 2: 67-72.
1903. Sakamoto Y, Takahashi M, Korogi Y, Bussaka H, Ushio Y (1991). Normal and abnormal pituitary glands: gadopentetate dimeglumine-enhanced MR imaging. Radiology 178: 441-445.
1904. Sakhuja P, Malhotra V, Gondal R, Dutt N, Choudhary A (2001). Periampullary gangliocytic paraganglioma. J Clin Gastroenterol 33: 154-156.
1905. Sakuishi K, Taguchi M, Takeshita A, Matsumoto T, Tanaka S, Matsushita T, Sano T, Ozawa Y (2003). Cushing's symdrome induced by ACTH production from the metastatic pancreatic gastrinoma in the liver. Hormones and Clinical Medicine (Hormone to Risho) 49 (Supple.): 178-185.
1906. Sakurai A, Katai M, Itakura Y, Ikeo Y, Hashizume K (1999). Premature centromere division in patients with multiple endocrine neoplasia type 1. Cancer Genet Cytogenet 109: 138-140.
1907. Sakurai A, Matsumoto K, Ikeo Y, Nishio SI, Kakizawa T, Arakura F, Ishihara Y, Saida T, Hashizume K (2000). Frequency of facial angiofibromas in Japanese patients with multiple endocrine neoplasia type 1. Endocr J 47: 569-573.
1908. Salassidis K, Bruch J, Zitzelsberger H, Lengfelder E, Kellerer AM, Bauchinger M (2000). Translocation t(10;14)(q11.2:q22.1) fusing the kinetin to the RET gene creates a novel rearranged form (PTC8) of the RET proto-oncogene in radiation-induced childhood papillary thyroid carcinoma. Cancer Res 60: 2786-2789.
1909. Salmenkivi K, Arola J, Voutilainen R, Ilvesmaki V, Haglund C, Kahri AI, Heikkila P, Liu J (2001). Inhibin/activin betaB-subunit expression in pheochromocytomas favors benign diagnosis. J Clin Endocrinol Metab 86: 2231-2235.
1910. Salmenkivi K, Haglund C, Arola J, Heikkila P (2001). Increased expression of tenascin in pheochromocytomas correlates with malignancy. Am J Surg Pathol 25: 1419-1423.
1911. Salmi J, Pelto-Huikko M, Auvinen O, Karvonen AL, Saaristo J, Paronen I, Poyhonen L, Seppanen S (1988). Adrenal pheochromocytoma-ganglioneuroma producing catecholamines and various neuropeptides. Acta Med Scand 224: 403-408.
1912. Salmon I, Kiss R, Segers V, Carroyer JM, Levivier M, Pasteels JL, Brotchi J, Flament-Durand J (1992). Characterization of nuclear size, ploidy, DNA histogram type and proliferation index in 79 nerve sheath tumors. Anticancer Res 12: 2277-2283.
1913. Salti IS, Mufarrij IS (1981). Familial Cushing Disease. Am J Med Genet 8: 91-94.
1914. Samaan NA, Hickey RC, Shutts PE (1988). Diagnosis, localization, and management of pheochromocytoma. Pitfalls and follow-up in 41 patients. Cancer 62: 2451-2460.
1915. Sambade C, Baldaque-Faria A, Cardoso-Oliveira M, Sobrinho-Simoes M (1988). Follicular and papillary variants of medullary carcinoma of the thyroid. Pathol Res Pract 184: 98-107.
1916. Sambade C, Franssila K, Basilio-de-Oliveira CA, Sobrinho-Simoes M (1990). Mucoepidermoid carcinoma of the thyroid revisited. Surg Pathol 3: 317-324.
1917. Sambade C, Franssila K, Cameselle-Teijeiro J, Nesland JM, Sobrinho-Simoes M (1991). Hyalinizing trabecular adenoma: a misnomer for a peculiar tumor of the thyroid gland. Endocr Pathol 2: 83-91.
1918. Sambade C, Sarabando F, Nesland JM, Sobrinho-Simoes M (1989). Hyalinizing trabecular adenoma of the thyroid (case of the Ullensvang course). Hyalinizing spindle cell tumor of the thyroid with dual differentiation (variant of the so-called hyalinizing trabecular adenoma). Ultrastruct Pathol 13: 275-280.
1919. Sameshima Y, Tsunematsu Y, Watanabe S, Tsukamoto T, Kawa-ha K, Hirata Y, Mizoguchi H, Sugimura T, Terada M, Yokota J (1992). Detection of novel germ-line p53 mutations in diverse-cancer-prone families identified by selecting patients with childhood adrenocortical carcinoma. J Natl Cancer Inst 84: 703-707.
1920. Samii M, Tatagiba M, Monteiro ML (1996). Meningiomas involving the parasellar region. Acta Neurochir Suppl (Wien) 65: 63-65.
1921. Samuels MH, Launder T (1998). Hyperthyroidism due to lymphoma involving the thyroid gland in a patient with acquired immunodeficiency syndrome: case report and review of the literature. Thyroid 8: 673-677.
1922. Samuelsson B, Axelsson R (1981). Neurofibromatosis. A clinical and genetic study of 96 cases in Gothenburg, Sweden. Acta Derm Venereol Suppl (Stockh) 95: 67-71.
1923. San-Juan J, Monteagudo C, Fraker D, Norton J, Merino MJ (1989). Significance of mitotic activity and other morphologic parameters in parathyroid adenomas and their correlation with clinical behavior. Am J Clin Pathol 92: 523.
1924. San Juan J, Monteagudo C, Navarro P, Terradez JJ (1999). Basal cell carcinoma with prominent central palisading of epithelial cells mimicking schwannoma. J Cutan Pathol 26: 528-532.
1925. Sandelin K, Auer G, Bondeson L, Grimelius L, Farnebo LO (1992). Prognostic factors in parathyroid cancer: a review of 95 cases. World J Surg 16: 724-731.
1926. Sanno N, Jin L, Qian X, Osamura RY, Scheithauer BW, Kovacs K, Lloyd RV (1997). Gonadotropin-releasing hormone and gonadotropin-releasing hormone receptor messenger ribonucleic acids expression in nontumorous and neoplastic pituitaries. J Clin Endocrinol Metab 82: 1974-1982.
1927. Sanno N, Teramoto A, Osamura RY (2000). Long-term surgical outcome in 16 patients with thyrotropin pituitary adenoma. J Neurosurg 93: 194-200.
1928. Sanno N, Teramoto A, Osamura RY, Genka S, Katakami H, Jin L, Lloyd RV, Kovacs K (1997). A growth hormone-releasing hormone-producing pancreatic islet cell tumor metastasized to the pituitary is associated with pituitary somatotroph hyperplasia and acromegaly. J Clin Endocrinol Metab 82: 2731-2737.
1929. Sano T, Asa SL, Kovacs K (1988). Growth hormone-releasing hormone-producing tumors: clinical, biochemical, and morphological manifestations. Endocr Rev 9: 357-373.
1930. Sano T, Kovacs K, Asa SL, Smyth HS (1990). Immunoreactive luteinizing hormone in functioning corticotroph adenomas of the pituitary. Immunohistochemical and tissue culture studies of two cases. Virchows Arch A Pathol Anat Histopathol 417: 361-367.
1931. Sano T, Ohshima T, Yamada S (1991). Expression of glycoprotein hormones and intracytoplasmic distribution of cytokeratin in growth hormone-producing pituitary adenomas. Pathol Res Pract 187: 530-533.
1932. Sano T, Yamada S (1994). Histologic and immunohistochemical study of clinically non-functioning pituitary adenomas: special reference to gonadotropin-positive adenomas. Pathol Int 44: 697-703.
1933. Santoro M, Carlomagno F, Hay ID, Herrmann MA, Grieco M, Melillo R, Pierotti MA, Bongarzone I, Della Porta G, Berger N, Peix JL, Paulin C, Fabien N, Vecchio G, Jenkins RB, Fusco A (1992). Ret oncogene activation in human thyroid neoplasms is restricted to the papillary cancer subtype. J Clin Invest 89: 1517-1522.
1934. Santoro M, Carlomagno F, Romano A, Bottaro DP, Dathan NA, Grieco M, Fusco A, Vecchio G, Matoskova B, Kraus MH, DiFiore PP (1995). Activation of RET as a dominant transforming gene by germline mutations of MEN2A and MEN2B. Science 267: 381-383.
1935. Santoro M, Chiappetta G, Cerrato A, Salvatore D, Zhang L, Manzo G, Picone A, Portella G, Santelli G, Vecchio G, Fusco A (1996). Development of thyroid papillary carcinomas secondary to tissue-specific expression of the RET/PTC1 oncogene in transgenic mice. Oncogene 12: 1821-1826.
1936. Santoro M, Dathan NA, Berlingieri MT, Bongarzone I, Paulin C, Grieco M, Pierotti MA, Vecchio G, Fusco A (1994). Molecular characterization of RET/PTC3; a novel rearranged version of the RETproto-oncogene in a human thyroid papillary carcinoma. Oncogene 9: 509-516.
1937. Santoro M, Papotti M, Chiappetta G, Garcia-Rostan G, Volante M, Johnson C, Camp RL, Pentimalli F, Monaco C, Herrero A, Carcangiu ML, Fusco A, Tallini G (2002). RET activation and clinicopathologic features in poorly differentiated thyroid tumors. J Clin Endocrinol Metab 87: 370-379.
1938. Sapino A, Papotti M, Macri L, Satolli MA, Bussolati G (1995). Intranodular reactive endothelial hyperplasia in adenomatous goitre. Histopathology 26: 457-462.
1939. Sardi A, Singer JA (1987). Insulinoma and gastrinoma in Wermer's disease (MEN I). Arch Surg 122: 835-836.
1940. Sarlis NJ, Chrousos GP, Doppman JL, Carney JA, Stratakis CA (1997). Primary pigmented nodular adrenocortical disease: reevaluation of a patient with carney complex 27 years after unilateral adrenalectomy. J Clin Endocrinol Metab 82: 1274-1278.
1941. Sarui H, Yoshimoto K, Okumura S, Kamura M, Takuno H, Ishizuka T, Takao H, Shimokawa K, Itakura M, Saji S, Yasuda K (1997). Cystic glucagonoma with loss of heterozygosity on chromosome 11 in multiple endocrine neoplasia type 1. Clin Endocrinol (Oxf) 46: 511-516.
1942. Sasaki A, Daa T, Kashima K, Yokoyama S, Nakayama I, Noguchi S (1996). Insular component as a risk factor of thyroid carcinoma. Pathol Int 46: 939-946.
1943. Sasano H (1994). Localization of steroidogenic enzymes in adrenal cortex and its disorders. Endocr J 41: 471-482.
1944. Sasano H, Sato F, Shizawa S, Nagura H, Coughtrie MW (1995). Immunolocalization of dehydroepiandrosterone sulfotransferase in normal and pathologic human adrenal gland. Mod Pathol 8: 891-896.
1945. Sasano H, Shizawa S, Suzuki T, Takayama K, Fukaya T, Morohashi K, Nagura H (1995). Ad4BP in the human adrenal cortex and its disorders. J Clin Endocrinol Metab 80: 2378-2380.
1946. Sasano H, Shizawa S, Suzuki T, Takayama K, Fukaya T, Morohashi K, Nagura H (1995). Transcription factor adrenal 4 binding protein as a marker of adrenocortical malignancy. Hum Pathol 26: 1154-1156.
1947. Sasano H, Suzuki T, Sano T, Kameya T, Sasano N, Nagura H (1991). Adrenocortical oncocytoma. A true nonfunctioning adrenocortical tumor. Am J Surg Pathol 15: 949-956.
1948. Sasano H, Suzuki T, Shizawa S, Kato K, Nagura H (1994). Transforming growth factor alpha, epidermal growth factor, and epidermal growth factor receptor expres-

sion in normal and diseased human adrenal cortex by immunohistochemistry and in situ hybridization. Mod Pathol 7: 741-746.
1949. Satake H, Inoue K, Kamada M, Watanabe H, Furihata M, Shuin T (2001). Malignant composite pheochromocytoma of the adrenal gland in a patient with von Recklinghausen's disease. J Urol 165: 1199-1200.
1950. Sato M, Kihara M, Nishitani A, Murao K, Kobayashi S, Miyauchi A, Takahara J (2000). Large and asymptomatic pancreatic islet cell tumor in a patient with multiple endocrine neoplasia type 1. Endocrine 13: 263-266.
1951. Saurenmann P, Binswanger R, Maurer R, Stamm B, Hegglin J (1987). [Somatostatin-producing endocrine pancreatic tumor in Recklinghausen's neurofibromatosis. Case report and literature review]. Schweiz Med Wochenschr 117: 1134-1139.
1952. Saw D, Wu D, Chess Q, Shemen L (1997). Spindle epithelial tumor with thymus-like element (SETTLE), a primary thyroid tumor. Int J Surg Pathol 4: 169-174.
1953. Sawka AM, Jaeschke R, Singh RJ, Young WFJr (2003). A comparison of biochemical tests for pheochromocytoma: measurement of fractionated plasma metanephrines compared with the combination of 24-hour urinary metanephrines and catecholamines. J Clin Endocrinol Metab 88: 553-558.
1954. Sayo Y, Murao K, Imachi H, Cao WM, Sato M, Dobashi H, Wong NC, Ishida T (2002). The multiple endocrine neoplasia type 1 gene product, menin, inhibits insulin production in rat insulinoma cells. Endocrinology 143: 2437-2440.
1955. Scarpulla RC (1996). Nuclear Respiratory Factors and the Pathways of Nuclear-Mitochondrial Interaction. Trends Cardiovasc Med 6: 39-45.
1956. Schaller B, Kirsch E, Tolnay M, Mindermann T (1998). Symptomatic granular cell tumor of the pituitary gland: case report and review of the literature. Neurosurgery 42: 166-170.
1957. Schantz A, Castleman B (1973). Parathyroid carcinoma. A study of 70 cases. Cancer 31: 600-605.
1958. Scheffler IE (1998). Molecular genetics of succinate:quinone oxidoreductase in eukaryotes. Prog Nucleic Acid Res Mol Biol 60: 267-315.
1959. Scheithauer BW, Fereidooni F, Horvath E, Kovacs K, Robbins P, Tews D, Henry K, Pernicone P, Gaffrey TAJr, Meyer FB, Young WFJr, Fahlbusch R, Buchfelder M, Lloyd RV (2001). Pituitary carcinoma: an ultrastructural study of eleven cases. Ultrastruct Pathol 25: 227-242.
1960. Scheithauer BW, Horvath E, Kovacs K, Laws ERJr, Randall RV, Ryan N (1986). Plurihormonal pituitary adenomas. Semin Diagn Pathol 3: 69-82.
1961. Scheithauer BW, Horvath E, Kovacs K, Lloyd RV (2000). Tumors of the adenohypophysis. In: Histological Typing of Endocrine Tumours, Solcia E, Kloppel G, Sobin LH, eds., 2nd ed. Springer: Geneva , pp. 15-28.
1962. Scheithauer BW, Horvath E, Kovacs K, Lloyd RV, Stefaneanu L, Buchfelder M, Fahlbusch R, von Werder K, Lyons DF (1999). Prolactin-producing pituitary adenoma and carcinoma with neuronal components—a metaplastic lesion. Pituitary 1: 197-205.
1963. Scheithauer BW, Horvath E, Lloyd RV, Kovacs K (2001). Pathology of pituitary adenomas and pituitary hyperplasia. In: Diagnosis and Management of Pituitary Tumors, Thapar K, Kovacs K, Scheithauer BW, Lloyd RV, eds., Humana Press: Totowa, NJ , pp. 91-154.
1964. Scheithauer BW, Jaap AJ, Horvath E, Kovacs K, Lloyd RV, Meyer FB, Laws ERJr, Young WFJr (2000). Clinically silent corticotroph tumors of the pituitary gland. Neurosurgery 47: 723-729.
1965. Scheithauer BW, Kovacs K, Randall RV, Ryan N (1985). Pituitary gland in hypothyroidism. Histologic and immunocytologic study. Arch Pathol Lab Med 109: 499-504.
1966. Scheithauer BW, Kovacs KT, Laws ERJr, Randall RV (1986). Pathology of invasive pituitary tumors with special reference to functional classification. J Neurosurg 65: 733-744.
1967. Scheithauer BW, Laws ERJr, Kovacs K, Horvath E, Randall RV, Carney JA (1987). Pituitary adenomas of the multiple endocrine neoplasia type I syndrome. Semin Diagn Pathol 4: 205-211.
1968. Scheithauer BW, Woodruff JM, Erlandson RA (1999). Tumors of the Peripheral Nervous System. Armed Forces Institute of Pathology: Washington, DC.
1969. Schelfhout LJ, Cornelisse CJ, Goslings BM, Hamming JF, Kuipers-Dijkshoorn NJ, van de Velde CJ, Fleuren GJ (1990). Frequency and degree of aneuploidy in benign and malignant thyroid neoplasms. Int J Cancer 45: 16-20.
1970. Schiemann U, Assert R, Moskopp D, Gellner R, Hengst K, Gullotta F, Domschke W, Pfeiffer A (1997). Analysis of a protein kinase C-alpha mutation in human pituitary tumours. J Endocrinol 153: 131-137.
1971. Schilling T, Burck J, Sinn HP, Clemens A, Otto HF, Hoppner W, Herfarth C, Ziegler R, Schwab M, Raue F (2001). Prognostic value of codon 918 (ATG—>ACG) RET proto-oncogene mutations in sporadic medullary thyroid carcinoma. Int J Cancer 95: 62-66.
1972. Schimke RN, Collins DL, Stolle CA (2000). von Hippel-Lindau syndrome. GeneReviews: genetic disease online reviews at GeneTests-GeneClinics http://www.geneclinics.org.
1973. Schlumberger HG (1946). Fibrous dysplasia of single bones (monostotic fibrous dysplasia). Milit Surg 99: 504-527.
1974. Schlumberger M, Gicquel C, Lumbroso J, Tenenbaum F, Comoy E, Bosq J, Fonseca E, Ghillani PP, Aubert B, Travagli JP, Gardet P, Parmentier C (1992). Malignant pheochromocytoma: clinical, biological, histologic and therapeutic data in a series of 20 patients with distant metastases. J Endocrinol Invest 15: 631-642.
1975. Schmid KW, Dockhorn-Dworniczak B, Fahrenkamp A, Kirchmair R, Totsch M, Fischer-Colbrie R, Bocker W, Winkler H (1993). Chromogranin A, secretogranin II and vasoactive intestinal peptide in phaeochromocytomas and ganglioneuromas. Histopathology 22: 527-533.
1976. Schmid M, Munscher A, Saeger W, Schreiber S, Ludecke DK (2001). Pituitary hormone mRNA in null cell adenomas and oncocytomas by in situ hybridization comparison with immunohistochemical and clinical data. Pathol Res Pract 197: 663-669.
1977. Schneider KA (2001). The cancer genetic counseling session. In: Counseling About Cancer: Strategies for Genetic Counseling, Schneider KA, ed., 2nd ed. John Wiley & Sons: New York , pp. 167-206.
1978. Schnitzer B, Smid D, Lloyd RV (1986). Primary T-cell lymphoma of the adrenal glands with adrenal insufficiency. Hum Pathol 17: 634-636.
1979. Schroder HD, Johannsen L (1986). Demonstration of S-100 protein in sustentacular cells of phaeochromocytomas and paragangliomas. Histopathology 10: 1023-1033.
1980. Schroder S, Bocker W (1986). Clear-cell carcinomas of thyroid gland: a clinicopathological study of 13 cases. Histopathology 10: 75-89.
1981. Schroder S, Bocker W, Baisch H, Burk CG, Arps H, Meiners I, Kastendieck H, Heitz PU, Kloppel G (1988). Prognostic factors in medullary thyroid carcinomas. Survival in relation to age, sex, stage, histology, immunocytochemistry, and DNA content. Cancer 61: 806-816.
1982. Schroder S, Husselmann H, Bocker W (1984). Lipid-rich cell adenoma of the thyroid gland. Report of a peculiar thyroid tumour. Virchows Arch A Pathol Anat Histopathol 404: 105-108.
1983. Schroder S, Niendorf A, Achilles E, Dietel M, Padberg BC, Beisiegel U, Dralle H, Bressel M, Kloppel G (1990). Immunocytochemical differential diagnosis of adrenocortical neoplasms using the monoclonal antibody D11. Virchows Arch A Pathol Anat Histopathol 417: 89-96.
1984. Schroder S, Padberg BC, Achilles E, Holl K, Dralle H, Kloppel G (1992). Immunocytochemistry in adrenocortical tumours: a clinicomorphological study of 72 neoplasms. Virchows Arch A Pathol Anat Histopathol 420: 65-70.
1985. Schuffenecker I, Billaud M, Calender A, Chambe B, Ginet N, Calmettes C, Modigliani E, Lenoir GM (1994). RET proto-oncogene mutations in French MEN 2A and FMTC families. Hum Mol Genet 3: 1939-1943.
1986. Schulte KM, Heinze M, Mengel M, Simon D, Scheuring S, Kohrer K, Roher HD (1999). MEN I gene mutations in sporadic adrenal adenomas. Hum Genet 105: 603-610.
1987. Schulte KM, Mengel M, Heinze M, Simon D, Scheuring S, Kohrer K, Roher HD (2000). Complete sequencing and messenger ribonucleic acid expression analysis of the MEN I gene in adrenal cancer. J Clin Endocrinol Metab 85: 441-448.
1988. Schulz-Ertner D, Haberer T, Jakel O, Thilmann C, Kramer M, Enghardt W, Kraft G, Wannenmacher M, Debus J (2002). Radiotherapy for chordomas and low-grade chondrosarcomas of the skull base with carbon ions. Int J Radiat Oncol Biol Phys 53: 36-42.
1989. Schussheim DH, Skarulis MC, Agarwal SK, Simonds WF, Burns AL, Spiegel AM, Marx SJ (2001). Multiple endocrine neoplasia type 1: new clinical and basic findings. Trends Endocrinol Metab 12: 173-178.
1990. Schutz W, Vogel E (1984). Pheochromocytoma of the urinary bladder—a case report and review of the literature. Urol Int 39: 250-255.
1991. Schwartz RA, Spicer MS, Leevy CB, Ticker JB, Lambert WC (1996). Cutaneous fibrous dysplasia: an incomplete form of the McCune-Albright syndrome. Dermatology 192: 258-261.
1992. Schwindinger WF, Francomano CA, Levine MA (1992). Identification of a mutation in the gene encoding the alpha subunit of the stimulatory G protein of adenylyl cyclase in McCune-Albright syndrome. Proc Natl Acad Sci U S A 89: 5152-5156.
1993. Sciubba JJ, Fantasia JE, Kahn LB (2001). Tumors and Cysts of the Jaw. 3rd ed. Armed Forces Institute of Pathology: Washington, DC.
1994. Sclafani LM, Woodruff JM, Brennan MF (1990). Extraadrenal retroperitoneal paragangliomas: natural history and response to treatment. Surgery 108: 1124-1129.
1995. Scopsi L, Castellani MR, Gullo M, Cusumano F, Camerini E, Pasini B, Orefice S (1996). Malignant pheochromocytoma in multiple endocrine neoplasia type 2B syndrome. Case report and review of the literature. Tumori 82: 480-484.
1996. Scopsi L, Cozzaglio L, Collini P, Gullo M, Bongarzone I, Giarola M, Radice P, Gennari L (1998). Concurrent Pheochromocytoma, Paraganglioma, Papillary Thyroid Carcinoma, and Desmoid Tumor: A Case Report with Analyses at the Molecular Level. Endocr Pathol 9: 79-90.
1997. Scott HWJr, Halter SA (1984). Oncologic aspects of pheochromocytoma: the importance of follow-up. Surgery 96: 1061-1066.
1998. Scott HWJr, Reynolds V, Green N, Page D, Oates JA, Robertson D, Roberts S (1982). Clinical experience with malignant pheochromocytomas. Surg Gynecol Obstet 154: 801-818.
1999. Sebastian JP, Williams SE, Wells M, Peake MD (1989). Familial malignant retroperitoneal paraganglioma. Postgrad Med J 65: 781-784.
2000. Seemann N, Kuhn D, Wrocklage C, Keyvani K, Hackl W, Buchfelder M, Fahlbusch R, Paulus W (2001). CDKN2A/p16 inactivation is related to pituitary adenoma type and size. J Pathol 193: 491-497.
2001. Segev DL, Saji M, Phillips GS, Westra WH, Takiyama Y, Piantadosi S, Smallridge RC, Nishiyama RH, Udelsman R, Zeiger MA (1998). Polymerase chain reaction-based microsatellite polymorphism analysis of follicular and Hurthle cell neoplasms of the thyroid. J Clin Endocrinol Metab 83: 2036-2042.
2002. Seidenwurm DJ, Elmer EB, Kaplan LM, Williams EK, Morris DG, Hoffman AR (1984). Metastases to the adrenal glands and the development of Addison's disease. Cancer 54: 552-557.
2003. Seizinger BR, Rouleau GA, Ozelius LJ, Lane AH, Faryniarz AG, Chao MV, Huson S, Korf BR, Parry DM, Pericak-Vance MA, Collins FS, Hobbs WJ, Falcone BG, Iannazzi JA, Roy JC, St George-Hyslop PH, Tanzi RE, Bothwell MA, Upadhyaya MN, Harper P, Goldstein AE, Hoover DL, Bader JL, Spence MA, Mulvihill JJ, Aylsworth AS, Vance JM, Rossenwasser GOD, Gaskell PC, Roses AD, Martuza RL, Breakefield XO, Gusella JF (1987). Genetic linkage of von Recklinghausen neurofibromatosis to the nerve growth factor receptor gene. Cell 49: 589-594.
2004. Selves J, Meggetto F, Brousset P, Voigt JJ, Pradere B, Grasset D, Icart J, Mariame B, Knecht H, Delsol G (1996). Inflammatory pseudotumor of the liver. Evidence for follicular dendritic reticulum cell proliferation associated with clonal Epstein-Barr virus. Am J Surg Pathol 20: 747-753.
2005. Semelka RC, Cumming MJ, Shoenut JP, Magro CM, Yaffe CS, Kroeker MA, Greenberg HM (1993). Islet cell tumors: comparison of dynamic contrast-enhanced CT and MR imaging with dynamic gadolinium enhancement and fat suppression. Radiology 186: 799-802.

2006. Sempoux C, Guiot Y, Dahan K, Moulin P, Stevens M, Lambot V, de Lonlay P, Fournet JC, Junien C, Jaubert F, Nihoul-Fekete C, Saudubray JM, Rahier J (2003). The focal form of persistent hyperinsulinemic hypoglycemia of infancy: morphological and molecular studies show structural and functional differences with insulinoma. Diabetes 52: 784-794.
2007. Seoane JM, Cameselle-Teijeiro J, Romero MA (2002). Poorly differentiated oxyphilic (Hurthle cell) carcinoma arising in lingual thyroid: a case report and review of the literature. Endocr Pathol 13: 353-360.
2008. Serrano J, Goebel SU, Peghini PL, Lubensky IA, Gibril F, Jensen RT (2000). Alterations in the p16INK4a/CDKN2A tumor suppressor gene in gastrinomas. J Clin Endocrinol Metab 85: 4146-4156.
2009. Serri O, Brazeau P, Kachra Z, Posner B (1992). Octreotide inhibits insulin-like growth factor-I hepatic gene expression in the hypophysectomized rat: evidence for a direct and indirect mechanism of action. Endocrinology 130: 1816-1821.
2010. Service FJ (1995). Hypoglycemic disorders. N Engl J Med 332: 1144-1152.
2011. Service FJ, Dale AJ, Elveback LR, Jiang NS (1976). Insulinoma: clinical and diagnostic features of 60 consecutive cases. Mayo Clin Proc 51: 417-429.
2012. Service FJ, McMahon MM, O'Brien PC, Ballard DJ (1991). Functioning insulinoma—incidence, recurrence, and long-term survival of patients: a 60-year study. Mayo Clin Proc 66: 711-719.
2013. Sgambati MT, Stolle C, Choyke PL, Walther MM, Zbar B, Linehan WM, Glenn GM (2000). Mosaicism in von Hippel-Lindau disease: lessons from kindreds with germline mutations identified in offspring with mosaic parents. Am J Hum Genet 66: 84-91.
2014. Shaha AR, Loree TR, Shah JP (1995). Prognostic factors and risk group analysis in follicular carcinoma of the thyroid. Surgery 118: 1131-1136.
2015. Shaha AR, Shah JP (1999). Parathyroid carcinoma: a diagnostic and therapeutic challenge. Cancer 86: 378-380.
2016. Shahedian B, Shi Y, Zou M, Farid NR (2001). Thyroid carcinoma is characterized by genomic instability: evidence from p53 mutations. Mol Genet Metab 72: 155-163.
2017. Shames JM, Dhurandhar NR, Blackard WG (1968). Insulin-secreting bronchial carcinoid tumor with widespread metastases. Am J Med 44: 632-637.
2018. Shan L, Nakamura Y, Nakamura M, Yokoi T, Tsujimoto M, Arima R, Kameya T, Kakudo K (1998). Somatic mutations of multiple endocrine neoplasia type 1 gene in the sporadic endocrine tumors. Lab Invest 78: 471-475.
2019. Shane E (2001). Clinical review 122: Parathyroid carcinoma. J Clin Endocrinol Metab 86: 485-493.
2020. Shane E, Bilezikian JP (1982). Parathyroid carcinoma: a review of 62 patients. Endocr Rev 3: 218-226.
2021. Shanks JH, Harris M, Howat AJ, Freemont AJ (1997). Angiotropic lymphoma with endocrine involvement. Histopathology 31: 161-166.
2022. Shannon KE, Gimm O, Hinze R, Dralle H, Eng C (1999). Germline V804M mutation in the RET proto-oncogene in two apparently sporadic cases of MTC presenting in the seventh decade of life. J Endocr Genet 1: 39-45.
2023. Shapiro B, Sisson JC, Lloyd R, Nakajo M, Satterlee W, Beierwaltes WH (1984). Malignant phaeochromocytoma: clinical, biochemical and scintigraphic characterization. Clin Endocrinol (Oxf) 20: 189-203.
2024. Shapiro B, Sisson JC, Wieland DM, Mangner TJ, Zempel SM, Mudgett E, Gross MD, Carey JE, Zasadny KR, Beierwaltes WH (1991). Radiopharmaceutical therapy of malignant pheochromocytoma with [131I]metaiodobenzylguanidine: results from ten years of experience. J Nucl Biol Med 35: 269-276.
2025. Shattuck TM, Costa J, Bernstein M, Jensen RT, Chung DC, Arnold A (2002). Mutational analysis of Smad3, a candidate tumor suppressor implicated in TGF-beta and menin pathways, in parathyroid adenomas and enteropancreatic endocrine tumors. J Clin Endocrinol Metab 87: 3911-3914.
2026. Shattuck TM, Valimaki S, Obara T, Gaz RD, Clark OH, Shoback D, Wierman ME, Tojo K, Robbins CM, Carpten JD, Farnebo LO, Larsson C, Arnold A (2003). Somatic and germ-line mutations of the HRPT2 gene in sporadic parathyroid carcinoma. N Engl J Med 349: 1722-1729.
2027. Sheehan JP, Kondziolka D, Flickinger J, Lunsford LD (2002). Radiosurgery for residual or recurrent nonfunctioning pituitary adenoma. J Neurosurg 97: 408-414.
2028. Sheehan T, Cuthbert RJ, Parker AC (1989). Central nervous system involvement in haematological malignancies. Clin Lab Haematol 11: 331-338.
2029. Sheeler LR, Myers JH, Eversman JJ, Taylor HC (1983). Adrenal insufficiency secondary to carcinoma metastatic to the adrenal gland. Cancer 52: 1312-1316.
2030. Shek TW, Luk IS, Ng IO, Lo CY (1996). Lymphoepithelioma-like carcinoma of the thyroid gland: lack of evidence of association with Epstein-Barr virus. Hum Pathol 27: 851-853.
2031. Shen T, Zhuang Z, Gersell DJ, Tavassoli FA (2000). Allelic Deletion of VHL Gene Detected in Papillary Tumors of the Broad Ligament, Epididymis, and Retroperitoneum in von Hippel-Lindau Disease Patients. Int J Surg Pathol 8: 207-212.
2032. Shenker A, Weinstein LS, Moran A, Pescovitz OH, Charest NJ, Boney CM, Van Wyk JJ, Merino MJ, Feuillan PP, Spiegel AM (1993). Severe endocrine and nonendocrine manifestations of the McCune-Albright syndrome associated with activating mutations of stimulatory G protein GS. J Pediatr 123: 509-518.
2033. Shenoy BV, Carpenter PC, Carney JA (1984). Bilateral primary pigmented nodular adrenocortical disease. Rare cause of the Cushing syndrome. Am J Surg Pathol 8: 335-344.
2034. Shepherd JJ (1991). The natural history of multiple endocrine neoplasia type 1. Highly uncommon or highly unrecognized? Arch Surg 126: 935-952.
2035. Sheps SG, Jiang NS, Klee GG, van Heerden JA (1990). Recent developments in the diagnosis and treatment of pheochromocytoma. Mayo Clin Proc 65: 88-95.
2036. Shetty MR, Boghossian HM, Duffell D, Freel R, Gonzales JC (1982). Tumor-induced hypoglycemia: a result of ectopic insulin production. Cancer 49: 1920-1923.
2037. Shi T, Farrell MA, Kaufmann JC (1984). Fibrosarcoma complicating irradiated pituitary adenoma. Surg Neurol 22: 277-284.
2038. Shi YF, Zou MJ, Schmidt H, Juhasz F, Stensky V, Robb D, Farid NR (1991). High rates of ras codon 61 mutation in thyroid tumors in an iodide-deficient area. Cancer Res 51: 2690-2693.
2039. Shields TW, Staley CJ (1961). Functioning parathyroid cysts. Arch Surg 82: 937-942.
2040. Shimaoka K, Tsukada Y (1980). Squamous cell carcinomas and adenosquamous carcinomas originating from the thyroid gland. Cancer 46: 1833-1842.
2041. Shin E, Fujita S, Takami K, Kurahashi H, Kurita Y, Kobayashi T, Mori T, Nishisho I, Takai S (1993). Deletion mapping of chromosome 1p and 22q in pheochromocytoma. Jpn J Cancer Res 84: 402-408.
2042. Shin JY, Lee SM, Hwang MY, Sohn CH, Suh SJ (2001). MR findings of the spinal paraganglioma : report of three cases. J Korean Med Sci 16: 522-526.
2043. Shin SJ, Hoda RS, Ying L, DeLellis RA (2000). Diagnostic utility of the monoclonal antibody A103 in fine-needle aspiration biopsies of the adrenal. Am J Clin Pathol 113: 295-302.
2044. Shintani Y, Yoshimoto K, Horie H, Sano T, Kanesaki Y, Hosoi E, Yokogoshi Y, Bando H, Iwahana H, Kannuki S, Matsumoto K, Itakura M, Saito S (1995). Two different pituitary adenomas in a patient with multiple endocrine neoplasia type 1 associated with growth hormone-releasing hormone-producing pancreatic tumor: clinical and genetic features. Endocr J 42: 331-340.
2045. Shirouzu K, Miyamoto Y, Shiramizu T, Morimatsu M (1985). Somatostatinoma of the pancreas. Acta Pathol Jpn 35: 1285-1292.
2046. Shono T, Sakai H, Minami Y, Suzu H, Kanetake H, Saito Y (1999). Paraganglioma of the urinary bladder: A case report and review of the Japanese literature. Urol Int 62: 102-105.
2047. Shore RE, Hildreth N, Dvoretsky P, Pasternack B, Andresen E (1993). Benign thyroid adenomas among persons X-irradiated in infancy for enlarged thymus glands. Radiat Res 134: 217-223.
2048. Shorter NA, Glick RD, Klimstra DS, Brennan MF, Laquaglia MP (2002). Malignant pancreatic tumors in childhood and adolescence: The Memorial Sloan-Kettering experience, 1967 to present. J Pediatr Surg 37: 887-892.
2049. Sidhu S, Marsh DJ, Theodosopoulos G, Philips J, Bambach CP, Campbell P, Magarey CJ, Russell CF, Schulte KM, Roher HD, Delbridge L, Robinson BG (2002). Comparative genomic hybridization analysis of adrenocortical tumors. J Clin Endocrinol Metab 87: 3467-3474.
2050. Siemeister G, Weindel K, Mohrs K, Barleon B, Martiny-Baron G, Marme D (1996). Reversion of deregulated expression of vascular endothelial growth factor in human renal carcinoma cells by von Hippel-Lindau tumor suppressor protein. Cancer Res 56: 2299-2301.
2051. Sikri KL, Varndell IM, Hamid QA, Wilson BS, Kameya T, Ponder BA, Lloyd RV, Bloom SR, Polak JM (1985). Medullary carcinoma of the thyroid. An immunocytochemical and histochemical study of 25 cases using eight separate markers. Cancer 56: 2481-2491.
2052. Silva ES, Lumbroso S, Medina M, Gillerot Y, Sultan C, Sokal EM (2000). Demonstration of McCune-Albright mutations in the liver of children with high gammaGT progressive cholestasis. J Hepatol 32: 154-158.
2053. Silverberg SJ, Shane E, Jacobs TP, Siris E, Bilezikian JP (1999). A 10-year prospective study of primary hyperparathyroidism with or without parathyroid surgery. N Engl J Med 341: 1249-1255.
2054. Sim SJ, Ro JY, Ordonez NG, Cleary KR, Ayala AG (1997). Sclerosing mucoepidermoid carcinoma with eosinophilia of the thyroid: report of two patients, one with distant metastasis, and review of the literature. Hum Pathol 28: 1091-1096.
2055. Simonds WF, James-Newton LA, Agarwal SK, Yang B, Skarulis MC, Hendy GN, Marx SJ (2002). Familial isolated hyperparathyroidism: clinical and genetic characteristics of 36 kindreds. Medicine (Baltimore) 81: 1-26.
2056. Simpson DJ, Bicknell JE, McNicol AM, Clayton RN, Farrell WE (1999). Hypermethylation of the p16/CDKN2A/MTSI gene and loss of protein expression is associated with nonfunctional pituitary adenomas but not somatotrophinomas. Genes Chromosomes Cancer 24: 328-336.
2057. Simpson DJ, Clayton RN, Farrell WE (2002). Preferential loss of Death Associated Protein kinase expression in invasive pituitary tumours is associated with either CpG island methylation or homozygous deletion. Oncogene 21: 1217-1224.
2058. Simpson DJ, Hibberts NA, McNicol AM, Clayton RN, Farrell WE (2000). Loss of pRb expression in pituitary adenomas is associated with methylation of the RB1 CpG island. Cancer Res 60: 1211-1216.
2059. Simpson DJ, Magnay J, Bicknell JE, Barkan AL, McNicol AM, Clayton RN, Farrell WE (1999). Chromosome 13q deletion mapping in pituitary tumors: infrequent loss of the retinoblastoma susceptibility gene (RB1) locus despite loss of RB1 protein product in somatotrophinomas. Cancer Res 59: 1562-1566.
2060. Simpson PR (1990). Adenomatoid tumor of the adrenal gland. Arch Pathol Lab Med 114: 725-727.
2061. Simpson WJ, Carruthers J (1988). Squamous cell carcinoma of the thyroid gland. Am J Surg 156: 44-46.
2062. Singhal S, Birch JM, Kerr B, Lashford L, Evans DG (2002). Neurofibromatosis type 1 and sporadic optic gliomas. Arch Dis Child 87: 65-70.
2063. Sinkre P, Lindberg G, Albores-Saavedra J (2001). Nasopharyngeal gangliocytic paraganglioma. Arch Pathol Lab Med 125: 1098-1100.
2064. Sipple JH (1961). The association of pheochromocytoma with carcinoma of the thyroid gland. Am J Med 31: 163-166.
2065. Skacel M, Ross CW, Hsi ED (2000). A reassessment of primary thyroid lymphoma: high-grade MALT-type lymphoma as a distinct subtype of diffuse large B-cell lymphoma. Histopathology 37: 10-18.
2066. Skogseid B, Oberg K, Benson L, Lindgren PG, Lorelius LE, Lundquist G, Wide L, Wilander E (1987). A standardized meal stimulation test of the endocrine pancreas for early detection of pancreatic endocrine tumors in multiple endocrine neoplasia type 1 syndrome: five years experience. J Clin Endocrinol Metab 64: 1233-1240.
2067. Skogseid B, Rastad J, Gobl A, Larsson C, Backlin K, Juhlin C, Akerstrom G, Oberg K (1995). Adrenal lesion in multiple endocrine neoplasia type 1. Surgery 118: 1077-1082.

2068. Smelka RC, Cumming MJ, Shoenut JP (1993). Islet cell tumors: comparison of dynamic contrast-enhanced CT and MR imaging with dynamic gadolinium enhancement and fat suppression. Radiology 186: 799-802.

2069. Smith DP, Houghton C, Ponder BA (1997). Germline mutation of RET codon 883 in two cases of de novo MEN 2B. Oncogene 15: 1213-1217.

2070. Smith JF, Coombs RR (1984). Histological diagnosis of carcinoma of the parathyroid gland. J Clin Pathol 37: 1370-1378.

2071. Smith SA, Gharib H, Goellner JR (1987). Fine-needle aspiration. Usefulness for diagnosis and management of metastatic carcinoma to the thyroid. Arch Intern Med 147: 311-312.

2072. Sneige N, Ordonez NG, Veanattukalathil S, Samaan NA (1987). Fine-needle aspiration cytology in pancreatic endocrine tumors. Diagn Cytopathol 3: 35-40.

2073. Snover DC, Foucar K (1981). Mitotic activity in benign parathyroid disease. Am J Clin Pathol 75: 345-347.

2074. Snyder PJ (1985). Gonadotroph cell adenomas of the pituitary. Endocr Rev 6: 552-563.

2075. Soares P, Berx G, van Roy F, Sobrinho-Simoes M (1997). E-cadherin gene alterations are rare events in thyroid tumors. Int J Cancer 70: 32-38.

2076. Soares P, Cameselle-Teijeiro J, Sobrinho-Simoes M (1994). Immunohistochemical detection of p53 in differentiated, poorly differentiated and undifferentiated carcinomas of the thyroid. Histopathology 24: 205-210.

2077. Soares P, Trovisco V, Rocha AS, Lima J, Castro P, Preto A, Maximo V, Botelho T, Seruca R, Sobrinho-Simoes M (2003). BRAF mutations and RET/PTC rearrangements are alternative events in the etiopathogenesis of papillary thyroid carcinoma. Oncogene 22: 4578-4580.

2078. Sobin LH, Wittekind C (2002). TNM Classification of Malignant Tumours. 6th ed. Wiley,John & Sons: Hoboken.

2079. Sobol SM, Dailey JC (1990). Familial multiple cervical paragangliomas: report of a kindred and review of the literature. Otolaryngol Head Neck Surg 102: 382-390.

2080. Sobrinho-Simoes M (1995). Tumours of the thyroid: A brief overview with emphasis on the most controversial issues. Current Diagnostic Pathology 2: 15-22.

2081. Sobrinho-Simoes M (1996). Poorly differentiated carcinomas of the thyroid. Endocr Pathol 7: 99-102.

2082. Sobrinho-Simoes M, Nesland JM, Johannessen JV (1988). Columnar-cell carcinoma. Another variant of poorly differentiated carcinoma of the thyroid. Am J Clin Pathol 89: 264-267.

2083. Sobrinho-Simoes M, Sambade C, Fonseca E, Soares P (2002). Poorly differentiated carcinomas of the thyroid gland: a review of the clinicopathologic features of a series of 28 cases of a heterogeneous, clinically aggressive group of thyroid tumors. Int J Surg Pathol 10: 123-131.

2084. Sobrinho-Simoes M, Sambade C, Nesland JM, Holm R, Damjanov I (1990). Lectin histochemistry and ultrastructure of medullary carcinoma of the thyroid gland. Arch Pathol Lab Med 114: 369-375.

2085. Sobrinho-Simoes M, Stenwig AE, Nesland JM, Holm R, Johannessen JV (1986). A mucinous carcinoma of the thyroid. Pathol Res Pract 181: 464-471.

2086. Sobrinho-Simoes MA, Nesland JM, Holm R, Sambade MC, Johannessen JV (1985). Hurthle cell and mitochondrion-rich papillary carcinomas of the thyroid gland: an ultrastructural and immunocytochemical study. Ultrastruct Pathol 8: 131-142.

2087. Sobrinho-Simoes MA, Nesland JM, Johannessen JV (1985). A mucin-producing tumor in the thyroid gland. Ultrastruct Pathol 9: 277-281.

2088. Sofferman RA, Randolph GW (2003). Intraoperative parathyroid hormone assessment during parathyroidectomy. In: Surgery of the Thyroid and Parathyroid Glands, Randolph GW, ed., Saunders: Philadelphia , pp. 557-563.

2089. Soga J, Yakuwa Y (1998). Glucagonomas/diabetico-dermatogenic syndrome (DDS): a statistical evaluation of 407 reported cases. J Hepatobiliary Pancreat Surg 5: 312-319.

2090. Soga J, Yakuwa Y (1998). Vipoma/diarrheogenic syndrome: a statistical evaluation of 241 reported cases. J Exp Clin Cancer Res 17: 389-400.

2091. Soga J, Yakuwa Y (1999). Somatostatinoma/inhibitory syndrome: a statistical evaluation of 173 reported cases as compared to other pancreatic endocrinomas. J Exp Clin Cancer Res 18: 13-22.

2092. Soga J, Yakuwa Y, Osaka M (1998). Insulinoma/hypoglycemic syndrome: a statistical evaluation of 1085 reported cases of a Japanese series. J Exp Clin Cancer Res 17: 379-388.

2093. Solcia E, Capella C, Fiocca R, Sessa F, LaRosa F, Rindi G (1988). Disorders of the endocrine system. In: Pathology of the Gastrointestinal Tract, Ming SC, Goldman H, eds., 2nd ed. Lippincott, Williams & Wilkins: Baltimore .

2094. Solcia E, Capella C, Kloppel G (1997). Tumors of the Pancreas. 3rd ed. Armed Forces Institute of Pathology: Washington, DC.

2095. Solcia E, Capella C, Riva C, Rindi G, Polak JM (1988). The morphology and neuroendocrine profile of pancreatic epithelial VIPomas and extrapancreatic, VIP-producing, neurogenic tumors. Ann N Y Acad Sci 527: 508-517.

2096. Solcia E, Dayal Y (1991). Endocrine Pathology of the Gut and the Pancreas. CRC Press: Boca Raton.

2097. Solcia E, Kloppel G, Sobin LH (2000). World Health Organization Histological Classification of Tumours. Histological Typing of Endocrine Tumours. 2nd ed. Springer Verlag: Berlin Heidelberg New York Geneva.

2098. Solica E, Capella C, Buffa R, Frigerio B, Fiocca R (1980). Pathology of the Zollinger-Ellison syndrome. In: Progress in Surgical Pathology, Fenoglio CM, Wolff M, eds., Masson: New York , pp. 119-133.

2099. Solomon AC, Baloch ZW, Salhany KE, Mandel S, Weber RS, LiVolsi VA (2000). Thyroid sclerosing mucoepidermoid carcinoma with eosinophilia: mimic of Hodgkin disease in nodal metastases. Arch Pathol Lab Med 124: 446-449.

2100. Songyang S, Carraway KLI, Eck MJ, Harrison SC, Feldman RA, Mohammadi M, Schlessinger J, Hubbard SR, Smith DP, Eng C, Lorenzo MJ, Ponder BA, Mayer BJ, Cantley LC (1995). Catalytic specificity of protein-tyrosine kinases is critical for selective signalling. Nature 373: 536-539.

2101. Sonneland PR, Scheithauer BW, LeChago J, Crawford BG, Onofrio BM (1986). Paraganglioma of the cauda equina region. Clinicopathologic study of 31 cases with special reference to immunocytology and ultrastructure. Cancer 58: 1720-1735.

2102. Sorensen SA, Mulvihill JJ, Nielsen A (1986). Long-term follow-up of von Recklinghausen neurofibromatosis. Survival and malignant neoplasms. N Engl J Med 314: 1010-1015.

2103. Sowa H, Kaji H, Canaff L, Hendy GN, Tsukamoto T, Yamaguchi T, Miyazono K, Sugimoto T, Chihara K (2003). Inactivation of menin, the product of the MEN1 gene, inhibits the commitment of multipotential Mesenchymal stem cells into the osteoblast lineage. J Biol Chem .

2104. Spada A, Vallar L, Faglia G (1992). G protein oncogenes in pituitary tumors. Trends Endocrinol Metab 73: 1302-1308.

2105. Speel EJ, Richter J, Moch H, Egenter C, Saremaslani P, Rutimann K, Zhao J, Barghorn A, Roth J, Heitz PU, Komminoth P (1999). Genetic differences in endocrine pancreatic tumor subtypes detected by comparative genomic hybridization. Am J Pathol 155: 1787-1794.

2106. Speel EJ, Saremaslani P, Roth J, Hopman AH, Komminoth P (1998). Improved mRNA in situ hybridization on formaldehyde-fixed and paraffin-embedded tissue using signal amplification with different haptenized tyramides. Histochem Cell Biol 110: 571-577.

2107. Speel EJ, Scheidweiler AF, Zhao J, Matter C, Saremaslani P, Roth J, Heitz PU, Komminoth P (2001). Genetic evidence for early divergence of small functioning and nonfunctioning endocrine pancreatic tumors: gain of 9Q34 is an early event in insulinomas. Cancer Res 61: 5186-5192.

2108. Spires JR, Schwartz MR, Miller RH (1988). Anaplastic thyroid carcinoma. Association with differentiated thyroid cancer. Arch Otolaryngol Head Neck Surg 114: 40-44.

2109. Stabile BE, Morrow DJ, Passaro EJ (1984). The gastrinoma triangle: operative implications. Am J Surg 147: 25-31.

2110. Stabile BE, Passaro EJ (1985). Benign and malignant gastrinoma. Am J Surg 149: 144-150.

2111. Stacpoole PW (1981). The glucagonoma syndrome: clinical features, diagnosis, and treatment. Endocr Rev 2: 347-361.

2112. Stacpoole PW, Jaspan J, Kasselberg AG, Halter SA, Polonsky K, Gluck FW, Liljenquist JE, Rabin D (1981). A familial glucagonoma syndrome: genetic, clinical and biochemical features. Am J Med 70: 1017-1026.

2113. Stadnik T, Stevenaert A, Beckers A, Luypaert R, Buisseret T, Osteaux M (1990). Pituitary microadenomas: diagnosis with two-and three-dimensional MR imaging at 1.5 T before and after injection of gadolinium. Radiology 176: 419-428.

2114. Stage JG, Stadil F (1979). The clinical diagnosis of the Zollinger-Ellison syndrome. Scand J Gastroenterol Suppl 53: 79-91.

2115. Stamm B, Hedinger CE, Saremaslani P (1986). Duodenal and ampullary carcinoid tumors. A report of 12 cases with pathological characteristics, polypeptide content and relation to the MEN I syndrome and von Recklinghausen's disease (neurofibromatosis). Virchows Arch A Pathol Anat Histopathol 408: 475-489.

2116. Starink TM, van der Veen JP, Arwert F, de Waal LP, de Lange GG, Gille JJ, Eriksson AW (1986). The Cowden syndrome: a clinical and genetic study in 21 patients. Clin Genet 29: 222-233.

2117. Staunton MD, Greening WP (1973). Clinical diagnosis of thyroid cancer. Br Med J 4: 532-535.

2118. Stebbins CE, Kaelin WGJr, Pavletich NP (1999). Structure of the VHL-ElonginC-ElonginB complex: implications for VHL tumor suppressor function. Science 284: 455-461.

2119. Stefaneanu L, Murray D, Kovacs K (1990). Comparative study of DNA content and interphase nucleolar organizer regions in human pituitary adenomas. Endocr Pathol 1: 182-187.

2120. Stefanini P, Carboni M, Patrassi N, Basoli A (1974). Beta-islet cell tumors of the pancreas: results of a study on 1,067 cases. Surgery 75: 597-609.

2121. Steiner AL, Goodman AD, Powers SR (1968). Study of a kindred with pheochromocytoma, medullary thyroid carcinoma, hyperparathyroidism and Cushing's disease: multiple endocrine neoplasia, type 2. Medicine (Baltimore) 47: 371-409.

2122. Stenstrom G, Heedman PA (1974). Clinical findings in patients with hypercalcaemia. A final investigation based on biochemical screening. Acta Med Scand 195: 473-477.

2123. Stenstrom G, Svardsudd K (1986). Pheochromocytoma in Sweden 1958-1981. An analysis of the National Cancer Registry Data. Acta Med Scand 220: 225-232.

2124. Stephens M, Williams GT, Jasani B, Williams ED (1987). Synchronous duodenal neuroendocrine tumours in von Recklinghausen's disease—a case report of co-existing gangliocytic paraganglioma and somatostatin-rich glandular carcinoid. Histopathology 11: 1331-1340.

2125. Stern J, Jakobiec FA, Housepian EM (1980). The architecture of optic nerve gliomas with and without neurofibromatosis. Arch Ophthalmol 98: 505-511.

2126. Steusloff K, Rocken C, Saeger W (1998). Basement membrane proteins, apolipoprotein E and glycosaminoglycans in pituitary adenomas and their correlation to amyloid. Virchows Arch 433: 29-34.

2127. Stevenaert A, Perrin G, Martin D, Beckers A (2002). [Cushing's disease and corticotrophic adenoma: results of pituitary microsurgery]. Neurochirurgie 48: 234-265.

2128. Stevens-Simon C, Stewart J, Nakashima II, White M (1991). Exacerbation of fibrous dysplasia associated with an adolescent pregnancy. J Adolesc Health 12: 403-405.

2129. Stewart BW, Kleihues P (2003). World Cancer Report. IARC Press: Lyon.

2130. Stewart C, Parente F, Piehl F, Farnebo F, Quincey D, Silins G, Bergman L, Carle GF, Lemmens I, Grimmond S, Xian CZ, Khodei S, Teh BT, Lagercrantz J, Siggers P, Calender A, Van de Vem V, Kas K, Weber G, Hayward N, Gaudray P, Larsson C (1998). Characterization of the mouse Men1 gene and its expression during development. Oncogene 17: 2485-2493.

2131. Stewart CJ, Imrie CW, Foulis AK (1994). Pancreatic islet cell tumour in a patient with familial adenomatous polyposis. J Clin Pathol 47: 860-861.

2132. Stewart PM (2002). The adrenal cortex. In: Williams Textbook of Endocrinology, Larsen PR, Kronenberg HM, Melmed S, Polonsky KS, eds., 10th ed. Saunders: Philadelphia , pp. 491-551.

2133. Stewart PM, Carey MP, Graham CT, Wright AD, London DR (1992). Growth hormone secreting pituitary carcinoma: a case report and literature review. Clin Endocrinol (Oxf) 37: 189-194.

2134. Stoffer SS, Van Dyke DL, Bach JV, Szpunar W, Weiss L (1986). Familial papillary carcinoma of the thyroid. Am J Med Genet 25: 775-782.

2135. Stojadinovic A, Ghossein RA, Hoos A, Nissan A, Marshall D, Dudas M, Cordon-Cardo C, Jaques DP, Brennan MF (2002). Adrenocortical carcinoma: clinical, morphologic, and molecular characterization. J Clin Oncol 20: 941-950.

2136. Stojadinovic A, Hoos A, Nissan A, Dudas ME, Cordon-Cardo C, Shaha AR, Brennan MF, Singh B, Ghossein RA (2003). Parathyroid neoplasms: clinical, histopathological, and tissue microarray-based molecular analysis. Hum Pathol 34: 54-64.

2137. Stolle C, Glenn G, Zbar B, Humphrey JS, Choyke P, Walther M, Pack S, Hurley K, Andrey C, Klausner R, Linehan WM (1998). Improved detection of germline mutations in the von Hippel-Lindau disease tumor suppressor gene. Hum Mutat 12: 417-423.

2138. Stork PJ, Herteaux C, Frazier R, Kronenburg H, Wolfe HJ (1989). Expression and distribution of parathyroid hormone and parathyroid messenger RNA in pathological conditions of the parathyroid. Lab Invest 60: 92A.

2139. Stratakis CA (2000). Genetics of Carney complex and related familial lentiginoses, and other multiple tumor syndromes. Pediatr Pathol Mol Med 19: 41-68.

2140. Stratakis CA (2002). Mutations of the gene encoding the protein kinase A type I-alpha regulatory subunit (PRKAR1A) in patients with the "complex of spotty skin pigmentation, myxomas, endocrine overactivity, and schwannomas" (Carney complex). Ann N Y Acad Sci 968: 3-21.

2141. Stratakis CA, Ball DW (2000). A concise genetic and clinical guide to multiple endocrine neoplasias and related syndromes. J Pediatr Endocrinol Metab 13: 457-465.

2142. Stratakis CA, Carney JA, Lin JP, Papanicolaou DA, Karl M, Kastner DL, Pras E, Chrousos GP (1996). Carney complex, a familial multiple neoplasia and lentiginosis syndrome. Analysis of 11 kindreds and linkage to the short arm of chromosome 2. J Clin Invest 97: 699-705.

2143. Stratakis CA, Cho-Chung YS (2002). Protein kinase A and human disease. Trends Endocrinol Metab 13: 50-52.

2144. Stratakis CA, Courcoutsakis NA, Abati A, Filie A, Doppman JL, Carney JA, Shawker T (1997). Thyroid gland abnormalities in patients with the syndrome of spotty skin pigmentation, myxomas, endocrine overactivity, and schwannomas (Carney complex). J Clin Endocrinol Metab 82: 2037-2043.

2145. Stratakis CA, Jenkins RB, Pras E, Mitsiadis CS, Raff SB, Stalboerger PG, Tsigos C, Carney JA, Chrousos GP (1996). Cytogenetic and microsatellite alterations in tumors from patients with the syndrome of myxomas, spotty skin pigmentation, and endocrine overactivity (Carney complex). J Clin Endocrinol Metab 81: 3607-3614.

2146. Stratakis CA, Kirschner LS, Carney JA (2001). Clinical and molecular features of the Carney complex: diagnostic criteria and recommendations for patient evaluation. J Clin Endocrinol Metab 86: 4041-4046.

2147. Stratakis CA, Papageorgiou T, Premkumar A, Pack S, Kirschner LS, Taymans SE, Zhuang Z, Oelkers WH, Carney JA (2000). Ovarian lesions in Carney complex: clinical genetics and possible

predisposition to malignancy. J Clin Endocrinol Metab 85: 4359-4366.

2148. Stratakis CA, Sarlis N, Kirschner LS, Carney JA, Doppman JL, Nieman LK, Chrousos GP, Papanicolaou DA (1999). Paradoxical response to dexamethasone in the diagnosis of primary pigmented nodular adrenocortical disease. Ann Intern Med 131: 585-591.

2149. Stratakis CA, Schussheim DH, Freedman SM, Keil MF, Pack SD, Agarwal SK, Skarulis MC, Weil RJ, Lubensky IA, Zhuang Z, Oldfield EH, Marx SJ (2000). Pituitary macroadenoma in a 5-year-old: an early expression of multiple endocrine neoplasia type 1. J Clin Endocrinol Metab 85: 4776-4780.

2150. Stratmann R, Krieg M, Haas R, Plate KH (1997). Putative control of angiogenesis in hemangioblastomas by the von Hippel-Lindau tumor suppressor gene. J Neuropathol Exp Neurol 56: 1242-1252.

2151. Straus C, Molcard S, Visot A, Epardeau B, le Parc JM (1997). Chemodectoma of the cauda equina. Rev Rhum Engl Ed 64: 345-347.

2152. Stringel G, Dalpe-Scott M, Perelman AH, Heick HM (1985). The occult insulinoma operative localization by quick insulin radioimmunoassay. J Pediatr Surg 20: 734-736.

2153. Studer H, Derwahl M (1995). Mechanisms of nonneoplastic endocrine hyperplasia—a changing concept: a review focused on the thyroid gland. Endocr Rev 16: 411-426.

2154. Stumpf E, Aalto Y, Hoog A, Kjellman M, Otonkoski T, Knuutila S, Andersson LC (2000). Chromosomal alterations in human pancreatic endocrine tumors. Genes Chromosomes Cancer 29: 83-87.

2155. Styne DM, Isaac R, Miller WL, Leisti S, Connors M, Conte FA, Grumbach MM (1983). Endocrine, histological, and biochemical studies of adrenocorticotropin-producing islet cell carcinoma of the pancreas in childhood with characterization of proopiomelanocortin. J Clin Endocrinol Metab 57: 723-731.

2156. Su L, Beals T, Bernacki EG, Giordano TJ (1997). Spindle epithelial tumor with thymus-like differentiation: a case report with cytologic, histologic, immunohistologic, and ultrastructural findings. Mod Pathol 10: 510-514.

2157. Suarez HG, du Villard JA, Severino M, Caillou B, Schlumberger M, Tubiana M, Parmentier C, Monier R (1990). Presence of mutations in all three ras genes in human thyroid tumors. Oncogene 5: 565-570.

2158. Sugg SL, Ezzat S, Rosen IB, Freeman JL, Asa SL (1998). Distinct multiple RET/PTC gene rearrangements in multifocal papillary thyroid neoplasia. J Clin Endocrinol Metab 83: 4116-4122.

2159. Sugita R, Nomura T, Yuda F (1998). Primary schwannoma of the thyroid gland: CT findings. AJR Am J Roentgenol 171: 528-529.

2160. Sugitani I, Kasai N, Fujimoto Y, Yanagisawa A (2001). Prognostic factors and therapeutic strategy for anaplastic carcinoma of the thyroid. World J Surg 25: 617-622.

2161. Sukhodolets KE, Hickman AB, Agarwal SK, Sukhodolets MV, Obungu VH, Novotny EA, Crabtree JS, Chandrasekharappa SC, Collins FS, Spiegel AM, Burns AL, Marx SJ (2003). The 32-kilodalton subunit of replication protein A interacts with menin, the product of the MEN1 tumor suppressor gene. Mol Cell Biol 23: 493-509.

2162. Sullivan M, Boileau M, Hodges CV (1978). Adrenal cortical carcinoma. J Urol 120: 660-665.

2163. Sutliff VE, Doppman JL, Gibril F, Venzon DJ, Yu F, Serrano J, Jensen RT (1997). Growth of newly diagnosed, untreated metastatic gastrinomas and predictors of growth patterns. J Clin Oncol 15: 2420-2431.

2164. Suzuki H, Matsuyama M (1971). Ultrastructure of functioning beta cell tumors of the pancreatic islets. Cancer 28: 1302-1313.

2165. Syed FA, Chalew SA (1999). Ketoconazole treatment of gonadotropin independent precocious puberty in girls with McCune-Albright syndrome: a preliminary report. J Pediatr Endocrinol Metab 12: 81-83.

2166. Szabo J, Heath B, Hill VM, Jackson CE, Zarbo RJ, Mallette LE, Chew SL, Besser GM, Thakker RV, Huff V, Leppert MF, Heath H (1995). Hereditary hyperparathyroidism-jaw tumor syndrome: the endocrine tumor gene HRPT2 maps to chromosome 1q21-q31. Am J Hum Genet 56: 944-950.

2167. Szinnai G, Meier C, Komminoth P, Zumsteg UW (2003). Review of multiple endocrine neoplasia type 2A in children: therapeutic results of early thyroidectomy and prognostic value of codon analysis. Pediatrics 111: E132-E139.

2168. Taccagni G, Sambade C, Nesland J, Terreni MR, Sobrinho-Simoes M (1993). Solitary fibrous tumour of the thyroid: clinicopathological, immunohistochemical and ultrastructural study of three cases. Virchows Arch A Pathol Anat Histopathol 422: 491-497.

2169. Tai P, Mould RF, Prysyazhnyuk AYe, Gristchenko VG, Obodovsky IA (2003). Descriptive epidemiology of thyroid carcinoma. Current Oncology 10: 54-65.

2170. Taira H, Takasita M, Yoshida S, Takita C, Tsumura H, Torisu T (2000). MR appearance of paraganglioma of the cauda equina. Case reports. Acta Radiol 41: 27-30.

2171. Takahashi H, Nakano K, Adachi Y, Aoki N, Hajiro K, Yamamoto T, Higashizawa T, Chikugo T, Suzuki T (1988). Multiple non-functional pancreatic islet cell tumor in multiple endocrine neoplasia type I. A case report. Acta Pathol Jpn 38: 667-682.

2172. Takahashi M, Buma Y, Iwamoto T, Inaguma Y, Ikeda H, Hiai H (1988). Cloning and expression of the ret proto-oncogene encoding a tyrosine kinase with two potential transmembrane domains. Oncogene 3: 571-578.

2173. Takahashi M, Iwashita T, Santoro M, Lyonnet S, Lenoir GM, Billaud M (1999). Co-segregation of MEN2 and Hirschsprung's disease: the same mutation of RET with both gain and loss-of-function? Hum Mutat 13: 331-336.

2174. Takahashi MH, Thomas GA, Williams ED (1995). Evidence for mutual interdependence of epithelium and stromal lymphoid cells in a subset of papillary carcinomas. Br J Cancer 72: 813-817.

2175. Takakuwa T, Dong Z, Takayama H, Matsuzuka F, Nagata S, Aozasa K (2001). Frequent mutations of Fas gene in thyroid lymphoma. Cancer Res 61: 1382-1385.

2176. Takami H, Ozaki O, Ito K (1996). Familial nonmedullary thyroid cancer: an emerging entity that warrants aggressive treatment. Arch Surg 131: 676.

2177. Takano T, Miyauchi A, Matsuzuka F, Yoshida H, Kuma K, Amino N (2000). Diagnosis of thyroid malignant lymphoma by reverse transcription-polymerase chain

reaction detecting the monoclonality of immunoglobulin heavy chain messenger ribonucleic acid. J Clin Endocrinol Metab 85: 671-675.

2178. Takashima S, Takayama F, Saito A, Wang Q, Hidaka K, Sone S (2000). Primary thyroid lymphoma: diagnosis of immunoglobulin heavy chain gene rearrangement with polymerase chain reaction in ultrasound-guided fine-needle aspiration. Thyroid 10: 507-510.

2179. Takaya K, Yoshimasa T, Arai H, Tamura N, Miyamoto Y, Itoh H, Nakao K (1996). Expression of the RET proto-oncogene in normal human tissues, pheochromocytomas, and other tumors of neural crest origin. J Mol Med 74: 617-621.

2180. Takayama F, Takashima S, Matsuba H, Kobayashi S, Ito N, Sone S (2001). MR imaging of primary leiomyosarcoma of the thyroid gland. Eur J Radiol 37: 36-41.

2181. Takehara K, Miyata Y, Matsuo M, Sakai H, Minami Y, Kanetake H (2001). [A case of malignant pheochromocytoma associated with von Recklinghausen's disease]. Hinyokika Kiyo 47: 257-260.

2182. Takei Y, Seyama S, Pearl GS, Tindall GT (1980). Ultrastructural study of the human neurohypophysis. II. Cellular elements of neural parenchyma, the pituicytes. Cell Tissue Res 205: 273-287.

2183. Takino H, Herman V, Weiss M, Melmed S (1995). Purine-binding factor (nm23) gene expression in pituitary tumors: marker of adenoma invasiveness. J Clin Endocrinol Metab 80: 1733-1738.

2184. Tallini G, Garcia-Rostan G, Herrero A, Zelterman D, Viale G, Bosari S, Carcangiu ML (1999). Downregulation of p27KIP1 and Ki67/Mib1 labeling index support the classification of thyroid carcinoma into prognostically relevant categories. Am J Surg Pathol 23: 678-685.

2185. Tallini G, Hsueh A, Liu S, Garcia-Rostan G, Speicher MR, Ward DC (1999). Frequent chromosomal DNA unbalance in thyroid oncocytic (Hurthle cell) neoplasms detected by comparative genomic hybridization. Lab Invest 79: 547-555.

2186. Tamimi DM (2002). The association between chronic lymphocytic thyroiditis and thyroid tumors. Int J Surg Pathol 10: 141-146.

2187. Tamouridis N, Deladetsima JK, Kastanias I, Delis S, Bramis J, Zerva CA, Anapliotou ML (1999). Cold thyroid nodule as the sole manifestation of Rosai-Dorfman disease with mild lymphadenopathy, coexisting with chronic autoimmune thyroiditis. J Endocrinol Invest 22: 866-870.

2188. Tanaka C, Yoshimoto K, Yamada S, Nishioka H, Ii S, Moritani M, Yamaoka T, Itakura M (1998). Absence of germ-line mutations of the multiple endocrine neoplasia type 1 (MEN1) gene in familial pituitary adenoma in contrast to MEN1 in Japanese. J Clin Endocrinol Metab 83: 960-965.

2189. Tanaka C, Yoshimoto K, Yang P, Kimura T, Yamada S, Moritani M, Sano T, Itakura M (1997). Infrequent mutations of p27Kip1 gene and trisomy 12 in a subset of human pituitary adenomas. J Clin Endocrinol Metab 82: 3141-3147.

2190. Tanaka S, Yamasaki S, Matsushita H, Ozawa Y, Kurosaki A, Takeuchi K, Hoshihara Y, Doi T, Watanabe G, Kawaminami K (2000). Duodenal somatostatinoma: a case report and review of 31 cases with special reference to the relationship between tumor size and metastasis. Pathol Int 50: 146-152.

2191. Tanaka T, Yoshimi N, Iwata H, Sugie S, Kato K, Sakamoto H, Mori H (1989). Fine-needle aspiration cytology of pheochromocytoma-ganglioneuroma of the organ of Zuckerkandl. Diagn Cytopathol 5: 64-68.

2192. Tanda F, Massarelli G, Bosincu L (1990). Primary mucoepidermoid carcinoma of the thyroid gland. Surg Pathol 3: 317-324.

2193. Tanda F, Massarelli G, Bosincu L, Cossu A (1988). Angiosarcoma of the thyroid: a light, electron microscopic and histoimmunological study. Hum Pathol 19: 742-745.

2194. Tanda F, Massarelli G, Mingioni V (1990). Mixed follicular-parafollicular carcinoma of the thyroid. A light, electron microscopic and histoimmunologic study. Surg Pathol 3: 65-74.

2195. Tang SH, Chen A, Lee CT, Yu DS, Chang SY, Sun GH (2003). Remote recurrence of malignant pheochromocytoma 14 years after primary operation. J Urol 169: 269.

2196. Tanimoto K, Makino Y, Pereira T, Poellinger L (2000). Mechanism of regulation of the hypoxia-inducible factor-1 alpha by the von Hippel-Lindau tumor suppressor protein. EMBO J 19: 4298-4309.

2197. Tanner HC, Dahlin DC, Childs DS (1961). Sarcoma complicating fibrous dysplasia: probably role of radiation therapy. Oral Surg 14: 837-846.

2198. Tano Assini MT, Oliva Otero G, Gomez SC (1968). [Visceral hemangiopericytoma. Presentation of 2 cases]. Prensa Med Argent 55: 996-1000.

2199. Tapper D, Lack EE (1983). Teratomas in infancy and childhood. A 54-year experience at the Children's Hospital Medical Center. Ann Surg 198: 398-410.

2200. Tartour E, Caillou B, Tenenbaum F, Schroder S, Luciani S, Talbot M, Schlumberger M (1993). Immunohistochemical study of adrenocortical carcinoma. Predictive value of the D11 monoclonal antibody. Cancer 72: 3296-3303.

2201. Taschner PE, Jansen JC, Baysal BE, Bosch A, Rosenberg EH, Brocker-Vriends AH, Der Mey AG, van Ommen GJ, Cornelisse CJ, Devilee P (2001). Nearly all hereditary paragangliomas in the Netherlands are caused by two founder mutations in the SDHD gene. Genes Chromosomes Cancer 31: 274-281.

2202. Tauchmanova L, Rossi R, Biondi B, Pulcrano M, Nuzzo V, Palmieri EA, Fazio S, Lombardi G (2002). Patients with subclinical Cushing's syndrome due to adrenal adenoma have increased cardiovascular risk. J Clin Endocrinol Metab 87: 4872-4878.

2203. Taylor RL, Singh RJ (2002). Validation of liquid chromatography-tandem mass spectrometry method for analysis of urinary conjugated metanephrine and normetanephrine for screening of pheochromocytoma. Clin Chem 48: 533-539.

2204. Taylor S (1982). High resolution computed tomography of the sella. Radiol Clin North Am 20: 207-236.

2205. Teears RJ, Silverman EM (1975). Clinicopathologic review of 88 cases of carcinoma metastatic to the putuitary gland. Cancer 36: 216-220.

2206. Teh BT, Esapa CT, Houlston R, Grandell U, Farnebo F, Nordenskjold M, Pearce CJ, Carmichael D, Larsson C, Harris PE (1998). A family with isolated hyperparathyroidism segregating a missense MEN1 mutation and showing loss of the wild-type alleles in the parathyroid tumors. Am J Hum Genet 63: 1544-1549.

2207. Teh BT, Farnebo F, Kristoffersson U, Sundelin B, Cardinal J, Axelson R, Yap A, Epstein M, Heath HI, Cameron D, Larsson C (1996). Autosomal dominant primary hyperparathyroidism and jaw tumor syndrome associated with renal hamartomas and cystic kidney disease: linkage to 1q21-q32 and loss of the wild type allele in renal hamartomas. J Clin Endocrinol Metab 81: 4204-4211.

2208. Teh BT, Kytola S, Farnebo F, Bergman L, Wong FK, Weber G, Hayward N, Larsson C, Skogseid B, Beckers A, Phelan C, Edwards M, Epstein M, Alford F, Hurley D, Grimmond S, Silins G, Walters M, Stewart C, Cardinal J, Khodaei S, Parente F, Tranebjaerg L, Jorde R, Menon J, Khir A, Tan TT, Chan SP, Zaini A, Khalid BAK, Sandelin K, Thompson N, Brandi ML, Warth M, Stock J, Leisti J, Cameron D, Shepherd JJ, Oberg K, Nordenskjold M, Salmela P (1998). Mutation analysis of the MEN1 gene in multiple endocrine neoplasia type 1, familial acromegaly and familial isolated hyperparathyroidism. J Clin Endocrinol Metab 83: 2621-2626.

2209. Teh BT, Zedenius J, Kytola S, Skogseid B, Trotter J, Choplin H, Twigg S, Farnebo F, Giraud S, Cameron D, Robinson B, Calender A, Larsson C, Salmela P (1998). Thymic carcinoids in multiple endocrine neoplasia type 1. Ann Surg 228: 99-105.

2210. Telander RL, Zimmerman D, Sizemore GW, van Heerden JA, Grant CS (1989). Medullary carcinoma in children. Results of early detection and surgery. Arch Surg 124: 841-843.

2211. Terada T, Kovacs K, Stefaneanu L, Horvath E (1995). Incidence, Pathology, and Recurrence of Pituitary Adenomas: Study of 647 Unselected Surgical Cases. Endocr Pathol 6: 301-310.

2212. Terada T, Matsunaga Y, Maeta H, Endo K, Horie S, Ohta T (1999). Mixed ductal-endocrine carcinoma of the pancreas presenting as gastrinoma with Zollinger-Ellison syndrome: an autopsy case with a 24-year survival period. Virchows Arch 435: 606-611.

2213. Terpstra L, Rauch F, Plotkin H, Travers R, Glorieux FH (2002). Bone mineralization in polyostotic fibrous dysplasia: histomorphometric analysis. J Bone Miner Res 17: 1949-1953.

2214. Terzolo M, Boccuzzi A, Bovio S, Cappia S, De Giuli P, Ali A, Paccotti P, Porpiglia F, Fontana D, Angeli A (2001). Immunohistochemical assessment of Ki-67 in the differential diagnosis of adrenocortical tumors. Urology 57: 176-182.

2215. Teyssier JR, Liautaud-Roger F, Ferre D, Patey M, Dufer J (1990). Chromosomal changes in thyroid tumors. Relation with DNA content, karyotypic features, and clinical data. Cancer Genet Cytogenet 50: 249-263.

2216. Thakker RV, Pook MA, Wooding C, Boscaro M, Scanarini M, Clayton RN (1993). Association of somatotrophinomas with loss of alleles on chromosome 11 and with gsp mutations. J Clin Invest 91: 2815-2821.

2217. Thannberger P, Wilhelm JM, Derragui A, Saraceni O, Kieffer P (2001). [Von Recklinghausen's disease associated with pancreatic somatostatinoma]. Presse Med 30: 1741-1743.

2218. Thapar K, Kovacs K (1998). Comments on: Symptomatic granular cell tumor of the pituitary gland: case report and review of the literature. Neurosurgery 42: 170-171.

2219. Thapar K, Kovacs K, Scheithauer BW, Stefaneanu L, Horvath E, Pernicone PJ, Murray D, Laws ERJr (1996). Proliferative activity and invasiveness among pituitary adenomas and carcinomas: an analysis using the MIB-1 antibody. Neurosurgery 38: 99-106.

2220. Thapar K, Kovacs K, Stefaneanu L, Scheithauer B, Killinger DW, Lioyd RV, Smyth HS, Barr A, Thorner MO, Gaylinn B, Laws ERJr (1997). Overexpression of the growth-hormone-releasing hormone gene in acromegaly-associated pituitary tumors. An event associated with neoplastic progression and aggressive behavior. Am J Pathol 151: 769-784.

2221. Thapar K, Laws ERJr (2001). Pituitary surgery. In: Diagnosis and Management of Pituitary Tumors, Thapar K, Kovacs K, Scheithauer BW, Lloyd RV, eds., Humana Press: Totowa, NJ , pp. 225-246.

2222. Thapar K, Scheithauer BW, Kovacs K, Pernicone PJ, Laws ERJr (1996). p53 expression in pituitary adenomas and carcinomas: correlation with invasiveness and tumor growth fractions. Neurosurgery 38: 763-770.

2223. The American Society of Clinical Oncology (1996). Statement of the American Society of Clinical Oncology: Genetic testing for cancer susceptibility. J Clinical Oncology 14: 1730-1736.

2224. The I, Murthy AE, Hannigan GE, Jacoby LB, Menon AG, Gusella JF, Bernards A (1993). Neurofibromatosis type 1 gene mutations in neuroblastoma. Nat Genet 3: 62-66.

2225. Thieblemont C, Mayer A, Dumontet C, Barbier Y, Callet-Bauchu E, Felman P, Berger F, Ducottet X, Martin C, Salles G, Orgiazzi J, Coiffier B (2002). Primary thyroid lymphoma is a heterogeneous disease. J Clin Endocrinol Metab 87: 105-111.

2226. Thodou E, Kontogeorgos G, Scheithauer BW, Lekka I, Tzanis S, Mariatos P, Laws ERJr (2000). Intrasellar chordomas mimicking pituitary adenoma. J Neurosurg 92: 976-982.

2227. Thom AK, Norton JA, Axiotis CA, Jensen RT (1991). Location, incidence, and malignant potential of duodenal gastrinomas. Surgery 110: 1086-1091.

2228. Thomas GA, Williams D, Williams ED (1989). The clonal origin of thyroid nodules and adenomas. Am J Pathol 134: 141-147.

2229. Thompson LD (2002). Pheochromocytoma of the Adrenal gland Scaled Score (PASS) to separate benign from malignant neoplasms: a clinicopathologic and immunophenotypic study of 100 cases. Am J Surg Pathol 26: 551-566.

2230. Thompson LD, Rosai J, Heffess CS (2000). Primary thyroid teratomas: a clinicopathologic study of 30 cases. Cancer 88: 1149-1158.

2231. Thompson LD, Wenig BM, Adair CF, Heffess CS (1996). Peripheral Nerve Sheath Tumors of the Thyroid Gland: A Series of Four Cases and a Review of the Literature. Endocr Pathol 7: 309-318.

2232. Thompson LD, Wenig BM, Adair CF, Shmookler BM, Heffess CS (1997). Primary smooth muscle tumors of the thyroid gland. Cancer 79: 579-587.

2233. Thompson LD, Wenig BM, Adair CF, Smith BC, Heffess CS (1996). Langerhans cell histiocytosis of the thyroid: a series of seven cases and a review of the literature. Mod Pathol 9: 145-149.

2234. Thompson NW, Dunn EL, Batsakis JG, Nishiyama RH (1974). Hurthle cell lesions of the thyroid gland. Surg Gynecol Obstet 139: 555-560.

2235. Thompson NW, Vinik AI, Eckhauser FE (1989). Microgastrinomas of the duodenum. A cause of failed operations for the Zollinger-Ellison syndrome. Ann Surg 209: 396-404.

2236. Thompson NW, Vinik AI, Eckhauser FE, Strodel WE (1985). Extrapancreatic gastrinomas. Surgery 98: 1113-1120.

2237. Thoren M, Rahn T, Guo WY, Werner S (1991). Stereotactic radiosurgery with the cobalt-60 gamma unit in the treatment of growth hormone-producing pituitary tumors. Neurosurgery 29: 663-668.

2238. Thorner MO, Vance ML (1988). Growth hormone, 1988. J Clin Invest 82: 745-747.

2239. Thurston V, Williams ED (1982). Experimental induction of C cell tumours in thyroid by increased dietary content of vitamin D3. Acta Endocrinol (Copenh) 100: 41-45.

2240. Tibbs REJr, Bowles APJr, Raila FA, Fratkin JD, Hutchins JB (1997). Should endolymphatic sac tumors be considered part of the von Hippel-Lindau complex? Pathology case report. Neurosurgery 40: 848-855.

2241. Tielens ET, Sherman SI, Hruban RH, Ladenson PW (1994). Follicular variant of papillary thyroid carcinoma. A clinicopathologic study. Cancer 73: 424-431.

2242. Tischler AS (1997). Paraganglia. In: Histology for Pathologists, Sternberg SS, ed., 2nd ed. Lippincott-Raven: Philadelphia , pp. 1153-1171.

2243. Tischler AS (1998). The adrenal medulla and extra-adrenal paraganglia. In: Functional Endocrine Pathology, Kovacs K, Asa SL, eds., Blackwell Science: Malden, MA , pp. 550-595.

2244. Tischler AS (2000). Divergent differentiation in neuroendocrine tumors of the adrenal gland. Semin Diagn Pathol 17: 120-126.

2245. Tischler AS, Dayal Y, Balogh K, Cohen RB, Connolly JL, Tallberg K (1987). The distribution of immunoreactive chromogranins, S-100 protein, and vasoactive intestinal peptide in compound tumors of the adrenal medulla. Hum Pathol 18: 909-917.

2246. Tischler AS, DeLellis RA, Biales B, Nunnemacher G, Carabba V, Wolfe HJ (1980). Nerve growth factor-induced neurite outgrowth from normal human chromaffin cells. Lab Invest 43: 399-409.

2247. Tischler AS, Lee YC, Perlman RL, Costopoulos D, Bloom SR (1985). Production of "ectopic" vasoactive intestinal peptide-like immunoreactivity in normal human chromaffin cell cultures. Life Sci 37: 1881-1886.

2248. Tischler AS, Lee YC, Perlman RL, Costopoulos D, Slayton VW, Bloom SR (1984). Production of "ectopic" vasoactive intestinal peptide-like and neurotensin-like immunoreactivity in human pheochromocytoma cell cultures. J Neurosci 4: 1398-1404.

2249. Tischler AS, Shih TS, Williams BO, Jacks T (1995). Characterization of Pheochromocytomas in a Mouse Strain with a Targeted Disruptive Mutation of the Neurofibromatosis Gene Nf1. Endocr Pathol 6: 323-335.

2250. Tisell LE, Carlsson S, Fjalling M, Hansson G, Lindberg S, Lundberg LM, Oden A (1985). Hyperparathyroidism subsequent to neck irradiation. Risk factors. Cancer 56: 1529-1533.

2251. Tomassetti P, Cometa G, Del Vecchio E, Baserga M, Faccioli P, Bosoni D, Paolucci G, Barbara L (1995). Chromosomal instability in multiple endocrine neoplasia type 1. Cytogenetic evaluation with DEB test. Cancer Genet Cytogenet 79: 123-126.
2252. Tomic S, Warner T (1996). Pancreatic somatostatin-secreting gangliocytic paraganglioma with lymph node metastases. Am J Gastroenterol 91: 607-608.
2253. Tomita T, Friesen SR, Kimmel JR (1986). Pancreatic polypeptide-secreting islet cell tumor. A follow-up report. Cancer 57: 129-133.
2254. Tomita T, Gates E (1999). Pituitary adenomas and granular cell tumors. Incidence, cell type, and location of tumor in 100 pituitary glands at autopsy. Am J Clin Pathol 111: 817-825.
2255. Tomita T, Kimmel JR, Friesen SR, Doull V, Pollock HG (1985). Pancreatic polypeptide in islet cell tumors. Morphologic and functional correlations. Cancer 56: 1649-1657.
2256. Tormey WP, Fitzgerald RJ, Thomas G, Kay EW, Leader MB (2000). Catecholamine secretion and ploidy in phaeochromocytoma. Int J Clin Pract 54: 520-523.
2257. Toth K, Peter I, Kremmer T, Sugar J (1990). Lipid-rich cell thyroid adenoma: histopathology with comparative lipid analysis. Virchows Arch A Pathol Anat Histopathol 417: 273-276.
2258. Tourniaire J, Chalendar D, Treluyer C, Trouillas J (1990). Les adénomes hypophysaires dit "silencieux". Rev Fr Endocrinol Clin 31: 303-308.
2259. Trautmann K, Thakker RV, Ellison DW, Ibrahim A, Lees PD, Harding B, Fischer C, Popp S, Bartram CR, Jauch A (2001). Chromosomal aberrations in sporadic pituitary tumors. Int J Cancer 91: 809-814.
2260. Travis WD, Lack EE, Azumi N, Tsokos M, Norton J (1990). Adenomatoid tumor of the adrenal gland with ultrastructural and immunohistochemical demonstration of a mesothelial origin. Arch Pathol Lab Med 114: 722-724.
2261. Triggs SM, Williams ED (1977). Experimental carcinogenesis in the thyroid follicular and C cells. A comparison of the effect of variation in dietary calcium and of radiation. Acta Endocrinol (Copenh) 85: 84-92.
2262. Trost BN, Koenig MP, Zimmermann A, Zachmann M, Muller J (1981). Virilization of a post-menopausal woman by a testosterone-secreting Leydig cell type adrenal adenoma. Acta Endocrinol (Copenh) 98: 274-282.
2263. Trouillas J (2002). [Pathology and pathogenesis of pituitary corticotroph adenoma]. Neurochirurgie 48: 149-162.
2264. Trouillas J, Daniel L, Guigard MP, Tong S, Gouvernet J, Jouanneau E, Jan M, Perrin G, Fischer G, Tabarin A, Rougon G, Figarella-Branger D (2003). Polysialylated neural cell adhesion molecules expressed in human pituitary tumors and related to extrasellar invasion. J Neurosurg 98: 1084-1093.
2265. Trouillas J, Delgrange E, Jouanneau E, Maiter D, Guigard MP, Donckier J, Perrin G, Jan M, Tourniaire J (2000). [Prolactinoma in man: clinical and histological characteristics]. Ann Endocrinol (Paris) 61: 253-257.
2266. Trouillas J, Girod C, Sassolas G, Vitte PA, Claustrat B, Perrin G, Lhéritier M, Fischer C, Dubois MP (1984). A human beta-endorphin pituitary adenoma. J Clin Endocrinol Metab 58: 242-249.
2267. Trouillas J, Guigard MP, Fonlupt P, Souchier C, Girod C (1996). Mapping of corticotropic cells in the normal human pituitary. J Histochem Cytochem 44: 473-479.
2268. Trovato M, Fraggetta F, Villari D, Batolo D, Mackey K, Trimarchi F, Benvenga S (1999). Loss of heterozygosity of the long arm of chromosome 7 in follicular and anaplastic thyroid cancer, but not in papillary thyroid cancer. J Clin Endocrinol Metab 84: 3235-3240.
2269. Trump D, Farren B, Wooding C, Pang JT, Besser GM, Buchanan KD, Edwards CR, Heath DA, Jackson CE, Jansen S, Lips K, Monson JP, O'Halloran D, Sampson J, Shalet SM, Wheeler MH, Zink A, Thakker RV (1996). Clinical studies of multiple endocrine neoplasia type 1 (MEN1). QJM 89: 653-669.
2270. Trump DL, Livingston JN, Baylin SB (1977). Watery diarrhea syndrome in an adult with ganglioneuroma-pheochromocytoma: identification of vasoactive intestinal peptide, calcitonin, and catecholamines and assessment of their biologic activity. Cancer 40: 1526-1532.
2271. Tscholl-Ducommun J, Hedinger CE (1982). Papillary thyroid carcinomas. Morphology and prognosis. Virchows Arch A Pathol Anat Histol 396: 19-39.
2272. Tulbah A, Al Dayel F, Fawaz I, Rosai J (1999). Epstein-Barr virus-associated leiomyosarcoma of the thyroid in a child with congenital immunodeficiency: a case report. Am J Surg Pathol 23: 473-476.
2273. Tung WS, Shevlin DW, Kaleem Z, Tribune DJ, Wells SAJr, Goodfellow PJ (1997). Allelotype of follicular thyroid carcinomas reveals genetic instability consistent with frequent nondisjunctional chromosomal loss. Genes Chromosomes Cancer 19: 43-51.
2274. Turner HE, Nagy Z, Esiri MM, Harris AL, Wass JA (2000). Role of matrix metalloproteinase 9 in pituitary tumor behavior. J Clin Endocrinol Metab 85: 2931-2935.
2275. Twomey P, Montgomery C, Clark O (1982). Successful treatment of adrenal metastases from large-cell carcinoma of the lung. JAMA 248: 581-583.
2276. Uchino S, Noguchi S, Kawamoto H, Yamashita H, Watanabe S, Yamashita H, Shuto S (2002). Familial nonmedullary thyroid carcinoma characterized by multifocality and a high recurrence rate in a large study population. World J Surg 26: 897-902.
2277. Uchino S, Noguchi S, Sato M, Yamashita H, Yamashita H, Watanabe S, Murakami T, Toda M, Ohshima A, Futata T, Mizukoshi T, Koike E, Takatsu K, Terao K, Wakiya S, Nagatomo M, Adachi M (2000). Screening of the Men1 gene and discovery of germ-line and somatic mutations in apparently sporadic parathyroid tumors. Cancer Res 60: 5553-5557.
2278. Uden P, Berglund J, Zederfeldt B, Aspelin P, Ljungberg O (1987). Parathyroid lipoadenoma: a rare cause of primary hyperparathyroidism. Case report. Acta Chir Scand 153: 635-639.
2279. Ueno NT, Amato RJ, Ro JJ, Weber RS (1998). Primary malignant teratoma of the thyroid gland: report and discussion of two cases. Head Neck 20: 649-653.
2280. Ulchaker JC, Goldfarb DA, Bravo EL, Novick AC (1999). Successful outcomes in pheochromocytoma surgery in the modern era. J Urol 161: 764-767.
2281. Unger P, Hoffman K, Pertsemlidis D, Thung S, Wolfe D, Kaneko M (1991). S100 protein-positive sustentacular cells in malignant and locally aggressive adrenal pheochromocytomas. Arch Pathol Lab Med 115: 484-487.
2282. Unger PD, Cohen JM, Thung SN, Gordon R, Pertsemlidis D, Dikman SH (1990). Lipid degeneration in a pheochromocytoma histologically mimicking an adrenal cortical tumor. Arch Pathol Lab Med 114: 892-894.
2283. Urbanski SJ, Bilbao JM, Horvath E, Kovacs K, So W, Ward JV (1980). Intrasellar solitary plasmacytoma terminating in multiple myeloma: a report of a case including electron microscopical study. Surg Neurol 14: 233-236.
2284. Urdaneta N, Chessin H, Fischer JJ (1976). Pituitary adenomas and craniopharyngiomas: analysis of 99 cases treated with radiation therapy. Int J Radiat Oncol Biol Phys 1: 895-902.
2285. Uribe M, Fenoglio-Preiser CM, Grimes M, Feind C (1985). Medullary carcinoma of the thyroid gland. Clinical, pathological, and immunohistochemical features with review of the literature. Am J Surg Pathol 9: 577-594.
2286. Vallar L, Spada A, Giannattasio G (1987). Altered Gs and adenylate cyclase activity in human GH-secreting pituitary adenomas. Nature 330: 566-568.
2287. Vallette-Kasic S, Dufour H, Mugnier M, Trouillas J, Valdes-Socin H, Caron P, Morange S, Girard N, Grisoli F, Jaquet P, Brue T (2000). Markers of tumor invasion are major predictive factors for the long-term outcome of corticotroph microadenomas treated by transsphenoidal adenomectomy. Eur J Endocrinol 143: 761-768.
2288. van Baars F, van den Broek P, Cremers C, Veldman J (1981). Familial nonchromaffinic paragangliomas (glomus tumors) : clinical aspects. Laryngoscope 91: 988-996.
2289. van der Harst E, Bruining HA, Jaap Bonjer H, van der Ham F, Dinjens WN, Lamberts SW, de Herder WW, Koper JW, Stijnen T, Proye C, Lecomte-Houcke M, Bosman FT, de Krijger RR (2000). Proliferative index in phaeochromocytomas: does it predict the occurrence of metastases? J Pathol 191: 175-180.
2290. van der Harst E, de Krijger RR, Bruining HA, Lamberts SW, Bonjer HJ, Dinjes WN, Proye C, Koper JW, Bosman FT, Roth J, Heitz PU, Komminoth P (1998). Prognostic value of RET proto-oncogene point mutations in malignant and benign, sporadic phaeochromocytomas. Int J Cancer 79: 537-540.
2291. van der Harst E, de Krijger RR, Dinjens WN, Weeks LE, Bonjer HJ, Bruining HA, Lamberts SW, Koper JW (1998). Germline mutations in the vhl gene in patients presenting with phaeochromocytomas. Int J Cancer 77: 337-340.
2292. van der Lely AJ, Hutson RK, Trainer PJ, Besser GM, Barkan AL, Katznelson L, Klibanski A, Herman-Bonert V, Melmed S, Vance ML, Freda PU, Stewart PM, Friend KE, Clemmons DR, Johannsson G, Stavrou S, Cook DM, Phillips LS, Strasburger CJ, Hackett S, Zib KA, Davis RJ, Scarlett JA, Thorner MO (2001). Long-term treatment of acromegaly with pegvisomant, a growth hormone receptor antagonist. Lancet 358: 1754-1759.
2293. van der Mey AG, Maaswinkel-Mooy PD, Cornelisse CJ, Schmidt PH, van de Kamp JJ (1989). Genomic imprinting in hereditary glomus tumours: evidence for new genetic theory. Lancet 2: 1291-1294.
2294. van der Sluys Veer J, Choufoer JC, Querido A, van der Heul RO, Hollander CF, van Rijssel TG (1964). Metastasising islet-cell tumour of the pancreas associated with hypoglycaemia and carcinoid syndrome. Lancet 1: 1416-1419.
2295. van Heerden JA, Edis AJ, Service FJ (1979). The surgical aspects of insulinomas. Ann Surg 189: 677-682.
2296. van Heerden JA, Roland CF, Carney JA, Sheps SG, Grant CS (1990). Long-term evaluation following resection of apparently benign pheochromocytoma(s)/paraganglioma(s). World J Surg 14: 325-329.
2297. van Heerden JA, Sheps SG, Hamberger B, Sheedy PF, Poston JG, ReMine WH (1982). Pheochromocytoma: current status and changing trends. Surgery 91: 367-373.
2298. van Schothorst EM, Beekman M, Torremans P, Kuipers-Dijkshoorn NJ, Wessels HW, Bardoel AF, van der Mey AG, van der Vijver MJ, van Ommen GJ, Devilee P, Cornelisse CJ (1998). Paragangliomas of the head and neck region show complete loss of heterozygosity at 11q22-q23 in chief cells and the flow-sorted DNA aneuploid fraction. Hum Pathol 29: 1045-1049.
2299. van Slooten H, Schaberg A, Smeenk D, Moolenaar AJ (1985). Morphologic characteristics of benign and malignant adrenocortical tumors. Cancer 55: 766-773.
2300. Vargas H, Mouzakes J, Purdy SS, Cohn AS, Parnes SM (2002). Follicular dendritic cell tumor: an aggressive head and neck tumor. Am J Otolaryngol 23: 93-98.
2301. Vargas MP, Vargas HI, Kleiner DE, Merino MJ (1997). The role of prognostic markers (MiB-1, RB, and bcl-2) in the diagnosis of parathyroid tumors. Mod Pathol 10: 12-17.
2302. Varghese JC, Hahn PF, Papanicolaou N, Mayo-Smith WW, Gaa JA, Lee MJ (1997). MR differentiation of phaeochromocytoma from other adrenal lesions based on qualitative analysis of T2 relaxation times. Clin Radiol 52: 603-606.
2303. Vasef MA, Brynes RK, Sturm M, Bromley C, Robinson RA (1999). Expression of cyclin D1 in parathyroid carcinomas, adenomas, and hyperplasias: a paraffin immunohistochemical study. Mod Pathol 12: 412-416.
2304. Vasiloff J, Chideckel EW, Boyd CB, Foshag LJ (1985). Testosterone-secreting adrenal adenoma containing crystalloids characteristic of Leydig cells. Am J Med 79: 772-776.
2305. Vassilopoulou-Sellin R, Palmer L, Taylor S, Cooksley CS (1999). Incidence of breast carcinoma in women with thyroid carcinoma. Cancer 85: 696-705.
2306. Vazquez-Ramirez F, Otal Salaverri C, Argueta Manzano O, Galera-Ruiz H, Gonzalez-Campora R (2000). Fine needle aspiration cytology of high grade mucoepidermoid carcinoma of the thyroid. A case report. Acta Cytol 44: 259-264.
2307. Venkatesh S, Ordonez NG, Ajani J, Schultz PN, Hickey RC, Johnston DA, Samaan NA (1990). Islet cell carcinoma of the pancreas. A study of 98 patients. Cancer 65: 354-357.
2308. Venkatesh YS, Ordonez NG, Schultz PN, Hickey RC, Goepfert H, Samaan NA (1990). Anaplastic carcinoma of the thyroid. A clinicopathologic study of 121 cases. Cancer 66: 321-330.
2309. Verdonk CA, Edis AJ (1981). Parathyroid "double adenomas": fact of fiction? Surgery 90: 523-526.

2310. Verges B, Boureille F, Goudet P, Murat A, Beckers A, Sassolas G, Cougard P, Chambe B, Montvernay C, Calender A (2002). Pituitary disease in MEN type 1 (MEN1): data from the France-Belgium MEN1 multicenter study. J Clin Endocrinol Metab 87: 457-465.
2311. Verhoef S, Diemen-Steenvoorde R, Akkersdijk WL, Bax NM, Ariyurek Y, Hermans CJ, van Nieuwenhuizen O, Nikkels PG, Lindhout D, Halley DJ, Lips K, van den Ouweland AM (1999). Malignant pancreatic tumour within the spectrum of tuberous sclerosis complex in childhood. Eur J Pediatr 158: 284-287.
2312. Verner JV, Morrison AB (1958). Islet cell tumor and a syndrome of refractory watery diarrhea and hypokalemia. Am J Med 25: 374-380.
2313. Verner JV, Morrison AB (1974). Endocrine pancreatic islet disease with diarrhea. Report of a case due to diffuse hyperplasia of nonbeta islet tissue with a review of 54 additional cases. Arch Intern Med 133: 492-499.
2314. Viale G, Doglioni C, Gambacorta M, Zamboni G, Coggi G, Bordi C (1992). Progesterone receptor immunoreactivity in pancreatic endocrine tumors. An immunocytochemical study of 156 neuroendocrine tumors of the pancreas, gastrointestinal and respiratory tracts, and skin. Cancer 70: 2268-2277.
2315. Vickery ALJr, Carcangiu ML, Johannessen JV, Sobrinho-Simoes M (1985). Papillary carcinoma. Semin Diagn Pathol 2: 90-100.
2316. Vidal S, Horvath E, Bonert V, Shahinian K, Kovacs K (2002). Neural transformation in a pituitary corticotroph adenoma. Acta Neuropathol (Berl) 104: 435-440.
2317. Vidal S, Kovacs K, Horvath E, Scheithauer BW, Kuroki T, Lloyd RV (2001). Microvessel density in pituitary adenomas and carcinomas. Virchows Arch 438: 595-602.
2318. Vierhapper H, Raber W, Bieglmayer C, Kaserer K, Weinhausl A, Niederle B (1997). Routine measurement of plasma calcitonin in nodular thyroid diseases. J Clin Endocrinol Metab 82: 1589-1593.
2319. Viglietto G, Chiappetta G, Martinez-Tello FJ, Fukunaga FH, Tallini G, Rigopoulou D, Visconti R, Mastro A, Santoro M, Fusco A (1995). RET/PTC oncogene activation is an early event in thyroid carcinogenesis. Oncogene 11: 1207-1210.
2320. Villablanca A, Calender A, Forsberg L, Hoog A, Cheng JD, Petillo D, Bauters C, Kahnoski K, Ebeling T, Salmela P, Richardson AL, Delbridge L, Meyrier A, Proye C, Carpten JD, Teh BT, Robinson B, Larsson C (2003). Germline and de novo mutations in the HRPT2 tumor suppressor gene in familial isolated hyperparathyroidism (FIHP). J Med Genet .
2321. Villaschi S, Macciomei MC (1996). Solitary fibrous tumor of the perithyroid soft tissue. Report of a case simulating a thyroid nodule. Ann Ital Chir 67: 89-91.
2322. Vinchon M, Soto-Ares G, Ruchoux MM, Dhellemmes P (2000). Cerebellar gliomas in children with NF1: pathology and surgery. Childs Nerv Syst 16: 417-420.
2323. Vinik AI, Strodel WE, Eckhauser FE, Moattari AR, Lloyd R (1987). Somatostatinomas, PPomas, neurotensinomas. Semin Oncol 14: 263-281.
2324. Vinores SA (1991). Demonstration of glial fibrillary acidic (GFA) protein by electron immunocytochemistry in the granular cells of a choristoma of the neurohypophysis. Histochemistry 96: 265-269.
2325. Viskochil D, Buchberg AM, Xu G, Cawthon RM, Stevens J, Wolff RK, Culver M, Carey JC, Copeland NG, Jenkins NA, White R, O'Connell P (1990). Deletions and a translocation interrupt a cloned gene at the neurofibromatosis type 1 locus. Cell 62: 187-192.
2326. Vodovnik A (2002). Fine needle aspiration cytology of primary thyroid paraganglioma. Report of a case with cytologic, histologic and immunohistochemical features and differential diagnostic considerations. Acta Cytol 46: 1133-1137.
2327. Vogelgesang S, Junge MH, Pahnke J, Gaab MR, Warzok RW (2002). August 2001: Sellar/suprasellar mass in a 59-year-old woman. Brain Pathol 12: 135-6, 139.
2328. Volante M, Allia E, Gugliotta P, Funaro A, Broglio F, Deghenghi R, Muccioli G, Ghigo E, Papotti M (2002). Expression of ghrelin and of the GH secretagogue receptor by pancreatic islet cells and related endocrine tumors. J Clin Endocrinol Metab 87: 1300-1308.
2329. Volante M, Papotti M, Roth J, Saremaslani P, Speel EJ, Lloyd RV, Carney JA, Heitz PU, Bussolati G, Komminoth P (1999). Mixed medullary-follicular thyroid carcinoma. Molecular evidence for a dual origin of tumor components. Am J Pathol 155: 1499-1509.
2330. von Herbay A, Sieg B, Schurmann G, Hofmann WJ, Betzler M, Otto HF (1991). Proliferative activity of neuroendocrine tumours of the gastroenteropancreatic endocrine system: DNA flow cytometric and immunohistological investigations. Gut 32: 949-953.
2331. von Werder K (1988). Physiologie und Pathophysiologie der Regulation der Prolactinsekretion. In: Hyperprolaktinamie-Prolaktinome. Physiologie-Klinik-Therapie, Jurgensen O, ed., Springer: Berlin , pp. 3-26.
2332. Vortmeyer AO, Lubensky IA, Fogt F, Linehan WM, Khettry U, Zhuang Z (1997). Allelic deletion and mutation of the von Hippel-Lindau (VHL) tumor suppressor gene in pancreatic microcystic adenomas. Am J Pathol 151: 951-956.
2333. Vortmeyer AO, Lubensky IA, Skarulis M, Li G, Moon YW, Park WS, Weil R, Barlow C, Spiegel AM, Marx SJ, Zhuang Z (1999). Multiple endocrine neoplasia type 1: atypical presentation, clinical course, and genetic analysis of multiple tumors. Mod Pathol 12: 919-924.
2334. Vos P, Croughs RJ, Thijssen JH, van 't Verlaat JW, van Ginkel LA (1988). Response of luteinizing hormone secreting pituitary adenoma to a long-acting somatostatin analogue. Acta Endocrinol (Copenh) 118: 587-590.
2335. Voutilainen PE, Multanen M, Haapiainen RK, Haglund CH, Sane T, Sivula AH (2000). Long term prognosis of medullary thyroid carcinoma in 39 patients. Ann Chir Gynaecol 89: 292-297.
2336. Voutilainen PE, Multanen M, Haapiainen RK, Leppaniemi AK, Sivula AH (1999). Anaplastic thyroid carcinoma survival. World J Surg 23: 975-978.
2337. Wachenfeld C, Beuschlein F, Zwermann O, Mora P, Fassnacht M, Allolio B, Reincke M (2001). Discerning malignancy in adrenocortical tumors: are molecular markers useful? Eur J Endocrinol 145: 335-341.
2338. Wagenmann A (1922). Multiple neurome des auges und der zunge. Ber Dtsch Ophthalmo Ges 43: 282-285.
2339. Wagner J, Portwine C, Rabin K, Leclerc JM, Narod SA, Malkin D (1994). High frequency of germline p53 mutations in childhood adrenocortical cancer. J Natl Cancer Inst 86: 1707-1710.
2340. Wahl HR, Robinson D (1943). Neuroblastoma of the mediastinum with pheochromoblastomatous elements. Arch Pathol 35: 571-578.
2341. Waisman M (1979). Patient encounters—patterns, perceptions, perplexities, precautions. J Am Acad Dermatol 1: 134-138.
2342. Wajchenberg BL, Albergaria Pereira MA, Medonca BB, Latronico AC, Campos Carneiro P, Alves VA, Zerbini MC, Liberman B, Carlos Gomes G, Kirschner MA (2000). Adrenocortical carcinoma: clinical and laboratory observations. Cancer 88: 711-736.
2343. Walker JD, Grossman A, Anderson JV, Ur E, Trainer PJ, Benn J, Lowy C, Sonksen PH, Plowman PN, Lowe DG, Doniach I, Wass JA, Besser GM (1993). Malignant prolactinoma with extracranial metastases: a report of three cases. Clin Endocrinol (Oxf) 38: 411-419.
2344. Walther MM, Choyke PL, Glenn G, Lyne JC, Rayford W, Venzon D, Linehan WM (1999). Renal cancer in families with hereditary renal cancer: prospective analysis of a tumor size threshold for renal parenchymal sparing surgery. J Urol 161: 1475-1479.
2345. Walther MM, Herring J, Enquist E, Keiser HR, Linehan WM (1999). von Recklinghausen's disease and pheochromocytomas. J Urol 162: 1582-1586.
2346. Walther MM, Keiser HR, Choyke PL, Rayford W, Lyne JC, Linehan WM (1999). Management of hereditary pheochromocytoma in von Hippel-Lindau kindreds with partial adrenalectomy. J Urol 161: 395-398.
2347. Walther MM, Lubensky IA, Venzon D, Zbar B, Linehan WM (1995). Prevalence of microscopic lesions in grossly normal renal parenchyma from patients with von Hippel-Lindau disease, sporadic renal cell carcinoma and no renal disease: clinical implications. J Urol 154: 2010-2014.
2348. Walther MM, Reiter R, Keiser HR, Choyke PL, Venzon D, Hurley K, Gnarra JR, Reynolds JC, Glenn GM, Zbar B, Linehan WM (1999). Clinical and genetic characterization of pheochromocytoma in von Hippel-Lindau families: comparison with sporadic pheochromocytoma gives insight into natural history of pheochromocytoma. J Urol 162: 659-664.
2349. Wan SK, Chan JK, Tang SK (1996). Paucicellular variant of anaplastic thyroid carcinoma. A mimic of Reidel's thyroiditis. Am J Clin Pathol 105: 388-393.
2350. Wang EH, Ebrahimi SA, Wu AY, Kashefi C, Passaro EJ, Sawicki MP (1998). Mutation of the MENIN gene in sporadic pancreatic endocrine tumors. Cancer Res 58: 4417-4420.
2351. Wang W, Johansson H, Bergholm U, Wilander E, Grimelius L (1996). Apoptosis and Expression of the Proto-Oncogenes bcl-2 and p53 and the Proliferation Factor Ki-67 in Human Medullary Thyroid Carcinoma. Endocr Pathol 7: 37-45.
2352. Wang WS, Liu JH, Chiou TJ, Hsieh RK, Yen CC, Chen PM (1997). Langerhans' cell histiocytosis with thyroid involvement masquerading as thyroid carcinoma. Jpn J Clin Oncol 27: 180-184.
2353. Ward LS, Brenta G, Medvedovic M, Fagin JA (1998). Studies of allelic loss in thyroid tumors reveal major differences in chromosomal instability between papillary and follicular carcinomas. J Clin Endocrinol Metab 83: 525-530.
2354. Warnakulasuriya S, Markwell BD, Williams DM (1985). Familial hyperparathyroidism associated with cementifying fibromas of the jaws in two siblings. Oral Surg Oral Med Oral Pathol 59: 269-274.
2355. Warner TF, Block M, Hafez GR, Mack E, Lloyd RV, Bloom SR (1983). Glucagonomas. Ultrastructure and immunocytochemistry. Cancer 51: 1091-1096.
2356. Wassif WS, Farnebo F, Teh BT, Moniz CF, Li FY, Harrison JD, Peters TJ, Larsson C, Harris P (1999). Genetic studies of a family with hereditary hyperparathyroidism-jaw tumour syndrome. Clin Endocrinol (Oxf) 50: 191-196.
2357. Watanobe H, Kawabe H (1997). Pituitary apoplexy developed in a patient with androgen insensitivity syndrome. J Endocrinol Invest 20: 497-500.
2358. Waterlot C, Porchet N, Bauters C, Decoulx M, Wemeau JL, Proye C, Degand PM, Aubert JP, Cortet C, Dewailly D (1999). Type 1 multiple endocrine neoplasia (MEN1): contribution of genetic analysis to the screening and follow-up of a large French kindred. Clin Endocrinol (Oxf) 51: 101-107.
2359. Watson JC, Stratakis CA, Bryant-Greenwood PK, Koch CA, Kirschner LS, Nguyen T, Carney JA, Oldfield EH (2000). Neurosurgical implications of Carney complex. J Neurosurg 92: 413-418.
2360. Watson KJ, Shulkes A, Smallwood RA, Douglas MC, Hurley R, Kalnins R, Moran L (1985). Watery diarrhea-hypokalemia-achlorhydria syndrome and carcinoma of the esophagus. Gastroenterology 88: 798-803.
2361. Wautot V, Khodaei S, Frappart L, Buisson N, Baro E, Lenoir GM, Calender A, Zhang CX, Weber G (2000). Expression analysis of endogenous menin, the product of the multiple endocrine neoplasia type 1 gene, in cell lines and human tissues. Int J Cancer 85: 877-881.
2362. Wautot V, Vercherat C, Lespinasse J, Chambe B, Lenoir GM, Zhang CX, Porchet N, Cordier M, Beroud C, Calender A (2002). Germline mutation profile of MEN1 in multiple endocrine neoplasia type 1: search for correlation between phenotype and the functional domains of the MEN1 protein. Hum Mutat 20: 35-47.
2363. Webb TA, Sheps SG, Carney JA (1980). Differences between sporadic pheochromocytoma and pheochromocytoma in multiple endocrine neoplasia, type 2. Am J Surg Pathol 4: 121-126.
2364. Weber CJ, Vansant J, Alazraki N, Christy J, Watts N, Phillips LS, Mansour K, Sewell W, McGarity WC (1993). Value of technetium 99m sestamibi iodine 123 imaging in reoperative parathyroid surgery. Surgery 114: 1011-1018.
2365. Weber HC, Venzon DJ, Lin JT, Fishbein VA, Orbuch M, Strader DB, Gibril F, Metz DC, Fraker DL, Norton JA, Jensen RT (1995). Determinants of metastatic rate and survival in patients with Zollinger-Ellison syndrome: a prospective long-term study. Gastroenterology 108: 1637-1649.
2366. Webster AR, Maher ER, Moore AT (1999). Clinical characteristics of ocular angiomatosis in von Hippel-Lindau disease and correlation with germline mutation. Arch Ophthalmol 117: 371-378.
2367. Webster AR, Richards FM, MacRonald FE, Moore AT, Maher ER (1998). An analysis of phenotypic variation

in the familial cancer syndrome von Hippel-Lindau disease: evidence for modifier effects. Am J Hum Genet 63: 1025-1035.

2368. Webster J, Page MD, Bevan JS, Richards SH, Douglas-Jones AG, Scanlon MF (1992). Low recurrence rate after partial hypophysectomy for prolactinoma: the predictive value of dynamic prolactin function tests. Clin Endocrinol (Oxf) 36: 35-44.

2369. Weigensberg C, Hubert D, Asa SL, Bedard YC, Mullen JBM (1990). Thyroid thymoma in childhood. Endocr Pathol 1: 123-127.

2370. Weiland AJ, Daniel RK (1980). Congenital pseudarthrosis of the tibia: treatment with vascularized autogenous fibular grafts. A preliminary report. Johns Hopkins Med J 147: 89-95.

2371. Weinstein LS, Shenker A, Gejman PV, Merino MJ, Friedman E, Spiegel AM (1991). Activating mutations of the stimulatory G protein in the McCune-Albright syndrome. N Engl J Med 325: 1688-1695.

2372. Weiss LM, Medeiros LJ, Vickery ALJr (1989). Pathologic features of prognostic significance in adrenocortical carcinoma. Am J Surg Pathol 13: 202-206.

2373. Wells SAJr, Chi DD, Toshima K, Dehner LP, Coffin CM, Dowton SB, Ivanovich JL, DeBenedetti MK, Dilley WG, Moley JF, Norton JA, Donis-Keller H (1994). Predictive DNA testing and prophylactic thyroidectomy in patients at risk for multiple endocrine neoplasia type 2A. Ann Surg 220: 237-247.

2374. Wells SAJr, Franz C (2000). Medullary carcinoma of the thyroid gland. World J Surg 24: 952-956.

2375. Wenig BM, Abbondanzo SL, Heffess CS (1994). Epithelioid angiosarcoma of the adrenal glands. A clinicopathologic study of nine cases with a discussion of the implications of finding "epithelial-specific" markers. Am J Surg Pathol 18: 62-73.

2376. Wenig BM, Adair CF, Heffess CS (1995). Primary mucoepidermoid carcinoma of the thyroid gland: a report of six cases and a review of the literature of a follicular epithelial-derived tumor. Hum Pathol 26: 1099-1108.

2377. Wenig BM, Thompson LD, Adair CF, Shmookler B, Heffess CS (1998). Thyroid papillary carcinoma of columnar cell type: a clinicopathologic study of 16 cases. Cancer 82: 740-753.

2378. Wermers RA, Khosla S, Atkinson EJ, Hodgson SF, O'Fallon WM, Melton LJI (1997). The rise and fall of primary hyperparathyroidism: a population-based study in Rochester, Minnesota, 1965-1992. Ann Intern Med 126: 433-440.

2379. Werness BA, Guccion JG (1997). Tumor of the broad ligament in von Hippel-Lindau disease of probable mullerian origin. Int J Gynecol Pathol 16: 282-285.

2380. Westfried M, Mandel D, Alderete MN, Groopman J, Minkowitz S (1978). Sipple's syndrome with a malignant pheochromocytoma presenting as a pericardial effusion. Cardiology 63: 305-311.

2381. Whalen RK, Althausen AF, Daniels GH (1992). Extra-adrenal pheochromocytoma. J Urol 147: 1-10.

2382. Wieneke JA, Thompson LD, Heffess CS (2001). Corticomedullary mixed tumor of the adrenal gland. Ann Diagn Pathol 5: 304-308.

2383. Wieneke JA, Thompson LD, Heffess CS (2003). Adrenal cortical neoplasms in the pediatric population: a clinicopathologic and immunophenotypic analysis of 83 patients. Am J Surg Pathol 27: 867-881.

2384. Wilander E, El Salhy M, Willen R, Grimelius L (1981). Immunocytochemistry and electron microscopy of an argentaffin endocrine tumour of the pancreas. Virchows Arch A Pathol Anat Histol 392: 263-269.

2385. Wild A, Langer P, Celik I, Chaloupka B, Bartsch DK (2002). Chromosome 22q in pancreatic endocrine tumors: identification of a homozygous deletion and potential prognostic associations of allelic deletions. Eur J Endocrinol 147: 507-513.

2386. Wilder RM, Allan FN, Power MH, Robertson HE (1927). Carcinoma of the islands of the pancreas; hyperinsulinism and hypoglycemia. JAMA 83: 348-355.

2387. Wilkens L, Benten D, Tchinda J, Brabant G, Potter E, Dralle H, von Wasielewski R (2000). Aberrations of chromosomes 5 and 8 as recurrent cytogenetic events in anaplastic carcinoma of the thyroid as detected by fluorescence in situ hybridisation and comparative genomic hybridisation. Virchows Arch 436: 312-318.

2388. Williams AJ, Coates PJ, Lowe DG, McLean C, Gale EA (1992). Immunochemical investigation of insulinomas for islet amyloid polypeptide and insulin: evidence for differential synthesis and storage. Histopathology 21: 215-223.

2389. Williams D (2002). Cancer after nuclear fallout: lessons from the Chernobyl accident. Nat Rev Cancer 2: 543-549.

2390. Williams ED (1966). Histogenesis of medullary carcinoma of the thyroid. J Clin Pathol 19: 114-118.

2391. Williams ED (2000). Guest Editorial: Two Proposals Regarding the Terminology of Thyroid Tumors. Int J Surg Pathol 8: 181-183.

2392. Williams ED, Doniach I, Bjarnason O, Michie W (1977). Thyroid cancer in an iodide rich area: a histopathological study. Cancer 39: 215-222.

2393. Williams ED, Toyn CE, Harach HR (1989). The ultimobranchial gland and congenital thyroid abnormalities in man. J Pathol 159: 135-141.

2394. Williamson EA, Johnson SJ, Foster S, Kendall-Taylor P, Harris PE (1995). G protein gene mutations in patients with multiple endocrinopathies. J Clin Endocrinol Metab 80: 1702-1705.

2395. Willis RA (1931). Metastatic tumors in the thyroid gland. Am J Pathol 7: 187-208.

2396. Willis RV (1973). The Spread of Tumours in the Human Body. 3rd ed. Butterworth: London.

2397. Willman CL (1994). Detection of clonal histiocytes in Langerhans cell histiocytosis: biology and clinical significance. Br J Cancer Suppl 23: S29-S33.

2398. Wilson SD (1982). The role of surgery in children with the Zollinger-Ellison syndrome. Surgery 92: 682-692.

2399. Wingrave SJ, Kay CR, Vessey MP (1980). Oral contraceptives and pituitary adenomas. Br Med J 280: 685-686.

2400. Winkler H (1997). Membrane composition of adrenergic large and small dense cored vesicles and of synaptic vesicles: consequences for their biogenesis. Neurochem Res 22: 921-932.

2401. Wirtzfeld DA, Winston JS, Hicks WLJr, Loree TR (2001). Clinical presentation and treatment of non-Hodgkin's lymphoma of the thyroid gland. Ann Surg Oncol 8: 338-341.

2402. Wittekind C, Henson DE, Hutter RVP, Sobin LH (2003). TNM Supplement:: a commentary on uniform use. 3rd ed. Wiley: Hoboken.

2403. Wizigmann-Voos S, Breier G, Risau W, Plate KH (1995). Up-regulation of vascular endothelial growth factor and its receptors in von Hippel-Lindau disease-associated and sporadic hemangioblastomas. Cancer Res 55: 1358-1364.

2404. Wohllk N, Cote GJ, Bugalho MM, Ordonez N, Evans DB, Goepfert H, Khorana S, Schultz P, Richards CS, Gagel RF (1996). Relevance of RET proto-oncogene mutations in sporadic medullary thyroid carcinoma. J Clin Endocrinol Metab 81: 3740-3745.

2405. Wolf EL, Sprayregen S, Frager D, Rifkin H, Gliedman ML (1984). Calcification in an insulinoma of the pancreas. Am J Gastroenterol 79: 559-561.

2406. Wolfe HJ, DeLellis RA (1981). Familial medullary thyroid carcinoma and C cell hyperplasia. Clin Endocrinol Metab 10: 351-365.

2407. Wolfe HJ, Melvin KE, Cervi-Skinner SJ, Saadi AA, Juliar JF, Jackson CE, Tashjian AHJr (1973). C-cell hyperplasia preceding medullary thyroid carcinoma. N Engl J Med 289: 437-441.

2408. Wolfe HJ, Voelkel EF, Tashjian AHJr (1974). Distribution of calcitonin-containing cells in the normal adult human thyroid gland: a correlation of morphology with peptide content. J Clin Endocrinol Metab 38: 688-694.

2409. Wolfe MM, Alexander RW, McGuigan JE (1982). Extrapancreatic, extraintestinal gastrinoma: effective treatment by surgery. N Engl J Med 306: 1533-1536.

2410. Wolff M, Goodman EN (1980). Functioning lipoadenoma of a supernumerary parathyroid gland in the mediastinum. Head Neck Surg 2: 302-307.

2411. Wollesen F, Andersen T, Karle A (1982). Size reduction of extrasellar pituitary tumors during bromocriptine treatment. Ann Intern Med 96: 281-286.

2412. Woloschak M, Yu A, Post KD (1997). Frequent inactivation of the p16 gene in human pituitary tumors by gene methylation. Mol Carcinog 19: 221-224.

2413. Woloschak M, Yu A, Xiao J, Post KD (1996). Frequent loss of the P16INK4a gene product in human pituitary tumors. Cancer Res 56: 2493-2496.

2414. Wolpert HR, Vickery ALJr, Wang CA (1989). Functioning oxyphil cell adenomas of the parathyroid gland. A study of 15 cases. Am J Surg Pathol 13: 500-504.

2415. Wolpert SM, Molitch ME, Goldman JA, Wood JB (1984). Size, shape, and appearance of the normal female pituitary gland. AJR Am J Roentgenol 143: 377-381.

2416. Woodruff JM, Perino G (1994). Non-germ-cell or teratomatous malignant tumors showing additional rhabdomyoblastic differentiation, with emphasis on the malignant Triton tumor. Semin Diagn Pathol 11: 69-81.

2417. Woodward ER, Buchberger A, Clifford SC, Hurst LD, Affara NA, Maher ER (2000). Comparative sequence analysis of the VHL tumor suppressor gene. Genomics 65: 253-265.

2418. Woodward ER, Eng C, McMahon R, Voutilainen R, Affara NA, Ponder BA, Maher ER (1997). Genetic predisposition to phaeochromocytoma: analysis of candidate genes GDNF, RET and VHL. Hum Mol Genet 6: 1051-1056.

2419. Woolner LB, Beahrs OH, Black BM, McConahey WM, Keating FRJr (1961). Classification and prognosis of thyroid carcinoma: A study of 885 cases observed in a thirty year period. Am J Surg 102: 354-387.

2420. Wooten MD, King DK (1993). Adrenal cortical carcinoma. Epidemiology and treatment with mitotane and a review of the literature. Cancer 72: 3145-3155.

2421. Wrabetz L, Feltri ML, Kim H, Daston M, Kamholz J, Scherer SS, Ratner N (1995). Regulation of neurofibromin expression in rat sciatic nerve and cultured Schwann cells. Glia 15: 22-32.

2422. Wreesmann VB, Ghossein RA, Patel SG, Harris CP, Schnaser EA, Shaha AR, Tuttle RM, Shah JP, Rao PH, Singh B (2002). Genome-wide appraisal of thyroid cancer progression. Am J Pathol 161: 1549-1556.

2423. Writing Group of the Histiocyte Society (1987). Histiocytosis syndromes in children. Writing Group of the Histiocyte Society. Lancet 1: 208-209.

2424. Wu Q, Fu WM, Liu WG, Zheng XJ, Yang XF (2002). [Clinical and pathological features of male pituitary prolactinoma]. Zhejiang Da Xue Xue Bao Yi Xue Ban 31: 299-301.

2425. Wu R, Lopez-Correa C, Rutkowski JL, Baumbach LL, Glover TW, Legius E (1999). Germline mutations in NF1 patients with malignancies. Genes Chromosomes Cancer 26: 376-380.

2426. Wynne AG, Gharib H, Scheithauer BW, Davis DH, Freeman SL, Horvath E (1992). Hyperthyroidism due to inappropriate secretion of thyrotropin in 10 patients. Am J Med 92: 15-24.

2427. Wynne AG, Scheithauer BW, Young WFJr, Kovacs K, Ebersold MJ, Horvath E (1992). Coexisting corticotroph and lactotroph adenomas: case report with reference to the relationship of corticotropin and prolactin excess. Neurosurgery 30: 919-923.

2428. Wynne AG, van Heerden J, Carney JA, Fitzpatrick LA (1992). Parathyroid carcinoma: clinical and pathologic features in 43 patients. Medicine (Baltimore) 71: 197-205.

2429. Xu B, Hirokawa M, Yoshimoto K, Miki H, Takahashi M, Kuma S, Sano T (2003). Spindle epithelial tumor with thymus-like differentiation of the thyroid: a case report with pathological and molecular genetics study. Hum Pathol 34: 190-193.

2430. Xu B, Yoshimoto K, Miyauchi A, Kuma S, Mizusawa N, Hirokawa M, Sano T (2003). Cribriform-morular variant of papillary thyroid carcinoma: a pathological and molecular genetic study with evidence of frequent somatic mutations in exon 3 of the beta-catenin gene. J Pathol 199: 58-67.

2431. Xu GF, Lin B, Tanaka K, Dunn D, Wood D, Gesteland R, White R, Weiss R, Tamanoi F (1990). The catalytic domain of the neurofibromatosis type 1 gene product stimulates ras GTPase and complements ira mutants of S. cerevisiae. Cell 63: 835-841.

2432. Xu H, Gutmann DH (1997). Mutations in the GAP-related domain impair the ability of neurofibromin to associate with microtubules. Brain Res 759: 149-152.

2433. Xu X, Quiros RM, Gattuso P, Ain KB, Prinz RA (2003). High prevalence of BRAF gene mutation in papillary thyroid carcinomas and thyroid tumor cell lines. Cancer Res 63: 4561-4567.

2434. Xu XC, el Naggar AK, Lotan R (1995). Differential expression of galectin-1 and galectin-3 in thyroid tumors. Potential diagnostic implications. Am J Pathol 147: 815-822.

2435. Yabut SMJr, Kenan S, Sissons HA, Lewis MM (1988). Malignant transformation of fibrous dysplasia. A case report and

review of the literature. Clin Orthop 281-289.
2436. Yaguchi H, Ohkura N, Tsukada T, Yamaguchi K (2002). Menin, the multiple endocrine neoplasia type 1 gene product, exhibits GTP-hydrolyzing activity in the presence of the tumor metastasis suppressor nm23. J Biol Chem 277: 38197-38204.
2437. Yamada M, Hashimoto K, Satoh T, Shibusawa N, Kohga H, Ozawa Y, Yamada S, Mori M (1997). A novel transcript for the thyrotropin-releasing hormone receptor in human pituitary and pituitary tumors. J Clin Endocrinol Metab 82: 4224-4228.
2438. Yamada M, Monden T, Satoh T, Satoh N, Murakami M, Iriuchijima T, Kakegawa T, Mori M (1993). Pituitary adenomas of patients with acromegaly express thyrotropin-releasing hormone receptor messenger RNA: cloning and functional expression of the human thyrotropin-releasing hormone receptor gene. Biochem Biophys Res Commun 195: 737-745.
2439. Yamada S, Asa SL, Kovacs K (1988). Oncocytomas and null cell adenomas of the human pituitary: morphometric and in vitro functional comparison. Virchows Arch A Pathol Anat Histopathol 413: 333-339.
2440. Yamada S, Kovacs K, Horvath E, Aiba T (1991). Morphological study of clinically nonsecreting pituitary adenomas in patients under 40 years of age. J Neurosurg 75: 902-905.
2441. Yamamoto T, Miyamoto KI, Ozono K, Taketani Y, Katai K, Miyauchi A, Shima M, Yoshikawa H, Yoh K, Takeda E, Okada S (2001). Hypophosphatemic rickets accompanying McCune-Albright syndrome: evidence that a humoral factor causes hypophosphatemia. J Bone Miner Metab 19: 287-295.
2442. Yamamoto T, Ozono K, Kasayama S, Yoh K, Hiroshima K, Takagi M, Matsumoto S, Michigami T, Yamaoka K, Kishimoto T, Okada S (1996). Increased IL-6-production by cells isolated from the fibrous bone dysplasia tissues in patients with McCune-Albright syndrome. J Clin Invest 98: 30-35.
2443. Yamamoto Y, Maeda T, Izumi K, Otsuka H (1990). Occult papillary carcinoma of the thyroid. A study of 408 autopsy cases. Cancer 65: 1173-1179.
2444. Yamauchi A, Tomita Y, Takakuwa T, Hoshida Y, Nakatsuka S, Sakamoto H, Aozasa K (2002). Polymerase chain reaction-based clonality analysis in thyroid lymphoma. Int J Mol Med 10: 113-117.
2445. Yang B, Ali SZ, Rosenthal DL (2002). CD10 facilitates the diagnosis of metastatic renal cell carcinoma from primary adrenal cortical neoplasm in adrenal fine-needle aspiration. Diagn Cytopathol 27: 149-152.
2446. Yang I, Park S, Ryu M, Woo J, Kim S, Kim J, Kim Y, Choi Y (1996). Characteristics of gsp-positive growth hormone-secreting pituitary tumors in Korean acromegalic patients. Eur J Endocrinol 134: 720-726.
2447. Yano T, Yamamoto N, Fujimori K, Inamori S, Hayashi H, Mizumoto R (1982). Glucagon-secreting pancreatic islet cell carcinoma, containing insulin and somatostatin, with hypoglycemic attack. Am J Gastroenterol 77: 387-391.
2448. Yantiss RK, Chang HK, Farraye FA, Compton CC, Odze RD (2002). Prevalence and prognostic significance of acinar cell differentiation in pancreatic endocrine tumors. Am J Surg Pathol 26: 893-901.
2449. Yap WM, Chuah KL, Tan PH (2001). Langerhans cell histiocytosis involving the thyroid and parathyroid glands. Mod Pathol 14: 111-115.
2450. Yashiro T, Hara H, Fulton NC, Obara T, Kaplan EL (1994). Point mutations of ras genes in human adrenal cortical tumors: absence in adrenocortical hyperplasia. World J Surg 18: 455-460.
2451. Yazawa K, Kuroda T, Watanabe H, Shimozawa N, Nimura Y, Nakata S, Fujimori Y, Koide N, Koike S, Kajikawa S, Adachi W, Kobayashi S, Ishii K, Amano J (1998). Multiple carcinoids of the duodenum accompanied by type I familial multiple endocrine neoplasia. Surg Today 28: 636-639.
2452. Yeh JJ, Lunetta KL, van Orsouw NJ, Moore FDJr, Mutter GL, Vijg J, Dahia PL, Eng C (2000). Somatic mitochondrial DNA (mtDNA) mutations in papillary thyroid carcinomas and differential mtDNA sequence variants in cases with thyroid tumours. Oncogene 19: 2060-2066.
2453. Yeh JJ, Marsh DJ, Zedenius J, Dwight T, Delbridge L, Robinson BG, Eng C (1999). Fine-structure deletion mapping of 10q22-24 identifies regions of loss of heterozygosity and suggests that sporadic follicular thyroid adenomas and follicular thyroid carcinomas develop along distinct neoplastic pathways. Genes Chromosomes Cancer 26: 322-328.
2454. Yla-Outinen H, Aaltonen V, Bjorkstrand AS, Hirvonen O, Lakkakorpi J, Vaha-Kreula M, Laato M, Peltonen J (1998). Upregulation of tumor suppressor protein neurofibromin in normal human wound healing and in vitro evidence for platelet derived growth factor (PDGF) and transforming growth factor-beta1 (TGF-beta1) elicited increase in neurofibromin mRNA steady-state levels in dermal fibroblasts. J Invest Dermatol 110: 232-237.
2455. Yla-Outinen H, Koivunen J, Nissinen M, Bjorkstrand AS, Paloniemi M, Korkiamaki T, Peltonen S, Karvonen SL, Peltonen J (2002). NF1 tumor suppressor mRNA is targeted to the cell-cell contact zone in Ca(2+)-induced keratinocyte differentiation. Lab Invest 82: 353-361.
2456. Yoshida K, Sumi S, Honda M, Hosoya Y, Yano M, Arai K, Ueda Y (1995). Serial lectin affinity chromatography demonstrates altered asparagine-linked sugar chain structures of gamma-glutamyltransferase in human renal cell carcinoma. J Chromatogr B Biomed Appl 672: 45-51.
2457. Yoshida SO, Imam A (1989). Monoclonal antibody to a proximal nephrogenic renal antigen: immunohistochemical analysis of formalin-fixed, paraffin-embedded human renal cell carcinomas. Cancer Res 49: 1802-1809.
2458. Yoshikawa K, Wakasa H (1980). Hypoglycemia associated with aberrant insulinoma: a case report of 16 years follow-up. Tohoku J Exp Med 132: 17-29.
2459. Yoshimi N, Tanaka T, Hara A, Bunai Y, Kato K, Mori H (1992). Extra-adrenal pheochromocytoma-ganglioneuroma. A case report. Pathol Res Pract 188: 1098-1100.
2460. Yoshimoto K, Iwahana H, Fukuda A, Sano T, Itakura M (1993). Rare mutations of the Gs alpha subunit gene in human endocrine tumors. Mutation detection by polymerase chain reaction-primer-introduced restriction analysis. Cancer 72: 1386-1393.
2461. Yoshimoto T, Naruse M, Zeng Z, Nishikawa T, Kasajima T, Toma H, Yamamori S, Matsumoto H, Tanabe A, Naruse K, Demura H (1998). The relatively high frequency of p53 gene mutations in multiple and malignant phaeochromocytomas. J Endocrinol 159: 247-255.
2462. Young AL, Baysal BE, Deb A, Young WFJr (2002). Familial malignant catecholamine-secreting paraganglioma with prolonged survival associated with mutation in the succinate dehydrogenase B gene. J Clin Endocrinol Metab 87: 4101-4105.
2463. Young WFJr (1997). Phaeochromocytoma: how to catch a moonbeam in your hand. Eur J Endocrinol 136: 28-29.
2464. Young WFJr (1999). Primary aldosteronism: A common and curable form of hypertension. Cardiol Rev 7: 207-214.
2465. Young WFJr (2000). Management approaches to adrenal incidentalomas. A view from Rochester, Minnesota. Endocrinol Metab Clin North Am 29: 159-185.
2466. Young WFJr, Maddox DE (1995). Spells: in search of a cause. Mayo Clin Proc 70: 757-765.
2467. Young WFJr, Scheithauer BW, Gharib H, Laws ERJr, Carpenter PC (1988). Cushing's syndrome due to primary multinodular corticotrope hyperplasia. Mayo Clin Proc 63: 256-262.
2468. Young WFJr, Scheithauer BW, Kovacs KT, Horvath E, Davis DH, Randall RV (1996). Gonadotroph adenoma of the pituitary gland: a clinicopathologic analysis of 100 cases. Mayo Clin Proc 71: 649-656.
2469. Yu F, Jensen RT, Lubensky IA, Mahlamaki EH, Zheng YL, Herr AM, Ferrin LJ (2000). Survey of genetic alterations in gastrinomas. Cancer Res 60: 5536-5542.
2470. Yumita W, Ikeo Y, Yamauchi K, Sakurai A, Hashizume K (2003). Suppression of insulin-induced AP-1 transactivation by menin accompanies inhibition of c-Fos induction. Int J Cancer 103: 738-744.
2471. Yun M, Kim W, Alnafisi N, Lacorte L, Jang S, Alavi A (2001). 18F-FDG PET in characterizing adrenal lesions detected on CT or MRI. J Nucl Med 42: 1795-1799.
2472. Zaatari GS, Saigo PE, Huvos AG (1983). Mucin production in medullary carcinoma of the thyroid. Arch Pathol Lab Med 107: 70-74.
2473. Zacharin M, O'Sullivan M (2000). Intravenous pamidronate treatment of polyostotic fibrous dysplasia associated with the McCune Albright syndrome. J Pediatr 137: 403-409.
2474. Zafar M, Ezzat S, Ramyar L, Pan N, Smyth HS, Asa SL (1995). Cell-specific expression of estrogen receptor in the human pituitary and its adenomas. J Clin Endocrinol Metab 80: 3621-3627.
2475. Zager EL, Hedley-Whyte ET (1987). Metastasis within a pituitary adenoma presenting with bilateral abducens palsies: case report and review of the literature. Neurosurgery 21: 383-386.
2476. Zahedi A, Booth GL, Smyth HS, Farrell WE, Clayton RN, Asa SL, Ezzat S (2001). Distinct clonal composition of primary and metastatic adrencorticotrophic hormone-producing pituitary carcinoma. Clin Endocrinol (Oxf) 55: 549-556.
2477. Zajac JD, Penschow J, Mason T, Tregear G, Coghlan J, Martin TJ (1986). Identification of calcitonin and calcitonin gene-related peptide messenger ribonucleic acid in medullary thyroid carcinomas by hybridization histochemistry. J Clin Endocrinol Metab 62: 1037-1043.
2478. Zak FG, Lawson W (1982). Anatomy and topography. In: Paraganglionic Chemoreceptor System: Physiology, Pathology, & Clinical Medicine, Zak FG, Lawson W, eds., Springer-Verlag: New York , pp. 15-49.
2479. Zak FG, Lawson W (1982). The Paraganglionic Chemoreceptor System: Physiology, Pathology, and Clinical Medicine. Springer Verlag: New York.
2480. Zanelli M, van der Walt JD (1996). Carotid body paraganglioma in von Hippel-Lindau disease: a rare association. Histopathology 29: 178-181.
2481. Zatyka M, da Silva NF, Clifford SC, Morris MR, Wiesener MS, Eckardt KU, Houlston RS, Richards FM, Latif F, Maher ER (2002). Identification of cyclin D1 and other novel targets for the von Hippel-Lindau tumor suppressor gene by expression array analysis and investigation of cyclin D1 genotype as a modifier in von Hippel-Lindau disease. Cancer Res 62: 3803-3811.
2482. Zatyka M, Morrissey C, Kuzmin I, Lerman MI, Latif F, Richards FM, Maher ER (2002). Genetic and functional analysis of the von Hippel-Lindau (VHL) tumour suppressor gene promoter. J Med Genet 39: 463-472.
2483. Zbar B, Kishida T, Chen F, Schmidt L, Maher ER, Richards FM, Crossey PA, Webster AR, Affara NA, Ferguson-Smith MA, Brauch H, Glavac D, Neumann HP, Tisherman S, Mulvihill JJ, Gross DJ, Shuin T, Whaley J, Seizinger B, Kley N, Olschwang S, Boisson C, Richard S, Lips CH, Linehan WM, Lerman M (1996). Germline mutations in the Von Hippel-Lindau disease (VHL) gene in families from North America, Europe, and Japan. Hum Mutat 8: 348-357.
2484. Zedenius J, Wallin G, Svensson A, Bovee J, Hoog A, Backdahl M, Larsson C (1996). Deletions of the long arm of chromosome 10 in progression of follicular thyroid tumors. Hum Genet 97: 299-303.
2485. Zee S, Hochwald S, Conlon K, Brennan M, Klimstra D (2001). Pleomorphic pancreatic endocrine neoplasms (PENs): a variant comonly confused with adenocarcinoma. Mod Pathol 14: 1212A.
2486. Zerella JT, Finberg FJ (1990). Obstruction of the neonatal airway from teratomas. Surg Gynecol Obstet 170: 126-131.
2487. Zhang JS, Nelson M, McIver B, Hay ID, Goellner JR, Grant CS, Eberhardt NL, Smith DI (1998). Differential loss of heterozygosity at 7q31.2 in follicular and papillary thyroid tumors. Oncogene 17: 789-793.
2488. Zhang X, Horwitz GA, Heaney AP, Nakashima M, Prezant TR, Bronstein MD, Melmed S (1999). Pituitary tumor transforming gene (PTTG) expression in pituitary adenomas. J Clin Endocrinol Metab 84: 761-767.
2489. Zhang X, Sun H, Danila DC, Johnson SR, Zhou Y, Swearingen B, Klibanski A (2002). Loss of expression of GADD45 gamma, a growth inhibitory gene, in human pituitary adenomas: implications for tumorigenesis. J Clin Endocrinol Metab 87: 1262-1267.
2490. Zhao J, Moch H, Scheidweiler AF, Baer A, Schaffer AA, Speel EJ, Roth J, Heitz PU, Komminoth P (2001). Genomic imbalances in the progression of endocrine pancreatic tumors. Genes Chromosomes Cancer 32: 364-372.
2491. Zhao J, Speel EJ, Muletta-Feurer S, Rutimann K, Saremaslani P, Roth J, Heitz PU, Komminoth P (1999). Analysis of genomic alterations in sporadic adreno-

cortical lesions. Gain of chromosome 17 is an early event in adrenocortical tumorigenesis. Am J Pathol 155: 1039-1045.

2492. Zhou XH (2002). Primary squamous cell carcinoma of the thyroid. Eur J Surg Oncol 28: 42-45.

2493. Zhou Y, Sun H, Danila DC, Johnson SR, Sigai DP, Zhang X, Klibanski A (2000). Truncated activin type I receptor Alk4 isoforms are dominant negative receptors inhibiting activin signaling. Mol Endocrinol 14: 2066-2075.

2494. Zhu Z, Gandhi M, Nikiforova MN, Fischer AH, Nikiforov YE (2003). Molecular profile and clinical-pathologic features of the follicular variant of papillary thyroid carcinoma. An unusually high prevalence of ras mutations. Am J Clin Pathol 120: 71-77.

2495. Zhuang Z, Vortmeyer AO, Pack S, Huang S, Pham TA, Wang C, Park WS, Agarwal SK, Debelenko LV, Kester M, Guru SC, Manickam P, Olufemi SE, Yu F, Heppner C, Crabtree JS, Skarulis MC, Venzon DJ, Emmert-Buck MR, Spiegel AM, Chandrasekharappa SC, Collins FS, Burns AL, Marx SJ, Jensen RT, Liotta LA, Lubensky IA (1997). Somatic mutations of the MEN1 tumor suppressor gene in sporadic gastrinomas and insulinomas. Cancer Res 57: 4682-4686.

2496. Zidan J, Karen D, Stein M, Rosenblatt E, Basher W, Kuten A (2003). Pure versus follicular variant of papillary thyroid carcinoma: clinical features, prognostic factors, treatment, and survival. Cancer 97: 1181-1185.

2497. Zimmer T, Stolzel U, Bader M, Koppenhagen K, Hamm B, Buhr H, Riecken EO, Wiedenmann B (1996). Endoscopic ultrasonography and somatostatin receptor scintigraphy in the preoperative localisation of insulinomas and gastrinomas. Gut 39: 562-568.

2498. Zollinger RM, Ellison EH (1955). Primary peptic ulcerations of the jejunum associated with islet cell tumors of the pancreas. Ann Surg 142: 709-728.

Subject index

Nesidioblastosis 185, 194, 223, 234
NESP55 255, 256
Neu 194
Neural crest-derived chromaffin cell tumour 137
Neuroblastoma 156, 157, 195, 214
NeuroD1 28
Neuroendocrine carcinoma 86, 88, 166, 207
Neuroendocrine carcinoma of the thyroid 86
Neuroendocrine tumours of the duodenum 245
Neurofibroma 170, 243-248, 250
Neurofibromatosis 138, 151, 155, 158, 164, 166, 242-244, 248, 249, 255
Neurofibromatosis type 1 (NF1) 147, 150, 151, 154, 155, 158, 161, 163, 186, 189, 190, 197, 198, 200, 243-248
Neurofibromin 247, 248
Neuroglucopenia 183
Neuromas of the tongue 211
Neuron specific enolase (NSE) 44, 178, 180, 207, 222
Neuronal choristoma 40
Neuron-specific enolase 163, 166, 213, 233, 235
Neuropeptide Y 241
Neurotensin 88, 177, 195
Nevus spilus 244
NF1 See Neurofibromatosis type 1 NF2 43, 243, 246
NF-KappaB family 225
NF-KappaB1 (p50) 225
NF-KappaB2 (p52) 225
NF-PETs 201-204
Nm23 225
NMTC, See Non-medullary thyroid cancer
NMTC1 gene, 257
Nocturia 143
Nodular (adenomatous) goiters 68, 70
Nodular goiter 57, 59, 81, 122
Nonchromaffin paraganglioma 159
Non-familial gastrinoma with ZES 191
Non-functioning pancreatic endocrine carcinoma 201
Non-functioning pancreatic endocrine neoplasm 201
Non-functioning pancreatic endocrine tumour (NF-PET) 201
Non-Hodgkin lymphoma 208
Non-medullary thyroid cancer (NMTC) 257, 258, 261
Non-secretory islet cell tumour 234
Nonsense-mediated decay (NMD) 252
Norepinephrine 138, 147, 163, 166, 213, 231, 240
Normetanephrine 147, 237

Normochromic and normocytic anaemia 187
N-RAS 65
NRF-1 241
NRF-2 241
NSE See Neuron specific enolase
NTRK1 75
Nucleoside diphosphate kinase ß isoform 1 225
Null cell adenoma 12, 33, 34

O

O13 208
Oat cell carcinoma 207
Occult hyperplasia 215, 218
Oesophageal leiomyoma 224
Oncocytic adenoma 100, 131
Oncocytic adrenal cortical adenoma 137
Oncocytic adrenal cortical carcinoma 137
Oncocytic carcinoma 67, 70, 72, 125
Oncocytic follicular carcinoma 67, 69, 71
Oncocytic papillary carcinoma 61, 65
Oncocytic variant of follicular carcinoma 69
Oncocytoma 33, 34, 145
Onocytic follicular carcinoma 69, 70
Onycholysis 187
Ophthalmopathy 24
Ophthalmoplegia 15, 46
Orbital paraganglioma 162
Ossifying fibroma 228, 255
Osteitis fibrosa cystica 55, 229, 255
Osteochondromyxoma 250
Osteomalacia 253, 254
Osteopenia 214
Osteopontin 254
Osteoporosis 26, 139, 143, 214
Osteosarcoma 122, 255
Ovarian cysts 250
Oxyphil cells 215, 219

P

P16^{INK4a} (CDKN2A) 12, 18, 22, 28, 79, 141, 154, 181, 182, 186, 204, 251
P21 81, 141
P27^{KIP1} 12, 19, 23, 29, 38, 47, 60, 64, 69, 79, 126, 130
P53 12, 18, 23, 29, 38, 39, 45, 47, 69, 74, 78, 81, 126, 130, 149, 208
P57 141, 142, 146
Pacinian corpuscles 244
Paget's disease 255
Pamidronate 255
Pancreatic cholera 195
Pancreatic cystic disease 234

Pancreatic endocrine tumour 177, 178, 181, 183, 184, 186-188, 190, 193, 194, 196, 202, 233
Pancreatic gastrinoma 191, 193
Pancreatic polypeptide (PP) 163, 177, 185, 193, 195, 203, 206, 221, 222, 234, 245
Pancreatitis 128, 177, 215, 223, 253
Pancreatoblastoma 180
Papillary adenocarcinoma 57
Papillary carcinoma 52-54, 57-67, 69, 71, 74, 75, 81, 82, 92, 93, 99, 100, 104, 105, 132, 249, 259, 260
Papillary carcinoma with fasciitis-like stroma 64
Papillary carcinoma with focal insular component 63
Papillary carcinoma with spindle and giant cell carcinoma 64
Papillary carcinoma with squamous cell or mucoepidermoid carcinoma 64
Papillary cystadenoma of the epididymis 234
Papillary cystadenoma of the broad ligament and mesosalpinx 235
Papillary microcarcinoma 64
Papillary microtumour 64
Papillary renal cell carcinoma 237
Papillary thyroid carcinoma 51-53, 57, 63-66, 84, 101, 105, 237, 257, 259
Paracrinopathy 215
Paradoxical hyperplasia 145
Paraganglioma 53, 88, 104, 117, 138, 151, 152, 154-166, 210, 231, 238-242, 245
Paraganglioma-like adenoma 104
Paraganglioma of the cauda equina 162
Paraganglioma of the urinary bladder 165
Paraganglioma producing excessive catecholamines 163
Paraganglioma, familial nonchromaffin, 3 (SDHC) 238
Paraganglioma, familial nonchromaffin 1 (SDHD) 238
Parasympathetic paragangliomas 117, 155, 159, 162, 163, 165, 239
Parathyroid adenoma 55, 56, 71, 124-130, 132, 215, 217, 219, 228, 256
Parathyroid carcinoma 55, 56, 124-128, 218, 130, 131, 228
Parathyroid hormone 55, 71, 100, 124, 126, 128-130, 132, 199, 214, 217, 227, 229
PDEC See Poorly differentiated endocrine carcinoma
Pem 225
Peptide histidine methionine (PHM) 195, 197
Peripheral nerve sheath tumours 116